Pathophysiology and Clinical Management of Pulmonary Fibrosis

Pathophysiology and Clinical Management of Pulmonary Fibrosis

Editor: Liam Lawrence

AMERICAN
MEDICAL PUBLISHERS
www.americanmedicalpublishers.com

AMERICAN
MEDICAL PUBLISHERS
www.americanmedicalpublishers.com

Cataloging-in-Publication Data

Pathophysiology and clinical management of pulmonary fibrosis / edited by Liam Lawrence.
p. cm.
Includes bibliographical references and index.
ISBN 979-8-88740-580-3
1. Pulmonary fibrosis. 2. Pulmonary fibrosis--Pathophysiology. 3. Pulmonary fibrosis--Treatment.
4. Lungs--Diseases. I. Lawrence, Liam.
RC776.F5 P38 2023
616.24--dc23

American Medical Publishers,
41 Flatbush Avenue,
1st Floor, New York,
NY 11217, USA

ISBN 979-8-88740-580-3 (Hardback)

Contents

Preface

This book was inspired by the evolution of our times; to answer the curiosity of inquisitive minds. Many developments have occurred across the globe in the recent past which has transformed the progress in the field.

Pulmonary fibrosis refers to a type of lung disease in which the lung tissue is scarred and injured. It also affects alveoli and connective tissue of the lungs. There are various symptoms of pulmonary fibrosis such as fatigue, shortness of breath, nail clubbing, dry cough and weight loss. Respiratory failure, lung cancer, pulmonary hypertension and pneumothorax are possible complications associated with it. The causes of pulmonary fibrosis include connective tissue diseases, interstitial lung diseases, environmental pollution, infections and certain medicines. Breathing tests, blood tests, biopsies, imaging tests and an oxygen desaturation study can be used to diagnose this medical condition. The treatment options of pulmonary fibrosis include pulmonary rehabilitation, lung transplantation and oxygen therapy. Medications can also be utilized to stop scarring from getting worse. This book brings forth some of the most innovative concepts and elucidates the unexplored aspects of the pathophysiology and clinical management of pulmonary fibrosis. It presents researches and studies performed by experts across the globe. The extensive content of this book provides the readers with a thorough understanding of pulmonary fibrosis.

This book was developed from a mere concept to drafts to chapters and finally compiled together as a complete text to benefit the readers across all nations. To ensure the quality of the content we instilled two significant steps in our procedure. The first was to appoint an editorial team that would verify the data and statistics provided in the book and also select the most appropriate and valuable contributions from the plentiful contributions we received from authors worldwide. The next step was to appoint an expert of the topic as the Editor-in-Chief, who would head the project and finally make the necessary amendments and modifications to make the text reader-friendly. I was then commissioned to examine all the material to present the topics in the most comprehensible and productive format.

I would like to take this opportunity to thank all the contributing authors who were supportive enough to contribute their time and knowledge to this project. I also wish to convey my regards to my family who have been extremely supportive during the entire project.

Editor

1

Impact of Transcriptomics on Our Understanding of Pulmonary Fibrosis

Milica Vukmirovic and Naftali Kaminski**

Section of Pulmonary, Critical Care and Sleep Medicine, Precision Pulmonary Medicine Center (P²MED), Yale University School of Medicine, New Haven, CT, United States

Correspondence:
Milica Vukmirovic
milica.vukmirovic@yale.edu;
Naftali Kaminski
naftali.kaminski@yale.edu

Idiopathic pulmonary fibrosis (IPF) is a lethal fibrotic lung disease characterized by aberrant remodeling of the lung parenchyma with extensive changes to the phenotypes of all lung resident cells. The introduction of transcriptomics, genome scale profiling of thousands of RNA transcripts, caused a significant inversion in IPF research. Instead of generating hypotheses based on animal models of disease, or biological plausibility, with limited validation in humans, investigators were able to generate hypotheses based on unbiased molecular analysis of human samples and then use animal models of disease to test their hypotheses. In this review, we describe the insights made from transcriptomic analysis of human IPF samples. We describe how transcriptomic studies led to identification of novel genes and pathways involved in the human IPF lung such as: matrix metalloproteinases, WNT pathway, epithelial genes, role of microRNAs among others, as well as conceptual insights such as the involvement of developmental pathways and deep shifts in epithelial and fibroblast phenotypes. The impact of lung and transcriptomic studies on disease classification, endotype discovery, and reproducible biomarkers is also described in detail. Despite these impressive achievements, the impact of transcriptomic studies has been limited because they analyzed bulk tissue and did not address the cellular and spatial heterogeneity of the IPF lung. We discuss new emerging technologies and applications, such as single-cell RNAseq and microenvironment analysis that may address cellular and spatial heterogeneity. We end by making the point that most current tissue collections and resources are not amenable to analysis using the novel technologies. To take advantage of the new opportunities, we need new efforts of sample collections, this time focused on access to all the microenvironments and cells in the IPF lung.

Keywords: interstitial lung diseases, idiopathic pulmonary fibrosis, transcriptomics, biomarkers, microenvironment, microarray, RNAseq

INTRODUCTION

Our understanding of idiopathic pulmonary fibrosis (IPF), a chronically progressive scarring lung disease, with a significant genetic component, has dramatically changed in the last two decades. This has happened because after years of formulating hypotheses based on animal models, or analogies from other diseases, pulmonary researchers shifted their focus to analyzing the human lung. The increased availability of well-characterized human tissues and the emergence of high throughput transcriptomic profiling technologies facilitated a new era in IPF research, one in which novel hypotheses are based on observations from human lungs. The sheer size of the data, and its unbiased nature, reintroduced serendipity in pulmonary fibrosis research, and thus led to numerous, previously unexpected observations, novel hypotheses and paradigm shifts. In this perspective, we provide an overview of the impact of transcriptomics on our understanding of IPF. We highlight the timeline of major discoveries (**Figure 1**) with a focus on mechanisms and pathways, novel biomarkers and disease classification, non-coding RNAs, and disease microenvironments.

BRIEF HISTORY

The history of transcriptomics in pulmonary fibrosis, is a story of ever increased technological throughput, enhanced sophistication of data analysis and availability of human samples. Gene expression microarrays, which allowed the parallel analysis of hundreds and later thousands of genes, emerged in the second half of the last decade of the twentieth century (1, 2). When the first publication of the application of microarray analysis to pulmonary fibrosis in mice was published in 2000 (3), microarrays could profile ~6,000 transcripts, the statistical approaches were not widely accepted, and human tissues were not available. Two years later, the first analysis of human lungs in 2002 included only eight samples, used a classification algorithm and did not mention a p-value (4). These papers were exciting and novel but very limited in numbers of samples and sophistication of analytical approaches.

Even several years later, studies that aimed at classifying disease included relatively low numbers of samples (5–10). These studies were more sophisticated in data normalization, visualization, and the wide adaptation of statistical approaches to address multiple testing (11, 12). Tissue availability has only increased when NIH-NHLBI established the Lung Tissue Research Consortium, a multicenter publicly available lung tissue repository (13). The expanded availability of tissues allowed application of microarray platforms to hundreds of samples (14, 15) as well the public availability of data through the Lung Genomics Research Consortium (16). Development of RNAseq for deeper sequencing than with microarray platforms resulted in routine profiling of the whole transcriptome including coding and non-coding RNAs, detection of larger dynamic ranges of transcripts, and identification of novel transcripts and variants (17, 18). This further allowed analysis of low-input and degraded RNA samples that enabled research on lung microenvironments and archived tissues (19, 20). Currently, when approaching a transcriptomic study, investigators do not have to be limited by sample or technological feasibility. Instead, they can follow a rational approach to design (**Figure 2**). The key insights below largely follow aspects of this outline.

MECHANISMS AND PATHWAYS

Transcriptomics studies revealed numerous novel molecules and pathways highly relevant for IPF pathogenesis. Here, we describe the most prominent findings, while a more complete list is available in **Table 1**.

Matrix Metalloproteinases

Development of IPF was initially explained as fibroblast proliferation, higher expression of tissue inhibitor proteinases (TIMPs), and reduced activity of matrix metalloproteases (MMP) (55). The

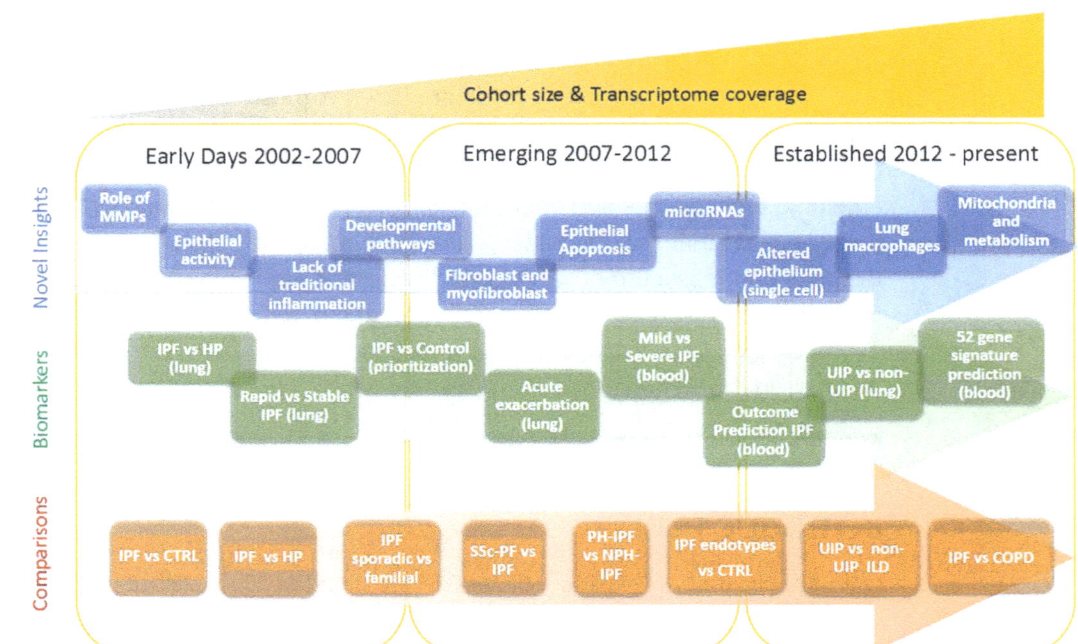

FIGURE 1 | Evolution of idiopathic pulmonary fibrosis (IPF) transcriptome analysis. The progression of IPF transcriptomic research is that of increased complexity, more genes studied, more sample studied, and more detailed phenotypes. In the early days, a few thousand genes were analyzed on a small number of samples and limited analytical approaches. During the emerging period investigators studied tens of samples, mostly on microarrays that profiled of all protein coding mRNAs. In the established period, the numbers of samples are in hundreds, all transcribed RNA is measured, and analytical methods are sophisticated.

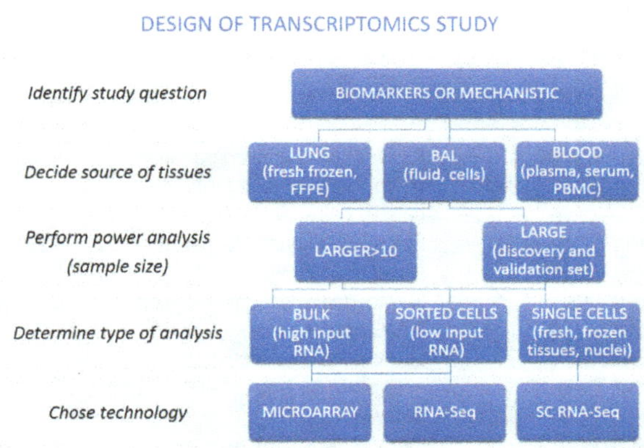

FIGURE 2 | A rational approach to design of transcriptomics study. An overview of steps to help researchers make appropriate study design is presented. First, distinguish whether study aims to identify biomarkers or mechanisms. Then, the source of tissues together with power analysis to calculate sample size to be able to answer research question should be performed. Decision about the type of analysis should be made (bulk, sorted cells, or single cells). Last, the technology to perform transcriptome analysis should be chosen.

first study that analyzed human lungs contradicted this paradigm (**Figure 1**; **Table 1**). Instead of the expected downregulation, authors found that MMPs were among the most increased genes in IPF lungs including MMP1, MMP2, MMP7, and MMP9 (4). MMP7 was localized predominantly in alveolar epithelium, and MMP7 knockout mice were relatively resistant to fibrosis (4). In addition to MMP7, MMP1 (4), MMP3 (28), MMP19 (29), and MMP28 (56) have been found to be increased in lung epithelial cells of patients with IPF, with diverse and sometimes opposing roles (57, 58).

While their exact roles have not been fully elucidated, the initial unexpected observation that MMPs are increased in the IPF lung, has been validated numerous times. It is now well accepted that MMPs affect numerous signaling pathways that together contribute to the profibrotic environment in the IPF lung and may also serve as effective biomarkers (see below).

Genes Expressed in Lung Epithelium

Transcriptomic analysis of bulk tissue depends on follow-up analyses to decipher the cellular origin of differentially expressed genes. One of the most surprising findings in IPF transcriptomics was that cellular origin of large number of genes that distinguish the IPF lung from controls ended up being the alveolar epithelium (59, 60) (**Figure 1**; **Table 1**). Among the first examples were MMP7, and later SPP1, a protein known to be expressed in inflammatory and bone cells, that in IPF is increased in the epithelial cells adjacent to myofibroblasts foci (22).

Other genes increased in IPF and unexpectedly localized to the alveolar epithelium adjacent to fibrotic regions include N-cadherin (5), HIF-1-alpha (31), IGFBP-4 (9), CCNA2 (10), TAGLN (33), CRLF1 (34), EGFR (35), and DIO2 (54). Among decreased genes, reduced expression of CAV1 (6) and AGER (52) in IPF compared with control lungs was thought to reflect changes in epithelial function or loss of type I alveolar epithelial cells (**Table 1**).

Of particular interest in this context, is a study that demonstrated that IPF patients with increased expression of cilia genes exhibited also increased MMP7 and MUC5B, as well as microscopic honeycombing but not myofibroblast foci on histological examination, suggesting that they represented a distinct IPF endophenotype (61) (**Table 1** and see below).

Fibroblasts and Fibroblast Foci Related Gene Expression

Genes associated with myofibroblasts, a hallmark of lung histology in IPF, have been described as early as 2002 in bulk tissue analysis (4). Analysis of lung fibroblasts treated with TGFB1 revealed responses to TGFB1 and smooth muscle like myofibroblast phenotype switching (62) that was similar to what was observed in the IPF lung. Fibroblasts isolated from IPF lungs exhibited increased expression of IGFBP3 and IGFBP5 (43), TWIST1 (48), WNT5A (45), COMP (63), and FOXF1 (38). Increased Vascular cell adhesion molecule 1 gene expression in IPF lungs negatively correlated with lung function (39). Another TGFB1 induced gene, FKBP10, a collagen chaperone, was also increased in IPF and IPF lung fibroblasts and contributed to Collagen synthesis (40). Recently, TAZ, a transcriptional coactivator important in development, was shown to be increased in the fibroblastic foci and to contribute to fibrotic response through TAZ-mediated regulation of CTGF (42) (**Figure 1**; **Table 1**).

Of particular interest are genes downregulated in IPF lungs and IPF fibroblasts, as they may represent key features lost during disease. RXFP1, a relaxin/insulin-like family peptide receptor is significantly decreased in IPF tissues and fibroblasts and correlates with disease severity. A relaxin-like peptide, CGEN25009 was effective at decreasing bleomycin-induced, fibrosis *in vivo* (41). Similarly, PTPN11, a ubiquitously expressed SH2 domain-containing tyrosine phosphatase, was decreased in IPF lungs and IPF fibroblasts. Overexpression of constitutively active PTPN11 reduced the responsiveness of fibroblasts to profibrotic stimuli, and viral delivery of PTPN11 to wild-type mice blunted bleomycin-induced pulmonary fibrosis (50) (**Figure 1**; **Table 1**).

The WNT Pathway in IPF

Perhaps, one of the most intriguing finding in IPF lungs gene expression was the aberrant activation of developmental pathways and especially the WNT/β-catenin pathway in IPF (**Figure 1**; **Table 1**) (64, 65). In 2003, the first observation of β-catenin expression in fibroblastic foci, as well as its expression and colocalization with WNT downstream target genes, CCND1 and MMP7 in adjacent proliferative bronchiolar lesions was reported (64). Subsequently, increased WNT1, WNT7b, WNT10b, FZD2 and FZD3, β-catenin, and LEF1 were found in IPF lungs (23). WNT1, WNT3a, β-catenin, and GSK3B were mainly localized to alveolar and bronchial epithelium with increased expression of WNT targets CCND1 and MMP7. Increased expression of WISP1, a WNT inducible signaling protein, was found in IPF lungs. WISP1 had profibrotic effects *in vitro*, and WISP1 neutralizing antibodies blunted fibrosis *in vivo* (47). Inhibition of WNT/β-catenin

TABLE 1 | Summary of relevant idiopathic pulmonary fibrosis (IPF) genes identified by transcriptome profiling.

Gene ID[a]	Gene name	Direction of expression	Tissue localization	Relevant pathway	Reference
Expressed in lung epithelium in IPF					
MMP7	Matrix metallopeptidase 7	Increased	Lung (alveolar epithelial cells and fibroblasts), peripheral blood and BAL	Extracellular matrix degradation, defensins, SPP1, and WNT/β-catenin pathway	(4, 5, 21–27)
MMP3	Matrix metallopeptidase 3	Increased	Lung, epithelial cells	Extracellular matrix degradation, β-catenin pathway	(28)
MMP19	Matrix metallopeptidase 19	Increased	Lung, epithelial cells	Extracellular matrix degradation, PTGS2 pathway	(29)
MMP1	Matrix metallopeptidase 1	Increased	Lung, epithelial cells	Extracellular matrix degradation, mitochondrial function/HIF-1-alpha pathway	(30)
SPP1	Osteopontin	Increased	Lung (epithelial cells)	Extracellular matrix degradation	(9, 22)
IGFBP-4	Insulin-like growth factor binding protein 4	Increased	Lung (alveolar and basal cells)	IGF1 pathway	(5, 24)
CCNA2	Cyclin A2	Increased	Lung (alveolar epithelial cells)	Cell cycle regulation	(10)
HIF1A	Hypoxia-inducible factor-1 alpha	Increased	Lung (alveolar epithelial cells)	Hypoxia, p53/VEGF pathways	(31)
CAV1	Caveolin-1	Decreased	Lung	Cell cycle regulation, TGF-b/JNK pathway	(6)
SYN-2	Syndecan-2	Increased	Lung, alveolar macrophages	TGF-b pathway	(32)
TAGLN	Transgelin	Increased	Lung, ATII cells	TGF-b pathway	(33)
CRLF 1	Cytokine receptor-like factor 1	Increased	Lung, ATII	Th1 cells inflammatory response	(34)
EGFR	Epidermal growth factor receptor	Increased	Lung, epithelial cells	Reepithelization	(35)
LYCAT	Lysocardiolipin acyltransferase	Decreased	Lung (epithelial cells), peripheral blood mononuclear cell (PBMC)	Mitochondrial membrane potential	(36)
SERPINF1 (PEDF)	Pigment epithelium-derived factor	Increased	Lung	Angiogenesis	(37)
Fibroblasts related gene expression in IPF					
FOXF1	Forkhead box F1	Increased	Lung	COL1/ARPC1 pathway	(38)
VCAM-1	Vascular cell adhesion molecule 1	Increased	Lung, fibroblast foci and blood vessels	TGF-b/ERK/Cyclin D pathway	(39)
FKBP10	FK506-binding protein 10	Increased	Lung, fibroblasts, and CD68 (+) macrophages	TGF-b/Col I synthesis	(40)
RXFP1	Relaxin/insulin-like family peptide receptor 1	Decreased	Lung	TGF-b	(41)
TAZ	Transcriptional coactivator with PDZ-binding motif	Increased	Lung	CTGF and Col1 pathways	(42)
IGFBP3, IGFBP5	Insulin-like growth factor binding proteins 3 and 5	Increased	Lung	IGF pathway	(43)
WNT pathway in IPF					
WNT1, 3a, 5a, 7b, 10b, Fzd2 and 3, β-catenin, Lef1, Gsk-3β	Wingless and others	Increased	Lung, fibroblasts, alveolar and bronchial epithelium	Wnt signaling	(23, 44, 45)
LRP5	Wnt co-receptor	Increased	Lung, PBMC	Wnt and TGF-b pathway	(46)
WISP1	Wnt1-inducible signaling protein-1	Increased	Lung	Wnt signaling	(47)
Apoptotic response in IPF					
TWIST1	Twist basic helix–loop–helix transcription factor 1	Increased	Lung—fibroblastic foci	Apoptosis/PDGF pathway	(48)
CXCL12	Chemokine ligand 12	Increased	Lung	Inflammation	(8)
TNSF10, BAX, CASP6	Apoptotic regulators	Altered expression	Lung	Apoptosis	(49)
SHP2 (PTPN11)	SH2 domain-containing tyrosine phosphatase-2	Decreased	Lung	Apoptosis/Tyr and Ser/Thr kinase pathways	(50)
Host defense implicated in IPF					
DEFA3–4	Defensin alpha 3 and 4	Increased	Lung and peripheral blood	Host defense	(10, 51)
AGER (RAGE)	Advanced glycosylation end product-specific receptor	Decreased	Lung and peripheral blood	Inflammation	(24, 52)
Mitochondria-related genes in IPF					
PINK1	PTEN-induced putative kinase 1	Decreased	Lung	Dysfunction of mitochondria	(53)
DIO2	Iodothyronine deiodinase 2	Increased	Lung	TH pathway/mitochondrial biogenesis	(54)

pathway attenuated lung fibrosis in mice, suggesting an essential role of WNT/β-catenin pathway in IPF development (46, 66).

While many of these observations were focused on epithelial cells, WNT5A, a member of the non-canonical signaling pathway was increased in IPF lung fibroblasts, with multiple observations suggesting its role in determining fibroblast phenotype in IPF (45, 67, 68).

Aging, Metabolism, and Mitochondria-Related Molecules

Mitochondrial dysfunction is emerging as one of the key features of IPF. Gene expression data revealed decreased PINK1, a key regulator of mitophagy, and analysis of IPF lungs revealed accumulation of dysfunctional mitochondria in alveolar epithelial cells. Findings from PINK1 knockout confirmed these results, and established a role for impaired mitophagy in IPF (53) potentially through TGFB1 effects (69).

High expression of DIO2, an enzyme that activates thyroid hormone in IPF lungs, and a predisposition to fibrosis among DIO2 knockout mice, led investigators to treat bleomycin treated mice with thyroid hormone or a small molecule agonist (54). Thyroid hormone reversed bleomycin-induced mitochondrial injury both *in vivo* and *in vitro* and augmented resolution of fibrosis in mouse models of pulmonary fibrosis. This effect was dependent on intact PPARGC1A and PINK1 pathways suggesting that the antifibrotic effect of thyroid hormone was mediated through restoration of mitochondrial homeostasis (54).

Changes in expression of genes encoding numerous metabolic enzymes from IPF lungs associated with glucose, fatty acid and citric acid metabolism suggesting on large alterations in mitochondria function (70). Similar findings were found in fibroblasts and alveolar macrophages (71, 72). More detailed review of age-related perturbations in genome and epigenome associating with plausible roles of mitochondria in pathogenesis were published elsewhere (73, 74).

GENE EXPRESSION PATTERNS AS TOOLS FOR DISEASE DIAGNOSIS, CLASSIFICATION, AND OUTCOME PREDICTORS

Transcriptomics studies have also been used to identify disease class related gene expression patterns in the lung, as well as to prioritize protein biomarkers found in the blood stream, or to identify peripheral blood mononuclear cells (PBMCs), gene expression patterns that correlate with disease clinical attributes. The studies are summarized in **Table 2**.

Disease Classification

An early suggestion that lung gene expression can be used to classify disease emerged from comparison of lungs of patients with IPF from those with fibrotic hypersensitivity pneumonitis (HP) using transcriptome analysis (5). The enrichment pathway analysis of the HP signature revealed T-cell activation, inflammation,

TABLE 2 | Summary of gene signatures that classify interstitial lung diseases.

# Genes	Tissue origin	Disease comparison	Sample size	Year	Reference
407	Lung	Idiopathic pulmonary fibrosis (IPF) vs HP	15 (IPF) 12 (HP)	2006	(5)
332/6	Lung	Sporadic IPF vs familial, IPF vs non-specific interstitial pneumonitis (NSIP)	16 sporadic IPF (2 NSIP) 10 familial (4 NSIP)	2007	(8)
242/335	Lung, fibroblasts	CTRL vs (SScPF; SScPAH; iPAH; IPF)	33 (15 severe PF, 6 moderate/severe PF and PAH, 4 moderate PF with PAH, 7 PAH), 10 IPF	2011	(75)
<50	Lung	SSc/IFP; IPF vs NSIP	≤10	2007, 2011	(8, 75)
22	Lung	IUP vs (non-IUP, sarc, HP)	77 training set (39 IUP, 38 non-IUP), validation set 48 (22 IUP, 26 non-IUP)	2015	(19)
4,734	Lung	PH-IPF and PAH vs CTRL	18 (PAH), 8 (PH-IPF)	2010	(76)
74	Lung	Chronic lung disease	13 data sets	2015	(77)
>1,500/32[a]	LCM lung	PH-IPF vs CTRL, PH-chronic obstructive pulmonary disease (COPD) vs CTRL, PH-IPF vs PH-COPD	LCM pulmonary arterioles (n = 8)	2014	(78)
255	LCM lung	PH-IPF vs NPH-IPF	8 PH-IPF, 8 NPH-IPF	2013	(79)
2,490[b] 337[c] 214[d]	Lung	IPF vs COPD vs CTRL	19 IPF, 49 COPD	2016	(18)
3 Gene clusters	Lung	IPF vs COPD vs CTRL	319 (3 data sets)[e]	2015	(15)

[a]*32 small DEGs overlap between PH-IPF and PH-COPD.*
[b]*2,490 DEGs between IPF and CTRL.*
[c]*DEGs between COPD and CTRL.*
[d]*DEGs overlap between IPF and COPD.*
[e]*4,259 mRNA and 438 microRNA and also includes 669 clinical variables.*

and humoral immune response pathways, whereas the IPF gene signature showed enrichment for cell adhesion, extracellular matrix, and lung development pathways (80).

Analysis of lung samples obtained from patients with sporadic IPF, familial pulmonary fibrosis with a usual interstitial pneumonia (UIP) pattern, and non-specific interstitial pneumonitis (NSIP) revealed similarities on gene expression patterns and pathways and a minimal difference between IPF and NSIP (**Table 2**) (5, 8). Similar findings were found when systemic sclerosis (SSc) associated pulmonary fibrosis and IPF were compared (75).

A recent study used supervised machine learning algorithms to distinguish lung biopsy samples with UIP from non-UIP (NSIP, sarcoidosis, and HP) identified a 22 gene signature (specificity 92%, sensitivity 64–82%). This approach was solely based on transcriptional data concordant with UIP pathological findings without integration of clinical information, or comparison to patient-level diagnoses by multidisciplinary teams, the current diagnostic gold standard (19). The same group continued improving genomic classifiers to differentiate UIP from non-UIP and demonstrate high robustness toward lung tissue collection using transbronchial biopsy (81, 82) (**Figure 1**; **Table 2**).

Lung Gene Expression Profiles Associated With Disease Activity and Severity

Idiopathic pulmonary fibrosis has different patterns of progression, from stable disease lasting for long periods of time to rapid progression, and acute exacerbations that are highly lethal. Despite a very small number of samples, differentially expressed genes were found in end-stage lungs obtained from patients with rapid and slow progression defined by length of symptoms (**Figures 1** and **2**; **Table 3**) (7). Similar findings were also found in a study aimed to identify genes that defined progression by rate of deterioration in pulmonary function tests (9). SFTPA1, SPP1, and HSPA1A were among top increased genes and correlated with worst survival in IPF in agreement with previous reports (83, 84).

The study of acute exacerbations of IPF has been limited, because of lack of tissue availability. Using a unique resource of rapid lung autopsies (88) investigators compared lung gene expression profiles of acute exacerbations, stable end-stage IPF, and controls (10). They did not find any significant evidence for infection or overt inflammation in acute exacerbation lungs, but they did find increased expression of CCNA2, and DEFA3 and DEFA4, antimicrobial proteins of the alpha-defensin family known to be cleaved by MMP7 (25) and evidence for widespread epithelial apoptosis.

A more sophisticated effort to identify disease endotypes based on tissue gene expression, incorporated clinical and histological information in the analysis (61). This determined that patients with increased expression of cilia-related genes, such as DNAH6, DNAH7, DNAI1, and RPGRIP1L, exhibited also increased expression of SPP1, MMP1, MMP7, PLUNC, MUC5B, as well as more microscopic honeycombing on histology but no myofibroblastic foci (61) (**Table 3**). Interestingly, MMP7 has previously been shown to attenuate ciliated cell differentiation during wound repair (27). Another effort to identify disease activity genes studied gene expression commonalities between IPF disease progression in humans and bleomycin-induced lung fibrosis in rats (14). They identified the largest overlap in differentially expressed genes between lung transcriptome of bleomycin-induced fibrosis and IPF human lungs and identified 12 genes (C6, CTHRC1, CTSE, FHL2, GAL, GREM1, LCN2, MMP7, NELL1, PCSK1, PLA2G2A, and SLC2A5) as translational markers of disease activity. Of those markers, four classified IPF patients based on disease severity (14).

Cross Disease Endotypes

The availability of large datasets such as the LGRC, allowed also analysis of multiple chronic lung disease in parallel. Recently, applying a novel computational approach named integrative phenotyping framework, investigators discovered novel endotypes of chronic obstructive pulmonary disease (COPD) and IPF (15). They integrated clinical phenotype data with mRNA and microRNA data and identified novel patient clusters. The genes that characterized the patients in the intermediate clusters were enriched with inflammatory and immune pathways, suggesting that patients from those clusters could have a mechanistically distinct autoimmune endotypes (15). Similarly, the same group integrated mRNA, microRNA, and splicing gene variants to identify convergent transcriptional regulatory networks in IPF and COPD (18). The p53/hypoxia pathway emerged as a convergent pathway in COPD and IPF. A recent study performed meta-analysis of 13 published data

TABLE 3 | Summary of gene signatures that predict idiopathic pulmonary fibrosis (IPF) progression [rapid vs slow (stable)].

# Genes	Tissue origin	Sample size (IPF)	Year	Reference
437	Lung	26 (rapid progressors), 88 (slow progressors)	2007	(7)
579	Lung	23 (stable), 8 (acute exacerbation)	2009	(10)
134	Lung	6 (stable), 6 (progressive)	2009	(9)
472	Lung	119 (training), 111 (validation)	2013	(61)
468/12[b]	Bleomycin rat/IPF human	100 (human), 73 (rats)	2015	(14)
1,428/2,790/13[a]	Peripheral blood mononuclear cell (PBMC)	130 (mild vs ctrl; severe vs ctrl; mild vs severe)	2012	(51)
118	PBMC	45 (training), 21 and 75 (validation)	2015	(85)
52	PBMC	45 (discovery), 75 (validation), and 425 (validation)	2013, 2017	(86, 87)

[a]*13 DEGs between mild and severe IPF.*
[b]*12 is set of translational markers.*

sets including cystic fibrosis, COPD, IPF and asthma, environmental conditions (smoking, epithelial injury), and control to identify general markers of chronic lung disease (77). Increased inflammatory, wounding, defense response and regulation of cell proliferation pathways, and decreased immune response pathways were observed (77). While intriguing, all of these studies were limited by lack of resolution with regard to cellular admixture and depth of clinical phenotyping (**Figure 1**; **Table 2**).

Prioritization of Protein Biomarkers

Genome scale transcriptome studies facilitated the development of protein-based biomarkers for IPF diagnosis (**Figures 1** and **2**; **Table 4**). A comparison of proteins in the blood flow of patients with IPF to control using a targeted proteomic approach identified a signature of MMP1, MMP7, MMP8, IGFBP1, and TNFRSA1F (24) that was able to distinguish IPF from controls with high sensitivity and specificity. MMP 1 and MMP 7 were also increased in the lungs of IPF patients and able to differentiate IPF patients from other chronic lung disease including hypersensitivity pneumonitis and sarcoidosis.

Indeed, MMP7, which emerged out of the first microarray analysis of human IPF lungs, was replicated as predictive of increased mortality in multiple cohorts of IPF patients (14, 26, 90–92, 95). Similar experimental strategy, following a lung gene expression finding with assessment of a protein in the peripheral blood, has been applied to many molecules including SPP1 (22), COMP (63), CXCL13 (93), CCL8 (94), and others (**Table 4**).

Peripheral Blood Gene Expression Patterns

The transcriptome of the peripheral blood is highly appealing because of information about disease presence and outcome. It represents a safe and accessible alternative to availability of samples from the lung. Microarray gene expression profiles of whole blood RNA (51) distinguished IPF patients from controls, and among IPF patients, 13 genes were changed with increased disease severity as assessed by DLCO but not FVC (**Figures 1** and **2**; **Table 3**) (51). Interestingly, alpha-defensins identified in acute exacerbations in the lung (10) were also associated with disease severity in the peripheral blood.

A subsequent study aimed to identify PBMC gene expression profiles predictive of increased mortality in patients with IPF (86). The authors performed microarray analysis on RNA isolated from PBMCs in discovery and replication cohorts of IPF patients. They identified a 52-gene outcome-predictive signature that distinguished two patient groups with significant differences in transplant free survival in both cohorts. Interestingly, increased mortality was associated with decreases in the T-cell co-stimulatory molecules CD28, ICOS, LCK, and ITK, potentially highlighting the role of potential T-cell aberrations and maybe the role of immunosenescence in IPF. Remarkably, the outcome-predictive accuracy of a score calculated based on the 52-gene signature was recently validated in a six cohorts study containing 425 IPF patients (87). Adding the 52-gene risk score to the Gender, Age, and Physiology index significantly improved its mortality predictive accuracy, suggesting that the genomic signature improved on the performance of validated clinical markers. Analysis of longitudinal changes in the signature revealed that while the 52-gene risk score tracked changes in FVC, patients never shifted their risk profile. However, in a subset of treated patients, a shift in the risk score was also accompanied by functional improvement, suggesting that the 52-gene signature may be indicative of response to the therapy. These datasets were also used in manuscripts that applied Weighted Gene Co-expression Network Analysis to identify gene expression modules that correlate with outcome (85) or microbiome changes (96) (**Table 3**). The impressive accuracy and replication should drive experiments that test the value of these biomarkers prospectively and assess in detail shift in circulating inflammatory cells in IPF using unbiased methods such as single-cell RNAseq.

ROLE OF NON-CODING RNAs IN IPF

Until recently considered the dark matter of the genome, the significant role of non-coding RNAs in human health and disease is increasingly appreciated (97). We will focus here on microRNAs, as their role has been extensively studied in pulmonary fibrosis.

MicroRNA Changes Reveal Loss of Differentiation

MicroRNAs are small non-coding RNAs that regulate gene expression by either initiating RNA degradation or inhibiting translation through binding to the 3′ UTR of their target gene. Acting as rheostats, many microRNAs regulate the general responsiveness of a cell to a certain stimulus by affecting numerous genes and frequently serving as gate keepers of feed forward

TABLE 4 | Summary of single genes—biomarkers of idiopathic pulmonary fibrosis (IPF) progression.

Gene ID	Gene name	Tissue origin	Sample size (IPF)	Year	Reference
MMP7	Matrix metallopeptidase 7	Lung, serum, plasma, BAL	13 (lung), 74 (plasma, lung, BAL)	2002, 2008	(4, 24)
			20 (BAL)	2009	(89)
			214 (plasma, 140 derivation and 101 validation)	2012	(26)
			65 (serum), 1,227 (serum), 97 (plasma)	2016, 2017	(90, 91, 92)
SPP1	Osteopontin	Lung, BAL	18	2005	(22)
COMP	Cartilage oligomeric matrix protein	Lung	115	2013	(63)
CXCL13	C–X–C motif chemokine 13	Lung, plasma	92, 94	2014	(93)
CCL8	Chemokine (C–C motif) ligand 8	Lung, BAL, plasma	8 (lung), 86 (BAL, plasma)	2017	(94)

loops. The expression of approximately 10% of the microRNAs is different in IPF compared with control lungs (98, 99). The microRNA expression patterns observed in IPF are similar to those observed in the developing lung. Comparison of fetal, IPF and control lungs revealed that miR-487b, miR-409-3p, miR-154, miR-154*, miR-134, miR-299–5p, miR-410, miR-382, miR-377, and miR-296 were increased in IPF or fetal lungs compared with controls (99). A time course systems biology analysis of microRNAs changed during postnatal lung development suggested that close to 40% were also changed in IPF (100). In the same vein, comparison of microRNA signatures in IPF and non-small cell lung cancer revealed significant similarities and numerous microRNAs that changed in the same direction. Notably, over 20 microRNAs including members of the miR-30, let-7, miR-29 families were decreased in IPF and lung cancer, commonly increased microRNAs included miR-155, miR-21, miR-205, and miR-31 (101). While the cellular origin and exact effects of all of these common microRNA changes are unclear, together with the observations about lung development, microRNA changes in the IPF lung suggest a loss of the differentiated organ regulatory networks potentially as a result of desynchronized aging (102, 103).

IPF MicroRNAs and TGFB1

One of the most recurrent themes in microRNAs in IPF, is that they are both regulated by and regulators of TGFB1 signaling. Thus, in many cases, a change in the expression of a microRNA disrupts the careful balance of self-limited activation of TGFB1. Let-7d, a microRNA known to regulate epithelial cell differentiation, is a good example. It is decreased in IPF lungs, it is inhibited by TGFB1 through direct effect of SMAD3, and when it is inhibited, it ceases to inhibit HMGA2, allowing amplification of TGFB1 signaling and early fibrotic changes *in vivo* and *in vitro* (98). Similarly, miR-21, a microRNA increased in IPF lungs, is induced by TGFB1 and is an inhibitor of SMAD7, a regulatory SMA that inhibits TGFB1 signaling pathways (104). A larger number of TGFB1 inducible microRNAs, localized to chromosome 14q32, were also increased in IPF lungs (99). Other microRNAs regulating or regulated by TGFB1 were found to be changed in IPF lungs include miR-30, miR-199, miR-29, miR-26, miR-155, miR-326, and others (105). While, it can be safely said that microRNA changes in IPF seem to result in lowering the cell profibrotic threshold, it has to be mentioned that they were obtained in isolation, for one microRNA at a time, but in the IPF lung, at least when analyzed in bulk, they happen simultaneously. To understand better the effects of microRNA perturbations, careful dissection of the cellular, spatial, and temporal changes, as well as their integrated effects is required.

miR-29, the Ultimate Antifibromir

Of microRNAs differentially expressed in IPF, the miR-29 family is probably the most extensively studied both mechanistically and as a therapeutic target, because of its known inhibitory effects on extracellular matrix proteins, and growth factors such CTGF and IGF1 (106). miR-29 family members are decreased in cardiac, renal and liver fibrosis, keloid, fibrotic Crohn's disease, and other fibrotic conditions (107–113). miR-29 family microRNAs are decreased in IPF lungs (114), they regulate numerous genes related to fibrosis (115) and seem to regulate profibrotic signals from the extracellular matrix to fibroblasts (116). Both gene delivery of miR-29 *via* a transposon method (117) or using a miR-29b mimic (118) augmented resolution of bleomycin-induced pulmonary fibrosis. While most of these studies focused on the role of miR-29 in fibroblasts, two recent studies suggested that miR-29 could be important in prevention of pulmonary fibrosis (119) or bronchopulmonary dysplasia (120) through beneficial effects on alveolar repair. Regardless of the cell specificity of the effect, miR-29 supplementation seems a viable option as an antifibrotic therapy.

TABLE 5 | Data and tissue repositories.

Name	Website	Reference
Lung Tissue Research Consortium	http://www.ltrcpublic.com/	(126)
Lung Genomics Research Consortium	http://www.lung-genomics.org/	(126)
Lung development map	https://www.lungmap.net/	(127, 128)
Cell differentiation analysis (scRNAseq)	http://www.cs.cmu.edu/~jund/scdiff/index.html	(129)

IPF MICROENVIRONMENTS

The IPF lung is characterized histologically by its regional, temporal and cellular heterogeneity, meaning that normal looking regions are interspersed with diseased regions, different regions may appear at different stages of disease (121, 122), and both the cellular content and the phenotype of known cells are dramatically altered in the IPF lung. Transcriptomic profiles of bulk tissue homogenates do not capture this complexity. They also do not allow understanding how cells influence each other in the remodeled IPF microenvironment. Improving the cellular and spatial resolution of transcriptomics using single cells and tissue microenvironments is critically important to decipher what happens in the IPF lung.

Tissue and Cellular Heterogeneity Are Starting to Emerge

Transcriptome analyses performed on bulk lung tissue detected strong gene expression signals, leading to discovery of IPF relevant signaling pathways (**Figures 1** and **2**). However, it is unclear whether alteration in transcriptome signals represented core features of disease or was dominated by changes in cellular admixture. Increased gene expression changes observed in the IPF lung were frequently assigned to cell types, based on prior knowledge or follow-up studies, as in the case of MMP7, SPP1, WISP1, COMP, TWIST1, PINK1, and the others mentioned earlier. In most cases, such analysis was done after the fact, using low throughput technologies such as immunohistochemistry, and was dependent on prior knowledge and availability of reagents. Only few studies analyzed transcriptomic gene expression

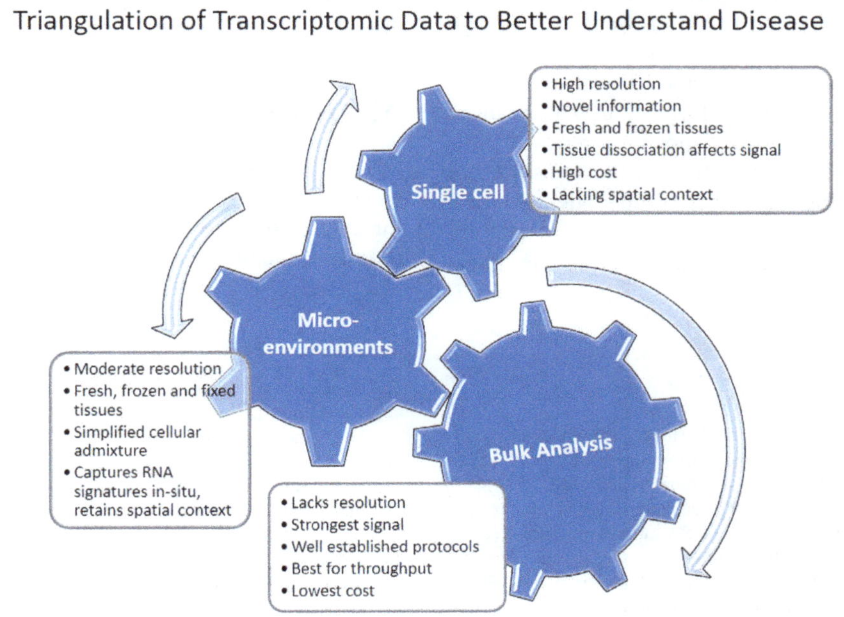

FIGURE 3 | Triangulation of transcriptomic data to understand disease. Single cell, microenvironment, and bulk tissue transcriptomic analysis have their advantages and disadvantages. When applied together, they can help in understanding regulatory networks in the tissue.

in well-defined IPF microenvironments. Comparison of the transcriptome of hyperplastic vs conserved epithelial cells and dense fibrotic lung regions, using laser capture microdissections identified previously unrecognized MMP19, as a molecule increased in hyperplastic epithelial cells, with an antifibrotic role (29). Two studies reported solely gene expression profiles of pulmonary vasculature and showed differential gene expression for IPF patients with and without coexistent PH (79) and for PH-IPF and COPD (78) (**Table 2**). Two clusters of co-regulated genes related to bronchiolar epithelium or lymphoid aggregates were identified when whole lung transcriptome was correlated with tissues histology and clinical variables (123). The first study to apply single-cell RNAseq of sorted epithelial cells from IPF patients or controls revealed distinct epithelial cell types in IPF lung and complete lack of some "normal" epithelial cells (124). Using transcriptomic profiling of flow-sorted cells, monocytes shown to differentiate into alveolar macrophages and continuously express profibrotic genes over the course of fibrosis. Thus, selective targeting of alveolar macrophage differentiation within the lung may decrease fibrosis and avoid global monocyte or tissue-resident alveolar macrophage depletion (125). Besides transcriptomics profiling of sorted and single cells isolated from fresh lung, the RNAseq of archival formalin-fixed paraffin-embedded lung biopsy from IPF patients is possible (20). This allows analysis of specific areas of lungs and their interaction observed microscopically (epithelium and fibroblastic foci), usage of clinical variables (survival) and overcoming the availability of fresh lung tissues.

While lung microenvironment studies are still rare, the rapid emergence of methods for high throughput sequencing of single cells, the improved ability to perform sequencing from IPF microenvironments, the improved analytical methods, and the success of old fashioned analyses of bulk tissue should encourage investigators to perform larger studies focusing on understanding temporo-spatial multicellular networks in IPF.

CONCLUSION AND FUTURE DIRECTIONS

The progress of transcriptomics in IPF is characterized by increased sophistication and complexity (**Figure 1**). Transcriptomics studies facilitated multiple shifts with regard to the role of MMPs, developmental pathways, microRNAs, and the importance of alveolar epithelial and myofibroblast regulatory networks in IPF. They have also had significant impact on the discovery and prioritization of validated biomarkers (**Figure 1**). However, most of these studies used low sample number and lack validation cohorts. NIH NHLBI funded efforts led to generation of publicly available datasets of multi-omics data generated from carefully characterized human and mouse samples (**Table 5**). They contain, mainly bulk tissue, but also limited amounts of sorted cells and single-cell transcriptomic profiles. With the advent of novel technologies for single cell and microenvironment transcriptomic profiling, we have a unique opportunity to triangulate IPF regulatory and transcriptional networks by analyzing the lung from a verity of perspectives, use available bulk data, as well as profiles of disease microenvironments and single cells (**Figure 3**). This will allow integration of information and resolution of the cellular, temporal, and spatial complexities of the IPF lungs and thus better therapeutics and diagnostics. In 2014 following a series of meetings sponsored by NIH-NHLBI, the Pulmonary Fibrosis Foundation and the American Thoracic Society Assembly of Respiratory, Cell and Molecular Biology convened a series of meetings that recommended among other things, an open access biorepository for IPF research (126). While various registries have been formed, new centralized efforts to obtain IPF lung tissues have not been renewed. This is a problem, because most current tissue collections are not amenable to analysis using the novel technologies. To take advantage of the new opportunities, to continue the momentum of transcriptomic success we need new efforts of sample collec tions, this time focused on access to all the microenvironments and cells in the IPF lung.

AUTHOR CONTRIBUTIONS

MV and NK substantially contributed to review design; data analysis and interpretation. Both the authors participated in writing and revising the review, approved the final work, and agreed to be accountable for all aspects of the review.

REFERENCES

1. Pease AC, Solas D, Sullivan EJ, Cronin MT, Holmes CP, Fodor SP. Light-generated oligonucleotide arrays for rapid DNA sequence analysis. *Proc Natl Acad Sci U S A* (1994) 91:5022–6. doi:10.1073/pnas.91.11.5022
2. Schena M, Shalon D, Davis RW, Brown PO. Quantitative monitoring of gene expression patterns with a complementary DNA microarray. *Science* (1995) 270:467–70. doi:10.1126/science.270.5235.467
3. Kaminski N, Allard JD, Pittet JF, Zuo F, Griffiths MJ, Morris D, et al. Global analysis of gene expression in pulmonary fibrosis reveals distinct programs regulating lung inflammation and fibrosis. *Proc Natl Acad Sci U S A* (2000) 97:1778–83. doi:10.1073/pnas.97.4.1778
4. Zuo F, Kaminski N, Eugui E, Allard J, Yakhini Z, Ben-Dor A, et al. Gene expression analysis reveals matrilysin as a key regulator of pulmonary fibrosis in mice and humans. *Proc Natl Acad Sci U S A* (2002) 99:6292–7. doi:10.1073/pnas.092134099
5. Selman M, Pardo A, Barrera L, Estrada A, Watson SR, Wilson K, et al. Gene expression profiles distinguish idiopathic pulmonary fibrosis from hypersensitivity pneumonitis. *Am J Respir Crit Care Med* (2006) 173:188–98. doi:10.1164/rccm.200504-644OC
6. Wang XM, Zhang Y, Kim HP, Zhou Z, Feghali-Bostwick CA, Liu F, et al. Caveolin-1: a critical regulator of lung fibrosis in idiopathic pulmonary fibrosis. *J Exp Med* (2006) 203:2895–906. doi:10.1084/jem.20061536
7. Selman M, Carrillo G, Estrada A, Mejia M, Becerril C, Cisneros J, et al. Accelerated variant of idiopathic pulmonary fibrosis: clinical behavior and gene expression pattern. *PLoS One* (2007) 2:e482. doi:10.1371/journal.pone.0000482
8. Yang IV, Burch LH, Steele MP, Savov JD, Hollingsworth JW, Mcelvania-Tekippe E, et al. Gene expression profiling of familial and sporadic interstitial pneumonia. *Am J Respir Crit Care Med* (2007) 175:45–54. doi:10.1164/rccm.200601-062OC
9. Boon K, Bailey NW, Yang J, Steel MP, Groshong S, Kervitsky D, et al. Molecular phenotypes distinguish patients with relatively stable from progressive idiopathic pulmonary fibrosis (IPF). *PLoS One* (2009) 4:e5134. doi:10.1371/journal.pone.0005134
10. Konishi K, Gibson KF, Lindell KO, Richards TJ, Zhang Y, Dhir R, et al. Gene expression profiles of acute exacerbations of idiopathic pulmonary fibrosis. *Am J Respir Crit Care Med* (2009) 180:167–75. doi:10.1164/rccm.200810-1596OC
11. Dave NB, Kaminski N. Analysis of microarray experiments for pulmonary fibrosis. *Methods Mol Med* (2005) 117:333–58. doi:10.1385/1-59259-940-0:333
12. Segal E, Friedman N, Kaminski N, Regev A, Koller D. From signatures to models: understanding cancer using microarrays. *Nat Genet* (2005) 37(Suppl):S38–45. doi:10.1038/ng1561
13. NIH-NHLBI. *Lung Tissue Resource Consortium*. (2005). Available from: https://ltrcpublic.com (Accessed: March 15, 2018).
14. Bauer Y, Tedrow J, De Bernard S, Birker-Robaczewska M, Gibson KF, Guardela BJ, et al. A novel genomic signature with translational significance for human idiopathic pulmonary fibrosis. *Am J Respir Cell Mol Biol* (2015) 52:217–31. doi:10.1165/rcmb.2013-0310OC
15. Kim S, Herazo-Maya JD, Kang DD, Juan-Guardela BM, Tedrow J, Martinez FJ, et al. Integrative phenotyping framework (iPF): integrative clustering of multiple omics data identifies novel lung disease subphenotypes. *BMC Genomics* (2015) 16:924. doi:10.1186/s12864-015-2170-4
16. Quackenbush J, Kaminski N, Schwartz DA, Spira A. *Lung Genomics Research Consoritum Download Page [Online]*. (2013). Available from: http://www.lung-genomics.org (Accessed: March 15, 2018).
17. Yang IV, Pedersen BS, Rabinovich E, Hennessy CE, Davidson EJ, Murphy E, et al. Relationship of DNA methylation and gene expression in idiopathic pulmonary fibrosis. *Am J Respir Crit Care Med* (2014) 190:1263–72. doi:10.1164/rccm.201408-1452OC
18. Kusko RL, Brothers JF II, Tedrow J, Pandit K, Huleihel L, Perdomo C, et al. Integrated genomics reveals convergent transcriptomic networks underlying chronic obstructive pulmonary disease and idiopathic pulmonary fibrosis. *Am J Respir Crit Care Med* (2016) 194:948–60. doi:10.1164/rccm.201510-2026OC
19. Kim SY, Diggans J, Pankratz D, Huang J, Pagan M, Sindy N, et al. Classification of usual interstitial pneumonia in patients with interstitial lung disease: assessment of a machine learning approach using high-dimensional transcriptional data. *Lancet Respir Med* (2015) 3:473–82. doi:10.1016/S2213-2600(15)00140-X
20. Vukmirovic M, Herazo-Maya JD, Blackmon J, Skodric-Trifunovic V, Jovanovic D, Pavlovic S, et al. Identification and validation of differentially expressed transcripts by RNA-sequencing of formalin-fixed, paraffin-embedded (FFPE) lung tissue from patients with idiopathic pulmonary fibrosis. *BMC Pulm Med* (2017) 17:15. doi:10.1186/s12890-016-0356-4
21. Cosgrove GP, Schwarz MI, Geraci MW, Brown KK, Worthen GS. Overexpression of matrix metalloproteinase-7 in pulmonary fibrosis. *Chest* (2002) 121:25s–6s. doi:10.1378/chest.121.3_suppl.25S-a
22. Pardo A, Gibson K, Cisneros J, Richards TJ, Yang Y, Becerril C, et al. Up-regulation and profibrotic role of osteopontin in human idiopathic pulmonary fibrosis. *PLoS Med* (2005) 2:e251. doi:10.1371/journal.pmed.0020251
23. Konigshoff M, Balsara N, Pfaff EM, Kramer M, Chrobak I, Seeger W, et al. Functional Wnt signaling is increased in idiopathic pulmonary fibrosis. *PLoS One* (2008) 3:e2142. doi:10.1371/journal.pone.0002142
24. Rosas IO, Richards TJ, Konishi K, Zhang Y, Gibson K, Lokshin AE, et al. MMP1 and MMP7 as potential peripheral blood biomarkers in idiopathic pulmonary fibrosis. *PLoS Med* (2008) 5:e93. doi:10.1371/journal.pmed.0050093
25. Wilson CL, Schmidt AP, Pirila E, Valore EV, Ferri N, Sorsa T, et al. Differential processing of {alpha}- and {beta}-defensin precursors by matrix metalloproteinase-7 (MMP-7). *J Biol Chem* (2009) 284:8301–11. doi:10.1074/jbc.M809744200
26. Richards TJ, Kaminski N, Baribaud F, Flavin S, Brodmerkel C, Horowitz D, et al. Peripheral blood proteins predict mortality in idiopathic pulmonary fibrosis. *Am J Respir Crit Care Med* (2012) 185:67–76. doi:10.1164/rccm.201101-0058OC
27. Gharib SA, Altemeier WA, Van Winkle LS, Plopper CG, Schlesinger SY, Buell CA, et al. Matrix metalloproteinase-7 coordinates airway epithelial injury response and differentiation of ciliated cells. *Am J Respir Cell Mol Biol* (2013) 48:390–6. doi:10.1165/rcmb.2012-0083OC
28. Yamashita CM, Dolgonos L, Zemans RL, Young SK, Robertson J, Briones N, et al. Matrix metalloproteinase 3 is a mediator of pulmonary fibrosis. *Am J Pathol* (2011) 179:1733–45. doi:10.1016/j.ajpath.2011.06.041
29. Yu G, Kovkarova-Naumovski E, Jara P, Parwani A, Kass D, Ruiz V, et al. Matrix metalloproteinase-19 is a key regulator of lung fibrosis in mice and humans. *Am J Respir Crit Care Med* (2012) 186:752–62. doi:10.1164/rccm.201202-0302OC
30. Herrera I, Cisneros J, Maldonado M, Ramirez R, Ortiz-Quintero B, Anso E, et al. Matrix metalloproteinase (MMP)-1 induces lung alveolar epithelial cell

migration and proliferation, protects from apoptosis, and represses mitochondrial oxygen consumption. *J Biol Chem* (2013) 288:25964–75. doi:10.1074/jbc.M113.459784
31. Tzouvelekis A, Harokopos V, Paparountas T, Oikonomou N, Chatziioannou A, Vilaras G, et al. Comparative expression profiling in pulmonary fibrosis suggests a role of hypoxia-inducible factor-1alpha in disease pathogenesis. *Am J Respir Crit Care Med* (2007) 176:1108–19. doi:10.1164/rccm.200705-683OC
32. Shi Y, Gochuico BR, Yu G, Tang X, Osorio JC, Fernandez IE, et al. Syndecan-2 exerts antifibrotic effects by promoting caveolin-1-mediated transforming growth factor-beta receptor I internalization and inhibiting transforming growth factor-beta1 signaling. *Am J Respir Crit Care Med* (2013) 188:831–41. doi:10.1164/rccm.201303-0434OC
33. Yu H, Konigshoff M, Jayachandran A, Handley D, Seeger W, Kaminski N, et al. Transgelin is a direct target of TGF-beta/Smad3-dependent epithelial cell migration in lung fibrosis. *FASEB J* (2008) 22:1778–89. doi:10.1096/fj.07-083857
34. Kass DJ, Yu G, Loh KS, Savir A, Borczuk A, Kahloon R, et al. Cytokine-like factor 1 gene expression is enriched in idiopathic pulmonary fibrosis and drives the accumulation of CD4+ T cells in murine lungs: evidence for an antifibrotic role in bleomycin injury. *Am J Pathol* (2012) 180:1963–78. doi:10.1016/j.ajpath.2012.01.010
35. Tzouvelekis A, Ntolios P, Karameris A, Vilaras G, Boglou P, Koulelidis A, et al. Increased expression of epidermal growth factor receptor (EGF-R) in patients with different forms of lung fibrosis. *Biomed Res Int* (2013) 2013:654354. doi:10.1155/2013/654354
36. Huang LS, Mathew B, Li H, Zhao Y, Ma SF, Noth I, et al. The mitochondrial cardiolipin remodeling enzyme lysocardiolipin acyltransferase is a novel target in pulmonary fibrosis. *Am J Respir Crit Care Med* (2014) 189:1402–15. doi:10.1164/rccm.201310-1917OC
37. Cosgrove GP, Brown KK, Schiemann WP, Serls AE, Parr JE, Geraci MW, et al. Pigment epithelium-derived factor in idiopathic pulmonary fibrosis: a role in aberrant angiogenesis. *Am J Respir Crit Care Med* (2004) 170:242–51. doi:10.1164/rccm.200308-1151OC
38. Melboucy-Belkhir S, Pradere P, Tadbiri S, Habib S, Bacrot A, Brayer S, et al. Forkhead Box F1 represses cell growth and inhibits COL1 and ARPC2 expression in lung fibroblasts in vitro. *Am J Physiol Lung Cell Mol Physiol* (2014) 307:L838–47. doi:10.1152/ajplung.00012.2014
39. Agassandian M, Tedrow JR, Sembrat J, Kass DJ, Zhang Y, Goncharova EA, et al. VCAM-1 is a TGF-beta1 inducible gene upregulated in idiopathic pulmonary fibrosis. *Cell Signal* (2015) 27:2467–73. doi:10.1016/j.cellsig.2015.09.003
40. Staab-Weijnitz CA, Fernandez IE, Knuppel L, Maul J, Heinzelmann K, Juan-Guardela BM, et al. FK506-binding protein 10, a potential novel drug target for idiopathic pulmonary fibrosis. *Am J Respir Crit Care Med* (2015) 192:455–67. doi:10.1164/rccm.201412-2233OC
41. Tan J, Tedrow JR, Dutta JA, Juan-Guardela B, Nouraie M, Chu Y, et al. Expression of RXFP1 is decreased in idiopathic pulmonary fibrosis. implications for relaxin-based therapies. *Am J Respir Crit Care Med* (2016) 194:1392–402. doi:10.1164/rccm.201509-1865OC
42. Noguchi S, Saito A, Mikami Y, Urushiyama H, Horie M, Matsuzaki H, et al. TAZ contributes to pulmonary fibrosis by activating profibrotic functions of lung fibroblasts. *Sci Rep* (2017) 7:42595. doi:10.1038/srep42595
43. Pilewski JM, Liu L, Henry AC, Knauer AV, Feghali-Bostwick CA. Insulin-like growth factor binding proteins 3 and 5 are overexpressed in idiopathic pulmonary fibrosis and contribute to extracellular matrix deposition. *Am J Pathol* (2005) 166:399–407. doi:10.1016/S0002-9440(10)62263-8
44. Studer SM, Kaminski N. Towards systems biology of human pulmonary fibrosis. *Proc Am Thorac Soc* (2007) 4:85–91. doi:10.1513/pats.200607-139JG
45. Vuga LJ, Ben-Yehudah A, Kovkarova-Naumovski E, Oriss T, Gibson KF, Feghali-Bostwick C, et al. WNT5A is a regulator of fibroblast proliferation and resistance to apoptosis. *Am J Respir Cell Mol Biol* (2009) 41:583–9. doi:10.1165/rcmb.2008-0201OC
46. Lam AP, Herazo-Maya JD, Sennello JA, Flozak AS, Russell S, Mutlu GM, et al. Wnt coreceptor Lrp5 is a driver of idiopathic pulmonary fibrosis. *Am J Respir Crit Care Med* (2014) 190:185–95. doi:10.1164/rccm.201401-0079OC
47. Konigshoff M, Kramer M, Balsara N, Wilhelm J, Amarie OV, Jahn A, et al. WNT1-inducible signaling protein-1 mediates pulmonary fibrosis in mice and is upregulated in humans with idiopathic pulmonary fibrosis. *J Clin Invest* (2009) 119:772–87. doi:10.1172/JCI33950
48. Bridges RS, Kass D, Loh K, Glackin C, Borczuk AC, Greenberg S. Gene expression profiling of pulmonary fibrosis identifies Twist1 as an antiapoptotic molecular "rectifier" of growth factor signaling. *Am J Pathol* (2009) 175:2351–61. doi:10.2353/ajpath.2009.080954
49. Emblom-Callahan MC, Chhina MK, Shlobin OA, Ahmad S, Reese ES, Iyer EP, et al. Genomic phenotype of non-cultured pulmonary fibroblasts in idiopathic pulmonary fibrosis. *Genomics* (2010) 96:134–45. doi:10.1016/j.ygeno.2010.04.005
50. Tzouvelekis A, Yu G, Lino Cardenas CL, Herazo-Maya JD, Wang R, Woolard T, et al. SH2 domain-containing phosphatase-2 is a novel antifibrotic regulator in pulmonary fibrosis. *Am J Respir Crit Care Med* (2017) 195:500–14. doi:10.1164/rccm.201602-0329OC
51. Yang IV, Luna LG, Cotter J, Talbert J, Leach SM, Kidd R, et al. The peripheral blood transcriptome identifies the presence and extent of disease in idiopathic pulmonary fibrosis. *PLoS One* (2012) 7:e37708. doi:10.1371/journal.pone.0037708
52. Englert JM, Hanford LE, Kaminski N, Tobolewski JM, Tan RJ, Fattman CL, et al. A role for the receptor for advanced glycation end products in idiopathic pulmonary fibrosis. *Am J Pathol* (2008) 172:583–91. doi:10.2353/ajpath.2008.070569
53. Bueno M, Lai YC, Romero Y, Brands J, St Croix CM, Kamga C, et al. PINK1 deficiency impairs mitochondrial homeostasis and promotes lung fibrosis. *J Clin Invest* (2015) 125:521–38. doi:10.1172/JCI74942
54. Yu G, Tzouvelekis A, Wang R, Herazo-Maya JD, Ibarra GH, Srivastava A, et al. Thyroid hormone inhibits lung fibrosis in mice by improving epithelial mitochondrial function. *Nat Med* (2018) 24:39–49. doi:10.1038/nm.4447
55. Selman M, Ruiz V, Cabrera S, Segura L, Ramirez R, Barrios R, et al. TIMP-1, -2, -3, and -4 in idiopathic pulmonary fibrosis. A prevailing nondegradative lung microenvironment? *Am J Physiol Lung Cell Mol Physiol* (2000) 279:L562–74. doi:10.1152/ajplung.2000.279.3.L562
56. Maldonado M, Salgado-Aguayo A, Herrera I, Cabrera S, Ortiz-Quintero B, Staab-Weijnitz CA, et al. Upregulation and nuclear location of MMP28 in alveolar epithelium of idiopathic pulmonary fibrosis. *Am J Respir Cell Mol Biol* (2018). doi:10.1165/rcmb.2017-0223OC
57. Pardo A, Selman M, Kaminski N. Approaching the degradome in idiopathic pulmonary fibrosis. *Int J Biochem Cell Biol* (2008) 40:1141–55. doi:10.1016/j.biocel.2007.11.020
58. Pardo A, Cabrera S, Maldonado M, Selman M. Role of matrix metalloproteinases in the pathogenesis of idiopathic pulmonary fibrosis. *Respir Res* (2016) 17:23. doi:10.1186/s12931-016-0343-6
59. Selman M, Pardo A. Idiopathic pulmonary fibrosis: an epithelial/fibroblastic cross-talk disorder. *Respir Res* (2002) 3:3. doi:10.1186/rr175
60. Selman M, Pardo A. Role of epithelial cells in idiopathic pulmonary fibrosis: from innocent targets to serial killers. *Proc Am Thorac Soc* (2006) 3:364–72. doi:10.1513/pats.200601-003TK
61. Yang IV, Coldren CD, Leach SM, Seibold MA, Murphy E, Lin J, et al. Expression of cilium-associated genes defines novel molecular subtypes of idiopathic pulmonary fibrosis. *Thorax* (2013) 68:1114–21. doi:10.1136/thoraxjnl-2012-202943
62. Chambers RC, Leoni P, Kaminski N, Laurent GJ, Heller RA. Global expression profiling of fibroblast responses to transforming growth factor-beta1 reveals the induction of inhibitor of differentiation-1 and provides evidence of smooth muscle cell phenotypic switching. *Am J Pathol* (2003) 162:533–46. doi:10.1016/S0002-9440(10)63847-3
63. Vuga LJ, Milosevic J, Pandit K, Ben-Yehudah A, Chu Y, Richards T, et al. Cartilage oligomeric matrix protein in idiopathic pulmonary fibrosis. *PLoS One* (2013) 8:e83120. doi:10.1371/journal.pone.0083120
64. Chilosi M, Poletti V, Zamo A, Lestani M, Montagna L, Piccoli P, et al. Aberrant Wnt/beta-catenin pathway activation in idiopathic pulmonary fibrosis. *Am J Pathol* (2003) 162:1495–502. doi:10.1016/S0002-9440(10)64282-4
65. Selman M, Pardo A, Kaminski N. Idiopathic pulmonary fibrosis: aberrant recapitulation of developmental programs? *PLoS Med* (2008) 5:e62. doi:10.1371/journal.pmed.0050062
66. Henderson WR Jr, Chi EY, Ye X, Nguyen C, Tien YT, Zhou B, et al. Inhibition of Wnt/beta-catenin/CREB binding protein (CBP) signaling reverses pulmonary fibrosis. *Proc Natl Acad Sci U S A* (2010) 107:14309–14. doi:10.1073/pnas.1001520107

67. Corbett L, Mann J, Mann DA. Non-canonical wnt predominates in activated rat hepatic stellate cells, influencing HSC survival and paracrine stimulation of Kupffer cells. *PLoS One* (2015) 10:e0142794. doi:10.1371/journal.pone.0142794
68. Guan S, Zhou J. Frizzled-7 mediates TGF-beta-induced pulmonary fibrosis by transmitting non-canonical Wnt signaling. *Exp Cell Res* (2017) 359:226–34. doi:10.1016/j.yexcr.2017.07.025
69. Patel AS, Song JW, Chu SG, Mizumura K, Osorio JC, Shi Y, et al. Epithelial cell mitochondrial dysfunction and PINK1 are induced by transforming growth factor-beta1 in pulmonary fibrosis. *PLoS One* (2015) 10:e0121246. doi:10.1371/journal.pone.0121246
70. Zhao YD, Yin L, Archer S, Lu C, Zhao G, Yao Y, et al. Metabolic heterogeneity of idiopathic pulmonary fibrosis: a metabolomic study. *BMJ Open Respir Res* (2017) 4:e000183. doi:10.1136/bmjresp-2017-000183
71. Xie N, Tan Z, Banerjee S, Cui H, Ge J, Liu RM, et al. Glycolytic reprogramming in myofibroblast differentiation and lung fibrosis. *Am J Respir Crit Care Med* (2015) 192:1462–74. doi:10.1164/rccm.201504-0780OC
72. Xie N, Cui H, Ge J, Banerjee S, Guo S, Dubey S, et al. Metabolic characterization and RNA profiling reveal glycolytic dependence of profibrotic phenotype of alveolar macrophages in lung fibrosis. *Am J Physiol Lung Cell Mol Physiol* (2017) 313:L834–44. doi:10.1152/ajplung.00235.2017
73. Budinger GRS, Kohanski RA, Gan W, Kobor MS, Amaral LA, Armanios M, et al. The intersection of aging biology and the pathobiology of lung diseases: a joint NHLBI/NIA workshop. *J Gerontol A Biol Sci Med Sci* (2017) 72:1492–500. doi:10.1093/gerona/glx090
74. Mora AL, Bueno M, Rojas M. Mitochondria in the spotlight of aging and idiopathic pulmonary fibrosis. *J Clin Invest* (2017) 127:405–14. doi:10.1172/JCI87440
75. Hsu E, Shi H, Jordan RM, Lyons-Weiler J, Pilewski JM, Feghali-Bostwick CA. Lung tissues in patients with systemic sclerosis have gene expression patterns unique to pulmonary fibrosis and pulmonary hypertension. *Arthritis Rheum* (2011) 63:783–94. doi:10.1002/art.30159
76. Rajkumar R, Konishi K, Richards TJ, Ishizawar DC, Wiechert AC, Kaminski N, et al. Genomewide RNA expression profiling in lung identifies distinct signatures in idiopathic pulmonary arterial hypertension and secondary pulmonary hypertension. *Am J Physiol Heart Circ Physiol* (2010) 298:H1235–48. doi:10.1152/ajpheart.00254.2009
77. Clarke LA, Botelho HM, Sousa L, Falcao AO, Amaral MD. Transcriptome meta-analysis reveals common differential and global gene expression profiles in cystic fibrosis and other respiratory disorders and identifies CFTR regulators. *Genomics* (2015) 106:268–77. doi:10.1016/j.ygeno.2015.07.005
78. Hoffmann J, Wilhelm J, Marsh LM, Ghanim B, Klepetko W, Kovacs G, et al. Distinct differences in gene expression patterns in pulmonary arteries of patients with chronic obstructive pulmonary disease and idiopathic pulmonary fibrosis with pulmonary hypertension. *Am J Respir Crit Care Med* (2014) 190:98–111. doi:10.1164/rccm.201401-0037OC
79. Patel NM, Kawut SM, Jelic S, Arcasoy SM, Lederer DJ, Borczuk AC. Pulmonary arteriole gene expression signature in idiopathic pulmonary fibrosis. *Eur Respir J* (2013) 41:1324–30. doi:10.1183/09031936.00084112
80. Kaminski N, Rosas IO. Gene expression profiling as a window into idiopathic pulmonary fibrosis pathogenesis: can we identify the right target genes? *Proc Am Thorac Soc* (2006) 3:339–44. doi:10.1513/pats.200601-011TK
81. Choi Y, Lu J, Hu Z, Pankratz DG, Jiang H, Cao M, et al. Analytical performance of Envisia: a genomic classifier for usual interstitial pneumonia. *BMC Pulm Med* (2017) 17:141. doi:10.1186/s12890-017-0485-4
82. Pankratz DG, Choi Y, Imtiaz U, Fedorowicz GM, Anderson JD, Colby TV, et al. Usual interstitial pneumonia can be detected in transbronchial biopsies using machine learning. *Ann Am Thorac Soc* (2017) 14:1646–54. doi:10.1513/AnnalsATS.201612-947OC
83. Greene KE, King TE Jr, Kuroki Y, Bucher-Bartelson B, Hunninghake GW, Newman LS, et al. Serum surfactant proteins-A and -D as biomarkers in idiopathic pulmonary fibrosis. *Eur Respir J* (2002) 19:439–46. doi:10.1183/09031936.02.00081102
84. Kahloon RA, Xue J, Bhargava A, Csizmadia E, Otterbein L, Kass DJ, et al. Patients with idiopathic pulmonary fibrosis with antibodies to heat shock protein 70 have poor prognoses. *Am J Respir Crit Care Med* (2013) 187:768–75. doi:10.1164/rccm.201203-0506OC
85. Huang Y, Ma SF, Vij R, Oldham JM, Herazo-Maya J, Broderick SM, et al. A functional genomic model for predicting prognosis in idiopathic pulmonary fibrosis. *BMC Pulm Med* (2015) 15:147. doi:10.1186/s12890-015-0142-8
86. Herazo-Maya JD, Noth I, Duncan SR, Kim S, Ma SF, Tseng GC, et al. Peripheral blood mononuclear cell gene expression profiles predict poor outcome in idiopathic pulmonary fibrosis. *Sci Transl Med* (2013) 5:205ra136. doi:10.1126/scitranslmed.3005964
87. Herazo-Maya JD, Sun J, Molyneaux PL, Li Q, Villalba JA, Tzouvelekis A, et al. Validation of a 52-gene risk profile for outcome prediction in patients with idiopathic pulmonary fibrosis: an international, multicentre, cohort study. *Lancet Respir Med* (2017) 5:857–68. doi:10.1016/S2213-2600(17)30349-1
88. Lindell KO, Erlen JA, Kaminski N. Lessons from our patients: development of a warm autopsy program. *PLoS Med* (2006) 3:e234. doi:10.1371/journal.pmed.0030234
89. Mckeown S, Richter AG, O'Kane C, Mcauley DF, Thickett DR. MMP expression and abnormal lung permeability are important determinants of outcome in IPF. *Eur Respir J* (2009) 33:77–84. doi:10.1183/09031936.00060708
90. Hamai K, Iwamoto H, Ishikawa N, Horimasu Y, Masuda T, Miyamoto S, et al. Comparative study of circulating MMP-7, CCL18, KL-6, SP-A, and SP-D as disease markers of idiopathic pulmonary fibrosis. *Dis Markers* (2016) 2016:4759040. doi:10.1155/2016/4759040
91. Armstrong HF, Podolanczuk AJ, Barr RG, Oelsner EC, Kawut SM, Hoffman EA, et al. Serum matrix metalloproteinase-7, respiratory symptoms, and mortality in community-dwelling adults: the multi-ethnic study of atherosclerosis. *Am J Respir Crit Care Med* (2017) 196:1311–7. doi:10.1164/rccm.201701-0254OC
92. Tzouvelekis A, Herazo-Maya JD, Slade M, Chu JH, Deiuliis G, Ryu C, et al. Validation of the prognostic value of MMP-7 in idiopathic pulmonary fibrosis. *Respirology* (2017) 22:486–93. doi:10.1111/resp.12920
93. Vuga LJ, Tedrow JR, Pandit KV, Tan J, Kass DJ, Xue J, et al. C-X-C motif chemokine 13 (CXCL13) is a prognostic biomarker of idiopathic pulmonary fibrosis. *Am J Respir Crit Care Med* (2014) 189:966–74. doi:10.1164/rccm.201309-1592OC
94. Lee JU, Cheong HS, Shim EY, Bae DJ, Chang HS, Uh ST, et al. Gene profile of fibroblasts identify relation of CCL8 with idiopathic pulmonary fibrosis. *Respir Res* (2017) 18:3. doi:10.1186/s12931-016-0493-6
95. Bauer Y, White ES, De Bernard S, Cornelisse P, Leconte I, Morganti A, et al. MMP-7 is a predictive biomarker of disease progression in patients with idiopathic pulmonary fibrosis. *ERJ Open Res* (2017) 3:00074–2016. doi:10.1183/23120541.00074-2016
96. Huang Y, Ma SF, Espindola MS, Vij R, Oldham JM, Huffnagle GB, et al. Microbes are associated with host innate immune response in idiopathic pulmonary fibrosis. *Am J Respir Crit Care Med* (2017) 196:208–19. doi:10.1164/rccm.201607-1525OC
97. Mestdagh P, Vandesompele J, Brusselle G, Vermaelen K. Non-coding RNAs and respiratory disease. *Thorax* (2015) 70:388–90. doi:10.1136/thoraxjnl-2014-206404
98. Pandit KV, Corcoran D, Yousef H, Yarlagadda M, Tzouvelekis A, Gibson KF, et al. Inhibition and role of let-7d in idiopathic pulmonary fibrosis. *Am J Respir Crit Care Med* (2010) 182:220–9. doi:10.1164/rccm.200911-1698OC
99. Milosevic J, Pandit K, Magister M, Rabinovich E, Ellwanger DC, Yu G, et al. Profibrotic role of miR-154 in pulmonary fibrosis. *Am J Respir Cell Mol Biol* (2012) 47:879–87. doi:10.1165/rcmb.2011-0377OC
100. Schulz MH, Pandit KV, Lino Cardenas CL, Ambalavanan N, Kaminski N, Bar-Joseph Z. Reconstructing dynamic microRNA-regulated interaction networks. *Proc Natl Acad Sci U S A* (2013) 110:15686–91. doi:10.1073/pnas.1303236110
101. Mizuno K, Mataki H, Seki N, Kumamoto T, Kamikawaji K, Inoue H. MicroRNAs in non-small cell lung cancer and idiopathic pulmonary fibrosis. *J Hum Genet* (2017) 62:57–65. doi:10.1038/jhg.2016.98
102. Nho RS. Alteration of aging-dependent microRNAs in idiopathic pulmonary fibrosis. *Drug Dev Res* (2015) 76:343–53. doi:10.1002/ddr.21272
103. Selman M, Lopez-Otin C, Pardo A. Age-driven developmental drift in the pathogenesis of idiopathic pulmonary fibrosis. *Eur Respir J* (2016) 48:538–52. doi:10.1183/13993003.00398-2016
104. Liu G, Friggeri A, Yang Y, Milosevic J, Ding Q, Thannickal VJ, et al. miR-21 mediates fibrogenic activation of pulmonary fibroblasts and lung fibrosis. *J Exp Med* (2010) 207:1589–97. doi:10.1084/jem.20100035

105. Pandit KV, Milosevic J. MicroRNA regulatory networks in idiopathic pulmonary fibrosis. *Biochem Cell Biol* (2015) 93:129–37. doi:10.1139/bcb-2014-0101
106. Deng Z, He Y, Yang X, Shi H, Shi A, Lu L, et al. MicroRNA-29: a crucial player in fibrotic disease. *Mol Diagn Ther* (2017) 21:285–94. doi:10.1007/s40291-016-0253-9
107. Van Rooij E, Sutherland LB, Thatcher JE, Dimaio JM, Naseem RH, Marshall WS, et al. Dysregulation of microRNAs after myocardial infarction reveals a role of miR-29 in cardiac fibrosis. *Proc Natl Acad Sci U S A* (2008) 105:13027–32. doi:10.1073/pnas.0805038105
108. Maurer B, Stanczyk J, Jungel A, Akhmetshina A, Trenkmann M, Brock M, et al. MicroRNA-29, a key regulator of collagen expression in systemic sclerosis. *Arthritis Rheum* (2010) 62:1733–43. doi:10.1002/art.27443
109. Qin W, Chung AC, Huang XR, Meng XM, Hui DS, Yu CM, et al. TGF-beta/Smad3 signaling promotes renal fibrosis by inhibiting miR-29. *J Am Soc Nephrol* (2011) 22:1462–74. doi:10.1681/ASN.2010121308
110. Roderburg C, Urban GW, Bettermann K, Vucur M, Zimmermann H, Schmidt S, et al. Micro-RNA profiling reveals a role for miR-29 in human and murine liver fibrosis. *Hepatology* (2011) 53:209–18. doi:10.1002/hep.23922
111. Wang B, Komers R, Carew R, Winbanks CE, Xu B, Herman-Edelstein M, et al. Suppression of microRNA-29 expression by TGF-beta1 promotes collagen expression and renal fibrosis. *J Am Soc Nephrol* (2012) 23:252–65. doi:10.1681/ASN.2011010055
112. Nijhuis A, Biancheri P, Lewis A, Bishop CL, Giuffrida P, Chan C, et al. In Crohn's disease fibrosis-reduced expression of the miR-29 family enhances collagen expression in intestinal fibroblasts. *Clin Sci (Lond)* (2014) 127:341–50. doi:10.1042/CS20140048
113. Zhang GY, Wu LC, Liao T, Chen GC, Chen YH, Zhao YX, et al. A novel regulatory function for miR-29a in keloid fibrogenesis. *Clin Exp Dermatol* (2016) 41:341–5. doi:10.1111/ced.12734
114. Pandit KV, Milosevic J, Kaminski N. MicroRNAs in idiopathic pulmonary fibrosis. *Transl Res* (2011) 157:191–9. doi:10.1016/j.trsl.2011.01.012
115. Cushing L, Kuang PP, Qian J, Shao F, Wu J, Little F, et al. miR-29 is a major regulator of genes associated with pulmonary fibrosis. *Am J Respir Cell Mol Biol* (2011) 45:287–94. doi:10.1165/rcmb.2010-0323OC
116. Parker MW, Rossi D, Peterson M, Smith K, Sikstrom K, White ES, et al. Fibrotic extracellular matrix activates a profibrotic positive feedback loop. *J Clin Invest* (2014) 124:1622–35. doi:10.1172/JCI71386
117. Xiao J, Meng XM, Huang XR, Chung AC, Feng YL, Hui DS, et al. miR-29 inhibits bleomycin-induced pulmonary fibrosis in mice. *Mol Ther* (2012) 20:1251–60. doi:10.1038/mt.2012.36
118. Montgomery RL, Yu G, Latimer PA, Stack C, Robinson K, Dalby CM, et al. MicroRNA mimicry blocks pulmonary fibrosis. *EMBO Mol Med* (2014) 6:1347–56. doi:10.15252/emmm.201303604
119. Xie T, Liang J, Geng Y, Liu N, Kurkciyan A, Kulur V, et al. MicroRNA-29c prevents pulmonary fibrosis by regulating epithelial cell renewal and apoptosis. *Am J Respir Cell Mol Biol* (2017) 57:721–32. doi:10.1165/rcmb.2017-0133OC
120. Durrani-Kolarik S, Pool CA, Gray A, Heyob KM, Cismowski MJ, Pryhuber G, et al. miR-29b supplementation decreases expression of matrix proteins and improves alveolarization in mice exposed to maternal inflammation and neonatal hyperoxia. *Am J Physiol Lung Cell Mol Physiol* (2017) 313:L339–49. doi:10.1152/ajplung.00273.2016
121. Katzenstein AL, Myers JL. Idiopathic pulmonary fibrosis: clinical relevance of pathologic classification. *Am J Respir Crit Care Med* (1998) 157:1301–15. doi:10.1164/ajrccm.157.4.9707039
122. Visscher DW, Myers JL. Histologic spectrum of idiopathic interstitial pneumonias. *Proc Am Thorac Soc* (2006) 3:322–9. doi:10.1513/pats.200602-019TK
123. Depianto DJ, Chandriani S, Abbas AR, Jia G, N'Diaye EN, Caplazi P, et al. Heterogeneous gene expression signatures correspond to distinct lung pathologies and biomarkers of disease severity in idiopathic pulmonary fibrosis. *Thorax* (2015) 70:48–56. doi:10.1136/thoraxjnl-2013-204596
124. Xu Y, Mizuno T, Sridharan A, Du Y, Guo M, Tang J, et al. Single-cell RNA sequencing identifies diverse roles of epithelial cells in idiopathic pulmonary fibrosis. *JCI Insight* (2016) 1:e90558. doi:10.1172/jci.insight.90558
125. Misharin AV, Morales-Nebreda L, Reyfman PA, Cuda CM, Walter JM, Mcquattie-Pimentel AC, et al. Monocyte-derived alveolar macrophages drive lung fibrosis and persist in the lung over the life span. *J Exp Med* (2017) 214:2387–404. doi:10.1084/jem.20162152
126. White ES, Brown KK, Collard HR, Conoscenti CS, Cosgrove GP, Flaherty KR, et al. Open-access biorepository for idiopathic pulmonary fibrosis. The way forward. *Ann Am Thorac Soc* (2014) 11:1171–5. doi:10.1513/AnnalsATS.201406-289OI
127. Ardini-Poleske ME, Clark RF, Ansong C, Carson JP, Corley RA, Deutsch GH, et al. LungMAP: the molecular atlas of lung development program. *Am J Physiol Lung Cell Mol Physiol* (2017) 313(5):L733–40. doi:10.1152/ajplung.00139.02017
128. Du Y, Kitzmiller JA, Sridharan A, Perl AK, Bridges JP, Misra RS, et al. Lung gene expression analysis (LGEA): an integrative web portal for comprehensive gene expression data analysis in lung development. *Thorax* (2017) 72:481–4. doi:10.1136/thoraxjnl-2016-209598
129. Ding J, Aronow B, Kaminski N, Kitzmiller J, Whitsett J, Bar-Joseph Z. Reconstructing differentiation networks and their regulation from time series single cell expression data. *Genome Res* (2018) 28:383–95. doi:10.1101/gr.225979.117

2

The NLRP3-Inflammasome-Caspase-1 Pathway is Upregulated in Idiopathic Pulmonary Fibrosis and Acute Exacerbations and is Inducible by Apoptotic A549 Cells

Benedikt Jäger[1,2,3†], Benjamin Seeliger[4†], Oliver Terwolbeck[1], Gregor Warnecke[5], Tobias Welte[4], Meike Müller[1], Christian Bode[6] and Antje Prasse[1,2,4]*

[1] Fraunhofer Institute for Toxicology and Experimental Medicine, Hannover, Germany, [2] Department of Respiratory Medicine, University Medical Center, Freiburg, Germany, [3] Faculty of Biology, Albert Ludwig University, Freiburg, Germany, [4] Department of Respiratory Medicine, Hannover Medical School and Biomedical Research in End-stage and Obstructive Lung Disease (BREATH), German Center for Lung Research (DZL), Hannover, Germany, [5] Department of Heart, Thoracic, Transplantation and Vascular Surgery, Hannover Medical School, Hannover, Germany, [6] Department of Anesthesiology and Intensive Care Medicine, University Hospital Bonn, Bonn, Germany

Correspondence:
Antje Prasse
prasse.antje@mh-hannover.de

[†]These authors have contributed equally to this work and share first authorship

Idiopathic pulmonary fibrosis (IPF) is a relentlessly progressive disease harboring significant morbidity and mortality despite recent advances in therapy. Regardless of disease severity acute exacerbations (IPF-AEs) may occur leading to considerable loss of function and are the leading cause of death in IPF. Histologic features of IPF-AE are very similar to acute respiratory distress syndrome (ARDS), but the underlying mechanisms are incompletely understood. We investigated the role of the NLRP3 inflammasome in IPF and IPF-AE. Bronchoalveolar lavage (BAL) cells were sampled from patients with IPF (n = 32), IPF-AE (n = 10), ARDS (n = 7) and healthy volunteers (HV, n = 37) and the NLRP3-inflammasome was stimulated *in-vitro*. We found the NLRP3 inflammasome to be hyper-inducible in IPF compared to HV with increased IL-1ß and pro-IL-1ß levels on ELISA upon stimulation as well as increased caspase-1 activity measured by caspase-1p20 immunoblotting. In IPF-AE, IL-1ß was massively elevated to an extent similar to ARDS. To evaluate potential mechanisms, we co-cultured BAL cells with radiated A549 cells (a model to simulate apoptotic alveolar epithelial cells), which led to increased NLRP3 mRNA expression and increased caspase-1 dependent IL-1ß production. In the presence of a reactive oxygen species (ROS) inhibitor (diphenyleneiodonium) and a cathepsin B inhibitor (E64D), NLRP3 expression was suppressed indicating that induction of NLRP3 activation following efferocytosis of apoptotic A549 cells is mediated *via* ROS and cathepsin-B. In summary, we present evidence of involvement of the NLRP3 inflammasome-caspase pathway in the pathogenesis of IPF-AE, similarly to ARDS, which may be mediated by efferocytosis of apoptotic alveolar epithelial cells in IPF.

Keywords: idiopathic pulmonary fibrosis, inflammasome, NLRP3, acute exacerbation, inflammation

INTRODUCTION

Idiopathic pulmonary fibrosis (IPF) is the most common of the idiopathic interstitial pneumonias and is characterized by its progressive nature and considerable mortality despite recent advances in antifibrotic therapy (1, 2). A severe complication of IPF may occur in the form of an acute exacerbation (IPF-AE), defined as unexplained worsening of the condition with new bilateral ground glass opacifications on chest computer tomography (CT) without evidence of pulmonary edema or lung embolism, overall sharing many features with acute respiratory distress syndrome (ARDS) (3, 4). Known triggers include lung injury due to thoracic surgery, chest trauma, invasive ventilation but also aspiration and infections (3). Notably, IPF-AE may occur irrespectively of disease severity and harbors a poor prognosis with in-hospital mortality of 50% (3). The most common histopathological pattern found in these patients is diffuse alveolar damage which is also found in ARDS (5, 6). The underlying pathomechanisms of IPF-AE are however, still poorly understood.

The NLRP3-inflammasome has been associated with various pulmonary diseases, including sarcoidosis (7), asbestosis and silicosis (8), rheumatoid arthritis associated interstitial lung disease and also IPF (9), but has not been studied in IPF-AE. Inflammasomes are multiprotein complexes which include a sensor, the adapter protein apoptosis-associated speck-like protein containing a CARD domain (ASC) and caspase-1 (10). Sensors include among others the nucleotide-binding oligomerization domain-like receptor (NLR) family, pyrin domain-containing 3 (NLRP3) (10). For the activation of caspase-1, two signals are necessary: signal 1 induces activation of pattern-recognition receptors (PRR) for example Toll-like receptors (TLRs) by pathogen associated molecular patterns (PAMPS) including lipopolysaccharides (LPS). This leads to nuclear factor kappa-light-chain-enhancer of activated B cells (NF-κB) regulated transcription of inflammasome components: pro-caspase-1, pro–IL-1β and NLRP3 (10). Signal 2 includes a magnitude of stimuli, including ATP and nigericin, which activate NLRP3 inducing inflammasome assembly *via* the oligomerization of ASC. This results in the activation of pro-caspase-1, which is spliced into its active forms caspase-1p10 and caspase 1p20 which in turn activate pro-IL-1β *via* proteolytic cleavage into the active cytokine IL-1β (10, 11). In ARDS, key cytokines include the caspase-1 dependent IL-1ß and IL-18 and the involvement of the NLRP3-inflammasome has been recently demonstrated (12, 13).

IPF pathogenesis is driven by dysfunctional repair mechanisms to microinjuries of the alveolar epithelium and especially of type II alveolar epithelial cells (AECs) (14). In the presence of persistent stress, the AEC-II dysfunctional response lead to cell apoptosis (15). These apoptotic cells are then ingested by alveolar macrophages (AMs), a process which is called efferocytosis (16), capable of providing a pro-fibrotic macrophage response which can induce pulmonary fibrosis (17). Dysregulated efferocytosis observed in IPF (18) can lead to increased production of reactive oxygen species (ROS). Interestingly also activation of the NLRP3 inflammasome by many trigger factors was shown to rely on ROS production (19–25) and cathepsin B leakage into the cytoplasm (26), suggesting a link between efferocytosis in IPF and NLRP3-inflammasome activation.

We aimed to examine the inducibility of the NLRP3-inflammasome in IPF, IPF-AE, and ARDS and the potential role of apoptotic epithelial cells in promoting NLRP3-inflammasome inducibility. We provide evidence of a hyper-inducible NLRP3-inflammasome-caspase 1 pathway which can be triggered by efferocytosis of apoptotic AECs.

MATERIAL AND METHODS

Patient Population and Bronchoalveolar Lavage Sample Preparation

BRONCHOALVEOLAR Lavage (BAL) sampling was performed in patients with acute respiratory distress syndrome (ARDS), idiopathic pulmonary fibrosis (IPF) with and without acute exacerbation (IPF-AE), and healthy volunteers (HV) at the University Medical Center in Freiburg im Breisgau (Germany) and at Hannover Medical School (Germany). Healthy volunteers were screened for pulmonary abnormalities by thorough medical history, physical examination, and pulmonary function testing. Diagnosis of ARDS was made in accordance with the Berlin 2012 definition (4), and a diagnosis of IPF was established per the practice guidelines issued by the American Thoracic Society and European Respiratory Society (1). The definition criteria of AE were: deterioration of dyspnoea >20% in <3 weeks, occurrence of new opacities, and absence of alternative cause (including infection, heart failure, or pulmonary embolism) (27). All IPF patients with suspicion of acute exacerbation received chest computed tomography.

All patients provided written informed consent, and collection of bio-samples was registered at the German Clinical Trials Register (DRKS00000017 and DRKS00000620). The respective institutional review boards approved of the bio-sampling (Freiburg 47/06 March 10th 2006, Hannover, #2923-2015 and #2516-2014, Nov 2nd 2015).

BAL was performed in the middle lobe or lingula. After BAL sampling, macro-impurities were removed by sample filtration through sterile gauze. Differential BAL total cell number was counted using May–Grunwald–Giemsa stain (Merck) on native sample. BAL samples were centrifuged at 500g for 10min at 4°C (28) and subsequently resuspended in Macrophage SFM Medium or DMEM medium. BALs were performed between 2010 and 2013 at the University Medical Center Freiburg and in 2017 and 2021 at Hannover Medical School.

Cell-Culture and NLRP3-Inflammasome Stimulation Protocol

The NLRP3 inflammasome was activated in accordance to our recently described protocol (7). In brief, 1×10^5 BAL cells derived from HV, IPF, and ARDS patients, were incubated with 100 µl of Macrophage SFM/Gibco Medium (Life Technologies, USA) with 1% penicillin and streptomycin (Biochrom, Germany) at 37°C and 5% CO_2 in a flat-bottom 96 well plate (**Figure 1A**). Two steps are needed for the activation of inflammasome-dependent caspase-1 activation: a first signal 1 such as an Toll-like-receptor agonist (LPS) and a second tissue damage signal such as ATP or Nigericin (29). BAL-cells were primed with 1 μM LPS (Fluka Biochemika, Switzerland) initially for 4h. Thereafter, 1 mM ATP (Sigma Aldrich, USA) or 10 μM Nigericin (Sigma Aldrich, USA) was added with incubation of another 2h. Supernatants were sampled and stored at −80°C until analysis. Cells were lysed with lysis buffer [PBS (Life Technologies, USA) with 0.5% triton X (Sigma Aldrich, USA) and 10% FCS (Biochrom, Germany)] for pro-IL-1ß ELISA and with 200 μl Trizol (Thermo Fisher Scientific, USA) for RNA isolation and stored at −80°C until analysis.

Cell Culture and Stimulation With Co-Culturing BAL Cells With Radiated A549 Cells

Since chronic cellular stress has been demonstrated to induce AEC apoptosis and consequently efferocytosis by alveolar macrophages, which is believed to contribute to IPF pathogenesis, we examined the effects of co-culturing alveolar macrophages with apoptotic A549 cells on NLRP3-inflammasome activation (15, 16). A549 cells were cultured in DMEM/Gibco medium (Life Technologies, USA) with 10% FCS and 1% penicillin/streptomycin at 37°C/5% CO_2 and radiated with 10 Gy and then incubated for additional 72h (30–32). Harvesting after 72h resulted in highest rate of apoptotic cells on viability testing. Viability was assessed *via* trypan blue staining and the FACS annexin V apoptosis detection Kit (BD, USA) as per manufacturer's instructions. 1×10^6 BAL-cells were then co-cultured w/wo 1×10^5 radiated A549 cells in 500 μl of macrophage/Gibco medium (serum free) in a 24-well cell culture plate and incubated for 1h at 37°C/5% CO_2 to allow for efferocytosis and consequently stimulated as described above.

To evaluate the effects of efferocytosis on NLRP3 mRNA expression, we co-cultured radiated, apoptotic A459 with normal BAL-cells for 1h. Following that, we stimulated BAL cells with 1 μM LPS in a 24-well cell culture plate for 2h at 37°C. Supernatants were discarded, and cells were lysed with 200 μl Trizol. In some experiments, we assessed the effect of the NADPH-Oxidase inhibitor [ROS-inhibitor; DPI; 20 μM (Sigma Aldrich, USA)] and of the cathepsin B inhibitor E64D (10 μM) (MCE, USA). Both compounds were added with the radiated A549 cells at baseline, and DMSO 0.2% was added as vehicle (both E64D and DPI were suspended in DMSO). Cell lysates were again sampled in 200 μl Trizol following 2h incubation at 37°C/5% CO_2. In another set of experiments, the effects of the selective NLRP3 inhibitor (MCC950) (33) and caspase-1 inhibitor VX-765 (both Invivogen, France) on IL-1ß and TNF-α production following inflammasome stimulation were

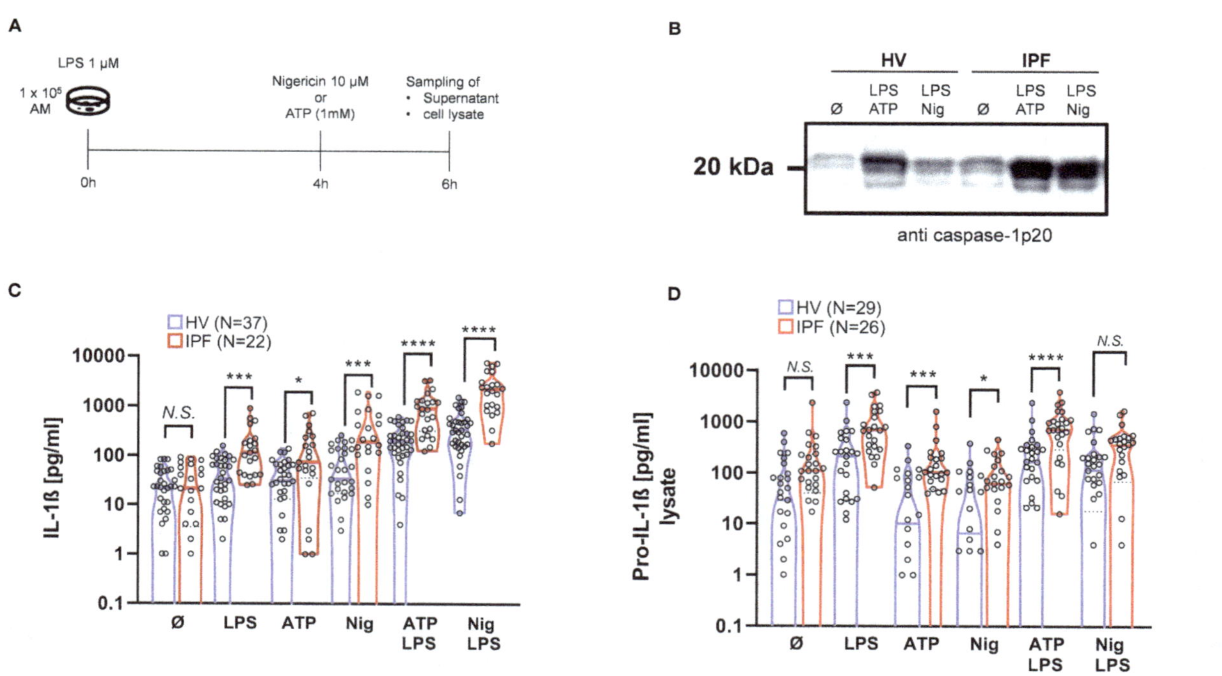

FIGURE 1 | The ability to activate the NLRP3 inflammasome is significantly increased in BAL cells from IPF patients. For NLRP3 stimulation, bronchoalveolar lavage (BAL) cells were incubated and stimulated with LPS at 0h, following Nigericin or ATP stimulation after 4h **(A)**. In both healthy volunteers (HVs) and idiopathic pulmonary fibrosis (IPF) there was a significant increase in IL-1ß production following NLRP3-inflammasome stimulation protocol **(B)**, with significant higher responses in IPF compared to HV. Caspase-1 activation is demonstrated by representative immunoblotting of cleaved caspase-1p20 (representative blot shown; total of n = 15 immunoblots performed). **(C)**. Pro-IL-1ß concentration in cell lysates was elevated in IPF patients compared to HV following stimulation with LPS, ATP, Nigericin, and LPS + ATP **(D)**. IL-1ß and Pro-IL-1ß values were compared using unpaired t-tests; *p < 0.05; ***p < 0.001; ****p < 0.0001, *N.S.* non-significant.

evaluated. Two different concentrations (1 + 10 μM and 25 + 75 μM, respectively) were added 30min before addition of radiated A549 cells.

Efferocytosis Assay

To demonstrate efferocytosis of radiated A549 cells by alveolar macrophages, 1×10^5 control BAL cells were incubated with 2 μM cytochalasin D (Sigma Aldrich #250255, USA), a known cytoskeletal disruptor of phagocytosis in macrophages, for 30min at 37°C. Radiated A549 cells were incubated with pHrodo (Red AM Intracellular pH Indicator, Thermo Fisher Scientific #P35372, USA) at a 1:100,000 dilution for 30min. Engulfment of A549 cells leads to a pH-shift in the alveolar macrophages inducing an increased pHrodo light emission (34). Afterwards 1×10^5 BAL cells were incubated with and without 3×10^5 pHrodo-labeled radiated A549 cells for 2h in a 96 well plate. All BAL cells with and without A549 cells were harvested with 100 μl PBS, and nuclear staining was performed with 1 μg/ml Hoechst-33342 dye solution (Thermo Fisher Scientific #H3570, USA) for 30min at RT. Immediately afterwards, a cytospin with 2×10^4 cells in 100 μl PBS was performed, and efferocytosis of macrophages was analyzed by fluorescence microscopy using Axio Observer Inverted microscope and ZEN navigation software (Zeiss, Germany). Percentage of pHrodo$^+$ and Hoechst-33342$^+$ cells was counted using ImageJ V.1.53e (NIH, USA) (35).

Immunoblot Analysis of Caspase-1p20 Activity

Supernatants collected after NLRP3-stimulation protocol were precipitated with methanol/chloroform. After initial centrifugation, the upper phase was discarded and methanol was added to the lower phase, followed by another centrifugation step. The supernatant was discarded, and the pellet was incubated at 55°C for 5min and resuspended in 20 μl Laemmli-buffer (Bio-Rad, USA). Samples were consequently cooked for 5min at 95°C. Samples were separated using 15% SDS-PAGE gels and transferred to polyvinylidene difluoride membranes. Cleaved caspase-1 (p20) was detected using primary antibody rabbit mAb cleaved caspase-1 (Asp297) (Cell Signaling Technology, USA) with the secondary antibody goat anti-rabbit (H + L) HRP conjugate (1:3,000) (Bio-Rad, USA). Enhanced chemiluminescence (Clarity™ Western ECL Substrate, Bio-Rad, USA) was used for detection with ChemiDoc™ MD Imaging System (BioRad, USA).

IL-1ß, pro-IL-1ß and TNF-α Measurement by ELISA

The concentration of both pro-IL-1ß and IL-1β was measured by ELISA (Human IL-1β/IL-1F2 DuoSet, R&D, USA) in the cell lysate and culture supernatant, respectively. (36). TNF-α concentration from culture supernatant was measured by ELISA (Human TNF-alpha DuoSet #DY210, R&D, USA).

RT-PCR for NLRP3

RNA was isolated *via* Trizol method (ThermoFisher Scientific, USA). 1×10^6 cells were lysed with 200 μl of Trizol. Extracted RNA was reverse-transcribed to cDNA using the iScript cDNA Synthesis kit (Bio-Rad, USA) as per manufacturer's instructions (7). The obtained cDNA was analyzed by Real-Time PCR (Light Cycler/Roche, Switzerland) with the following primers: huNLRP3 (5′-AGAATGCCTTGGGAGACTCA-3′ and 5′-CAGAATTCACCAACCCCAGT-3′), resulting in a 93 bp product, exon 6/7 overlapping; GAPDH (5′-ACAGTCAGCC GCATCTTCTT-3′ and 5′-GTTAAAAGCAGCCCTGGTGA-3′) as reference (7). The expression of huNLRP3 was normalized to GAPDH expression. A cycle threshold value was calculated and used to ascertain the relative level of huNLRP3 messenger RNA by the following formula: relative expression = [2 (cycle threshold of glyceraldehyde 3-phosphate dehydrogenase- ycle threshold of huNLRP3)] × 10,000 for each complementary DNA sample.

Statistical Analysis

Statistical analyses were performed using GraphPad Prism 9 Software (La Jolla, USA) and RStudio version 1.3.1093 (RStudio Inc., USA). Variables were compared by unpaired t-test. All data are expressed as mean + SD unless stated otherwise. A two-tailed p-value of <0.05 was considered to statistically significant.

RESULTS

Study Population

A total of 86 BALs were used in this study from patients with IPF (n = 32), IPF/AE (n = 10), ARDS (n = 7), and HV (n = 37) with demographics, pulmonary function tests (in IPF), and BAL cell counts shown in **Table 1**. All patients were naïve to antifibrotic therapy, since the majority of patients were recruited prior to the widespread introduction of antifibrotics. At the time of BAL, 41% of IPF and 60% of IPF-AE patients were receiving triple-therapy with n-acetylcystein, prednisolone, and azathioprine. In 2021, additional BALs in three IPF patients were performed (two female; mean age 71 years, mean forced vital capacity 70% of predicted, mean diffusion capacity for carbon monoxide 52% of predicted; mean alveolar macrophages in BAL 87%, mean neutrophils in BAL 4%).

The NLRP3 Inflammasome Activation Is Significantly Increased in AM From IPF Patients Compared to HV

In a first step, the IL-1ß production of normal BAL cells derived from HV was tested following NLRP3-inflammasome stimulation (**Figure 1A**). Normal BAL cells did not spontaneously produce IL-1ß, which production is tightly regulated (37). Mean basal IL-1ß production without stimulation was increased with LPS alone ($p = 0.002$), Nigericin alone ($p = 0.0002$), and with ATP alone ($p = 0.0005$) (**Figure 1B**). Most pronounced IL-1ß production was seen with co-stimulation of LPS + ATP ($p < 0.0001$) and LPS + Nigericin ($p < 0.0001$). Evidence of caspase-1 activation by NLRP3 inflammasome was seen by increased protein band intensity of the caspase-1p20 fragment by immunoblot with stimulation by LPS + ATP and LPS + Nigericin (**Figure 1C**).

TABLE 1 | Study population and BAL differential cell counts.

Characteristics	IPF (n = 32)	IPF/AE (n = 10)	ARDS (n = 7)	HV (n = 37)
Age, years (SD)	68 ± 10	68 ± 10	52 ± 15	29 ± 8
Sex (male), N (%)	30 (94)	9 (90)	6 (86)	20 (54)
Forced vital capacity, % of predicted, mean (SD)	64 ± 16	–	–	–
Diffusion capacity for carbon monoxide (single breath), % of predicted, mean (SD)	36 ± 20	–	–	–
Invasive ventilation, n (%)	0	2 (20)	7 (100)	0
Received n-acetylcysteine, prednisolone, and azathioprine	13 (41)	6 (60)	0	0
BAL cell count, × 10^6/100ml (SD)	14.6 ± 7.8	18.0 ± 7.5	32.4 ± 30.7	7.0 ± 3.2
Alveolar macrophages, % (SD)	65.1 ± 21.2	59.1 ± 15.5	32.7 ± 19.5	86.0 ± 5.2
Lymphocytes, % (SD)	12.1 ± 12.8	4.0 ± 3.0	8.5 ± 3.6	10.5 ± 5.2
Neutrophils, % (SD)	18.9 ± 22.0	30.8 ± 17.3	56.2 ± 20.9	2.3 ± 1.8
Eosinophils, % (SD)	3.4 ± 4.7	6.3 ± 4.4	2.0 ± 3.9	0.3 ± 0.7

ARDS, acute respiratory distress syndrome; BAL, bronchoalveolar lavage; HVs, healthy volunteers; IPF, idiopathic pulmonary fibrosis; IPF/AE, acute exacerbation of idiopathic pulmonary fibrosis.

Compared to BAL cells from IPF patients, basal (unstimulated) IL-1ß production was similar compared to HV. Of note, there was a consistently higher IL-1ß production in BAL cells from IPF patients after stimulation with LPS ($p = 0.0002$), Nigericin: ($p = 0.0001$), and ATP ($p = 0.0002$). With the combined stimulation with LPS + ATP and LPS + Nigericin, discrepancies were even more pronounced (both $p < 0.0001$).

In line with this, there was a significant increase in caspase-1 activation determined by caspase-1p20 protein-band intensity after co-stimulations in IPF patients compared to HV (**Figure 1C**).

Intracellular Pro-IL-1ß Protein Expression Following Stimulation Is Increased in BAL-Cells From IPF Patients Compared to HV, but Not Without Stimulation

In order to test whether the NLRP3 inflammasome is already primed (signal 1 activated) in BAL cells derived from IPF patients, we analyzed intracellular pro-IL-1ß levels. Notably, baseline (unstimulated) pro-IL-1ß levels were not statistically significantly elevated in IPF compared to HV, indicating that NLRP3 inflammasome is rather hyper-inducible than primed. As expected, intracellular pro-IL-1ß levels increased following priming with LPS; LPS + ATP and LPS + Nigericin, but not with ATP and Nigericin alone (**Figure 1D**). Compared to HV, pro-IL-1ß production was significantly increased following stimulation with LPS + ATP ($p < 0.0001$) and LPS alone ($p = 0.0003$), as well as ATP ($p = 0.03$) and Nigericin ($p = 0.005$) in IPF (**Figure 1D**).

NLRP3 Inflammasome Is Markedly Upregulated in Patients With Acute Exacerbation of IPF to Similar Extent as Patients With Primary ARDS

To see how the NLRP3 inflammasome contributes to IPF/AE, we stimulated BAL cells from patients with IPF/AE (n = 10) with the same protocol as described above. As shown in **Figure 2**, there was a markedly elevated IL-1ß production of BAL cells from patients with both IPF/AE and ARDS following singular and combined stimulation and without stimulation (compared to HV). With IPF/AE and ARDS, the fold-change for IL-1ß production compared to IPF (without AE) for the combined stimuli was 3–4 and 15–20 compared to HV (**Figure 2F**).

Co-Culturing BAL Cells From HV With Radiated A549 Cells Results in Efferocytosis and Increases NLRP3-Inflammasome Activation. Selective NLRP3 and Caspase-1 Inhibition Suppresses IL-1ß Production Following Co-Incubation

To further investigate potential mechanisms behind the increased NLRP3 inflammasome activation in IPF patients *vs* HV, AECs (A549) were radiated with 10 Gy and harvested 72h after radiation (**Figure 3A**). Radiation induced apoptosis in the majority of cells, while a small proportion was double positive for annexin V and propidium iodide (**Figure 3C**). To verify if efferocytosis was actually performed, we labeled radiated A549 cells with pHrodo before co-incubation with BAL cells. Following co-incubation with A549 cells, alveolar macrophages became pHrodo$^+$ in 83% of all Hoechst-33342$^+$ cells, indicating efferocytosis of A549 cells. Following pre-treatment with cytochalasin-D (2 μM), this effect was almost completely inhibited (9% pHrodo$^+$/H-33342$^+$ cells) (**Figure 4**).

BAL cells of HV were co-incubated with radiated A549 cells for 1h before running the NLRP3 stimulation protocol. There was a significant 2.2-fold increase in IL-1ß production in BAL cells co-cultured with radiated A549 at baseline (without stimulation; $p = 0.031$) and following stimulation with LPS + Nigericin (3.5-fold; $p = 0.025$) (**Figure 3B**). With the other stimulations, IL-1ß production was increased but did not reach statistical significance. Equally, on immunoblotting there was an increased protein band both with caspase 1-p20 with co-culturing of radiated A549 (**Figure 3D**). There was no difference in pro-IL-1ß concentration in the cell lysates with or without co-culturing of A549 (**Figure 3E**).

To evaluate if the IL-1ß response was mainly mediated *via* the NLRP3 inflammasome, we pre-treated BAL cells with a selective NLRP3-inhibitor (MCC-950) or caspase-1 inhibitor (VX-765) before co-culturing the A549 cells (**Figure 3A**). Both agents

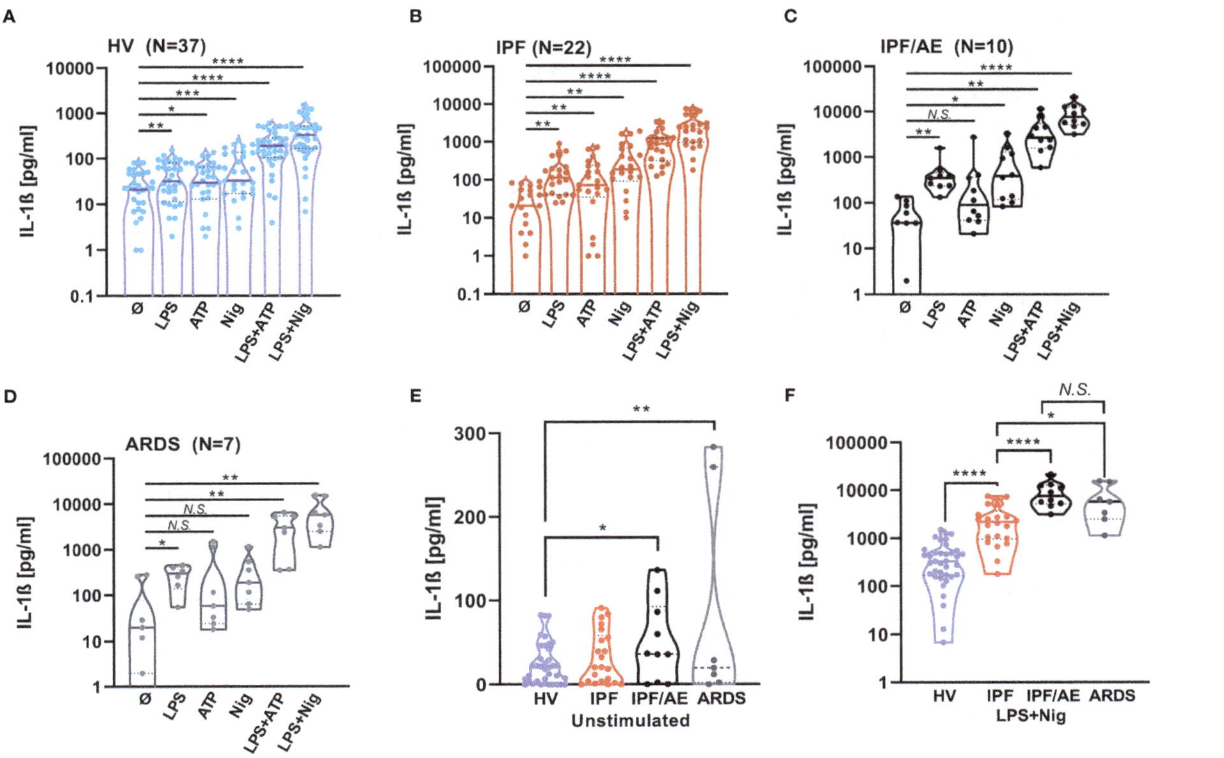

FIGURE 2 | IL-1β production after NLRP3 inflammasome stimulation is highest in BAL cells from patients with an acute exacerbation during IPF and BAL cells from patients with ARDS. IL-1ß production was detected by ELISA and is inducible by NLRP3 stimulation in alveolar macrophages of patients with acute exacerbation of idiopathic pulmonary fibrosis **(C)** and acute respiratory distress syndrome **(D)**. IL-1ß values for healthy volunteers (HVs) and IPF are shown for comparison **(A, B)**. IL-1ß production in these two cohorts is significantly increased compared to healthy volunteers (HVs) to a similar extent at baseline and following stimulation **(E, F)**. IL-1ß levels with stimulation compared to baseline and unstimulated IL-1ß levels between groups and LPS/Nigericin stimulation were compared using unpaired t-tests; *$p < 0.05$; **$p < 0.01$; *** $p < 0.001$; ****$p < 0.0001$, *N.S.* non-significant.

suppressed IL-1ß production >90% (**Figure 3H**), while TNF-α production remained largely (**Figure 3I**). These results indicate the increased IL-1ß response following efferocytosis of A549 cells is primarily mediated *via* the NLRP3/caspase-1 pathway.

NLRP3-Gene Expression Is Increased by Co-Culturing With Apoptotic A549 Cells and Attenuated by Inhibition of ROS and Cathepsin B

Acute lung injury and consecutive epithelial cell death trigger AE-IPF and ARDS. On this background we got interested in the role of efferocytosis in NLRP3 inflammasome activation. We therefore induced apoptosis of the AEC line A549 using radiation. Indeed, 72h after radiation 67% of A549 cells were apoptotic and only 14% necrotic (**Figure 3C**). These apoptotic A549 cells were then co-cultured with normal BAL cells for 1h and resulted in their phagocytosis by AM (**Figure 4**). Co-culturing with radiated A549 cells induced NLRP3 mRNA expression relative to GAPDH in a similar magnitude compared to stimulation with LPS and was significantly increased compared to baseline NLRP3 expression (**Figure 3F**). Combined stimulation with radiated A549 and LPS induced high NLRP3 gene expression. To evaluate possible mechanisms for the increased NLRP3 mRNA expression *via* radiated A549 cells, we tested a ROS and cathepsin B inhibitor. In the presence of a ROS inhibitor (DPI) or a cathepsin B inhibitor (E64D), the NRLP3 mRNA expression in response to co-culturing with radiated A549 cells was completely suppressed (**Figure 3G**), while GAPDH expression was maintained.

DISCUSSION

Although IPF-AE is the leading cause of death in IPF, underlying mechanisms are poorly understood (38). In this study we demonstrate that the NLRP3-inflammasome is hyper-inducible in BAL cells from IPF patients compared to HV. BAL cells harvested during IPF-AE produced extraordinarily high IL-1ß levels in a similar range as BAL cells of ARDS patients. We found that one potential mechanism driving NLRP3 hyperactivation in IPF-AE may be efferocytosis of apoptotic cells which led to increased NLRP3 expression and caspase-1 activation. The IL-1ß response could be almost completely suppressed by specific inhibition of NLRP3 and caspase-1-activity. Inhibition of ROS

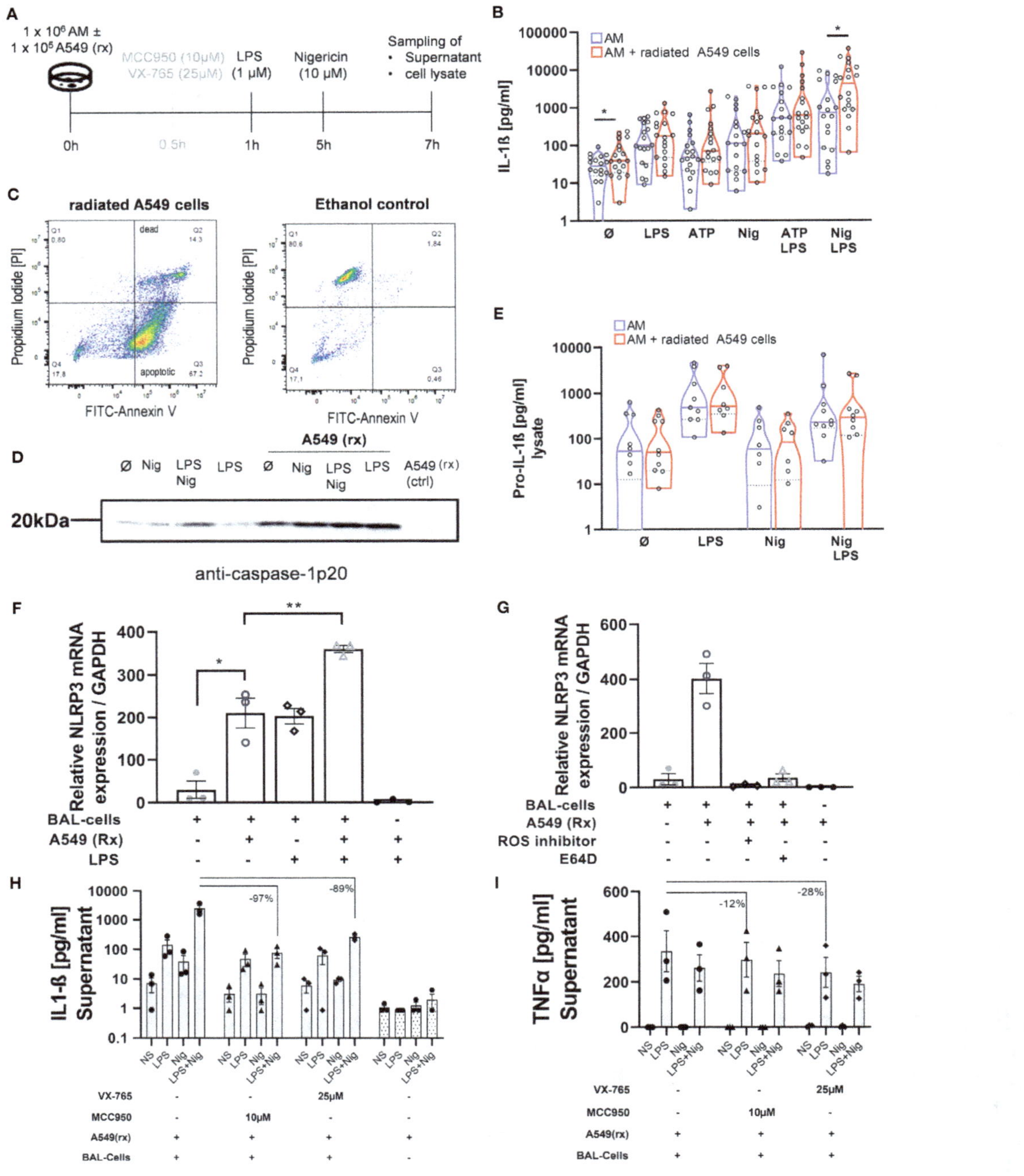

FIGURE 3 | Efferocytosis of apoptotic alveolar epithelial cells activates the NLRP3 inflammasome in AM. BAL cells were co-cultured with the radiated (rx) A549 cells, and the NLRP3 inflammasome was additionally stimulated **(A)**. A549 cells were radiated with 10 Gy and incubated for 72h, following which the majority of the cells were apoptotic demonstrated by Annexin-V staining **(C)**. There were increased IL-1ß levels with all stimulations, which were statistically significant at baseline and following LPS + Nigericin (Nig) stimulation **(B)**. Increased caspase-1 activation with A549(rx) co-culture was demonstrated by immunoblotting of cleaved caspase-1p20 subsegment (representative blot shown; total of n = 3 immunoblots performed) **(D)**. Pro-IL-1ß levels in cell lysate were not different between BAL cells and BAL cells co-cultured with A549(rx) cells **(E)**. NLRP3 mRNA expression was assessed after 2h of stimulation, w/wo the presence of A549(rx). BAL cells cocultured with A459(rx) expressed NLRP3-mRNA in a similar range as BAL cells stimulated with LPS alone **(F)**. Combined stimulation of LPS and A549(rx) resulted in a marked increase in NLRP3-mRNA expression. The effect on NRLP3-mRNA expression (relative to GAPDH) by efferocytosis was inhibited by either a NADPH-Oxidase inhibitor (ROS-inhibitor; DPI) or a cathepsin inhibitor (E64D) **(G)**. IL-1ß production could be inhibited by inhibition of NLRP3 (MCC950) and also caspase-1 (VX-765) **(H)**, while TNF-α levels were largely retained **(I)**. IL-1ß levels and NLRP3 mRNA levels were compared using unpaired t-tests; *$p < 0.05$; **$p < 0.01$; *N.S.* non-significant.

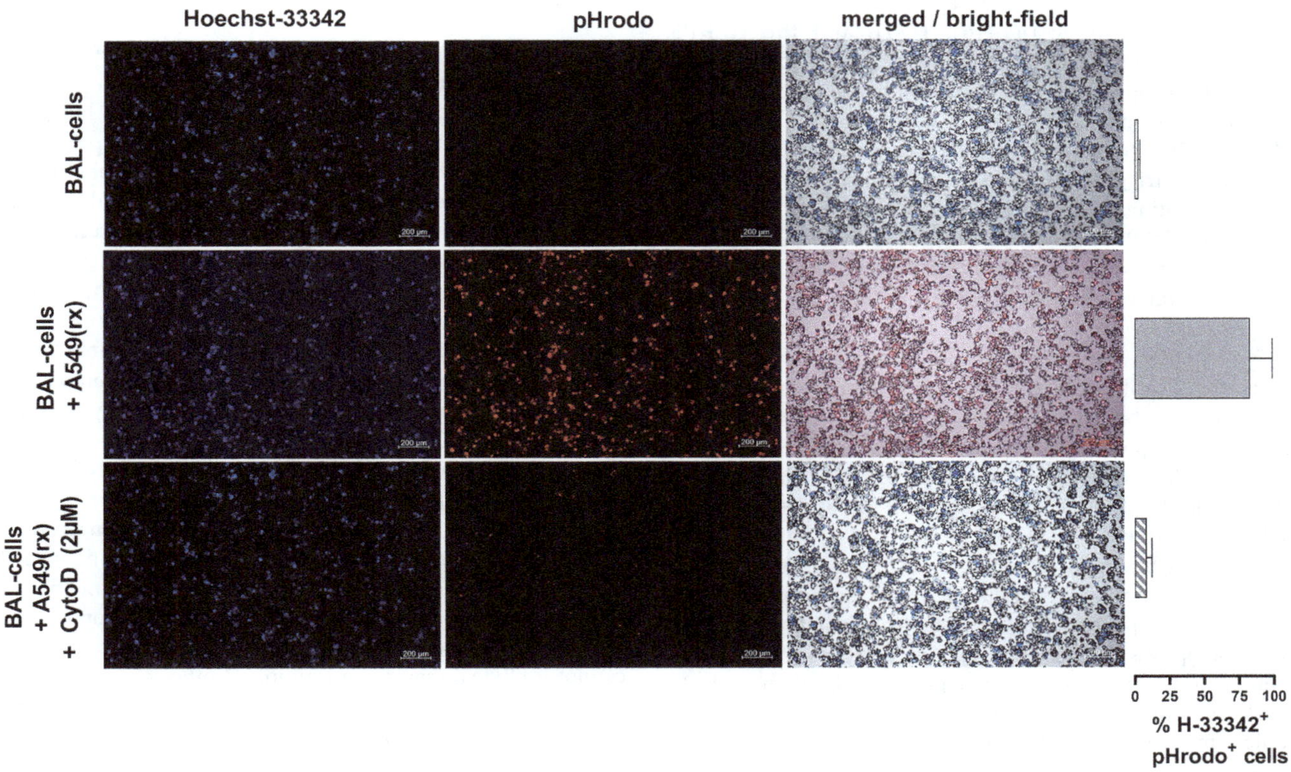

FIGURE 4 | Co-incubation of alveolar macrophages with pHrodo-labeled radiated A549 cells leads to efferocytosis of A549 cells. Nucleolar staining with Hoechst-33342 of BAL cells was performed. Following co-incubation with pHrodo labeled radiated A549 cells, pHrodo positive alveolar macrophages were detected, indicating efferocytosis of A549 cells. Following pre-treatment with cytochalasin-D (2 µM), this effect was almost completely inhibited. Exemplary fluorescence microscopy images (5x magnification) of BAL cells with and without co-incubation and pre-treatment of cytochalasin D are shown, and the percentages of Hoechst$^+$/pHrodo$^+$ cells of all Hoechst$^+$ cells are shown in the right hand panel. Bronchoalveolar lavages from three patients were used and measured in triplicates for each condition.

or cathepsin B signaling blocked the effect of co-culturing with radiated A549 cells on NLRP3-mRNA transcription in BAL cells.

Our data indicate that the NLRP3 inflammasome is hyper-inducible in IPF BAL cells and especially during acute exacerbation. BAL cells harvested at the time of IPF-AE produced tremendously high levels of IL-1ß and in a similar range as AMs of patients with ARDS. While the role and significant involvement of the NLRP3-inflammasome in ARDS are well documented, activation of the NLRP3 inflammasome pathway in IPF-AE is a novel finding. Our observations in BAL cells from IPF patients are in line with previous observations of elevated IL-1ß and IL-1ß mRNA in IPF (10, 35–37). Activation of the NLRP3-inflammasome pathway has been demonstrated to induce IL-1ß and IL-18 production of BAL cells and is tightly regulated (11). Although we have not purified macrophages from BAL prior to inflammasome stimulation protocol and therefore cannot exclude contribution of other cell types, we think, in line with the literature, that our experiments mainly reflect inflammasome activation of alveolar macrophages. In addition, the relatively short incubation time of 6h used in this study render cell–cell contact dependent mechanisms unlikely as the primary driver for increased NLRP3 activation and IL-1ß production. Furthermore, the neutrophil count between IPF patients with and without AE was relatively small owing to inclusion of IPF patients with advanced disease (39), while the changes in NLRP3-inflammasome inducibility between these groups were considerable.

Several factors have been shown to activate the NLRP3 inflammasome such as phagocytosis of crystalline substances such as silicates or cholesterol but is also triggered by viral and bacterial infection releasing LPS and other TLR ligands as well as DNA and RNA (12, 40). Of note, mechanical ventilation and ventilation induced lung injury also activated the NLRP3-inflammasome in murine models (41, 42). These triggers are also commonly reported to precede acute exacerbation in IPF (3, 27), and it is thus conceivable that elevated inflammasome inducibility in IPF patients (such as the increased pro-IL-1ß an IL-1ß production shown herein upon signal 1 or signal 2 stimulation) predisposes them to increased risk of acute exacerbation when exposed to these stimuli. Notably, in a multicentric BAL gene expression analysis in IPF, a gene set was identified to carry poor prognosis, among which the IL-1ß gene and the NLRP3 gene were included (43). Thus, our data indicate a role of NLRP3 inflammasome signaling in acute exacerbation of IPF.

The NLRP3 inflammasome and IL-1ß signaling are closely linked to neutrophil influx and represent a key pathway in response to cell injury (44–46). IL-1ß and the NLRP3 inflammasome activation also are part of an acute injury response and promote fibrosis and pro-fibrotic pathways such as transforming growth factor (TGF)-*ß* signaling in animal models (47–50). Inflammation caused by bleomycin induced lung injury is triggered by NLRP3 inflammasome activation, while the resulting inflammation and fibrosis were completely prevented by NLRP3 inhibitors (48). Moreover, asbestos and silica, which are known inducers of pulmonary fibrosis, are capable of activating the NLRP3 inflammasome with subsequent IL-1ß production (51). IL-1ß itself can promote TGF-*ß* responses, considered as a key driver in pulmonary fibrosis *via* fibroblast activation (52). Interestingly, both approved antifibrotic agents for the treatment of IPF (nintedanib and pirfenidone) have been shown to reduce IL-1ß expression in lung tissues (53, 54), which might be a mechanism for the reduced risk of acute exacerbation in patients receiving antifibrotic treatment (55, 56).

Another key finding of our study is that co-incubation of BAL cells with apoptotic AEC (A549) and their phagocytosis increase inflammasome-dependent caspase-1 activation. Our model for inducing apoptosis in A549 AECs is well accepted (30–32), and we demonstrated apoptosis in the majority of cells *via* annexin-V expression, and we also demonstrate their efferocytosis by alveolar macrophages. Phagocytosis and generation of phagolysosomes are linked to ROS production and lysosomal stress. Interestingly also activation of the NLRP3 inflammasome by many trigger factors was shown to rely on ROS production (19–25) and cathepsin B leakage into the cytoplasm (26). Based on these findings we tested the effects of ROS or cathepsin B inhibition and found that both of them completely attenuated NLRP3 expression in the context of efferocytosis (16). Studies suggest that ROS, among other direct effects on inflammasome assembly, also upregulates NLRP3 gene expression *via* TLR-4 signaling (57), providing a potential mechanisms for the reduction in NLRP3-mRNA expression observed in this study. A recent murine model showed that apoptotic AEC-II induce a pro-fibrotic gene expression signature in AM following efferocytosis, which on repeated exposure can induce pulmonary fibrosis (17), a process which may be equally important in IPF. Previous animal studies have also implicated that impaired autophagy mechanisms in IPF and aging result in deranged mitochondrial turnover resulting in mitochondria-generated reactive oxygen species (ROS) leading to caspase-1 activation (19–25, 50). Equally, recent reports demonstrated a dependency on cathepsin B (which is also induced by nigericin used in our model) for NLRP3-inflammasome assembly (58, 59). Cathepsin B is released into the cytoplasm upon lysosomal membrane permeabilization (26). Thus, efferocytosis triggers NLRP3 inflammasome activation in alveolar macrophages. While ROS inhibitors convey multifactorial effects, the possibility to suppress the observed IL-1ß response by the specific NLRP3-inhibitor MCC950 (33) carries potential treatment options for IPF-AE and other forms of acute respiratory failure such as COVID-19 (60), which remain to be clinically studied.

Our study has significant limitations to consider: Our data derived from human samples demonstrates evidence for an increased activation of the NLRP3 inflammasome, but given a limited number of measured inflammasome components, we cannot exclude that additional inflammasome subtypes may have equally been activated. Age, comorbidities, and respiratory failure in patients with IPF-AE often preclude these patients from undergoing bronchoscopy which primary function lies in exclusion of infection, rendering these bio samples available only in few cases recruited in the era before antifibrotic treatment was available. The considerable younger age of the recruited healthy volunteers also limits comparability to IPF patients since inflammasome activation may also occur with aging alone (61). Although the differences observed in the present study appear unlikely to be explained solely by age, at least a contributory effect can be assumed. Another important limitation of this study is that we did not purify macrophages prior to the described *in vitro* experiments. On one side this experimental protocol leaves cells untouched since methods for cell purification have been shown to activate macrophages. On the other hand, because we studied BAL cells in complete, we cannot exclude a major contribution of other cell types such as neutrophils (62). Neutrophils have been recently shown to activate NLRP3 inflammasome upon respiratory infections (63) which can be achieved *via* production of neutrophil extracellular traps (44, 45). Compared with macrophages, neutrophils are however short-lived and difficult to study *in vitro* because most of the neutrophils are lost within 2h of cell culture.

In conclusion, our study demonstrates in human BAL cells the hyper-inducibility of the NLRP3-inflammasome in IPF and particularly at acute exacerbation. We identified efferocytosis of apoptotic cells caused by lung injury as one responsible mechanism. The activated NLRP3 inflammasome in IPF-AE may be of potential therapeutic value, and compounds blocking NLRP3-inflammasome activation might be of potential benefit for this fatal condition (53). Future research is needed to explore the clinical role of inflammasome inhibitors on the course of pulmonary fibrosis and acute exacerbation in particular.

ETHICS STATEMENT

The studies involving human participants were reviewed and approved by the Ethics committee of The University of Freiburg im Breisgau. The patients/participants provided their written informed consent to participate in this study.

AUTHOR CONTRIBUTIONS

BJ and BS wrote the first draft of the manuscript, conducted the experiments, contributed to the study design, and interpreted the data. OT conducted the experiments, provided technical support, and revised the manuscript. GW, TW, and CB interpreted the data, critically revised the manuscript, and supervised the project. MM conducted the experiments, provided technical support, and interpreted the data. AP designed the study, supervised the project, interpreted the data, and critically revised the manuscript. All authors contributed to the article and approved the submitted version. All authors take responsibility for the integrity of the data.

REFERENCES

1. Raghu G, Remy-Jardin M, Myers JL, Richeldi L, Ryerson CJ, Lederer DJ, et al. Diagnosis of Idiopathic Pulmonary Fibrosis. An Official Ats/Ers/Jrs/Alat Clinical Practice Guideline. *Am J Respir Crit Care Med* (2018) 198(5):e44–68. doi: 10.1164/rccm.201807-1255ST
2. Khor YH, Ng Y, Barnes H, Goh NSL, McDonald CF, Holland AE. Prognosis of Idiopathic Pulmonary Fibrosis Without Anti-Fibrotic Therapy: A Systematic Review. *Eur Respir Rev* (2020) 29(157). doi: 10.1183/16000617.0158-2019
3. Collard HR, Ryerson CJ, Corte TJ, Jenkins G, Kondoh Y, Lederer DJ, et al. Acute Exacerbation of Idiopathic Pulmonary Fibrosis. An International Working Group Report. *Am J Respir Crit Care Med* (2016) 194(3):265–75. doi: 10.1164/rccm.201604-0801CI
4. Ranieri VM, Rubenfeld GD, Thompson BT, Ferguson ND, Caldwell E, Fan E, et al. Acute Respiratory Distress Syndrome: The Berlin Definition. *JAMA* (2012) 307(23):2526–33. doi: 10.1001/jama.2012.5669
5. de Hemptinne Q, Remmelink M, Brimioulle S, Salmon I, Vincent J-L. ARDS: A Clinicopathological Confrontation. *Chest* (2009) 135(4):944–9. doi: 10.1378/chest.08-1741
6. Ferguson ND, Frutos-Vivar F, Esteban A, Fernández-Segoviano P, Aramburu JA, Nájera L, et al. Acute Respiratory Distress Syndrome: Underrecognition by Clinicians and Diagnostic Accuracy of Three Clinical Definitions. *Crit Care Med* (2005) 33(10):2228–34. doi: 10.1097/01.CCM.0000181529.08630.49
7. Huppertz C, Jäger B, Wieczorek G, Engelhard P, Oliver SJ, Bauernfeind F-G, et al. The NLRP3 Inflammasome Pathway is Activated in Sarcoidosis and Involved in Granuloma Formation. *Eur Respir J* (2020) 55(3). doi: 10.1183/13993003.00119-2019
8. Dostert C, Pétrilli V, van Bruggen R, Steele C, Mossman BT, Tschopp J. Innate Immune Activation Through Nalp3 Inflammasome Sensing of Asbestos and Silica. *Science* (2008) 320(5876):674–7. doi: 10.1126/science.1156995
9. Lasithiotaki I, Giannarakis I, Tsitoura E, Samara KD, Margaritopoulos GA, Choulaki C, et al. NLRP3 Inflammasome Expression in Idiopathic Pulmonary Fibrosis and Rheumatoid Lung. *Eur Respir J* (2016) 47(3):910–8. doi: 10.1183/13993003.00564-2015
10. Latz E, Xiao TS, Stutz A. Activation and Regulation of the Inflammasomes. *Nat Rev Immunol* (2013) 13(6):397–411. doi: 10.1038/nri3452
11. Bauernfeind F, Hornung V. Of Inflammasomes and Pathogens–Sensing of Microbes by the Inflammasome. *EMBO Mol Med* (2013) 5(6):814–26. doi: 10.1002/emmm.201201771
12. Dolinay T, Kim YS, Howrylak J, Hunninghake GM, An CH, Fredenburgh L, et al. Inflammasome-Regulated Cytokines are Critical Mediators of Acute Lung Injury. *Am J Respir Crit Care Med* (2012) 185(11):1225–34. doi: 10.1164/rccm.201201-0003OC
13. de Nardo D, de Nardo CM, Latz E. New Insights Into Mechanisms Controlling the NLRP3 Inflammasome and its Role in Lung Disease. *Am J Pathol* (2014) 184(1):42–54. doi: 10.1016/j.ajpath.2013.09.007
14. Sgalla G, Iovene B, Calvello M, Ori M, Varone F, Richeldi L. Idiopathic Pulmonary Fibrosis: Pathogenesis and Management. *Respir Res* (2018) 19 (1):32. doi: 10.1186/s12931-018-0730-2
15. Wolters PJ, Collard HR, Jones KD. Pathogenesis of Idiopathic Pulmonary Fibrosis. *Annu Rev Pathol* (2014) 9:157–79. doi: 10.1146/annurev-pathol-012513-104706
16. McCubbrey AL, Curtis JL. Efferocytosis and Lung Disease. *Chest* (2013) 143 (6):1750–7. doi: 10.1378/chest.12-2413
17. Kim KK, Dotson MR, Agarwal M, Yang J, Bradley PB, Subbotina N, et al. Efferocytosis of Apoptotic Alveolar Epithelial Cells is Sufficient to Initiate Lung Fibrosis. *Cell Death Dis* (2018) 9(11):1056. doi: 10.1038/s41419-018-1074-z
18. Morimoto K, Janssen WJ, Terada M. Defective Efferocytosis by Alveolar Macrophages in IPF Patients. *Respir Med* (2012) 106(12):1800–3. doi: 10.1016/j.rmed.2012.08.020
19. Shimada K, Crother TR, Karlin J, Dagvadorj J, Chiba N, Chen S, et al. Oxidized Mitochondrial DNA Activates the NLRP3 Inflammasome During Apoptosis. *Immunity* (2012) 36(3):401–14. doi: 10.1016/j.immuni.2012.01.009
20. Nakahira K, Haspel JA, Rathinam VAK, Lee S-J, Dolinay T, Lam HC, et al. Autophagy Proteins Regulate Innate Immune Responses by Inhibiting the Release of Mitochondrial DNA Mediated by the NALP3 Inflammasome. *Nat Immunol* (2011) 12(3):222–30. doi: 10.1038/ni.1980
21. van der Burgh R, Nijhuis L, Pervolaraki K, Compeer EB, Jongeneel LH, van Gijn M, et al. Defects in Mitochondrial Clearance Predispose Human Monocytes to Interleukin-1β Hypersecretion. *J Biol Chem* (2014) 289 (8):5000–12. doi: 10.1074/jbc.M113.536920
22. Margaritopoulos GA, Tsitoura E, Tzanakis N, Spandidos DA, Siafakas NM, Sourvinos G, et al. Self-Eating: Friend or Foe? The Emerging Role of Autophagy in Idiopathic Pulmonary Fibrosis. *BioMed Res Int* (2013) 2013:420497. doi: 10.1155/2013/420497
23. Araya J, Kojima J, Takasaka N, Ito S, Fujii S, Hara H, et al. Insufficient Autophagy in Idiopathic Pulmonary Fibrosis. *Am J Physiol Lung Cell Mol Physiol* (2013) 304(1):L56–69. doi: 10.1152/ajplung.00213.2012
24. Bueno M, Lai Y-C, Romero Y, Brands J, St Croix CM, Kamga C, et al. PINK1 Deficiency Impairs Mitochondrial Homeostasis and Promotes Lung Fibrosis. *J Clin Invest* (2015) 125(2):521–38. doi: 10.1172/JCI74942
25. Katzen J, Beers MF. Contributions of Alveolar Epithelial Cell Quality Control to Pulmonary Fibrosis. *J Clin Invest* (2020) 130(10):5088–99. doi: 10.1172/JCI139519
26. Hook G, Yu J, Toneff T, Kindy M, Hook V. Brain Pyroglutamate Amyloid-β is Produced by Cathepsin B and is Reduced by the Cysteine Protease Inhibitor E64d, Representing a Potential Alzheimer's Disease Therapeutic. *J Alzheimers Dis* (2014) 41(1):129–49. doi: 10.3233/JAD-131370
27. Kolb M, Bondue B, Pesci A, Miyazaki Y, Song JW, Bhatt NY, et al. Acute Exacerbations of Progressive-Fibrosing Interstitial Lung Diseases. *Eur Respir Rev* (2018) 27(150). doi: 10.1183/16000617.0071-2018
28. Prasse A, Georges CG, Biller H, Hamm H, Matthys H, Luttmann W, et al. Th1 Cytokine Pattern in Sarcoidosis is Expressed by Bronchoalveolar CD4+ and CD8+ T Cells. *Clin Exp Immunol* (2000) 122(2):241–8. doi: 10.1046/j.1365-2249.2000.01365.x
29. Netea MG, Nold-Petry CA, Nold MF, Joosten LAB, Opitz B, van der Meer JHM, et al. Differential Requirement for the Activation of the Inflammasome for Processing and Release of IL-1beta in Monocytes and Macrophages. *Blood* (2009) 113(10):2324–35. doi: 10.1182/blood-2008-03-146720
30. Pinar B, Henríquez-Hernández LA, Lara PC, Bordon E, Rodriguez-Gallego C, Lloret M, et al. Radiation Induced Apoptosis and Initial DNA Damage are Inversely Related in Locally Advanced Breast Cancer Patients. *Radiat Oncol* (2010) 5:85. doi: 10.1186/1748-717X-5-85
31. Henríquez-Hernández LA, Carmona-Vigo R, Pinar B, Bordón E, Lloret M, Núñez MI, et al. Combined Low Initial DNA Damage and High Radiation-Induced Apoptosis Confers Clinical Resistance to Long-Term Toxicity in Breast Cancer Patients Treated With High-Dose Radiotherapy. *Radiat Oncol* (2011) 6:60. doi: 10.1186/1748-717X-6-60
32. Dewey WC, Ling CC, Meyn RE. Radiation-Induced Apoptosis: Relevance to Radiotherapy. *Int J Radiat OncologyBiologyPhysics* (1995) 33(4):781–96. doi: 10.1016/0360-3016(95)00214-8
33. Coll RC, Robertson AAB, Chae JJ, Higgins SC, Muñoz-Planillo R, Inserra MC, et al. A Small-Molecule Inhibitor of the NLRP3 Inflammasome for the Treatment of Inflammatory Diseases. *Nat Med* (2015) 21(3):248–55. doi: 10.1038/nm.3806
34. Aziz M, Yang W-L, Wang P. Measurement of Phagocytic Engulfment of Apoptotic Cells by Macrophages Using pHrodo Succinimidyl Ester. *Curr Protoc Immunol* (2013) 14(1):14.31. doi: 10.1002/0471142735.im1431s100

35. Schneider CA, Rasband WS, Eliceiri KW. Nih Image to ImageJ: 25 Years of Image Analysis. *Nat Methods* (2012) 9(7):671–5. doi: 10.1038/nmeth.2089
36. Lopez-Castejon G, Brough D. Understanding the Mechanism of IL-1β Secretion. *Cytokine Growth Factor Rev* (2011) 22(4):189–95. doi: 10.1016/j.cytogfr.2011.10.001
37. Madej MP, Töpfer E, Boraschi D, Italiani P. Different Regulation of Interleukin-1 Production and Activity in Monocytes and Macrophages: Innate Memory as an Endogenous Mechanism of IL-1 Inhibition. *Front Pharmacol* (2017) 8:335. doi: 10.3389/fphar.2017.00335
38. Natsuizaka M, Chiba H, Kuronuma K, Otsuka M, Kudo K, Mori M, et al. Epidemiologic Survey of Japanese Patients With Idiopathic Pulmonary Fibrosis and Investigation of Ethnic Differences. *Am J Respir Crit Care Med* (2014) 190(7):773–9. doi: 10.1164/rccm.201403-0566OC
39. Ziegenhagen MW, Zabel P, Zissel G, Schlaak M, Müller-Quernheim J. Serum Level of Interleukin 8 is Elevated in Idiopathic Pulmonary Fibrosis and Indicates Disease Activity. *Am J Respir Crit Care Med* (1998) 157(3 Pt 1):762–8. doi: 10.1164/ajrccm.157.3.9705014
40. Grailer JJ, Canning BA, Kalbitz M, Haggadone MD, Dhond RM, Andjelkovic AV, et al. Critical Role for the NLRP3 Inflammasome During Acute Lung Injury. *J Immunol* (2014) 192(12):5974–83. doi: 10.4049/jimmunol.1400368
41. Jones HD, Crother TR, Gonzalez-Villalobos RA, Jupelli M, Chen S, Dagvadorj J, et al. The NLRP3 Inflammasome is Required for the Development of Hypoxemia in LPS/mechanical Ventilation Acute Lung Injury. *Am J Respir Cell Mol Biol* (2014) 50(2):270–80. doi: 10.1165/rcmb.2013-0087OC
42. Kuipers MT, Aslami H, Janczy JR, van der Sluijs KF, Vlaar APJ, Wolthuis EK, et al. Ventilator-Induced Lung Injury is Mediated by the NLRP3 Inflammasome. *Anesthesiology* (2012) 116(5):1104–15. doi: 10.1097/ALN.0b013e3182518bc0
43. Prasse A, Binder H, Schupp JC, Kayser G, Bargagli E, Jaeger B, et al. Bal Cell Gene Expression is Indicative of Outcome and Airway Basal Cell Involvement in Idiopathic Pulmonary Fibrosis. *Am J Respir Crit Care Med* (2019) 199 (5):622–30. doi: 10.1164/rccm.201712-2551OC
44. Liu D, Yang P, Gao M, Yu T, Shi Y, Zhang M, et al. NLRP3 Activation Induced by Neutrophil Extracellular Traps Sustains Inflammatory Response in the Diabetic Wound. *Clin Sci (Lond)* (2019) 133(4):565–82. doi: 10.1042/CS20180600
45. Desai O, Winkler J, Minasyan M, Herzog EL. The Role of Immune and Inflammatory Cells in Idiopathic Pulmonary Fibrosis. *Front Med* (2018) 5:43. doi: 10.3389/fmed.2018.00043
46. Miller EJ, Nagao S, Carr FK, Noble JM, Cohen AB. Interleukin-8 (IL-8) is a Major Neutrophil Chemotaxin From Human Alveolar Macrophages Stimulated With Staphylococcal Enterotoxin A (Sea). *Inflammation Res* (1996) 45(8):386–92. doi: 10.1007/BF02252933
47. Prasse A, Pechkovsky DV, Toews GB, Jungraithmayr W, Kollert F, Goldmann T, et al. A Vicious Circle of Alveolar Macrophages and Fibroblasts Perpetuates Pulmonary Fibrosis Via CCL18. *Am J Respir Crit Care Med* (2006) 173 (7):781–92. doi: 10.1164/rccm.200509-1518OC
48. Xu J-F, Washko GR, Nakahira K, Hatabu H, Patel AS, Fernandez IE, et al. Statins and Pulmonary Fibrosis: The Potential Role of NLRP3 Inflammasome Activation. *Am J Respir Crit Care Med* (2012) 185(5):547–56. doi: 10.1164/rccm.201108-1574OC
49. Stout-Delgado HW, Cho SJ, Chu SG, Mitzel DN, Villalba J, El-Chemaly S, et al. Age-Dependent Susceptibility to Pulmonary Fibrosis Is Associated With NLRP3 Inflammasome Activation. *Am J Respir Cell Mol Biol* (2016) 55 (2):252–63. doi: 10.1165/rcmb.2015-0222OC
50. Gasse P, Riteau N, Charron S, Girre S, Fick L, Pétrilli V, et al. Uric Acid is a Danger Signal Activating NALP3 Inflammasome in Lung Injury Inflammation and Fibrosis. *Am J Respir Crit Care Med* (2009) 179(10):903–13. doi: 10.1164/rccm.200808-1274OC
51. Hosseinian N, Cho Y, Lockey RF, Kolliputi N. The Role of the NLRP3 Inflammasome in Pulmonary Diseases. *Ther Adv Respir Dis* (2015) 9(4):188–97. doi: 10.1177/1753465815586335
52. Liu R-M. Oxidative Stress, Plasminogen Activator Inhibitor 1, and Lung Fibrosis. *Antioxid Redox Signal* (2008) 10(2):303–19. doi: 10.1089/ars.2007.1903
53. Wollin L, Maillet I, Quesniaux V, Holweg A, Ryffel B. Antifibrotic and Anti-Inflammatory Activity of the Tyrosine Kinase Inhibitor Nintedanib in Experimental Models of Lung Fibrosis. *J Pharmacol Exp Ther* (2014) 349 (2):209–20. doi: 10.1124/jpet.113.208223
54. Oku H, Shimizu T, Kawabata T, Nagira M, Hikita I, Ueyama A, et al. Antifibrotic Action of Pirfenidone and Prednisolone: Different Effects on Pulmonary Cytokines and Growth Factors in Bleomycin-Induced Murine Pulmonary Fibrosis. *Eur J Pharmacol* (2008) 590(1-3):400–8. doi: 10.1016/j.ejphar.2008.06.046
55. Maher TM, Strek ME. Antifibrotic Therapy for Idiopathic Pulmonary Fibrosis: Time to Treat. *Respir Res* (2019) 20(1):205. doi: 10.1186/s12931-019-1161-4
56. Richeldi L, Du Bois RM, Raghu G, Azuma A, Brown KK, Costabel U, et al. Efficacy and Safety of Nintedanib in Idiopathic Pulmonary Fibrosis. *N Engl J Med* (2014) 370(22):2071–82. doi: 10.1056/NEJMoa1402584
57. Sarir H, Mortaz E, Karimi K, Kraneveld AD, Rahman I, Caldenhoven E, et al. Cigarette Smoke Regulates the Expression of TLR4 and IL-8 Production by Human Macrophages. *J Inflammation (Lond)* (2009) 6:12. doi: 10.1186/1476-9255-6-12
58. Chevriaux A, Pilot T, Derangère V, Simonin H, Martine P, Chalmin F, et al. Cathepsin B is Required for NLRP3 Inflammasome Activation in Macrophages, Through NLRP3 Interaction. *Front Cell Dev Biol* (2020) 8:167. doi: 10.3389/fcell.2020.00167
59. Amaral EP, Riteau N, Moayeri M, Maier N, Mayer-Barber KD, Pereira RM, et al. Lysosomal Cathepsin Release Is Required for NLRP3-Inflammasome Activation by Mycobacterium Tuberculosis in Infected Macrophages. *Front Immunol* (2018) 9:1427. doi: 10.3389/fimmu.2018.01427
60. de Rivero Vaccari JC, Dietrich WD, Keane RW, de Rivero Vaccari JP. The Inflammasome in Times of COVID-19. *Front Immunol* (2020) 11:583373. doi: 10.3389/fimmu.2020.583373
61. Latz E, Duewell P. NLRP3 Inflammasome Activation in Inflammaging. *Semin Immunol* (2018) 40:61–73. doi: 10.1016/j.smim.2018.09.001
62. Surabhi S, Cuypers F, Hammerschmidt S, Siemens N. The Role of NLRP3 Inflammasome in Pneumococcal Infections. *Front Immunol* (2020) 11:614801. doi: 10.3389/fimmu.2020.614801
63. Hassane M, Demon D, Soulard D, Fontaine J, Keller LE, Patin EC, et al. Neutrophilic NLRP3 Inflammasome-Dependent IL-1β Secretion Regulates the γδt17 Cell Response in Respiratory Bacterial Infections. *Mucosal Immunol* (2017) 10(4):1056–68. doi: 10.1038/mi.2016.113

3

Pirfenidone in the Treatment of Post-COVID-19 Pulmonary Fibrosis

Xianglin Zhou [1,2,3†], Danhui Yang [1,2,3†], Xianglong Kong [4], Chengli Wei [1,2,3], Siqi LvQiu [1,2,3], Lin Wang [1,2,3], Yongkang Lin [1,2,3], Zhilan Yin [5], Zhiguo Zhou [4] and Hong Luo [1,2,3*]*

[1] Department of Pulmonary and Critical Care Medicine, the Second Xiangya Hospital, Central South University, Changsha, China, [2] Research Unit of Respiratory Disease, Central South University, Changsha, China, [3] Hunan Diagnosis and Treatment Center of Respiratory Disease, Changsha, China, [4] Respiratory Medicine, The First Hospital of Changsha, Changsha, China, [5] Department of Radiology, The Second Xiangya Hospital, Central South University, Changsha, China

***Correspondence:**
Hong Luo
luohonghuxi@csu.edu.cn
Zhiguo Zhou
13807311490@163.com

† These authors have contributed equally to this work

Background: Pulmonary fibrosis is one of the sequelae of the COVID-19, which seriously affects the quality of life of survivors. Currently, there are no optimal evidence based guidelines targeting this population.

Case Presentation: We report a 66-year-old female patient without underlying comorbidities admitted to Changsha Public Health Center because of COVID-19. During hospitalization, she developed co-bacterial infection and acute respiratory distress syndrome, and received broad-spectrum antibacterial therapy, invasive mechanical ventilation and extracorporeal membrane oxygenation. After the acute phase, she developed post-COVID-19 pulmonary fibrosis subsequently treated with pirfenidone. Over 96 weeks after pirfenidone treatment, her modified Medical Research Council Dyspnea level improved to 2 from 4 at discharge. Her 6 minutes walk test distance, total lung capacity, and diffusion capacity for carbon monoxide all increased. Chest CT performed on 2 years after illness onset showed regressing fibrosis. The Hospital Anxiety and Depression Scale, Athens Insomnia Scale, and 36-Item Short Form Health Survey questionnaire all improved.

Conclusion: Post-COVID-19 pulmonary fibrosis is a challenging consequence of COVID-19, and our case suggests that pirfenidone may be an effective treatment option.

Keywords: pulmonary fibrosis, post-COVID-19, pirfenidone, long COVID, sequelae

INTRODUCTION

Since the first report of the Coronavirus disease 2019 (COVID-19) caused by the Severe Acute Respiratory Syndrome Coronavirus 2 (SARS-CoV-2) in Wuhan city on December 2019, the COVID-19 pandemic has lasted more than 2 years. As of March 29, 2022, more than 480 million confirmed cases and 6 million deaths had been reported worldwide according to the World Health Organization (WHO) (1). The clinical manifestations, pathophysiology, and treatment during the acute phase of COVID-19 are well described (2, 3). Several long-term longitudinal follow-up cohorts of patients recovered from COVID-19 have shown that although most patients recover well, up to 57.7–100% of patients still have persistent lung structural abnormalities and pulmonary function impairment (4–6). The common pattern of pulmonary interstitial lesions, also known as post-COVID-19 pulmonary fibrosis or COVID-19 pulmonary fibrosis-like (7), were ground glass opacities (GGOs), ground-glass attenuation and reticular abnormalities (8). At the same time, chest imaging showed bilateral diffuse interstitial lung disease among patients who complicated acute respiratory distress syndrome (ARDS) during acute phase (9). Relatedly, these survivals suffered from more serious 'Long COVID' (10, 11), a condition described by signs and symptoms of COVID-19 that last longer than 12 weeks and are not explained by an alternative diagnosis, with the most common symptoms of dyspnea, fatigue and 'brain fog'. However, there was no definite long-term medical advice or treatment to reverse pulmonary fibrosis for this population.

Pirfenidone, one of only two drugs approved for the treatment of idiopathic pulmonary fibrosis (IPF) in the world, is a class of pleiotropic pyridine compounds with anti-inflammatory, anti-fibrotic and antioxidant properties. Another drug is nintedanib, which can significantly reduce the absolute value of the drop in forced vital capacity (FVC) among IPF patients (12). The results of a multi-center, double-blind, randomized controlled phase 3 clinical study (ASCEND study) suggest that pirfenidone significantly delayed the decline in FVC in patients with IPF at 52 weeks compared with placebo (−235 ml vs. −428 ml, $P < 0.001$) (13). Besides, at 52 weeks, pirfenidone can reduce all-cause mortality in patients with IPF according to a pooled analyse and meta-analyses (14). To our knowledge, the effectiveness of pirfenidone in the treatment of post-COVID-19 pulmonary fibrosis is unclear. Here, we report a case of post-COVID-19 pulmonary fibrosis treated with pirfenidone over 96 weeks. During the 2-year follow-up period, the patient's symptoms, diffusing function, and interstitial lesions showed continuous improvement.

CASE DESCRIPTION

A previously healthy, 66-year-old female patient presented to the emergency department of Xiangya Hospital on February 2, 2020 (day 2 of illness onset) with a 1-day history of dizziness, nausea and diarrhea. There were no background of pulmonary problems and impaired physical capacity. She underwent a quantitative Real-time Reverse Transcription-Polymerase Chain Reaction (RT-PCR) test for SARS-CoV-2 and a chest computed tomography (CT) examination because of a travel history from Wuhan City within 14 days. The results showed positive to SARS-CoV-2 and multiple GGOs in the right lower lobe (**Figure 1**). Consequently, she was referred to the Changsha Public Health Center for isolation and hospitalization (day 3).

On admission, physical examination showed a body temperature of 37.3°C, a level at 98% of resting finger oxygen saturation without additional oxygen supplement, overweight with a body mass index (BMI) of 25.3 kg/m^2, and moist rales in bilateral lower lungs. The laboratory examination results were as follows: white blood cell (WBC) count was 2.79×10^9/L, with a lymphocyte percentage of 22.2%, the procalcitonin concentration was 0.054 ng/mL, the level of C-reactive protein was 65.7 mg/L, the erythrocyte sedimentation rate was 106 mm/h, the ferritin level was 505.5 ng/mL. The serum β-(1,3)-glucan, galactomannan, RT-PCR results for influenza A and B viruses were normal. A reviewed chest high resolution CT taken on February 3 (day3) presented new and progressive, diffuse, peripheral GGOs in the right upper lobe, right middle lobe and left lower lobe, and consolidation in the right lower lobe (**Figure 1**), typical of acute COVID-19. She was diagnosed with COVID-19 (common type) according to the Chinese Clinical Guidance for COVID-19 Pneumonia Diagnosis and Treatment (4th edition) (15), and received oral antiviral drugs Arbidol and low dose intravenous methylprednisolone hemisuccinate. From day 9, she developed progressive hypoxemia due to suspected co-bacterial infection and COVID-19 aggravation. She was treated with empirical broad-spectrum antibiotics (moxifloxacin, piperacillin tazobactam, meropenem), intravenous immunoglobulin convalescent serum and supported by non-invasive high concentration oxygen. On day 31, she became critically ill and invasive mechanical ventilation (IMV) was conducted because of refractory hypoxemia and progressive lung shadows. Immediately, she was commenced on extracorporeal membrane oxygenation (ECMO) on the next day after IMV. The antibiotics were adjusted to polymyxin B sulfate combined with linezolid, based on a report of bronchoalveolar lavage fluid metagenomic next-generation sequencing which detected 2,55,418 sequences mapped to *Actinomyces odontolyticus* and 3,897 sequences mapped to *Staphylococcus aureus*. Her hypoxia was improved on day 37. She was weaned off ECMO support, meanwhile, de-escalation of antibiotic therapy was conducted. On day 89, she was extubated and freed from IMV.

Chest CT scanned on day 61 showed diffuse interstitial changes, with extensive areas of subpleural and peribronchovascular septal thickening, subpleural reticular abnormalities, traction bronchiectasis, and honeycomb-like changes under the subpleura in both lung fields, which manifested as interstitial lung disease (ILD) (**Figure 2**), and she started taking pirfenidone (Initially 600 mg per day, after 1 week maintain 1,800 mg per day). After 2 months of therapy, her dyspnea and pulmonary fibrosis improved (**Figure 2**), and subsequently, the patient was discharged on day 130, with a level of modified Medical Research Council Dyspnea Scale (mMRC) at 4 (**Table 1**). The patient maintained long-term pirfenidone therapy at home without any liver function damage and hematological complications, and she was followed up on the 7th (1 year after onset) and 20th (2 year after onset) month after discharge. The patient's symptoms and physical capacity had improved with the mMRC scores improved from 4 to 2 and 6-min walking test distance (6-MWD) recovered to 309 meters from 188 meters during treatment. Similarly, the Hospital Anxiety and Depression Scale (HADS), Athens Insomnia Scale (AIS), and Chinese vision of the 36-Item Short Form Health Survey questionnaire (SF-36) all improved on 2 year after initial insult. Pulmonary function tests showed improvement in restrictive ventilatory and diffusing function, with FVC improved from 1.98 liters to 2.30 liters, total lung capacity (TLC) improved from 61.7% of predict to 72.3% and diffusion capacity for carbon monoxide (DLCO) improved from 30.3% of predict to 47.9%. Reticular abnormalities, interlobular septal thickening and honeycomb-like changes were reduced in bilateral lung fields on chest CT screened on day 758 (**Figure 2**).

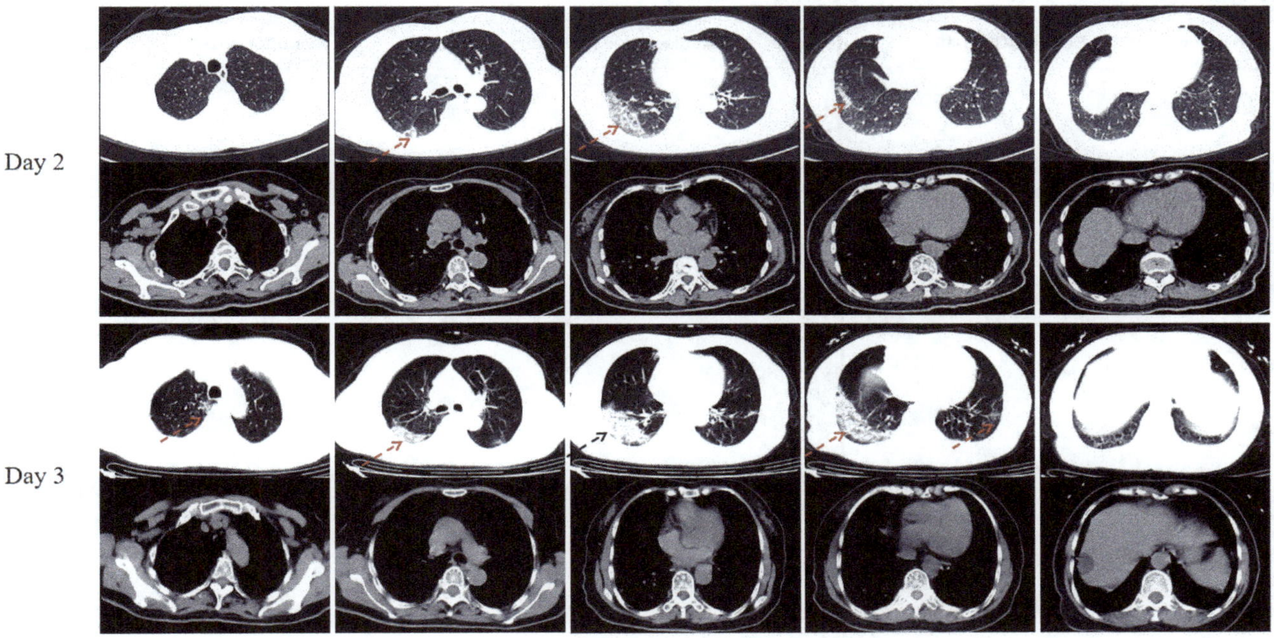

FIGURE 1 | Chest CT of the patient on day 2 and day 3 (On admission) after illness onset. Red dotted arrow: multiple ground glass opacities (GGOs); Black dotted arrow: consolidation.

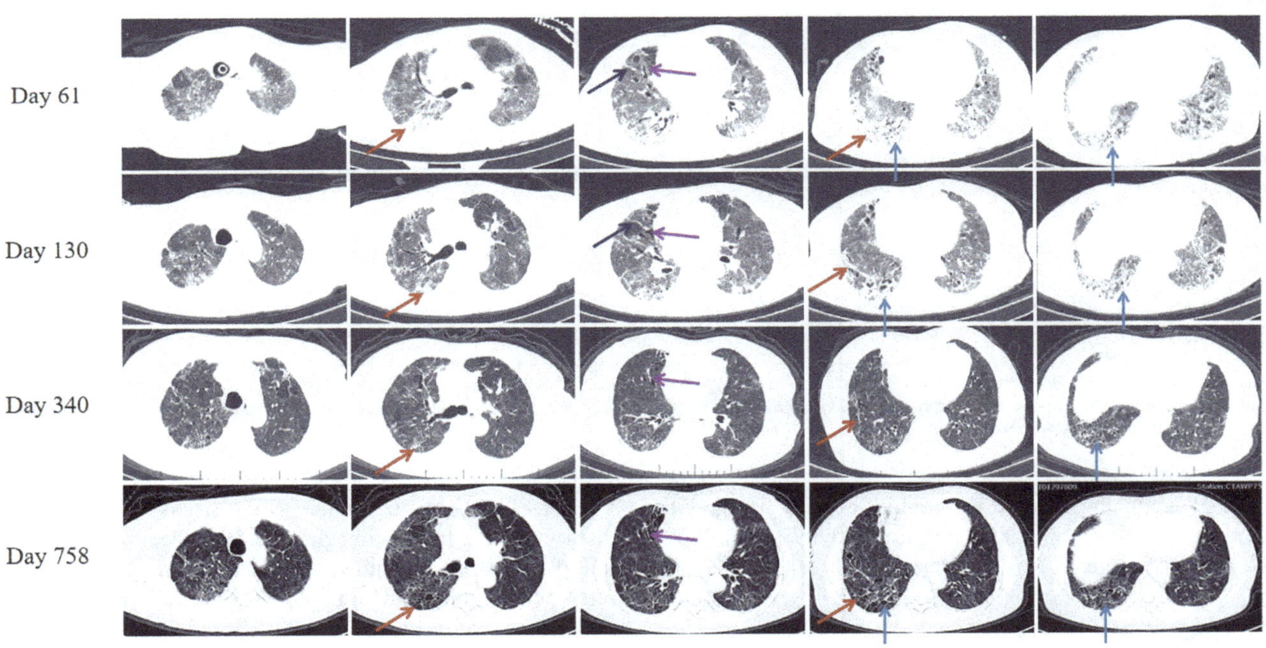

FIGURE 2 | Chest CT on day 61 (Starting taking pirfenidone), day 130 (At discharge), day 340 and day 758 after illness onset. Red solid arrows: subpleural reticular abnormalities and fibrous cords. Black solid arrow: interlobular septal thickening. Purple solid arrow: traction bronchiectasis. Blue solid arrow: honeycomb-like change under the subpleura.

TABLE 1 | Evolution of clinical features from illness onset and taking pirfenidone (2 months after onset).

Clinical features	Before COVID-19	Acute stage	At discharge (4 months after onset)	1 year after onset	2 years after onset
Symptoms					
Fever		√			
Cough		√	√	√	√
Dyspnoea		√	√	√	√
Headache		√			
Fatigue		√	√	√	√
Myalgia		√	√	√	
Nausea/Vomiting		√			
Diarrhea		√			
Chest pain		√	√	√	√
Anosmia		√	√		
Dysgeusia		√	√		
Other		√	√		
Pulmonary rale	/	Moist rale	Velcro rale	Velcro rale	Velcro rale
mMRC, level	0	/	4	3	2
6-MWD, m	/	/	/*	188	309
HADS score					
Anxiety	/	/	/	1	0
Depression	/	/	/	0	0
AIS Score	/	/	/	10	2
SF-36 score					
Physical functioning	/	/	/	25	85
Role-physical	/	/	/	0	100
Bodily pain	/	/	/	72	74
General health	/	/	/	35	55
Vitality	/	/	/	55	85
Social functioning	/	/	/	37.5	87.5
Role-emotional	/	/	/	100	100
Mental health	/	/	/	84	92
Health transition	/	/	/	75	75
Pulmonary function					
FVC, L	/	/	/*	1.98	2.30
FEV1, L	/	/	/*	1.64	1.80
FEV1/FVC	/	/	/*	0.82	0.83
TLC, % of predict	/	/	/*	61.7	72.3
DLCO, % of predict	/	/	/*	30.3	47.9

**The patient can't tolerate it. mMRC, modified Medical Research Council Dyspnea Scale; 6-MWD, 6 Minutes Walk Test Distance; HADS, Hospital Anxiety and Depression Scale; AIS, Athens Insomnia Scale; SF-36, Chinese vision of the 36-Item Short Form Health Survey questionnaire; FVC, Forced Vital Capacity; FEV1, Forced Expiratory Volume in 1 s; TLC, Total Lung Capacity; DLCO, Diffusion Capacity for Carbon monoxide.*

The patient gradually returned to activities of daily living, with self-care on the 7th month and physical activity on the 20th month after discharge.

DISCUSSION

The developing and toughest challenge is how to manage COVID-19 sequelae, in view of our greater understanding of the consequences of post-COVID-19 infection (11). A cohort study of 2,73,168 discharged patients from the United Kingdom showed that 36.5% of patients recorded one or more symptoms between 3 and 6 months after discharge (16).

Post-COVID-19 pulmonary fibrosis is a heterogeneous disease with different imaging performance. The researchers found that residual changes after acute stage vary over time. A retrospective study shown that (17), 3 months after acute phase, pulmonary fibrosis was clinically confirmed in 56% and 71% of the patients with moderate and severe COVID-19 symptoms respectively. In a prospective study (4), Wu et al. found that 78% of patients (65/83) had residual changes on CT at 3 months after discharge and the most common CT features were GGO (78%), interlobular septal thickening (34%), reticular opacity (33%), and subpleural curvilinear opacity (11%). In the same study, 24% of patients (20/83) had persistent imaging abnormalities

TABLE 2 | Clinical trials[a] of pirfenidone and deupirfenidone[b] for the treatment of post-COVID-19 pulmonary fibrosis.

Identifier		Start time	Study design	Phase	Objects	Number enrolled and distribution	Intervention	Primary outcome
NCT04607928 (26)		29-Oct-20	Multicenter, randomized, placebo-controlled	II	Patients with fibrotic lung sequelae after recovery from acute phase of severe COVID pneumonia	148 2:1 (Pirfenidone: Placebo)	Pirfenidone: 2403 mg/day for 24weeks; Controlled: placebo for 24 weeks;	Change from baseline in % in forced vital capacity (FVC) and % fibrosis in high resolution computed tomography of the lung
NCT04856111 (27)		22-Apr-21	Singlecenter, randomized	IV	Patients with fibrotic lung disease after COVID-19	48 1:1 (Pirfenidone: Nintedanib)	Pirfenidone: 2,400 mg/day for 24 weeks; Nintedanib: 300 mg/day for 24 weeks;	Change in the forced vital capacity (FVC)
NCT04652518 (28)	Part A	3-Dec-20	Multicenter, randomized, double-blind, placebo-controlled	II	Adults with post-acute COVID-19 respiratory complications	168 1:1 (Deupirfenidone: Placebo)	Deupirfenidone: 500 mg for 91 days; Controlled: placebo for 91 days	Change in distance walked on the 6-minutes walk test (6 MWT)
	Part B	-	Open label extension study	II	Eligible patients who completed part A	-	Deupirfenidone: an additional 91 days	Assess the longer-term safety, tolerability, and efficacy of Deupirfenidone through up to 182 days of treatment; (One of the secondary objective: Inflammatory, fibrosis and other biomarkers;)
ChiCTR2000030892 (29)		16-Mar-20	Parallel	-	Patients with severe post-COVID-19 fibrosis	40 1:1 (Pirfenidone: blank control)	-	Change in HRCT pulmonary fibrosis score

[a]*Data retrieved from ClinicalTrials.gov and chictr.org;* [b]*Deupirfenidone: a selectively deuterated form of pirfenidone.*

during the 1-year follow-up, without progressive interstitial changes and definite intervention. However, another prospective study presented higher proportion. According to Huang and his colleagues (6), the rate of persisting imaging abnormalities at 12 months after discharged was 76% among patients with severity scale 5 to 6. The phenomenon was similar to severe acute respiratory syndrome (SARS) and Middle East respiratory syndrome (MERS) survivors. In a retrospective study (18), 21.5% (67/311) of SARS patients had radiographic pulmonary fibrosis at discharge and 40 patients exhibited improvement of fibrosis at one-year follow-up. Analogously, a study of MERS (19) survivors revealed 33% of patients presented chest radiological abnormalities at 80 days after discharge.

In our case, the patient presented with marked restrictive ventilatory dysfunction and impaired diffusing function, which is consistent with previous studies. Mo et al. (20) reported abnormal diffusion function and decreased TLC in 47.2 and 25.0% of patients at discharge. Although this percentage was undoubtedly underestimated, disease severity in the acute phase was inextricably linked to pulmonary function at discharge. Significant difference in impaired diffusing capacity among the different groups of severity, which accounted for 30.4% in mild and 84.2% in severe illness, respectively (20). Meanwhile, the proportion of anomalies gradually decreased over time. Follow-up studies revealed that the proportion of survivors with abnormal pulmonary diffusing function decreased to 35–55% and 21–33% at 3 and 12 months after discharge respectively (4, 6, 21). In a 12-month longitudinal follow-up study, GGO and irregular lines were positively associated with risk of lung diffusion impairment at 12 months (6). This suggested that further reductions in pulmonary fibrosis could improve their lung function and quality of life.

The treatment strategy, oral pirfenidone, 1,800 mg per day (22), for post-COVID-19 pulmonary fibrosis, was bold, novel and aggressive, given there was no reliable evidence of effectiveness of pirfenidone in this population. This protocol was developed because her chest imaging changes were consistent with ILD, including common IPF. In the CAPACITY-004 study (23), pirfenidone reduced decline in FVC with a mean FVC change at −8.0% in the pirfenidone (2,403 mg/day) group and −12.4% in the placebo group at week 72. However, in another concurrent RCT study (CAPACITY-006), the difference between groups in FVC change at week 72 was not significant. More attention should be paid to the application of pirfenidone in interstitial lung diseases other than IPF. A multi-center, double-blind, randomized controlled phase 2 clinical study (uILD study) (24) reported that, for unclassifiable interstitial pneumonia, the use of pirfenidone (2,403 mg/d) for 24 weeks significantly delayed the decline in FVC (−17.8 vs. −113 ml, $P = 0.002$). Although evidence shown that pirfenidone could alleviate inflammatory responses in hospitalized adult patients with severe COVID-19 (25), its effectiveness in post-COVID-19 pulmonary fibrosis is still unknown.

Surprisingly, encouraging effectiveness was observed in our patient. Fibrotic lesions gradually subsided, lung diffusing function improved and she returned to normal daily life after pirfenidone therapy. However, this study has some limitations. First, there is reporting bias and it was unclear whether her improvement was benefited from pirfenidone or a natural regression of the disease course. Second, this study is not general, and the effect of pirfenidone in patients with other lung diseases is still unknown. Ongoing clinical trials (26–29) about pirfenidone and deupirfenidone in the treatment of post-COVID-19 pulmonary fibrosis may be able to provide a clear answer (**Table 2**).

CONCLUSION

In summary, our study reported a case of post-COVID-19 pulmonary fibrosis treated with long-term oral pirfenidone and the patient recovered well in terms of symptoms, pulmonary function and chest CT images. Pirfenidone may be an effective therapeutic strategy for post-COVID-19 pulmonary fibrosis. RCTs are needed for validation.

ETHICS STATEMENT

The studies involving human participants were reviewed and approved by the Review Board of the Second Xiangya Hospital of Central South University. The patients/participants provided their written informed consent to participate in this study.

AUTHOR CONTRIBUTIONS

XZ and DY collected the data and wrote the manuscript. XK, CW, SQ, LW, YL, and ZY analyzed, interpreted the data, and performed the clinical assessment. ZZ and HL designed the study and performed the clinical assessment. All authors reviewed, edited, and approved the final manuscript.

FUNDING

This study was supported by the National Natural Science Foundation of China (82070003 to HL), Natural Science Foundation of Hunan Province, China (2021JJ30943 to HL), the Science and Technology Program of Changsha, China (kq1901120 to HL), Xiangya Clinical Big Data System Construction Project in Pulmonary Inflammatory Disease of Central South University, and the National Key Clinical Specialty Construction Projects of China.

ACKNOWLEDGMENTS

We thank the Respiratory Rehabilitation Room, Pulmonary Function Test Room and Radiology Center of the Second Xiangya Hospital of Central South University for technical support of this manuscript.

REFERENCES

1. World Health Organization. Coronavirus disease 2019 (COVID-19) situation report. 2022. https://www.who.int/emergencies/diseases/novel-coronavirus-2019/situation-reports (accessed April 2, 2022).
2. Wiersinga WJ, Rhodes A, Cheng AC, Peacock SJ, Prescott HC. Pathophysiology, transmission, diagnosis, and treatment of coronavirus disease 2019 (COVID-19): a review. *JAMA.* (2020) 324:782–93. doi: 10.1001/jama.2020.12839
3. Guan WJ Ni ZY, Hu Y, Liang WH, Ou CQ, He JX, et al. Clinical characteristics of coronavirus disease 2019 in China. *N Engl J Med.* (2020) 382:1708–20. doi: 10.1056/NEJMoa2002032
4. Wu X, Liu X, Zhou Y, Yu H, Li R, Zhan Q, et al. 3-month, 6-month, 9-month, and 12-month respiratory outcomes in patients following COVID-19-related hospitalisation: a prospective study. *Lancet Respir Med.* (2021) 9:747–54. doi: 10.1016/S2213-2600(21)00174-0
5. Yin X, Xi X, Min X, Feng Z, Li B, Cai W, et al. Long-term chest CT follow-up in COVID-19 Survivors: 102-361 days after onset. *Ann Transl Med.* (2021) 9:1231. doi: 10.21037/atm-21-1438
6. Huang L, Yao Q, Gu X, Wang Q, Ren L, Wang Y, et al. 1-year outcomes in hospital survivors with COVID-19: a longitudinal cohort study. *Lancet.* (2021) 398:747–58. doi: 10.1016/S0140-6736(21)01755-4
7. Lei P, Fan B, Mao J, Wei J, Wang P. The progression of computed tomographic (CT) images in patients with coronavirus disease (COVID-19) pneumonia: running title: The CT progression of COVID-19 pneumonia, *J Infect.* (2020) 80:e30–1. doi: 10.1016/j.jinf.2020.03.020
8. Faverio P, Luppi F, Rebora P, Andrea G, Stainer A, et al. 1-year pulmonary impairment after severe COVID-19: a prospective, multicenter follow-up study. *Respir Res.* (2022) 23:65. doi: 10.1186/s12931-022-01994-y
9. Cocconcelli E, Bernardinello N, Giraudo C, Castelli G, Giorgino A, Leoni D, et al. Characteristics and prognostic factors of pulmonary fibrosis after COVID-19 pneumonia. *Front Med.* (2021) 8:823600. doi: 10.3389/fmed.2021.823600
10. Naeije R, Caravita S. Phenotyping long COVID. *Eur Respir J.* (2021) 58:1763. doi: 10.1183/13993003.01763-2021
11. Crook H, Raza S, Nowell J, Young M. Edison P. Long covid-mechanisms, risk factors, and management. *BMJ.* (2021) 374:n1648. doi: 10.1136/bmj.n1648
12. Richeldi L, du Bois RM, Raghu G, Azuma A, Brown KK, Costabel U, et al. Efficacy and safety of nintedanib in idiopathic pulmonary fibrosis. *N Engl J Med.* (2014) 370:2071–82. doi: 10.1056/NEJMoa1402584
13. King TE Jr, Bradford WZ, Castro-Bernardini S, Fagan EA, Glaspole I, Glassberg MK, et al. A phase 3 trial of pirfenidone in patients with idiopathic pulmonary fibrosis. *N Engl J Med.* (2014) 370:2083–92. doi: 10.1056/NEJMoa1402582
14. Nathan SD, Albera C, Bradford WZ, Costabel U, Glaspole I, Glassberg MK, et al. Effect of pirfenidone on mortality: pooled analyses and meta-analyses of clinical trials in idiopathic pulmonary fibrosis. *Lancet Respir Med.* (2017) 5:33–41. doi: 10.1016/S2213-2600(16)30326-5
15. China National Health Commission (NHC). Chinese Clinical Guidance for COVID-19 Pneumonia Diagnosis and Treatment (4th edition). Available online at: http://www.nhc.gov.cn/ (accessed April 2, 2022).
16. Taquet M, Dercon Q, Luciano S, Geddes JR, Husain M, Harrison PJ. Incidence, co-occurrence, and evolution of long-COVID features: A 6-month retrospective cohort study of 273,618 survivors of COVID-19. *PLoS Med.* (2021) 18:e1003773. doi: 10.1371/journal.pmed.10 03773
17. Fu Z, Tang N, Chen Y, Ma L, Wei Y, Lu Y, et al. CT features of COVID-19 patients with two consecutive negative RT-PCR tests after treatment. *Sci Rep.* (2020) 10:11548. doi: 10.1038/s41598-020-6 8509-x
18. Xie L, Liu Y, Fan B, Xiao Y, Tian Q, Chen L, et al. Dynamic changes of serum SARS-coronavirus IgG, pulmonary function and radiography in patients recovering from SARS after hospital discharge. *Respir Res.* (2005) 6:5. doi: 10.1186/1465-9921-6-5
19. Das KM, Lee EY, Singh R, Enani MA, Al Dossari K, Van Gorkom K, et al. Follow-up chest radiographic findings in patients with MERS-CoV after recovery. *Indian J Radiol Imaging.* (2017) 27:342–9. doi: 10.4103/ijri.IJRI_469_16
20. Mo X, Jian W, Su Z, Chen M, Peng H, Peng P, et al. Abnormal pulmonary function in COVID-19 patients at time of hospital discharge. *Eur Respir J.* (2020) 2020:55. doi: 10.1183/13993003.01217-2020
21. Frija-Masson J, Debray MP, Gilbert M, Lescure FX, Travert F, Borie R, et al. Functional characteristics of patients with SARS-CoV-2 pneumonia at 30 days post-infection. *Eur Respir J.* (2020) 2020:56. doi: 10.1183/13993003.01754-2020
22. Taniguchi H, Ebina M, Kondoh Y, Ogura T, Azuma A, Suga M, et al. Pirfenidone in idiopathic pulmonary fibrosis. *Eur Respir J.* (2010) 35:821–9. doi: 10.1183/09031936.00005209
23. Noble PW, Albera C, Bradford WZ, Costabel U, Glassberg MK, Kardatzke D, et al. Pirfenidone in patients with idiopathic pulmonary fibrosis (CAPACITY): two randomised trials. *Lancet.* (2011) 377:1760–9. doi: 10.1016/S0140-6736(11)60405-4
24. Maher TM, Corte TJ, Fischer A, Kreuter M, Lederer DJ, Molina-Molina M, et al. Pirfenidone in patients with unclassifiable progressive fibrosing interstitial lung disease: a double-blind, randomised, placebo-controlled, phase 2 trial. *Lancet Respir Med.* (2020) 8:147–57. doi: 10.1016/S2213-2600(19)30341-8
25. Zhang F, Wei Y, He L, Zhang H, Hu Q, Yue H, et al. A trial of pirfenidone in hospitalized adult patients with severe coronavirus disease 2019. *Chin Med J.* (2021) 135:368–70. doi: 10.1097/CM9.0000000000001614
26. Phase-II Randomized Clinical Trial to Evaluate the Effect of Pirfenidone Compared to Placebo in Post-COVID19 Pulmonary Fibrosis; Identifier NCT04607928; Available online at: https://clinicaltrials.gov/ (accessed April 2, 2022).
27. A Study of the Efficacy and Safety of Pirfenidone vs. Nintedanib in the Treatment of Fibrotic Lung Disease After Coronavirus Disease-19 Pneumonia; Identifier NCT04856111; Available online at: https://clinicaltrials.gov/ (accessed April 2, 2022).
28. A Phase 2 Randomized, Double-blind, Placebo-controlled Trial and Open Label Extension to Evaluate the Safety and Efficacy of Deupirfenidone (LYT-100) in Post-acute COVID-19 Respiratory Disease; Identifier NCT04652518; Available online at: https://clinicaltrials.gov/ (accessed April 2, 2022).
29. Efficacy and Safety of Pirfenidone in the Treatment of Severe Post-Novel Coronavirus Pneumonia (COVID-19) Fibrosis:a prospective exploratory experimental medical study; Identifier ChiCTR2000030892; Available online at: https://www.chictr.org.cn (accessed April 2, 2022).

4

Exploring Animal Models that Resemble Idiopathic Pulmonary Fibrosis

Jun Tashiro[1], Gustavo A. Rubio[1], Andrew H. Limper[2], Kurt Williams[3], Sharon J. Elliot[1], Ioanna Ninou[4], Vassilis Aidinis[4], Argyrios Tzouvelekis[4†] and Marilyn K. Glassberg[1,5†]*

[1] Department of Surgery, University of Miami Miller School of Medicine, Miami, FL, United States, [2] Department of Medicine, Mayo Clinic College of Medicine, Rochester, MN, United States, [3] Department Pathobiology and Diagnostic Investigations, College of Veterinary Medicine, Michigan State University, East Lansing, MI, United States, [4] Division of Immunology, Biomedical Sciences Research Center "Alexander Fleming", Athens, Greece, [5] Department of Medicine, University of Miami Miller School of Medicine, Miami, FL, United States

***Correspondence:**
Marilyn K. Glassberg
mglassbe@med.miami.edu

†These authors have contributed equally to this work.

Large multicenter clinical trials have led to two recently approved drugs for patients with idiopathic pulmonary fibrosis (IPF); yet, both of these therapies only slow disease progression and do not provide a definitive cure. Traditionally, preclinical trials have utilized mouse models of bleomycin (BLM)-induced pulmonary fibrosis—though several limitations prevent direct translation to human IPF. Spontaneous pulmonary fibrosis occurs in other animal species, including dogs, horses, donkeys, and cats. While the fibrotic lungs of these animals share many characteristics with lungs of patients with IPF, current veterinary classifications of fibrotic lung disease are not entirely equivalent. Additional studies that profile these examples of spontaneous fibroses in animals for similarities to human IPF should prove useful for both human and animal investigators. In the meantime, studies of BLM-induced fibrosis in aged male mice remain the most clinically relevant model for preclinical study for human IPF. Addressing issues such as time course of treatment, animal size and characteristics, clinically irrelevant treatment endpoints, and reproducibility of therapeutic outcomes will improve the current status of preclinical studies. Elucidating the mechanisms responsible for the development of fibrosis and disrepair associated with aging through a collaborative approach between researchers will promote the development of models that more accurately represent the realm of interstitial lung diseases in humans.

Keywords: bleomycin, idiopathic pulmonary fibrosis, murine model, asbestosis, aged mice

BACKGROUND

Idiopathic pulmonary fibrosis (IPF) is a devastating chronic lung disease, primarily affecting middle aged and older adults (1, 2). Lung function decline is gradual, with the potential for intermittent, unpredictable, acute exacerbations and the development of associated pulmonary hypertension (3). Disease diagnosis is primarily based on a typical radiology pattern (high-resolution computed tomography—HRCT) of usual interstitial pneumonia (UIP) characterized by reticulation and honeycomb cysts of subpleural and bibasilar distribution coupled with exclusion of other known causes of lung fibrosis as assessed by absence of exposures (occupational, environmental, drug), a negative immunologic profile and compatible bronchoalveolar lavage fluid (BALF) findings (i.e., absence

TABLE 1 | Selected pulmonary fibrosis conditions in animal species.

Selected pulmonary fibrosis conditions in animal species

Species	**Model/disease**	**Features**	**Histology**
Mouse (C57BL/6J)	Bleomycin (BLM) (experimental)	Increased collagen deposition Patchy fibrosis associated with inflammatory infiltrates Resolution in young mice starting at 3 weeks	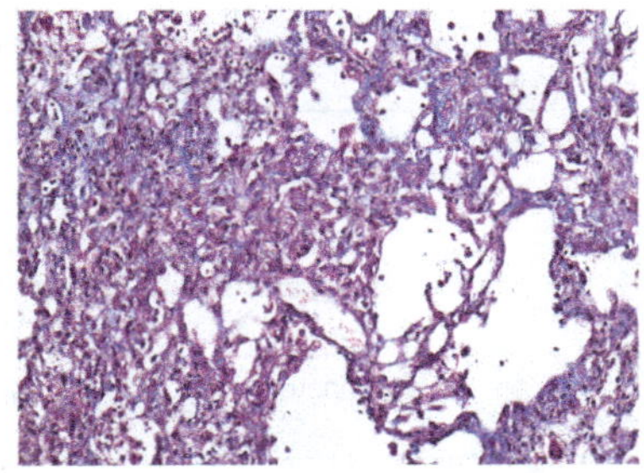
Dog (West Highland Terrier)	Interstitial lung disease (ILD)	Septal widening and collagen deposition Normal alveolar cells	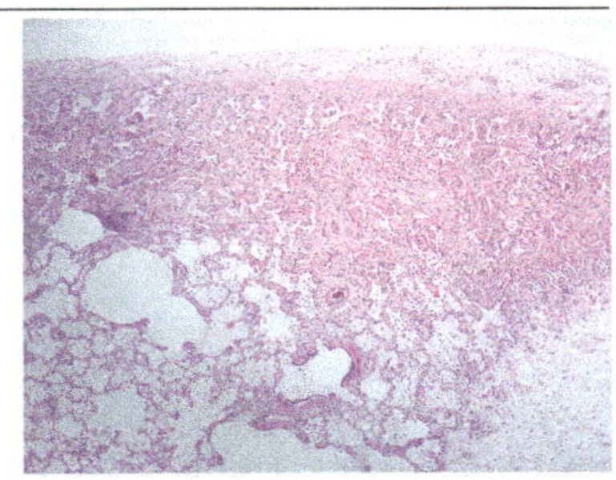
Donkey	Chronic pleuropulmonary fibrosis	Associated with asinine herpesvirus 5 infection Pleural, subpleural, and septal fibrosis extending to interstitium Intra-alveolar fibrosis and alveolar septal elastosis	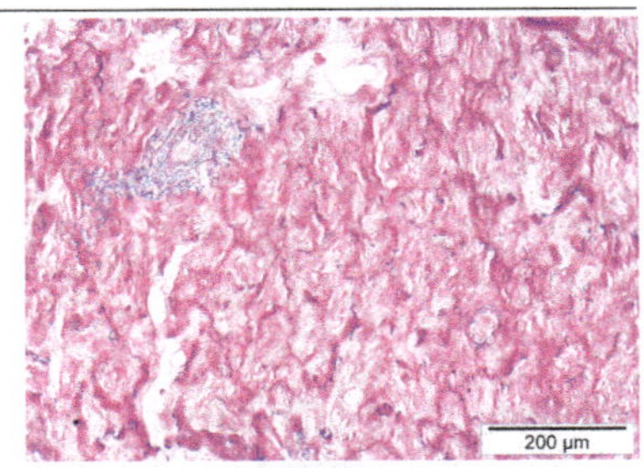
Horses	Equine multinodular pulmonary fibrosis	Associated with equine herpesvirus 5 infection Multifocal coalescing nodules within parenchyma, centered on alveoli	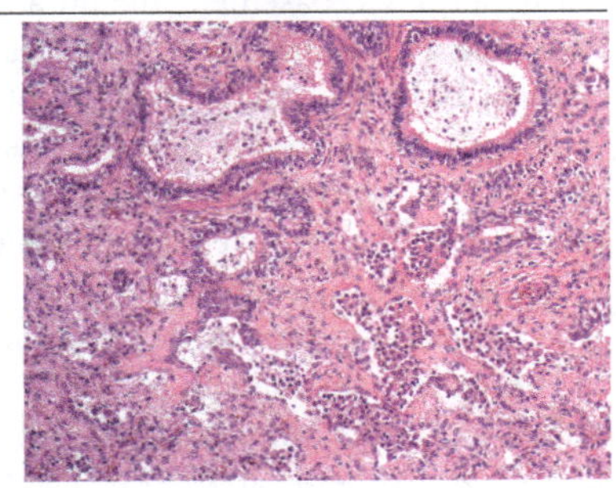
Cats	Idiopathic pulmonary fibrosis	Temporally heterogeneous fibrosis without inflammation Patchy remodeling leading to honeycomb lung in late disease	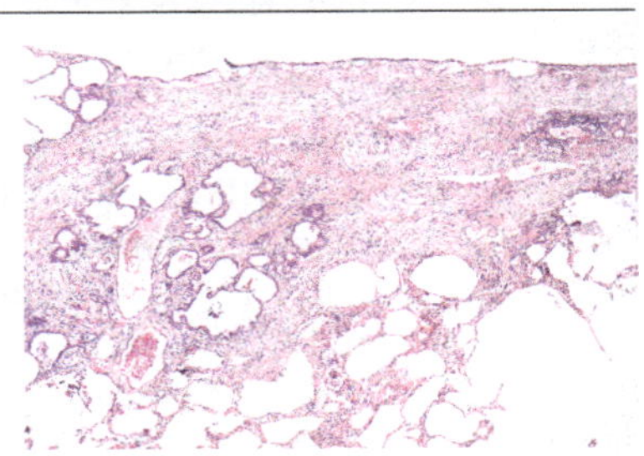

A variety of animal species exhibit pulmonary fibrosis conditions with characteristics similar to idiopathic pulmonary fibrosis (IPF) in humans. ILD has been studied as fibrosis occurs spontaneously in many animals, including West Highland Terriers, donkeys, cats, and horses. Mice have been used as experimental models with BLM-induced pulmonary fibrosis. Histologic images are provided at 10–20× magnification on Trichrome stain to display representative characteristics and similarities. Reproduced with permission, from Dr. Paul Mercer. Clin Sci (2015) 128:235–256, © The Biochemical Society (97).

TABLE 2 | Pros/cons of animal models for studying pulmonary fibrosis.

Murine models	Pros	Cons
Bleomycin	Early molecular signature most similar to accelerated acute phase of IPF in humans	Patchy, young mice resolve spontaneously unless repeatedly doses
Silica	Good model of lung injury in humans and persistence of fibrotic lesions	Lack of reproducibility, difficult delivery, prolonged time to fibrosis, absence of usual interstitial pneumonia (UIP)-like lesions
Asbestosis	Recapitulates asbestos exposure in human lung fibrosis	Inhalation model requires at least a month for fibrosis to develop. Single intratracheal dose leads to central fibrosis rather than subpleural, unevenly distributed between lungs
Cytokine overexpressing	Ability to dissect downstream signaling events relevant to specific fibrotic-inducing cytokines	Models limited to dissecting specific pathways, rather than recapitulating the complexity of human disease
Fluorescent isothiocyanate	Relatively reproducible and persistent fibrotic phenotypes	Lack representative UIP and inflammatory infiltrates preceding fibrosis
Radiation induced	Results in fibrosis, not pneumonitis if B6 mice are used	Need to wait a long time for development of fibrosis
Familial models	Gave insight on telomere and telomerase gene involvement in IPF	May produce a susceptible phenotype, requiring a second hit
Humanized (NOD/SCID mice)	Can afford insight into role of different fibroblast populations, dissects the contribution of epithelial-fibroblast crosstalk in the absence of immune cells	May not be representative of human disease where immune cells play a role. Expensive and requires specialized housing
Domestic animals	**Pros**	**Cons**
Dogs	Usually present in middle to old age. IPF in Westies shares some features of human disease; foci with severe lesions, histological criteria more typical for UIP may be present. Spontaneously develop ILD	The diffuse interstitial lesion, present in all affected Westies, histologically resembles fibrotic NSIP in man
Cats	Anatomy of distal lung similar to humans. UIP-like disease. Spontaneously develop ILD	Strain-dependent
Donkeys	Spontaneously develop ILD	Majority of cases of APF share key pathological features with human pleuroparenchymal fibroelastosis not IPF
Horses	Spontaneously develop ILD. Overlapping features of pulmonary fibrosis including weight loss and characteristic radiologic findings	Pathology not the same as IPF

of lymphocytosis). Hallmark features of UIP include epithelial cell hyperplasia, basement membrane denudation, honeycomb cysts, and accumulation of myofibroblasts foci in a pattern with regional and temporal heterogeneity (4).

Disease pathogenesis still remains elusive and controversial. Currently, the prevailing hypothesis assumes an ineffective wound healing response to alveolar epithelial cell injury (5, 6). Injury magnitude and susceptibility appears to be related to aging and genetic predisposition, with subsequent innate immune system and fibroblast activation (3, 5, 7). The overall prognosis of patients with IPF is highly unpredictable and poor with median survival after diagnosis being approximately 3.8 years (3, 8, 9). Attempts to understand disease pathogenesis, identify prognosticators, and unravel novel therapeutic targets (10–14) have relied on animal models. Unfortunately, no animal model fully recapitulates the histologic pattern of UIP or exhibits features of progressive disease. This, however, should not underestimate the fact that animal models are essential prerequisites for the subsequent application of prognostic tests and therapeutic interventions. Numerous clinical trials have been completed based on preclinical studies in animals and have led to the FDA approval of two drugs, pirfenidone and nintedanib (15, 16). Although these drugs slow disease progression, they do not cure IPF (5, 17), thus at the best case leaving patients with significant pulmonary disability. Therefore, further studies in animal models that more closely mimic human IPF are needed to investigate potentially curative therapies. Although it is recognized that the spontaneous development of lung fibrosis in domestic animals (cats, dogs, etc.) can be informative, the most indispensable models for studies of pathogenesis and preclinical therapeutic assessment involve rodents. Many traditional and newly developed experimental models have provided us with valuable insights into disease pathogenesis and helped us to identify novel therapeutic targets to assess and validate in clinical trials (18–20). For a tabular representation of these models, see **Table 1**. This review aims to summarize current state of knowledge on animal modeling of lung fibrosis, mainly focusing on rodents, including environmental and genetic models, highlight limitations, and suggest future potentials.

MURINE MODELS

Bleomycin (BLM)

The model of BLM-induced lung fibrosis represents the most commonly applied experimental model. BLM is a chemotherapeutic antibiotic that has been identified as a pro-fibrotic agent when lymphoma patients developed pulmonary fibrosis after intravenous administration of BLM. It has been used in multiple species including mice, rats, guinea pigs, hamsters, dogs, and primates; yet, mice are most common (21). A sheep model is also currently under development (22). A recent ATS workshop report confirmed that there is a consensus view of the intratracheal BLM model as "the best-characterized animal model available for preclinical testing" (23).

Mechanism of Action and Kinetics of Injury

It is believed that BLM acts by causing single and double-strand DNA breaks in tumor cells and thereby interrupting cell cycle leading to apoptosis. BLM hydrolase, a BLM-inactivating enzyme, majorly affects drug effects on a tissue-specific basis. The lungs maintain low levels of the enzyme, as compared to liver, and therefore are more susceptible to BLM-induced injury. An overproduction of reactive oxygen species, due to chelation of metal ions and reaction of the formed pseudoenzyme with oxygen, leads to epithelial cell death (days 1–3), excessive inflammatory infiltrates (days 3–9, neutrophils found in the BALF at day 3 and lymphocytes at day 6), and ultimately to fibroblasts activation, extracellular matrix deposition, and development of fibrosis (days 10–21 with a peak around day 14), at the molecular (24–26) and histologic (21, 24, 25, 27) levels. Relative to IPF, it has been shown that the early molecular signature in mice is most similar to the accelerated acute phase of IPF in humans (28). Measurements of alveolar septal thickening, intra-alveolar fibrosis, increases in alveolar macrophages, and dilation of bronchioles and alveolar ducts demonstrated a rather uniform fibrotic state in a large sample size (29). Nevertheless, BLM-induced lung fibrosis has been severely criticized for not being representative of IPF due to the rapidity of its development, inflammation preceding fibrosis, and self-resolution nature usually after 21–28 days following BLM challenge.

Strains, Gender, and Age

C57BL/6J mice have been the predominant animal model, as this particular strain is highly susceptible to lung injury following intratracheal BLM administration (30, 31). Conversely, the BALB/c or SV129 strains confer resistance to BLM-induced pulmonary fibrosis, presumably due to alterations in transforming growth factor (TGF)-β expression (31). This phenomenon parallels the experience in humans regarding genetic susceptibility and other potential risk factors for development of fibrosis in end organs following exposure to BLM. The majority of studies investigating BLM-induced pulmonary fibrosis to date have used young male mouse models, aged 8–12 weeks (28, 29, 32). Young mice, however, have been shown to undergo spontaneous resolution of BLM-induced pulmonary fibrosis, a phenomenon not observed in aged mice (24, 33, 34). Whether sex differences in mice parallel human IPF, which exhibits a tendency toward male predominance has not been fully determined. However, the use of aged male mice may provide a more clinically relevant model of IPF (33).

Route of Delivery and Dose Regimens

So far, BLM has been delivered by multiple methods including intratracheal, intraperitoneal, subcutaneous, intravenous, and inhalational. However, intratracheal is the most commonly route of administration (21, 24, 26, 28, 29, 32, 35–39). It is believed that intratracheal administration better recapitulates the human phenotype that is limited to the lungs. However, it requires a surgical incision at the level of the trachea, and thus, it is associated with considerable peri-operative mortality. To this end, investigators are now applying the orotracheal route of delivery that exhibits similar kinetics of injury as intratracheal administration with significantly less side effects.

Another issue identified in studies using the BLM mouse model is the wide range of dosing regimens used (40). In mouse studies, weight-based dosing is most common, beginning at 1.25 U/kg (39) and up to a maximum of 4 U/kg (35, 36). This dose is usually suspended in 50–100 μL of phosphate-buffered saline for intratracheal instillation. Peng et al. performed BLM dose-escalation experiments with mortality rates of 19% with 3 U/kg and 50% with 5 U/kg (28). A slightly lower dose of 2.0–2.5 U/kg appears to provide the most effective model of lung fibrosis, while reducing sample loss due to high mortality. With regard to frequency of dosing, Degryse and colleagues directly addressed the issue of single versus repetitive dosing to model IPF using BLM-induced pulmonary fibrosis (24). Results from their investigation in young mice found that repetitive dosing of BLM promoted persistent fibrosis, evidenced by measures of hydroxyproline content and inflammatory cell infiltrates, in contrast to single dose experiments that demonstrated spontaneous resolution in young mice (24, 34). Most studies evaluating therapeutic interventions have not used repetitive dosing; rather, the use of a single dose of intratracheal BLM is usually followed shortly by administration of the therapy under investigation (35–38). Potential therapies are usually administered within 1–7 days following BLM exposure, leading to the conclusion that the therapeutic measures may provide benefit primarily through prevention of the inflammatory cascade rather than reversal of fibrosis, thus limiting their applicability to human IPF (40). More recent studies have begun to explore administration of drugs after 7 days (41, 42). To our knowledge, only two studies to date have evaluated repetitive BLM injury (43, 44). Lee et al. administered intratracheal BLM (0.04 U) biweekly for a total of 4 months in young mice (43). They reported that in response to repeated BLM administration, mice developed hyperplasia of Club cells (Clara cells) and cuboidal alveolar epithelial cells, infiltration of the perialveolar ducts by inflammatory cells, septal thickening, enlarged alveoli, and extensive fibrosis (43).

Silica

Silica administration into murine lungs leads to the development of fibrotic nodules that resemble lesions that develop in humans following exposure to mineral fibers and particulate aerosols (45). Silica delivery presents with many variations including aerosolization, intratracheal, or orotracheal instillation (46–50). The fibrotic response is strain dependent with C57BL/6 mice found to be more susceptible than CBA/J mice after intratracheal delivery of silica fibers. Nodules develop around silica deposits and silica fibers are easily identified both by histology and polarization microscopy (47). The fibrotic response is associated with limited inflammation and enhanced fibrotic lesions mediated by increased production of pro-fibrotic growth factors and cytokines including PDGF, TGF-β, TNFa, and IL-10 (51–53). Kinetics of injury is highly heterogeneous and dependent upon route of administration, dose regimens, and formulations of silica particles (45). In particular, intratracheal models are easier, shorter (fibrosis develops within 14–28 days), and cost-efficient, while aerosolized route of delivery takes longer to produce fibrotic lesions (40–120 days) (45). Heating preparation procedures before instillation are mandatory in order to inactivate any trace endotoxin (45). The greatest advantage of the silica model of lung fibrosis is the persistence of fibrotic lesions due to diminished clearance of silica particles from the lungs (51, 52, 54). However, the model presents with major caveats including problematic and highly expensive equipment for aerosolized delivery, prolonged waiting periods until development of fibrosis (4–16 weeks), lack of reproducibility of fibrotic pattern, and absence of characteristic UIP-like lesions such as fibroblastic foci, regional heterogeneity, and hyperplastic epithelium. These have severely limited its widespread applicability in the preclinical setting (20).

Asbestosis

Another model that recapitulates an important form of human lung fibrosis is that of asbestos exposure. Asbestos-induced model of lung fibrosis is clearly distinguished from IPF by several histologic findings including asbestos bodies embedded within the fibrous tissue, fewer myofibroblasts foci and bronchial wall fibrosis. In some cases, the pattern of UIP can be also present (55, 56). Some of these features are recapitulated in inhalation models in animals and have helped us understand the pathogenesis of both asbestosis and IPF (57–61). A single intratracheal administration of asbestos fibers mediates development of fibrosis; however, the model presents with several caveats since fibrosis that tends to be central rather than subpleural and is quite often unevenly distributed between lungs. Inhalation models develop a more peripheral pattern; yet, disease development can be prolonged, especially if using chrysotile fibers. The intratracheal animal models with amphibole fibers follow the kinetics of BLM models, with fibrosis development at day 7 and peak at day 14. Inhalation models may take up to a month for establishment of fibrotic injuries. Mechanistically, the deposition of asbestos fibers triggers fibrosis through alveolar epithelial cell apoptosis, M2 polarization of macrophages, and overproduction of pro-fibrotic cytokines by activated T lymphocytes, all events leading to myofibroblast differentiation and extracellular matrix production (57–61).

Age-Related Models

IPF is an age-related disease paradigm, and more recently, it has been proposed that many of the hallmarks of aging including genomic instability, telomere attrition, epigenetic alterations, deregulated cellular bioenergetics, and cellular senescence, can be considered characteristics of the fibrotic lung (62–64). Studies have shown that older mice are more susceptible than younger mice to pro-fibrotic stimuli including BLM (26). This is of particular interest given that IPF is predominant in older individuals. Transgenic deletion of senescence-related genes including RAGE, and relaxin has been associated with spontaneous age-dependent development of lung fibrosis indicating the cardinal role of aging in disease susceptibility (65–67). On the other hand, the role of "virome" as a pro-fibrotic mediator has been further dissected in the context of aged-related development of lung fibrosis by demonstrating that only aged mice (>15 months) develop γ-herpesvirus-68-induced lung fibrosis through a mechanism that involved alveolar epithelial cell reprogramming to produce pro-fibrotic factors and enhanced TGF-β signaling in lung fibroblasts (68). In addition, Torres-Gonzalez et al. (69) reported that aging mice receiving gamma herpesvirus responded with endoplasmic reticulum stress, apoptosis of type II lung epithelial cells, and activation of profibrotic pathways.

This evidence could be reminiscent to the presence of herpes viral genomes within IPF lungs and the epidemiological association between viral infections and IPF acute exacerbations (70).

Cytokine Overexpression

During the past two decades, more sophisticated and advanced methods have been widely used to study the features of lung fibrosis on an experimental setting. Both gene transfer *via* adenoviral or lentiviral vectors and transgenic approaches have been used to overexpress pro-fibrotic cytokines including TGF-β, TNF-α, IL-1β, and IL-13 and promote fibrotic phenotypes by dissecting downstream signaling pathways that are highly relevant to human lung fibrosis (71–73). The overexpression of TGF-β can be produced via adenoviral intranasal delivery or doxycycline-induced transgenic overexpression in CC-10-positive lung epithelial cells. Both models are strain dependent with C57BL/6 mice being more susceptible that BALB/c. In the doxycycline-inducible Clara cell (CC10)-promoter driven model of TGF-β-induced lung fibrosis, addition of doxycycline to the water of animals leads to release of the tetracycline-controlled transcriptional suppressor allowing the reverse tetracycline transactivator to bind to the transgene (TGF-β) and promote its acute expression even 12 h after treatment with doxycycline (74). That leads to alveolar epithelial apoptosis and myofibroblast accumulation leading to airway and parenchymal fibrotic response starting at day 7 and peaking at days 14–21. Fibrosis may persist and progress over the duration of doxycycline exposure for up to 2 months (74). Similar kinetics are also observed with adenoviral delivery of TGF-β through the intranasal route leading to epithelial cell apoptosis (day 1), mononuclear cell infiltration (days 3–7), and fibrotic scarring that tends to be more persistent than those produced by BLM exposure and thus tend to mimic better human disease features (71). Nevertheless, both models quite often produce highly variable and heterogeneous kinetics of injury with regards to severity and extent of lesions and lack of major reproducibility. A similar concept has been also applied for adenoviral-mediated gene transfer of IL-1β (75) and TNF-α (76, 77) or lung-specific transgenic overexpression of IL-13 (78), thereby resulting in an early inflammatory response and later collagen deposition through activation of TGF-β signaling pathway. Nonetheless, these models are not well established and thus can only be used to dissect relevant pathogenic pathways and not on a general basis to recapitulate the complexity of human disease.

Other Models

Fluorescent isothiocyanate (FITC) is another chemical compound used to induce experimental lung fibrosis (79). Fluorescein acts as a hapten and binds to airway proteins, thus acting as a depot for prolonged exposure to the injurious stimulus leading to fibrotic responses within 2–4 weeks that persist up to 24 weeks (79, 80). The model produces relatively reproducible and persistent fibrotic phenotypes in both BALB/c and C57BL/6 mice. Disadvantages include absence of representative UIP findings and predominant inflammatory infiltrates that precede fibrosis (80). The model is mostly dependent on Th2 cytokines (IL-13) and was seminally discovered to explore the relationship between the chemokine signaling receptor 2 (CCR2) and its ligand CCL12 for recruitment of fibrocytes during progression of fibrosis (81). It offers the advantage of easily trackable fluorescence-labeled fibrotic tissues. Nevertheless, model robustness is largely dependent on technical issues that are highly variable including the batch of FITC and the size of the particles formulated through sonication (20). Smaller particle sizes due to prolonged sonication may lead to acute toxicity and death (20). Finally and most important, FITC is an artificial chemical compound with limited human relevance since this type of injurious stimulus has never been described in humans (20).

Radiation-induced fibrosis represents a human relevant injury that leads to development of fibrosis which is strain dependent (C57BL/6 are the most susceptible) and can be local or systemic if other organs are not shielded (82–87). It is a relatively slow procedure that results in mature fibrosis after 24 weeks; yet, fibrosis is majorly dependent on inflammation and free-radical-mediated DNA damage and less on TGF-β (84).

Familial models of IPF have been also used to study the contribution of the disease genetic background that significantly altered our perspective regarding disease pathogenesis and treatment response. Mice with targeted deletion of shelterin, a six-protein complex that binds and preserves telomeric repeats, from type alveolar epithelial cells, have been shown to develop spontaneous fibrosis (88, 89).

Mutations in the telomere and telomerase genes have been associated with familial IPF (90). Telomere dysfunction results in alveolar epithelial stem cell senescence, which is sufficient to drive lung remodeling and recruit inflammation. Telomerase reverse transcriptase has been reported to be transiently increased in BLM, hypoxic, or silica-induced lung injury (91–93). On the other hand, telomerase-deficient mice, despite significant telomere shortening, did not present with enhanced BLM-induced fibrotic responses (94).

Although mutations resulting in SP-C deficiencies are linked to a small subset of spontaneous and familial cases of interstitial lung disease (ILD) and interstitial pulmonary fibrosis (95, 96), SP-C-deficient mice do not fully recapitulate familial interstitial pulmonary fibrosis (97) as they develop mild ILD and an emphysematous phenotype. It is more than evident that these mutations may generate a susceptible phenotype; yet, a second hit of environmental origin is needful to partially recapitulate human phenotype.

Finally, humanized models of lung fibrosis involving the intravenous instillation of human IPF lung fibroblasts into immunodeficient non-obese diabetic mice (NOD/SCID) have recently garnered much attention (98–100). This model allows for cell trafficking during different stages of fibrosis development and progression, offers unique insights into different fibroblast populations that reflect IPF heterogeneity, and dissects the contribution of epithelial–fibroblast crosstalk into the disease pathogenesis considering the absence of immune cells (99). Nevertheless, the latter is not representative of human disease where immune cells appear to play cardinal role. Another major disadvantage that limits its widespread applicability is the high cost and the specialized housing that is required (101). The use of animals with humanized immune system may also provide unique insights and fully recapitulate features of IPF (101).

DOMESTIC ANIMALS

The field of comparative oncology has set the stage for collaborations that utilize spontaneous models of progressive fibrotic lung diseases of mutual interest to veterinary and human medicine. The results of these kinds of studies promise to enhance the understanding of common factors important to disease development in a variety of species and to refine treatments for both humans and animals. Moreover, they may provide insights into unanswered questions involving naturally occurring models of pulmonary fibrosis.

In contrast to the six million dogs and cats that develop cancers, the incidence and prevalence of pulmonary fibrosis in animals is not known (102). West Highland Terriers (Westies), cats, donkeys, and horses develop ILD (102–107). There is limited information on the spectrum of clinical parameters (e.g., radiology) and pathology of these lung diseases leading to the classification of "idiopathic pulmonary fibrosis" being applied to such cases, without using the same strict clinical criteria that have been developed for human IPF. Recent evidence suggests that in contrast to IPF in humans, applying the term "idiopathic" in animals may be premature because of more non-specific features in lung interstitial disease in animals. The American Thoracic Society/European Respiratory Society definition of IPF incorporates histology, radiographic, and clinical course in the definition and the exclusion of other known causes of ILD, including environmental exposures, connective tissue disease, and drug toxicity (108). Further studies using multidisciplinary classification of veterinary lung disease to better characterize the disease in animals will help to define their relation to human disease and their potential role as models to develop treatments for both human and veterinary medical practice.

A study on Westies (109) found that the majority of dogs with IPF showed multifocal areas of accentuated subpleural and peribronchiolar fibrosis with occasional "honeycombing" and profound alveolar epithelial changes, reminiscent of human UIP and not commonly seen in NSIP. Interstitial fibroblastic foci, characteristic of UIP, were not seen in WHWTs with IPF. Progressive fibrosis, with intra-alveolar organizing fibrosis alongside interstitial mature collagen deposition, was present within the more severely affected areas of lung in WHWTs with IPF. Severe pulmonary lesions were seen more commonly in the caudal than in the cranial lung lobes.

A more recent study correlating CT scans and course of disease in Westies found a generalized ground-glass pattern was determined to be a sign of a mild form of canine idiopathic pulmonary fibrosis, whereas mosaic ground-glass and mild honeycombing patterns was identified in moderate and severe forms of the disease (110).

The ubiquitous gammaherpesvirus equine herpesvirus 5 (EHV 5) has been detected in lung tissue from horses that develop progressive pulmonary fibrosis and is now considered to be the likely cause of this disease in these animals (111). The pathology of this disease is distinct from human IPF, demonstrating multiple nodules and is therefore termed equine multinodular pulmonary fibrosis (111). Although the pathology is not the same as IPF, there are striking overlapping features including weight loss and gradual exercise intolerance, accompanied by characteristic radiologic features (111). Temporal heterogeneity or fibroblast foci, hallmarks of human disease, are not present in the disease in horses, though these characteristics have been described in feline pulmonary fibrosis (111, 112). Similar to EBV in humans, which has been associated with IPF, EHV 5 is a ubiquitous subclinical gammaherpesviral infection in horses (113). Considered largely non-pathogenic in the natural host, some strains of EHV5 appear to be pathogenic and capable of inducing lung fibrosis (103). While EHV5 was isolated from horses with spontaneous disease, the virus was not isolated from dead inoculated horses that developed lung fibrosis (111). This model raises interesting questions regarding induction of lung fibrosis by EHV 5 during viral latency versus lytic infection.

For a tabular representation of the overall advantages and disadvantages of each model, see **Table 2**.

Read-Out Assays for Assessment of Fibrotic Injury

Each experimental model presents with its own kinetics of fibrotic injury; however, investigators have applied standard operating procedures for reproducible evaluations of lung fibrosis. In view of the pathologic hallmarks of IPF, appropriate read-out assays include assessment of collagen deposition, alveolar epithelial cell apoptosis, and BALF complemented by survival analysis and respiratory mechanics. These are achieved with the following modalities: (1) histological analysis with Masson trichrome and H&E staining coupled with Aschroft score that quantifies extent of fibrotic changes, (2) hydroxyproline or total collagen content for quantification of lung collagen deposition, (3) TUNEL assay for the identification of apoptotic cells, (4) BALF analysis to assess changes in differential cell count and levels of inflammatory and fibrotic markers, (5) survival analysis with Kaplan–Meier plots, (6) *in vivo* lung function measurements (elastance and compliance) using the Flexi-vent ventilator, and (7) micro-CT imaging which provides state-of-the art multidimensional imaging of the injured lung that is reminiscent of HRCT applied for IPF diagnosis (19).

Limitations

The past 35 years more than 500 experimental studies have been performed describing therapeutic efficacy of novel compounds in the BLM model. Unfortunately, less than 5% have applied a therapeutic protocol indicated by drug administration at >7 days following BLM challenge (18, 114). Even day 7 in most of the experimental models represents a stage of inflammation or early fibrosis, evidence that comes in contrast to the clinical situation in which treatment is initiated after onset of symptoms and when fibrosis has already been established. Intriguingly, pirfenidone and nintedanib received approval to proceed to clinical trials based on preventive protocols or even therapeutic protocols targeting the inflammatory or the early-fibrotic phase of the BLM model (115–117). In addition, most of the therapeutic compounds have been preclinically tested in young animals while it has been clearly shown that aged mice are more susceptible to fibrotic injury (26), which is in accordance with patients with IPF. Importantly, preclinical efficacy of the majority of anti-fibrotic agents was tested in a single model, majorly the BLM-induced model, and based on histologic end points, such as collagen deposition that are not clinically relevant, at least to the extent of lung function tests or survival analysis. Moreover, many of the therapeutic outcomes were subject to evaluation bias considering that most of the preclinical studies were not blinded and the investigator was aware of the animals' treatment. Reproducibility issues arising from different experimental settings between different labs could also account for discrepancies in treatment effects and lack of generalizable results. Finally, it is worth mentioning that animal size needs to be balanced with the statistical power needed to generate robust data and that insufficient reporting of experimental animal data or unpublished negative therapeutic results severely hamper the validity of experimental studies.

Conclusion and Personal View

An animal model is a simple representation of a complex biology system. Critics focusing on the reasons why an animal model cannot fully reproduce human disease are not helpful and do not elicit a solution. The role of an animal model is to recapitulate specific aspects of a disease. Consequently, animal models should be carefully selected, designed, and conducted in order to bridge translational gaps between bench and bedside. Currently, the BLM model of lung fibrosis represents the cheapest, easiest, fastest, most reproducible, and thus most extensively used animal model of IPF; advantages that overcome the handicap of minimal representation of human disease. So far, it has provided us with invaluable insights into IPF pathogenesis, prognosis, and treatment. We recommend the use of the male aged BLM mouse model as the first-line animal model to test safety and efficacy of a therapeutic compound administered during the stage of established fibrosis. Nevertheless, efficacy preclinical studies should be enriched with two or even three animal models including clinically relevant end points such as lung function mechanics, survival analysis as well as biomarkers (28). Collaboration between veterinary and human clinical researchers must be encouraged in order to establish and solidify a common language, and common diagnostic criteria and nomenclature, thus strengthening the opportunity for advancements toward a cure for lung fibrosis in both animal and humans. Humanization of animal models, spontaneous fibroses animals and application of high-throughput "omics" tools may help us improve the clinical translation in the near future.

AUTHOR CONTRIBUTIONS

Conception and study oversight: MG, AL, VA, and AT. Drafting manuscript: JT, GR, KW, SJ, and IN. Critical revision of manuscript: MG, AL, VA, and AT. Final approval: all authors.

ACKNOWLEDGMENTS

The authors acknowledge the Lester and Sue Smith Foundation, Coalition for Pulmonary Fibrosis, and the Pulmonary Fibrosis Foundation for their support. The authors also acknowledge Amy Miele, BVM&S MRCVS (University of Edinburgh) for her contributions in providing veterinary histopathology images used in the construction of **Table 1**. AT is a recipient of a Marie Curie/Sklodowska ERS/RESPIRE 2 fellowship (8860-2015). All authors have no financial affiliations or conflicts of interest to disclose.

REFERENCES

1. Raghu G, Rochwerg B, Zhang Y, Garcia CA, Azuma A, Behr J, et al. An official ATS/ERS/JRS/ALAT clinical practice guideline: treatment of idiopathic pulmonary fibrosis. An update of the 2011 clinical practice guideline. *Am J Respir Crit Care Med* (2015) 192(2):e3–19. doi:10.1164/rccm.201506-1063ST
2. Travis WD, Costabel U, Hansell DM, King TE Jr, Lynch DA, Nicholson AG, et al. An official American Thoracic Society/European Respiratory Society statement: update of the international multidisciplinary classification of the idiopathic interstitial pneumonias. *Am J Respir Crit Care Med* (2013) 188(6):733–48. doi:10.1164/rccm.201308-1483ST
3. Ryu JH, Moua T, Daniels CE, Hartman TE, Yi ES, Utz JP, et al. Idiopathic pulmonary fibrosis: evolving concepts. *Mayo Clin Proc* (2014) 89(8):1130–42. doi:10.1016/j.mayocp.2014.03.016
4. Blackwell TS, Tager AM, Borok Z, Moore BB, Schwartz DA, Anstrom KJ, et al. Future directions in idiopathic pulmonary fibrosis research: an NHLBI workshop report. *Am J Respir Crit Care Med* (2014) 189(2):214–22. doi:10.1164/rccm.201306-1141WS
5. Ahluwalia N, Shea BS, Tager AM. New therapeutic targets in idiopathic pulmonary fibrosis. Aiming to rein in runaway wound-healing responses. *Am J Respir Crit Care Med* (2014) 190(8):867–78. doi:10.1164/rccm.201403-0509PP
6. Chilosi M, Carloni A, Rossi A, Poletti V. Premature lung aging and cellular senescence in the pathogenesis of idiopathic pulmonary fibrosis and COPD/emphysema. *Transl Res* (2013) 162(3):156–73. doi:10.1016/j.trsl.2013.06.004
7. Tzouvelekis A, Kaminski N. Epigenetics in idiopathic pulmonary fibrosis. *Biochem Cell Biol* (2015) 93(2):159–70. doi:10.1139/bcb-2014-0126
8. Jones MG, Fletcher S, Richeldi L. Idiopathic pulmonary fibrosis: recent trials and current drug therapy. *Respiration* (2013) 86(5):353–63. doi:10.1159/000356958
9. Raghu G, Chen SY, Yeh WS, Maroni B, Li Q, Lee YC, et al. Idiopathic pulmonary fibrosis in US Medicare beneficiaries aged 65 years and older: incidence, prevalence, and survival, 2001-11. *Lancet Respir Med* (2014) 2(7):566–72. doi:10.1016/S2213-2600(14)70101-8
10. Spagnolo P, Tzouvelekis A, Maher TM. Personalized medicine in idiopathic pulmonary fibrosis: facts and promises. *Curr Opin Pulm Med* (2015) 21(5):470–8. doi:10.1097/MCP.0000000000000187
11. Tzouvelekis A, Bonella F, Spagnolo P. Update on therapeutic management of idiopathic pulmonary fibrosis. *Ther Clin Risk Manag* (2015) 11:359–70. doi:10.2147/TCRM.S69716
12. Tzouvelekis A, Herazo-Maya J, Sakamoto K, Bouros D. Biomarkers in the evaluation and management of idiopathic pulmonary fibrosis. *Curr Top Med Chem* (2016) 16(14):1587–98. doi:10.2174/1568026616666150930120959
13. Tzouvelekis A, Tzilas V, Papiris S, Aidinis V, Bouros D. Diagnostic and prognostic challenges in Idiopathic Pulmonary Fibrosis: a patient's "Q and A" approach. *Pulm Pharmacol Ther* (2017) 42:21–24. doi:10.1016/j.pupt.2016.12.002
14. Tzouvelekis A, Yu G, Lino Cardenas C, Herazo-Maya JD, Wang R, Woolard T, et al. SH2 domain-containing phosphatase-2 is a novel antifibrotic regulator in pulmonary fibrosis. *Am J Respir Crit Care Med* (2017) 195(4):500–514. doi:10.1164/rccm.201602-0329OC
15. King TE Jr, Bradford WZ, Castro-Bernardini S, Fagan EA, Glaspole I, Glassberg MK, et al. A phase 3 trial of pirfenidone in patients with idiopathic pulmonary fibrosis. *N Engl J Med* (2014) 370(22):2083–92. doi:10.1056/NEJMoa1402582
16. Richeldi L, du Bois RM, Raghu G, Azuma A, Brown KK, Costabel U, et al. Efficacy and safety of nintedanib in idiopathic pulmonary fibrosis. *N Engl J Med* (2014) 370(22):2071–82. doi:10.1056/NEJMoa1402584
17. Bouros D, Tzouvelekis A. Idiopathic pulmonary fibrosis: on the move. *Lancet Respir Med* (2014) 2(1):17–9. doi:10.1016/S2213-2600(13)70240-6
18. Moeller A, Ask K, Warburton D, Gauldie J, Kolb M. The bleomycin animal model: a useful tool to investigate treatment options for idiopathic pulmonary fibrosis? *Int J Biochem Cell Biol* (2008) 40(3):362–82. doi:10.1016/j.biocel.2007.08.011
19. Mouratis MA, Aidinis V. Modeling pulmonary fibrosis with bleomycin. *Curr Opin Pulm Med* (2011) 17(5):355–61. doi:10.1097/MCP.0b013e328349ac2b
20. Moore BB, Lawson WE, Oury TD, Sisson TH, Raghavendran K, Hogaboam CM. Animal models of fibrotic lung disease. *Am J Respir Cell Mol Biol* (2013) 49(2):167–79. doi:10.1165/rcmb.2013-0094TR
21. Moore BB, Hogaboam CM. Murine models of pulmonary fibrosis. *Am J Physiol Lung Cell Mol Physiol* (2008) 294(2):L152–60. doi:10.1152/ajplung.00313.2007
22. Organ L, Bacci B, Koumoundouros E, Barcham G, Kimpton W, Nowell CJ, et al. A novel segmental challenge model for bleomycin-induced pulmonary fibrosis in sheep. *Exp Lung Res* (2015) 41(3):115–34. doi:10.3109/01902148.2014.985806
23. Jenkins RG, Moore BB, Chambers RC, Eickelberg O, Konigshoff M, Kolb M, et al. An official American Thoracic Society workshop report: use of animal models for the preclinical assessment of potential therapies for pulmonary fibrosis. *Am J Respir Cell Mol Biol* (2017) 56(5):667–79. doi:10.1165/rcmb.2017-0096ST
24. Degryse AL, Tanjore H, Xu XC, Polosukhin VV, Jones BR, McMahon FB, et al. Repetitive intratracheal bleomycin models several features of idiopathic pulmonary fibrosis. *Am J Physiol Lung Cell Mol Physiol* (2010) 299(4):L442–52. doi:10.1152/ajplung.00026.2010
25. Cai Y, Zhu L, Zhang F, Niu G, Lee S, Kimura S, et al. Noninvasive monitoring of pulmonary fibrosis by targeting matrix metalloproteinases (MMPs). *Mol Pharm* (2013) 10(6):2237–47. doi:10.1021/mp300613x
26. Sueblinvong V, Neujahr DC, Mills ST, Roser-Page S, Ritzenthaler JD, Guidot D, et al. Predisposition for disrepair in the aged lung. *Am J Med Sci* (2012) 344(1):41–51. doi:10.1097/MAJ.0b013e318234c132
27. Naik PK, Moore BB. Viral infection and aging as cofactors for the development of pulmonary fibrosis. *Expert Rev Respir Med* (2010) 4(6):759–71. doi:10.1586/ers.10.73
28. Peng R, Sridhar S, Tyagi G, Phillips JE, Garrido R, Harris P, et al. Bleomycin induces molecular changes directly relevant to idiopathic pulmonary fibrosis: a model for "active" disease. *PLoS One* (2013) 8(4):e59348. doi:10.1371/journal.pone.0059348
29. Izbicki G, Segel MJ, Christensen TG, Conner MW, Breuer R. Time course of bleomycin-induced lung fibrosis. *Int J Exp Pathol* (2002) 83(3):111–9. doi:10.1046/j.1365-2613.2002.00220.x
30. Stefanov AN, Fox J, Depault F, Haston CK. Positional cloning reveals strain-dependent expression of Trim16 to alter susceptibility to bleomycin-induced pulmonary fibrosis in mice. *PLoS Genet* (2013) 9(1):e1003203. doi:10.1371/journal.pgen.1003203
31. Hoyt DG, Lazo JS. Alterations in pulmonary mRNA encoding procollagens, fibronectin and transforming growth factor-beta precede bleomycin-induced pulmonary fibrosis in mice. *J Pharmacol Exp Ther* (1988) 246(2):765–71.
32. Aguilar S, Scotton CJ, McNulty K, Nye E, Stamp G, Laurent G, et al. Bone marrow stem cells expressing keratinocyte growth factor via an inducible lentivirus protects against bleomycin-induced pulmonary fibrosis. *PLoS One* (2009) 4(11):e8013. doi:10.1371/journal.pone.0008013
33. Redente EF, Jacobsen KM, Solomon JJ, Lara AR, Faubel S, Keith RC, et al. Age and sex dimorphisms contribute to the severity of bleomycin-induced lung injury and fibrosis. *Am J Physiol Lung Cell Mol Physiol* (2011) 301(4):L510–8. doi:10.1152/ajplung.00122.2011
34. Chung MP, Monick MM, Hamzeh NY, Butler NS, Powers LS, Hunninghake GW. Role of repeated lung injury and genetic background in bleomycin-induced fibrosis. *Am J Respir Cell Mol Biol* (2003) 29(3 Pt 1):375–80. doi:10.1165/rcmb.2003-0029OC

35. Ortiz LA, Gambelli F, McBride C, Gaupp D, Baddoo M, Kaminski N, et al. Mesenchymal stem cell engraftment in lung is enhanced in response to bleomycin exposure and ameliorates its fibrotic effects. *Proc Natl Acad Sci U S A* (2003) 100(14):8407–11. doi:10.1073/pnas.1432929100
36. Rojas M, Xu J, Woods CR, Mora AL, Spears W, Roman J, et al. Bone marrow-derived mesenchymal stem cells in repair of the injured lung. *Am J Respir Cell Mol Biol* (2005) 33(2):145–52. doi:10.1165/rcmb.2004-0330OC
37. Ortiz LA, Dutreil M, Fattman C, Pandey AC, Torres G, Go K, et al. Interleukin 1 receptor antagonist mediates the antiinflammatory and antifibrotic effect of mesenchymal stem cells during lung injury. *Proc Natl Acad Sci U S A* (2007) 104(26):11002–7. doi:10.1073/pnas.0704421104
38. Foskett AM, Bazhanov N, Ti X, Tiblow A, Bartosh TJ, Prockop DJ. Phase-directed therapy: TSG-6 targeted to early inflammation improves bleomycin-injured lungs. *Am J Physiol Lung Cell Mol Physiol* (2014) 306(2):L120–31. doi:10.1152/ajplung.00240.2013
39. Hecker L, Logsdon NJ, Kurundkar D, Kurundkar A, Bernard K, Hock T, et al. Reversal of persistent fibrosis in aging by targeting Nox4-Nrf2 redox imbalance. *Sci Transl Med* (2014) 6(231):231ra47. doi:10.1126/scitranslmed.3008182
40. Srour N, Thebaud B. Mesenchymal stromal cells in animal bleomycin pulmonary fibrosis models: a systematic review. *Stem Cells Transl Med* (2015) 4(12):1500–10. doi:10.5966/sctm.2015-0121
41. Cross J, Stenton GR, Harwig C, Szabo C, Genovese T, Di Paola R, et al. AQX-1125, a small molecule SHIP1 activator, inhibits bleomycin-induced pulmonary fibrosis. *Br J Pharmacol* (2017). doi:10.1111/bph.13934
42. Tanaka KI, Niino T, Ishihara T, Takafuji A, Takayama T, Kanda Y, et al. Protective and therapeutic effect of felodipine against bleomycin-induced pulmonary fibrosis in mice. *Sci Rep* (2017) 7(1):3439. doi:10.1038/s41598-017-03676-y
43. Lee SH, Lee EJ, Lee SY, Kim JH, Shim JJ, Shin C, et al. The effect of adipose stem cell therapy on pulmonary fibrosis induced by repetitive intratracheal bleomycin in mice. *Exp Lung Res* (2014) 40(3):117–25. doi:10.3109/01902148.2014.881930
44. Moodley Y, Vaghjiani V, Chan J, Baltic S, Ryan M, Tchongue J, et al. Anti-inflammatory effects of adult stem cells in sustained lung injury: a comparative study. *PLoS One* (2013) 8(8):e69299. doi:10.1371/journal.pone.0069299
45. Davis GS, Leslie KO, Hemenway DR. Silicosis in mice: effects of dose, time, and genetic strain. *J Environ Pathol Toxicol Oncol* (1998) 17(2):81–97.
46. Davis GS, Pfeiffer LM, Hemenway DR. Interferon-gamma production by specific lung lymphocyte phenotypes in silicosis in mice. *Am J Respir Cell Mol Biol* (2000) 22(4):491–501. doi:10.1165/ajrcmb.22.4.3599
47. Antonini JM, Hemenway DR, Davis GS. Quantitative image analysis of lung connective tissue in murine silicosis. *Exp Lung Res* (2000) 26(2):71–88. doi:10.1080/019021400269880
48. Davis GS, Pfeiffer LM, Hemenway DR. Expansion of interferon-gamma-producing lung lymphocytes in mouse silicosis. *Am J Respir Cell Mol Biol* (1999) 20(4):813–24. doi:10.1165/ajrcmb.20.4.3407
49. Davis GS, Pfeiffer LM, Hemenway DR. Persistent overexpression of interleukin-1beta and tumor necrosis factor-alpha in murine silicosis. *J Environ Pathol Toxicol Oncol* (1998) 17(2):99–114.
50. Lakatos HF, Burgess HA, Thatcher TH, Redonnet MR, Hernady E, Williams JP, et al. Oropharyngeal aspiration of a silica suspension produces a superior model of silicosis in the mouse when compared to intratracheal instillation. *Exp Lung Res* (2006) 32(5):181–99. doi:10.1080/01902140600817465
51. Barbarin V, Arras M, Misson P, Delos M, McGarry B, Phan SH, et al. Characterization of the effect of interleukin-10 on silica-induced lung fibrosis in mice. *Am J Respir Cell Mol Biol* (2004) 31(1):78–85. doi:10.1165/rcmb.2003-0299OC
52. Barbarin V, Xing Z, Delos M, Lison D, Huaux F. Pulmonary overexpression of IL-10 augments lung fibrosis and Th2 responses induced by silica particles. *Am J Physiol Lung Cell Mol Physiol* (2005) 288(5):L841–8. doi:10.1152/ajplung.00329.2004
53. Davis GS, Holmes CE, Pfeiffer LM, Hemenway DR. Lymphocytes, lymphokines, and silicosis. *J Environ Pathol Toxicol Oncol* (2001) 20(Suppl 1):53–65. doi:10.1615/JEnvironPatholToxicolOncol.v20.iSuppl.1.50
54. Misson P, van den Brule S, Barbarin V, Lison D, Huaux F. Markers of macrophage differentiation in experimental silicosis. *J Leukoc Biol* (2004) 76(5):926–32. doi:10.1189/jlb.0104019
55. Baur X, Woitowitz HJ, Budnik LT, Egilman D, Oliver C, Frank A, et al. Asbestos, asbestosis, and cancer: the Helsinki criteria for diagnosis and attribution. Critical need for revision of the 2014 update. *Am J Ind Med* (2017) 60(5):411–21. doi:10.1002/ajim.22709
56. Roggli V, Gibbs AR, Attanoos R, Churg A, Popper H, Corrin B, et al. Pathology of asbestosis: an update of the diagnostic criteria response to a critique. *Arch Pathol Lab Med* (2016) 140(9):950–2. doi:10.5858/arpa.2015-0503-SA
57. Kim SJ, Cheresh P, Jablonski RP, Williams DB, Kamp DW. The role of mitochondrial DNA in mediating alveolar epithelial cell apoptosis and pulmonary fibrosis. *Int J Mol Sci* (2015) 16(9):21486–519. doi:10.3390/ijms160921486
58. Cyphert JM, Padilla-Carlin DJ, Schladweiler MC, Shannahan JH, Nyska A, Kodavanti UP, et al. Long-term response of rats to single intratracheal exposure of Libby amphibole or amosite. *J Toxicol Environ Health A* (2012) 75(3):183–200. doi:10.1080/15287394.2012.641203
59. Rasmussen DL, Pfau JC. Asbestos activates CH12.LX B-lymphocytes via macrophage signaling. *J Immunotoxicol* (2012) 9(2):129–40. doi:10.3109/1547691X.2011.631953
60. Padilla-Carlin DJ, Schladweiler MC, Shannahan JH, Kodavanti UP, Nyska A, Burgoon LD, et al. Pulmonary inflammatory and fibrotic responses in Fischer 344 rats after intratracheal instillation exposure to Libby amphibole. *J Toxicol Environ Health A* (2011) 74(17):1111–32. doi:10.1080/15287394.2011.586940
61. Li J, Poovey HG, Rodriguez JF, Brody A, Hoyle GW. Effect of platelet-derived growth factor on the development and persistence of asbestos-induced fibroproliferative lung disease. *J Environ Pathol Toxicol Oncol* (2004) 23(4):253–66. doi:10.1615/JEnvPathToxOncol.v23.i4.20
62. Selman M, Buendia-Roldan I, Pardo A. Aging and pulmonary fibrosis. *Rev Invest Clin* (2016) 68(2):75–83.
63. Meiners S, Eickelberg O, Konigshoff M. Hallmarks of the ageing lung. *Eur Respir J* (2015) 45(3):807–27. doi:10.1183/09031936.00186914
64. Thannickal VJ, Murthy M, Balch WE, Chandel NS, Meiners S, Eickelberg O, et al. Blue journal conference. Aging and susceptibility to lung disease. *Am J Respir Crit Care Med* (2015) 191(3):261–9. doi:10.1164/rccm.201410-1876PP
65. Englert JM, Hanford LE, Kaminski N, Tobolewski JM, Tan RJ, Fattman CL, et al. A role for the receptor for advanced glycation end products in idiopathic pulmonary fibrosis. *Am J Pathol* (2008) 172(3):583–91. doi:10.2353/ajpath.2008.070569
66. Samuel CS, Zhao C, Bond CP, Hewitson TD, Amento EP, Summers RJ. Relaxin-1-deficient mice develop an age-related progression of renal fibrosis. *Kidney Int* (2004) 65(6):2054–64. doi:10.1111/j.1523-1755.2004.00628.x
67. Samuel CS, Zhao C, Bathgate RA, Bond CP, Burton MD, Parry LJ, et al. Relaxin deficiency in mice is associated with an age-related progression of pulmonary fibrosis. *FASEB J* (2003) 17(1):121–3. doi:10.1096/fj.02-0449fje
68. Naik PN, Horowitz JC, Moore TA, Wilke CA, Toews GB, Moore BB. Pulmonary fibrosis induced by gamma-herpesvirus in aged mice is associated with increased fibroblast responsiveness to transforming growth factor-beta. *J Gerontol A Biol Sci Med Sci* (2012) 67(7):714–25. doi:10.1093/gerona/glr211
69. Torres-Gonzalez E, Bueno M, Tanaka A, Krug LT, Cheng DS, Polosukhin VV, et al. Role of endoplasmic reticulum stress in age-related susceptibility to lung fibrosis. *Am J Respir Cell Mol Biol* (2012) 46(6):748–56. doi:10.1165/rcmb.2011-0224OC
70. Egan JJ, Adamali HI, Lok SS, Stewart JP, Woodcock AA. Ganciclovir antiviral therapy in advanced idiopathic pulmonary fibrosis: an open pilot study. *Pulm Med* (2011) 2011:240805. doi:10.1155/2011/240805
71. Sime PJ, Xing Z, Graham FL, Csaky KG, Gauldie J. Adenovector-mediated gene transfer of active transforming growth factor-beta1 induces prolonged severe fibrosis in rat lung. *J Clin Invest* (1997) 100(4):768–76. doi:10.1172/JCI119590
72. Lee CG, Kang HR, Homer RJ, Chupp G, Elias JA. Transgenic modeling of transforming growth factor-beta(1): role of apoptosis in fibrosis and alveolar remodeling. *Proc Am Thorac Soc* (2006) 3(5):418–23. doi:10.1513/pats.200602-017AW

73. Vicencio AG, Lee CG, Cho SJ, Eickelberg O, Chuu Y, Haddad GG, et al. Conditional overexpression of bioactive transforming growth factor-beta1 in neonatal mouse lung: a new model for bronchopulmonary dysplasia? *Am J Respir Cell Mol Biol* (2004) 31(6):650–6. doi:10.1165/rcmb.2004-0092OC
74. Lee CG, Cho SJ, Kang MJ, Chapoval SP, Lee PJ, Noble PW, et al. Early growth response gene 1-mediated apoptosis is essential for transforming growth factor beta1-induced pulmonary fibrosis. *J Exp Med* (2004) 200(3):377–89. doi:10.1084/jem.20040104
75. Kolb M, Margetts PJ, Anthony DC, Pitossi F, Gauldie J. Transient expression of IL-1beta induces acute lung injury and chronic repair leading to pulmonary fibrosis. *J Clin Invest* (2001) 107(12):1529–36. doi:10.1172/JCI12568
76. Sime PJ, Marr RA, Gauldie D, Xing Z, Hewlett BR, Graham FL, et al. Transfer of tumor necrosis factor-alpha to rat lung induces severe pulmonary inflammation and patchy interstitial fibrogenesis with induction of transforming growth factor-beta1 and myofibroblasts. *Am J Pathol* (1998) 153(3):825–32. doi:10.1016/S0002-9440(10)65624-6
77. Xing Z, Tremblay GM, Sime PJ, Gauldie J. Overexpression of granulocyte-macrophage colony-stimulating factor induces pulmonary granulation tissue formation and fibrosis by induction of transforming growth factor-beta 1 and myofibroblast accumulation. *Am J Pathol* (1997) 150(1): 59–66.
78. Lee CG, Homer RJ, Zhu Z, Lanone S, Wang X, Koteliansky V, et al. Interleukin-13 induces tissue fibrosis by selectively stimulating and activating transforming growth factor beta(1). *J Exp Med* (2001) 194(6):809–21. doi:10.1084/jem.194.6.809
79. Roberts SN, Howie SE, Wallace WA, Brown DM, Lamb D, Ramage EA, et al. A novel model for human interstitial lung disease: hapten-driven lung fibrosis in rodents. *J Pathol* (1995) 176(3):309–18. doi:10.1002/path.1711760313
80. Christensen PJ, Goodman RE, Pastoriza L, Moore B, Toews GB. Induction of lung fibrosis in the mouse by intratracheal instillation of fluorescein isothiocyanate is not T-cell-dependent. *Am J Pathol* (1999) 155(5):1773–9. doi:10.1016/S0002-9440(10)65493-4
81. Moore BB, Paine R III, Christensen PJ, Moore TA, Sitterding S, Ngan R, et al. Protection from pulmonary fibrosis in the absence of CCR2 signaling. *J Immunol* (2001) 167(8):4368–77. doi:10.4049/jimmunol.167.8.4368
82. Karvonen RL, Fernandez-Madrid F, Maughan RL, Palmer KC, Fernandez-Madrid I. An animal model of pulmonary radiation fibrosis with biochemical, physiologic, immunologic, and morphologic observations. *Radiat Res* (1987) 111(1):68–80. doi:10.2307/3577022
83. Paun A, Haston CK. Genomic and genome-wide association of susceptibility to radiation-induced fibrotic lung disease in mice. *Radiother Oncol* (2012) 105(3):350–7. doi:10.1016/j.radonc.2012.08.004
84. Haston CK. Mouse genetic approaches applied to the normal tissue radiation response. *Front Oncol* (2012) 2:94. doi:10.3389/fonc.2012.00094
85. Paun A, Fox J, Balloy V, Chignard M, Qureshi ST, Haston CK. Combined Tlr2 and Tlr4 deficiency increases radiation-induced pulmonary fibrosis in mice. *Int J Radiat Oncol Biol Phys* (2010) 77(4):1198–205. doi:10.1016/j.ijrobp.2009.12.065
86. Haston CK, Travis EL. Murine susceptibility to radiation-induced pulmonary fibrosis is influenced by a genetic factor implicated in susceptibility to bleomycin-induced pulmonary fibrosis. *Cancer Res* (1997) 57(23): 5286–91.
87. Haston CK, Amos CI, King TM, Travis EL. Inheritance of susceptibility to bleomycin-induced pulmonary fibrosis in the mouse. *Cancer Res* (1996) 56(11):2596–601.
88. Naikawadi RP, Disayabutr S, Mallavia B, Donne ML, Green G, La JL, et al. Telomere dysfunction in alveolar epithelial cells causes lung remodeling and fibrosis. *JCI Insight* (2016) 1(14):e86704. doi:10.1172/jci.insight.86704
89. Povedano JM, Martinez P, Flores JM, Mulero F, Blasco MA. Mice with pulmonary fibrosis driven by telomere dysfunction. *Cell Rep* (2015) 12(2):286–99. doi:10.1016/j.celrep.2015.06.028
90. Armanios M. Telomerase and idiopathic pulmonary fibrosis. *Mutat Res* (2012) 730(1–2):52–8. doi:10.1016/j.mrfmmm.2011.10.013
91. Driscoll B, Buckley S, Bui KC, Anderson KD, Warburton D. Telomerase in alveolar epithelial development and repair. *Am J Physiol Lung Cell Mol Physiol* (2000) 279(6):L1191–8.
92. Kim JK, Lim Y, Kim KA, Seo MS, Kim JD, Lee KH, et al. Activation of telomerase by silica in rat lung. *Toxicol Lett* (2000) 111(3):263–70. doi:10.1016/S0378-4274(99)00195-2
93. Liu T, Chung MJ, Ullenbruch M, Yu H, Jin H, Hu B, et al. Telomerase activity is required for bleomycin-induced pulmonary fibrosis in mice. *J Clin Invest* (2007) 117(12):3800–9. doi:10.1172/JCI32369
94. Degryse AL, Xu XC, Newman JL, Mitchell DB, Tanjore H, Polosukhin VV, et al. Telomerase deficiency does not alter bleomycin-induced fibrosis in mice. *Exp Lung Res* (2012) 38(3):124–34. doi:10.3109/01902148.2012.658148
95. Nogee LM, Dunbar AE III, Wert S, Askin F, Hamvas A, Whitsett JA. Mutations in the surfactant protein C gene associated with interstitial lung disease. *Chest* (2002) 121(3 Suppl):20S–1S. doi:10.1378/chest.121.3_suppl.20S
96. Nogee LM, Dunbar AE III, Wert SE, Askin F, Hamvas A, Whitsett JA. A mutation in the surfactant protein C gene associated with familial interstitial lung disease. *N Engl J Med* (2001) 344(8):573–9. doi:10.1056/NEJM200102223440805
97. Glasser SW, Detmer EA, Ikegami M, Na CL, Stahlman MT, Whitsett JA. Pneumonitis and emphysema in sp-C gene targeted mice. *J Biol Chem* (2003) 278(16):14291–8. doi:10.1074/jbc.M210909200
98. Pierce EM, Carpenter K, Jakubzick C, Kunkel SL, Flaherty KR, Martinez FJ, et al. Therapeutic targeting of CC ligand 21 or CC chemokine receptor 7 abrogates pulmonary fibrosis induced by the adoptive transfer of human pulmonary fibroblasts to immunodeficient mice. *Am J Pathol* (2007) 170(4):1152–64. doi:10.2353/ajpath.2007.060649
99. Trujillo G, Meneghin A, Flaherty KR, Sholl LM, Myers JL, Kazerooni EA, et al. TLR9 differentiates rapidly from slowly progressing forms of idiopathic pulmonary fibrosis. *Sci Transl Med* (2010) 2(57):57ra82. doi:10.1126/scitranslmed.3001510
100. Fujii H, Luo ZJ, Kim HJ, Newbigging S, Gassas A, Keating A, et al. Humanized chronic graft-versus-host disease in NOD-SCID il2rgamma-/- (NSG) mice with G-CSF-mobilized peripheral blood mononuclear cells following cyclophosphamide and total body irradiation. *PLoS One* (2015) 10(7):e0133216. doi:10.1371/journal.pone.0133216
101. Shultz LD, Ishikawa F, Greiner DL. Humanized mice in translational biomedical research. *Nat Rev Immunol* (2007) 7(2):118–30. doi:10.1038/nri2017
102. Roman J, Brown KK, Olson A, Corcoran BM, Williams KJ; ATS Comparative Biology of Lung Fibrosis Working Group. An official American thoracic society workshop report: comparative pathobiology of fibrosing lung disorders in humans and domestic animals. *Ann Am Thorac Soc* (2013) 10(6):S224–9. doi:10.1513/AnnalsATS.201309-321ST
103. Williams KJ, Maes R, Del Piero F, Lim A, Wise A, Bolin DC, et al. Equine multinodular pulmonary fibrosis: a newly recognized herpesvirus-associated fibrotic lung disease. *Vet Pathol* (2007) 44(6):849–62. doi:10.1354/vp.44-6-849
104. Norris AJ, Naydan DK, Wilson DW. Interstitial lung disease in West Highland White Terriers. *Vet Pathol* (2005) 42(1):35–41. doi:10.1354/vp.42-1-35
105. Miele A, Dhaliwal K, Du Toit N, Murchison JT, Dhaliwal C, Brooks H, et al. Chronic pleuropulmonary fibrosis and elastosis of aged donkeys: similarities to human pleuroparenchymal fibroelastosis. *Chest* (2014) 145(6):1325–32. doi:10.1378/chest.13-1306
106. Wong DM, Belgrave RL, Williams KJ, Del Piero F, Alcott CJ, Bolin SR, et al. Multinodular pulmonary fibrosis in five horses. *J Am Vet Med Assoc* (2008) 232(6):898–905. doi:10.2460/javma.232.6.898
107. Mercer PF, Abbott-Banner K, Adcock IM, Knowles RG. Translational models of lung disease. *Clin Sci* (2015) 128(4):235–56. doi:10.1042/CS20140373
108. Raghu G, Collard HR, Egan JJ, Martinez FJ, Behr J, Brown KK, et al. An official ATS/ERS/JRS/ALAT statement: idiopathic pulmonary fibrosis: evidence-based guidelines for diagnosis and management. *Am J Respir Crit Care Med* (2011) 183(6):788–824. doi:10.1164/rccm.2009-040GL
109. Syrjä P, Heikkilä HP, Lilja-Maula L, Krafft E, Clercx C, Day MJ, et al. The histopathology of idiopathic pulmonary fibrosis in West Highland White Terriers shares features of both non-specific interstitial pneumonia and usual interstitial pneumonia in man. *J Comp Pathol* (2013) 149(2):303–13. doi:10.1016/j.jcpa.2013.03.006
110. Thierry F, Handel I, Hammond G, King LG, Corcoran BM, Schwarz T. Further characterization of computed tomographic and clinical features for staging and prognosis of idiopathic pulmonary fibrosis in West Highland

White Terriers. *Vet Radiol Ultrasound* (2017) 58(4):381–8. doi:10.1111/vru.12491

111. Williams KJ, Robinson NE, Lim A, Brandenberger C, Maes R, Behan A, et al. Experimental induction of pulmonary fibrosis in horses with the gammaherpesvirus equine herpesvirus 5. *PLoS One* (2013) 8(10):e77754. doi:10.1371/journal.pone.0077754
112. Williams K, Malarkey D, Cohn L, Patrick D, Dye J, Toews G. Identification of spontaneous feline idiopathic pulmonary fibrosis: morphology and ultrastructural evidence for a type II pneumocyte defect. *Chest* (2004) 125(6):2278–88. doi:10.1378/chest.125.6.2278
113. Back H, Ullman K, Leijon M, Soderlund R, Penell J, Stahl K, et al. Genetic variation and dynamics of infections of equid herpesvirus 5 in individual horses. *J Gen Virol* (2016) 97(1):169–78. doi:10.1099/jgv.0.000332
114. Antoniu SA, Kolb MR. Update on models of pulmonary fibrosis therapy for preclinical drug research. *Expert Opin Drug Discov* (2009) 4(9):939–46. doi:10.1517/17460440903186100
115. Schaefer CJ, Ruhrmund DW, Pan L, Seiwert SD, Kossen K. Antifibrotic activities of pirfenidone in animal models. *Eur Respir Rev* (2011) 20(120):85–97. doi:10.1183/09059180.00001111
116. Huang J, Beyer C, Palumbo-Zerr K, Zhang Y, Ramming A, Distler A, et al. Nintedanib inhibits fibroblast activation and ameliorates fibrosis in preclinical models of systemic sclerosis. *Ann Rheum Dis* (2016) 75(5):883–90. doi:10.1136/annrheumdis-2014-207109
117. Wollin L, Maillet I, Quesniaux V, Holweg A, Ryffel B. Antifibrotic and anti-inflammatory activity of the tyrosine kinase inhibitor nintedanib in experimental models of lung fibrosis. *J Pharmacol Exp Ther* (2014) 349(2):209–20. doi:10.1124/jpet.113.208223

5

Roles of Macrophage Polarization and Macrophage-Derived miRNAs in Pulmonary Fibrosis

Amit Kishore[1,2*] *and Martin Petrek*[1,3,4*]

[1] *Department of Pathological Physiology, Faculty of Medicine and Dentistry, Palacky University, Olomouc, Czechia,* [2] *Accuscript Consultancy, Ludhiana, India,* [3] *Institute of Molecular and Translational Medicine, Faculty of Medicine and Dentistry, Palacky University, Olomouc, Czechia,* [4] *Departments of Experimental Medicine, and Immunology, University Hospital Olomouc, Olomouc, Czechia*

Correspondence:
Amit Kishore
amitkishore.bio@gmail.com
Martin Petrek
martin.petrek2@fnol.cz

This mini-review summarizes the current evidence for the role of macrophage activation and polarization in inflammation and immune response pertinent to interstitial lung disease, specifically pulmonary fibrosis. In the fibrosing lung, the production and function of inflammatory and fibrogenic mediators involved in the disease development have been reported to be regulated by the effects of polarized M1/M2 macrophage populations. The M1 and M2 macrophage phenotypes were suggested to correspond with the pro-inflammatory and pro-fibrogenic signatures, respectively. These responses towards tissue injury followed by the development and progression of lung fibrosis are further regulated by macrophage-derived microRNAs (miRNAs). Besides cellular miRNAs, extracellular exosomal-miRNAs derived from M2 macrophages have also been proposed to promote the progression of pulmonary fibrosis. In a future perspective, harnessing the noncoding miRNAs with a key role in the macrophage polarization is, therefore, suggested as a promising therapeutic strategy for this debilitating disease.

Keywords: macrophage plasticity, M1/M2 polarization, MicroRNAs, exosomes, pulmonary fibrosis

INTRODUCTION

Pulmonary fibrosis (PF) is a progressive, irreversible and lethal lung disease and has remained a challenge for clinicians and researchers. The tissue injury accompanied by cellular inflammation in the lungs drives fibrotic response and thus, plays a crucial role in the pathogenesis of fibrosis. Inflammatory cells release TGF-β, the key regulator of several profibrotic cytokines/chemokines, their receptors/subunits, and growth factors inducing epithelial-mesenchymal transition (EMT) (1–3). The pro-inflammatory and profibrotic cytokines involved in PF promote inflammation and irreversible damage to lung architecture with the loss of alveolar-capillary barrier basal membrane leading to persistent fibrosis (4). These pathogenic factors for PF have further been reported as associated with genetic factors including gene variants and non-coding regulatory microRNAs (3–7).

The tissue-resident macrophages (M0) are versatile cells that exhibit a high degree of plasticity represented by classically activated M1 (pro-inflammatory) or alternatively activated M2 (anti-inflammatory/pro-fibrotic) macrophages (8). The macrophage polarization is extremely variable and switching of one "activation-type" to another, stimulated by appropriate factors or tissue microenvironment, is a rapid and reversible process. The cross-talk between macrophages and the microenvironment regulates tissue regeneration, flagged with key surface markers in both pro-regenerative and profibrotic environments (9).

Thus, besides the development of tissue homeostasis, these cells are suggested with sequential roles in both induction and resolution of inflammation. The M0 macrophages can polarize to M1 or M2 (M2a, M2b, M2c, and M2d) in response to different activators, such as LPS/IFNγ and IL4/IL13, respectively (10). The M1 macrophage phenotype can also be stimulated without the presence of lymphocytes, for example, by inflammatory cytokines and microorganism-derived molecules (10–13). The anti-inflammatory or immune-compromised state associated with the M2 macrophage phenotype is also supported with suppressed multiple interferon-associated pathways as one of the most prominent signals common among all M2-polarizing stimuli (14). The M1 macrophage can readily repolarize to M2a (stimulated with reduced IL10 and TNFα, and increased Ym1 level) and M2b (increased IL10 and reduced TNFα) subpopulations (13). Similarly, macrophage M2b can convert to other M2 subtypes in response to different stimuli (15). The different approaches to macrophage polarization have been associated with both the demerits and benefits influencing their utility for specific tissues. Where possible, future therapeutic approaches are suggested to consider tailoring of strategy towards the formation of a specific tissue-microenvironment, as well as promotion of specific disease-associated cell subsets, to improve efficacy and minimize off-target effect (11).

In deciphering pathomechanisms of lung fibrosis, pulmonary macrophages have been implicated with a key role in the fibrogenic process. The PF has been proposed to be regulated by macrophage plasticity (M1/M2 polarization) with an immunogenic signature network of chemokines such as MCP-1, MIP-1α, CCL18, and cytokines such as TNFα, TGFβ1, and their respective signaling pathways (16–18). The pro-inflammatory M1 macrophage polarization with overexpression of iNOS, TNFα, IL1, IL6, IL12, IL23, MCP-1, and IFNγ is associated with inflammation, antitumoral functions and graft rejection (**Table 1**). The anti-inflammatory M2 macrophage polarization, characterised by overexpression of signature proteins such as TGFβ1, IL10, Arginase1, CD204, CD206, VEGF, Ym1, PDGF, MMPs, and IL4Ralpha, was associated with immune regulation, matrix deposition, tissue remodelling, protumoral functions, and graft acceptance (17, 19). The antitumoral and protumoral role of M1 and M2 macrophages, respectively, are further supported with longer survival outcomes among patients with a high M1/M2 ratio in cancers such as ovarian (20, 21) and breast (22) cancer.

ROLE OF LUNG MACROPHAGE POLARIZATION IN PULMONARY FIBROSIS

Macrophages are innate immune cells with antimicrobial phagocytic activity and also play a key role in the pathogenesis of fibrotic disease of pulmonary interstitium. Macrophages are involved at all stages of lung injury and repair, and can promote as well as inhibit fibrosis (16, 23). Airway lumen-based Alveolar macrophages (AM) with surface markers $CD11b^{low}$ $CD11c^{++}$

TABLE 1 | Macrophage subtypes, its activators and implication of cytokines and chemokines in functional response that is also regulated by microRNAs-mediated macrophage plasticity.

M1 and M2 subtypes	Polarization activators	Cytokines and chemokines	Functional response	MicroRNAs expression and its role in M1/M2 macrophage polarization
M1	LPS, IFNγ, TNFα and GM-CSF	Cytokines: TNFα, IL1β, IL6, IL8/CXCL8, IL12, IL23 Chemokines: CCL2, CCL3, CCL4, CCL5, CCL8, CCL9, CCL10, CCL11, CXCL1	Th1 response to infection; produces pro-inflammatory molecules, including TNFα and IL1, IL6, IL12, IL23	↑: miR-21 (M1⊣; M2→), -33 (M1→; M2⊣), -34a (M1→; M2⊣), -101 (M1→; M2⊣), -125b-5p (M1→; M2⊣), -146b (M1⊣), -155 (M1→; M2⊣), -342-5p (M1→) ↓: miR-125b-5p (M1⊣), let-7e (M1⊣)
M2a	IL4, IL13	Cytokines: IL10, TGFβ, IL1Rα Chemokines: CCL17, CCL22, CCL24	Th2 cells, eosinophils, basophils, and macrophages produce IL4. Facilitation of parasite encapsulation	↑: miR-124 (M1⊣; M2→), -125a-5p (M1→), -135b (M2↑), -146a (M1⊣; M2→), let-7c (M1⊣; M2→), -511-3p (M2→), -378-3p (M2→), -223 (M1⊣; M2→), ↓: miR-140 (M2→)
M2b	Immune complexes plus TLR or IL1R ligands	Cytokines: TNF, IL1β, IL6, IL10 Chemokines: CCL1	Immunoregulation with up-regulated IL10 and antigen presentation (MHC II, CD86), and down-regulated IL12	
M2c	IL10, TGFβ1 and glucocorticoids	Cytokines: IL10, TGFβ	Tissue remodelling and extracellular matrix production	
M2d	IL6 and adenosine	–	Tumour-associated immune regulation	

TNF-α, Tumour necrosis factor-α; IFN-γ, Interferon-γ, LPS, lipopolysaccharide; GM-CSF, granulocyte-macrophage colony stimulation factor; IL, interleukin; miR, microRNA.
Symbols for MicroRNA expression level: ↑, up-regulation; ↓, down-regulation.
Symbols for M1/M2 macrophage polarization: →, progression; ⊣, inhibition.

CD169$^+$, and lung parenchymal interstitial macrophages (IM) with CD11b$^+$ CD11c^{lo} CD169$^-$ are the two major distinct macrophage populations contributing to lung homeostasis (24). During the development processes of tissue injury and inflammatory reaction and their subsequent progression to PF, AM and IM are polarized to different cell phenotypes - M1 and M2 macrophages, respectively (16, 25). During tissue damage and the early inflammatory phase, activation of M1 macrophages clears the pathogenic microorganisms and promotes inflammation through extracellular matrix degrading matrix metalloproteases (MMPs) and pro-inflammatory cytokines. The active cytokine milieu, including elevated Th1 cytokines, IL2, IFNγ, and TNFα, is believed to drive the classical pro-inflammatory (M1) macrophage activation, while a proportion of anti-inflammatory M2 macrophages tends to be higher in other types of interstitial lung diseases (ILDs), including idiopathic pulmonary fibrosis (IPF) (26).

The enhanced M2 macrophage polarization has been suggested to inhibit the inflammatory reaction and/or directly regulate the development and progression of fibrotic lung diseases through the production of chemokines, MMPs, tissue inhibitor of metalloproteinases (TIMPs), and fibronectin as well as, the capability of M2 to differentiate into fibrocyte-like cells that express collagen (27–30). Among ILDs, an increased proportion of M2 macrophages has been observed in granulomas of patients with sarcoidosis as compared with tuberculous granulomas (31). It still needs to be established if a higher proportion of M2 macrophages identifies a profibrotic mechanism inherent to the pathogenesis of sarcoidosis rather than as a part of a generalized wound-healing mechanism to lung inflammation and injury (30, 31). Further, activated macrophages secrete cytokines that attract and stimulate proliferation, promote survival and migration of fibroblast mediated by platelet-derived growth factor (PDGF) (32). In a recent study, inhibition of M2 macrophage polarization has been shown to inhibit bleomycin-induced IPF in rats (33). Similarly, Wang et al. reported that treatment with microcystin-leucine arginine ameliorates PF through suppressed CD206$^+$ M2-like macrophage polarization by blocking EMT and fibroblast-myofibroblast transition (FMT), and also substantial reduction of TGFβ1/Smad signaling in rat pulmonary tissues (34). Thus, pro-fibrotic processes such as EMT, FMT, and TGFβ1/Smad signaling represent potential targets in mitigating the development and/or progression of PF (**Figure 1**). Supporting the profibrotic role of M2, a recent study showed attenuation of M2 macrophage infiltration in the lung to significantly protect mice against bleomycin-induced lung injury and fibrosis through suppression of Sart1 by small interfering RNA-loaded liposomes (35).

The macrophage-based pathways implicated in PF majorly include signaling pathways such as TGFβ/Smad (36–39), Wnt/beta-catenin (37, 40–42) and interleukin signaling (43–45). Other signaling pathways reported in a limited number of studies include Lrp5/beta-Catenin (46), MAPK (23), Notch (47), PI3K-AKT-mTOR (48, 49), STAT1 and NF-kappaB (50), IGF-1 receptor (51), 4-1BB (52), NRG-1/ErbB4 (53) and M-CSF/M-CSFR (54). Deciphering the molecular mechanisms of macrophage involved in the development of PF, M2 macrophage was shown to promote EMT through the TGFβ1/Smad2 pathway in bleomycin-induced PF mouse model (39). The PF has been alleviated by pirfenidone through suppressed Wnt/GSK-3beta/beta-catenin and TGFβ1/Smad2/3 signaling pathways (37), and by neohesperidin through TGFβ1/Smad3 inhibition (36); whereas, multiwall carbon nanotubes has been reported to mediate macrophage activation and PF progression through induced TGF-beta/Smad signaling pathway (38).

Macrophage M2 promotes myofibroblast differentiation and is associated with pulmonary fibrogenesis. This process is mitigated by suppressed Wnt/beta-catenin signaling through pirfenidone (37), salinomycin administration (40), and targeted inhibition by PRI-724 (41) and ICG-001 (42). The IL signaling is implicated in PF by IL-4–mediated M2 polarization with elevated Gab 1/2 docking proteins (43), by IL-4Ralpha pathway through crystalline silica exposure (45), or by IL-13 pathway in macrophages induced through sphingosine-1-phosphate receptor-2 (44). Also, activation of p38 MAPK signaling pathway mediated through loss of a transcription factor Forkhead box M1 (FOXM1) in macrophages was shown to promote PF. Regarding its molecular substance, activation of p38 MAPK pathway in macrophages was reported with the production of pro-fibrotic mediators IL1β, IL6, and TNFα that stimulated fibroblast activation and survival, thus, exacerbating PF (23). Thus, the interplay between M1/M2 macrophage phenotypes has been suggested to play a key role in the development and progression of lung fibrosis (**Figure 1**).

MICRORNA-BASED REGULATION OF MACROPHAGE POLARIZATION IN IMMUNE RESPONSE, INFLAMMATION, AND FIBROSIS

miRNAs and Their Regulatory Role Towards Macrophage Phenotypes

MicroRNAs (miRNAs) are transcriptional regulators that participate in lung inflammatory responses (5, 55) and are also shown to mediate macrophage polarization. The macrophage subtypes release a various spectrum of cytokines and chemokines that are either pro-inflammatory (M1 phenotypes) and sometimes pro-inflammatory with enhanced tissue destruction, or wound healing and tissue repair (M2 phenotypes), both of which are also regulated through miRNAs (**Table 1**). As an example, miRNA-regulated macrophage polarization is strongly related to miRNA-124, miRNA-155, and miRNA-223. Briefly, higher expression of miRNA-124 attenuates M1 macrophage, whereas miRNA-155 promotes M1 and miRNA-223 depletion also produces M1 polarization (56) (**Supplementary Table S1**). The **Supplementary Table S1** lists a wide spectrum of miRNAs involved in macrophage polarization along with their target proteins and their plausible roles in regulating lung fibrosis.

The regulatory roles of microRNA-mediated macrophage activation and polarization in immune response and inflammation have been extensively reviewed (57–59).

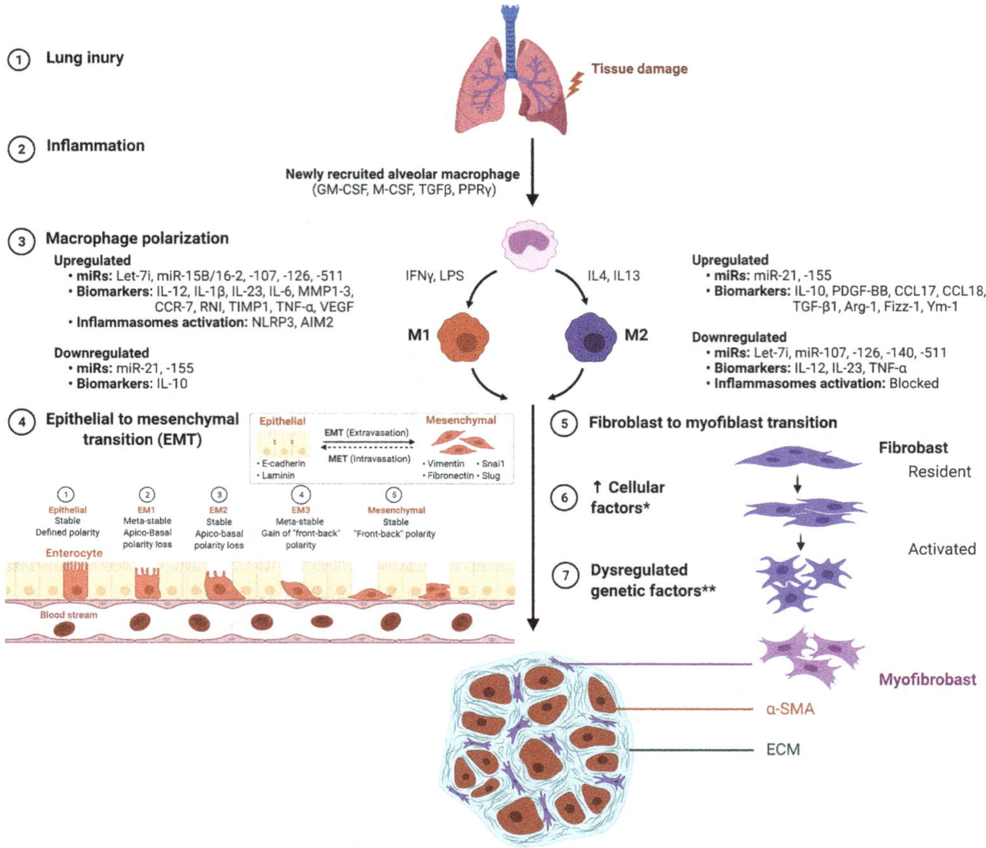

FIGURE 1 | M1 macrophage and M2 macrophage polarization during the development of pulmonary fibrosis. *Increased cellular factors include proliferation, α-smooth muscle actin (α-SMA), matrix factors, collagen, growth factors and cytokines. **Dysregulated genetic factors include upregulated miR-21 and miR-155 and down-regulated Let-7i, miR-107, mir-126, miR-140 and miR-511. Figure created with BioRender. *AIM2*, absent in melanoma 2; *ARG1*, Arginase 1; *Fizz1/RETNLB*, resistin like beta; *Ym1/Chil3*, chitinase-like 3.

This and the following section, therefore, updates the findings of miRNA-mediated macrophage polarization and modulation of pro-inflammatory M1 and/or pro-fibrotic M2 phenotypes in lung disease, in particular, lung fibrosis.

MicroRNA-17, miR-20a, and miR-106a (miR-17/20a/106a) have been shown to effectively regulate alveolar macrophage inflammatory responses such as macrophage infiltration, phagocytosis, and proinflammatory cytokine secretion through targeting leukocyte signal-regulatory protein-α (SIRPα) in both *in-vitro* and *in-vivo* assays (60). The up-regulation of miR-33 in alveolar macrophages exhibited the M1 phenotype with elevated pro-inflammatory cytokines and was demonstrated to promote granuloma formation in a murine model of chronic granulomatous disease, resembling human sarcoidosis pathology, through the suppression of anti-inflammatory lipid transporters (61). An over-expression of macrophage miR-34a has been demonstrated to favour pro-inflammatory M1 phenotype and inhibition of M2 polarization in lipopolysaccharides (LPS) induced acute lung injury (ALI) in mice (62). Similarly, miR-155 was shown to be induced during the macrophage inflammatory response and it orchestrated inflammatory cytokine production in tumour-associated macrophages (TAM). The pro-inflammatory effect of miR-155 has been indicated to promote fibrosis mediated by cross-signaling between macrophages and fibroblasts that governed upregulation of collagen synthesis through TGFβ1 signaling (63). Jaiswal et al., (64) reported overexpression of Let-7c and miR-99a miRNAs in murine bone marrow-derived macrophages (BMDMs) to mitigate Angiotensin-II-induced M1 phenotype activation and to promote M2 phenotype. This inhibition of miR-99a was further shown to reduce ovalbumin-induced Th2 dominance and alleviate allergic airways inflammation (64).

There have also been reports of miR-124 acting to attenuate M1 macrophages as a universal regulator of macrophage into the M2 subtype by decreasing NFκB activity in various subsets of monocytic cells and tissue-resident macrophages including lung macrophages (65, 66). The dysregulation of miR-142-5p and miR-130a-3p was characterised as an important factor governing the polarization of macrophages with higher levels of M2-like phenotypic markers and was associated with airway remodelling in ovalbumin-sensitized mice (67). Another miRNA, miR-146a has been reported to modulate macrophage polarization by inhibiting Notch pathways in RAQ264.7 macrophage cell lines (68). In this context, we observed an elevated level of miR-146a in pulmonary sarcoidosis inflammation (69). Concerning miRNAs involvement in TAM polarization miR-146a-5p, miR-324-5p, miR-223-3p, miR-223-5p, miR-21, miR-125a, miR-130a, and miR-155a were characterized as oncogenic miRNA, while, miR-1207 and miR-320a as a tumour suppressor miRNA in lung cancer including non-small-cell lung carcinoma (NSCLC) (70). These reports thus emphasize the important role of miRNAs in regulating M1/M2 macrophage polarization in lung diseases in general.

Potential Role of Macrophage-Derived microRNAs in Pulmonary Fibrosis

The microRNA crosstalk influences epithelial-to-mesenchymal and fibroblast-to-myofibroblast transitions implicated in process of macrophage polarization. However, to date, only limited studies have explored the miRNA-based genetic regulation of macrophage polarization and its role in lung fibrosis. An overexpression of let-7c was reported in alveolar macrophages from fibrotic lungs in a bleomycin-induced mouse model as compared with normal lungs, and thus, indicated upregulation of let-7c in macrophages to mitigate M1 phenotype while promoting M2 phenotype polarization (71). Duru et al., (72) reviewed the miRNA-based regulation of macrophage polarization with M2 predominant population in radiation-induced lung fibrosis (RILF) and characterized miR-21 and miR-155 as pro-fibrotic, while let-7i, miR-107, mir-126, miR-140, and miR-511 as anti-fibrotic (72). The IL4 and IL13 induced increased expression of miR-142-5p and downregulated miR-130a-3p transcripts were reported to regulate macrophage profibrogenic expression in tissue samples of patients with IPF (73). The macrophage miR-155 was reported to promote lipopolysaccharide-induced ALI in mice and rats (74). Similarly, miR-155$^{-/-}$ in murine lung macrophages and fibroblasts, and in human IPF lung fibroblasts was implicated in exacerbated pathogenic PF (75). In another study, miR-140 was reported with a key protective role against RILF by inhibiting myofibroblast differentiation and inflammation, and its loss was suggested to induce lung fibrosis through reprogramming fibroblasts and M2 macrophages (76). The role of non-coding RNAs in modulating macrophage phenotypic plasticity and functional heterogeneity among different fibrotic diseases has been recently reviewed (77). These reports further highlight the plausible role of macrophage-derived microRNAs in PF.

Macrophage-Derived Exosomal miRNAs Mediate Pulmonary Fibrosis

Exosomes are cell-derived vesicles produced by several cell types that function in signaling between cells. Exosomes carry a variety of different biomolecules, such as cytokines and microRNAs, and their content may vary from progenitor or target cells. Exosomal miRNAs have also been implicated in interstitial lung diseases including pulmonary sarcoidosis (55) and IPF (78). Recently, interest has also been gained to decipher the role of macrophage-derived exosomal microRNA (miRNA) in lung fibrosis. Exosomal miRNA-328 from M2 macrophages was shown to enhance pulmonary interstitial fibroblast proliferation and promote the progression of PF in a rat model (78). Besides, macrophage-derived exosomes have been recently suggested to mitigate PF progression *via* delivery of antifibrotic miR-142-3p to alveolar epithelial cells and lung fibroblasts by repressing transforming growth factor β receptor 1 (TGFβ-R1) (79). Another study demonstrated that miRNAs contained in alveolar epithelial type-I cells derived-EVs are actively delivered into alveolar macrophages, subsequently promoting inflammasome activation, neutrophil recruitment, and M1-macrophage polarization and thus endorse pro-inflammatory responses in bacterial lung infection (80). In ALI, young mesenchymal stem cells-derived extracellular vesicles (MSC-EVs) showed higher expression of miR-223-5p and lower levels of miR-127-3p and miR-125b-5p compared with aging MSC-EVs. Further, inhibition of miR-127-3p and miR-125b-5p in BMDMs was reported to downregulate M1 and thus, supported their role in M1 macrophage polarization (81). Besides, MSC-EVs were reported to mitigate ALI at least partially through the transfer of miR-27a-3p to alveolar macrophages and promoted M2 macrophage polarization (34). MiR-27a-3p was also shown to target NFKB1 and thus, was suggested as a key regulator of M2 macrophage polarization (34). Recently, a study investigated the potential connections between arsenic and epigenetic changes that mediate M2 macrophage polarization in the development of PF and reported arsenite, elevated LncRNA H19, c-Myc, and Arg1 along with decreased let-7a to be associated with PF in mice (82). Another recent study in a mouse model reported MSC –derived exosomal miR–135b to promote M2 polarization of synovial macrophage by targeting MAPK6, thus mitigating cartilage injury (83). Thus, evidence supports the role of M2 macrophage-derived exosomal miRNA in pulmonary interstitial fibroblast proliferation and in promoting the progression of lung fibrosis. This is further supported by MSC–EVs-derived miRNAs that are suggested to mediate M2 macrophage polarization in the development of PF (34). In ALI, young and aging MSC-EVs harbours differentially expressed miRNAs associated with M1/M2 macrophage polarization (81).

CONCLUSION

The present minireview summarizes major findings on the role of macrophage polarization in diseases, in particular, PF. The non-coding regulatory miRNAs are also discussed in the context of their modulation of M1/M2 macrophage phenotypes in the development and progression of IPF. Further, exosomal miRNA from M2 macrophages favouring pulmonary interstitial fibroblast proliferation and promoting the progression of PF are also described.

In summary, the regulation of macrophage polarization by miRNA is suggested to represent one of the key pathogenetic factors in the development and progression of PF. Further research focused on distinct levels of these processes will undoubtedly provide updated information. Apart from detailing our current theoretical knowledge, it could be translated into future diagnostic approaches and/or designing novel therapeutic strategies helping to combat IPF, which despite the advancements still constitutes a major debilitating disease.

AUTHOR CONTRIBUTIONS

AK and MP contributed to the conception and writing of this review. All authors contributed to the article and approved the submitted version.

REFERENCES

1. Martinez FJ, Collard HR, Pardo A, Raghu G, Richeldi L, Selman M, et al. Idiopathic Pulmonary Fibrosis. *Nat Rev Dis Primers* (2017) 3:17074. doi: 10.1038/nrdp.2017.74
2. Pardo A, Selman M. The Interplay of the Genetic Architecture, Aging, and Environmental Factors in the Pathogenesis of Idiopathic Pulmonary Fibrosis. *Am J Respir Cell Mol Biol* (2021) 64(2):163–72. doi: 10.1165/rcmb.2020-0373PS
3. Barros A, Oldham J, Noth I. Genetics of Idiopathic Pulmonary Fibrosis. *Am J Med Sci* (2019) 357(5):379–83. doi: 10.1016/j.amjms.2019.02.009
4. Kishore A, Zizkova V, Kocourkova L, Petrek M. A Dataset of 26 Candidate Gene and Pro-Inflammatory Cytokine Variants for Association Studies in Idiopathic Pulmonary Fibrosis: Frequency Distribution in Normal Czech Population. *Front Immunol* (2015) 6:476. doi: 10.3389/fimmu.2015.00476
5. Kishore A, Borucka J, Petrkova J, Petrek M. Novel Insights Into miRNA in Lung and Heart Inflammatory Diseases. *Mediators Inflamm* (2014) 2014:259131. doi: 10.1155/2014/259131
6. Kishore A, Zizkova V, Kocourkova L, Petrkova J, Bouros E, Nunes H, et al. Association Study for 26 Candidate Loci in Idiopathic Pulmonary Fibrosis Patients From Four European Populations. *Front Immunol* (2016) 7:274. doi: 10.3389/fimmu.2016.00274
7. Allen RJ, Guillen-Guio B, Oldham JM, Ma SF, Dressen A, Paynton ML, et al. Genome-Wide Association Study of Susceptibility to Idiopathic Pulmonary Fibrosis. *Am J Respir Crit Care Med* (2020) 201(5):564–74. doi: 10.1164/rccm.201905-1017OC
8. Vasse GF, Nizamoglu M, Heijink IH, Schleputz M, van Rijn P, Thomas MJ, et al. Macrophage-Stroma Interactions in Fibrosis: Biochemical, Biophysical, and Cellular Perspectives. *J Pathol* (2021) 254(4):344–57. doi: 10.1002/path.5632
9. Perciani CT, MacParland SA. Lifting the Veil on Macrophage Diversity in Tissue Regeneration and Fibrosis. *Sci Immunol* (2019) 4(40):eaaz0749. doi: 10.1126/sciimmunol.aaz0749
10. Tarique AA, Logan J, Thomas E, Holt PG, Sly PD, Fantino E. Phenotypic, Functional, and Plasticity Features of Classical and Alternatively Activated Human Macrophages. *Am J Respir Cell Mol Biol* (2015) 53(5):676–88. doi: 10.1165/rcmb.2015-0012OC
11. Bart VMT, Pickering RJ, Taylor PR, Ipseiz N. Macrophage Reprogramming for Therapy. *Immunology* (2020) 163(2):128–44. doi: 10.1111/imm.13300
12. Porcheray F, Viaud S, Rimaniol AC, Leone C, Samah B, Dereuddre-Bosquet N, et al. Macrophage Activation Switching: An Asset for the Resolution of Inflammation. *Clin Exp Immunol* (2005) 142(3):481–9. doi: 10.1111/j.1365-2249.2005.02934.x
13. Kudlik G, Hegyi B, Czibula A, Monostori E, Buday L, Uher F. Mesenchymal Stem Cells Promote Macrophage Polarization Toward M2b-Like Cells. *Exp Cell Res* (2016) 348(1):36–45. doi: 10.1016/j.yexcr.2016.08.022
14. Gharib SA, McMahan RS, Eddy WE, Long ME, Parks WC, Aitken ML, et al. Transcriptional and Functional Diversity of Human Macrophage Repolarization. *J Allergy Clin Immunol* (2019) 143(4):1536–48. doi: 10.1016/j.jaci.2018.10.046
15. Wang LX, Zhang SX, Wu HJ, Rong XL, Guo J. M2b Macrophage Polarization and Its Roles in Diseases. *J Leukoc Biol* (2019) 106(2):345–58. doi: 10.1002/JLB.3RU1018-378RR
16. Liu G, Zhai H, Zhang T, Li S, Li N, Chen J, et al. New Therapeutic Strategies for IPF: Based on the "Phagocytosis-Secretion-Immunization" Network Regulation Mechanism of Pulmonary Macrophages. *BioMed Pharmacother* (2019) 118:109230. doi: 10.1016/j.biopha.2019.109230
17. Lee KY. M1 and M2 Polarization of Macrophages: A Mini-Review. *Med Biol Sci Eng* (2019) 2(1):1–5. doi: 10.30579/mbse.2019.2.1.1
18. Murray PJ. Macrophage Polarization. *Annu Rev Physiol* (2017) 79:541–66. doi: 10.1146/annurev-physiol-022516-034339
19. Mantovani A, Locati M. Tumor-Associated Macrophages as a Paradigm of Macrophage Plasticity, Diversity, and Polarization: Lessons and Open Questions. *Arterioscler Thromb Vasc Biol* (2013) 33(7):1478–83. doi: 10.1161/ATVBAHA.113.300168
20. Maccio A, Gramignano G, Cherchi MC, Tanca L, Melis L, Madeddu C. Role of M1-Polarized Tumor-Associated Macrophages in the Prognosis of Advanced Ovarian Cancer Patients. *Sci Rep* (2020) 10(1):6096. doi: 10.1038/s41598-020-63276-1
21. Zhang M, He Y, Sun X, Li Q, Wang W, Zhao A, et al. A High M1/M2 Ratio of Tumor-Associated Macrophages Is Associated With Extended Survival in Ovarian Cancer Patients. *J Ovarian Res* (2014) 7:19. doi: 10.1186/1757-2215-7-19
22. Suarez-Arriaga MC, Mendez-Tenorio A, Perez-Koldenkova V, Fuentes-Panana EM. Claudin-Low Breast Cancer Inflammatory Signatures Support Polarization of M1-Like Macrophages With Protumoral Activity. *Cancers (Basel)* (2021) 13(9):2248. doi: 10.3390/cancers13092248
23. Goda C, Balli D, Black M, Milewski D, Le T, Ustiyan V, et al. Loss of FOXM1 in Macrophages Promotes Pulmonary Fibrosis by Activating P38 MAPK Signaling Pathway. *PloS Genet* (2020) 16(4):e1008692. doi: 10.1371/journal.pgen.1008692
24. Byrne AJ, Maher TM, Lloyd CM. Pulmonary Macrophages: A New Therapeutic Pathway in Fibrosing Lung Disease? *Trends Mol Med* (2016) 22(4):303–16. doi: 10.1016/j.molmed.2016.02.004
25. Zhang L, Wang Y, Wu G, Xiong W, Gu W, Wang CY. Macrophages: Friend or Foe in Idiopathic Pulmonary Fibrosis? *Respir Res* (2018) 19(1):170. doi: 10.1186/s12931-018-0864-2
26. Wojtan P, Mierzejewski M, Osinska I, Domagala-Kulawik J. Macrophage Polarization in Interstitial Lung Diseases. *Cent Eur J Immunol* (2016) 41 (2):159–64. doi: 10.5114/ceji.2016.60990
27. Byrne AJ, Mathie SA, Gregory LG, Lloyd CM. Pulmonary Macrophages: Key Players in the Innate Defence of the Airways. *Thorax* (2015) 70(12):1189–96. doi: 10.1136/thoraxjnl-2015-207020
28. Gharib SA, Johnston LK, Huizar I, Birkland TP, Hanson J, Wang Y, et al. MMP28 Promotes Macrophage Polarization Toward M2 Cells and Augments Pulmonary Fibrosis. *J Leukoc Biol* (2014) 95(1):9–18. doi: 10.1189/jlb.1112587
29. Medbury HJ, James V, Ngo J, Hitos K, Wang Y, Harris DC, et al. Differing Association of Macrophage Subsets With Atherosclerotic Plaque Stability. *Int Angiol* (2013) 32(1):74–84.
30. Polverino F, Balestro E, Spagnolo P. Clinical Presentations, Pathogenesis, and Therapy of Sarcoidosis: State of the Art. *J Clin Med* (2020) 9(8):2363. doi: 10.3390/jcm9082363
31. Shamaei M, Mortaz E, Pourabdollah M, Garssen J, Tabarsi P, Velayati A, et al. Evidence for M2 Macrophages in Granulomas From Pulmonary Sarcoidosis: A New Aspect of Macrophage Heterogeneity. *Hum Immunol* (2018) 79(1):63–9. doi: 10.1016/j.humimm.2017.10.009
32. Partida-Zavala N, Antonio Ponce-Gallegos M, Buendia-Roldan I, Falfan-Valencia R. Type 2 Macrophages and Th2 CD4+ Cells in Interstitial Lung Diseases (ILDs): An Overview. *Sarcoidosis Vasc Diffuse Lung Dis* (2018) 35 (2):98–108. doi: 10.36141/svdld.v35i2.6691
33. Guo Z, Li S, Zhang N, Kang Q, Zhai H. Schisandra Inhibit Bleomycin-Induced Idiopathic Pulmonary Fibrosis in Rats *via* Suppressing M2 Macrophage Polarization. *BioMed Res Int* (2020) 2020:5137349. doi: 10.1155/2020/5137349
34. Wang J, Xu L, Xiang Z, Ren Y, Zheng X, Zhao Q, et al. Microcystin-LR Ameliorates Pulmonary Fibrosis *via* Modulating CD206(+) M2-Like Macrophage Polarization. *Cell Death Dis* (2020) 11(2):136. doi: 10.1038/s41419-020-2329-z
35. Pan T, Zhou Q, Miao K, Zhang L, Wu G, Yu J, et al. Suppressing Sart1 to Modulate Macrophage Polarization by siRNA-Loaded Liposomes: A

Promising Therapeutic Strategy for Pulmonary Fibrosis. *Theranostics* (2021) 11(3):1192–206. doi: 10.7150/thno.48152
36. Guo J, Fang Y, Jiang F, Li L, Zhou H, Xu X, et al. Neohesperidin Inhibits TGF-Beta1/Smad3 Signaling and Alleviates Bleomycin-Induced Pulmonary Fibrosis in Mice. *Eur J Pharmacol* (2019) 864:172712. doi: 10.1016/j.ejphar.2019.172712
37. Lv Q, Wang J, Xu C, Huang X, Ruan Z, Dai Y. Pirfenidone Alleviates Pulmonary Fibrosis *In Vitro* and *In Vivo* Through Regulating Wnt/GSK-3beta/Beta-Catenin and TGF-Beta1/Smad2/3 Signaling Pathways. *Mol Med* (2020) 26(1):49. doi: 10.1186/s10020-020-00173-3
38. Wang P, Nie X, Wang Y, Li Y, Ge C, Zhang L, et al. Multiwall Carbon Nanotubes Mediate Macrophage Activation and Promote Pulmonary Fibrosis Through TGF-Beta/Smad Signaling Pathway. *Small* (2013) 9(22):3799–811. doi: 10.1002/smll.201300607
39. Zhu L, Fu X, Chen X, Han X, Dong P. M2 Macrophages Induce EMT Through the TGF-Beta/Smad2 Signaling Pathway. *Cell Biol Int* (2017) 41(9):960–8. doi: 10.1002/cbin.10788
40. Hou J, Shi J, Chen L, Lv Z, Chen X, Cao H, et al. M2 Macrophages Promote Myofibroblast Differentiation of LR-MSCs and are Associated With Pulmonary Fibrogenesis. *Cell Commun Signal* (2018) 16(1):89. doi: 10.1186/s12964-018-0300-8
41. Okazaki H, Sato S, Koyama K, Morizumi S, Abe S, Azuma M, et al. The Novel Inhibitor PRI-724 for Wnt/beta-Catenin/CBP Signaling Ameliorates Bleomycin-Induced Pulmonary Fibrosis in Mice. *Exp Lung Res* (2019) 45 (7):188–99. doi: 10.1080/01902148.2019.1638466
42. Cao H, Wang C, Chen X, Hou J, Xiang Z, Shen Y, et al. Inhibition of Wnt/beta-Catenin Signaling Suppresses Myofibroblast Differentiation of Lung Resident Mesenchymal Stem Cells and Pulmonary Fibrosis. *Sci Rep* (2018) 8(1):13644. doi: 10.1038/s41598-018-28968-9
43. Guo X, Li T, Xu Y, Xu X, Zhu Z, Zhang Y, et al. Increased Levels of Gab1 and Gab2 Adaptor Proteins Skew Interleukin-4 (IL-4) Signaling Toward M2 Macrophage-Driven Pulmonary Fibrosis in Mice. *J Biol Chem* (2017) 292 (34):14003–15. doi: 10.1074/jbc.M117.802066
44. Zhao J, Okamoto Y, Asano Y, Ishimaru K, Aki S, Yoshioka K, et al. Sphingosine-1-Phosphate Receptor-2 Facilitates Pulmonary Fibrosis Through Potentiating IL-13 Pathway in Macrophages. *PloS One* (2018) 13 (5):e0197604. doi: 10.1371/journal.pone.0197604
45. Migliaccio CT, Buford MC, Jessop F, Holian A. The IL-4Ralpha Pathway in Macrophages and Its Potential Role in Silica-Induced Pulmonary Fibrosis. *J Leukoc Biol* (2008) 83(3):630–9. doi: 10.1189/jlb.0807533
46. Sennello JA, Misharin AV, Flozak AS, Berdnikovs S, Cheresh P, Varga J, et al. Lrp5/beta-Catenin Signaling Controls Lung Macrophage Differentiation and Inhibits Resolution of Fibrosis. *Am J Respir Cell Mol Biol* (2017) 56(2):191–201. doi: 10.1165/rcmb.2016-0147OC
47. Zhang N, Yang K, Bai J, Yi J, Gao C, Zhao J, et al. Myeloid-Specific Blockade of Notch Signaling Alleviates Murine Pulmonary Fibrosis Through Regulating Monocyte-Derived Ly6c(lo) MHCII(hi) Alveolar Macrophages Recruitment and TGF-Beta Secretion. *FASEB J* (2020) 34(8):11168–84. doi: 10.1096/fj.201903086RR
48. Han B, Chu C, Su X, Zhang N, Zhou L, Zhang M, et al. N(6)-Methyladenosine-Dependent Primary microRNA-126 Processing Activated PI3K-AKT-mTOR Pathway Drove the Development of Pulmonary Fibrosis Induced by Nanoscale Carbon Black Particles in Rats. *Nanotoxicology* (2020) 14(1):1–20. doi: 10.1080/17435390.2019.1661041
49. Tsitoura E, Wells AU, Karagiannis K, Lasithiotaki I, Vasarmidi E, Bibaki E, et al. MiR-185/AKT and miR-29a/Collagen 1a Pathways Are Activated in IPF BAL Cells. *Oncotarget* (2016) 7(46):74569–81. doi: 10.18632/oncotarget.12740
50. Haydar D, Cory TJ, Birket SE, Murphy BS, Pennypacker KR, Sinai AP, et al. Azithromycin Polarizes Macrophages to an M2 Phenotype *via* Inhibition of the STAT1 and NF-kappaB Signaling Pathways. *J Immunol* (2019) 203 (4):1021–30. doi: 10.4049/jimmunol.1801228
51. Chung EJ, Kwon S, Reedy JL, White AO, Song JS, Hwang I, et al. IGF-1 Receptor Signaling Regulates Type II Pneumocyte Senescence and Resulting Macrophage Polarization in Lung Fibrosis. *Int J Radiat Oncol Biol Phys* (2021) 110(2):526–38. doi: 10.1016/j.ijrobp.2020.12.035
52. Lu Y, Li C, Du S, Chen X, Zeng X, Liu F, et al. 4-1bb Signaling Promotes Alveolar Macrophages-Mediated Pro-Fibrotic Responses and Crystalline Silica-Induced Pulmonary Fibrosis in Mice. *Front Immunol* (2018) 9:1848. doi: 10.3389/fimmu.2018.01848
53. Vermeulen Z, Hervent AS, Dugaucquier L, Vandekerckhove L, Rombouts M, Beyens M, et al. Inhibitory Actions of the NRG-1/ErbB4 Pathway in Macrophages During Tissue Fibrosis in the Heart, Skin, and Lung. *Am J Physiol Heart Circ Physiol* (2017) 313(5):H934–H45. doi: 10.1152/ajpheart.00206.2017
54. Joshi N, Watanabe S, Verma R, Jablonski RP, Chen CI, Cheresh P, et al. A Spatially Restricted Fibrotic Niche in Pulmonary Fibrosis Is Sustained by M-CSF/M-CSFR Signalling in Monocyte-Derived Alveolar Macrophages. *Eur Respir J* (2020) 55(1):1900646. doi: 10.1183/13993003.00646-2019
55. Kishore A, Navratilova Z, Kolek V, Novosadova E, Cepe K, du Bois RM, et al. Expression Analysis of Extracellular microRNA in Bronchoalveolar Lavage Fluid From Patients With Pulmonary Sarcoidosis. *Respirology* (2018) 23 (12):1166–72. doi: 10.1111/resp.13364
56. Self-Fordham JB, Naqvi AR, Uttamani JR, Kulkarni V, Nares S. MicroRNA: Dynamic Regulators of Macrophage Polarization and Plasticity. *Front Immunol* (2017) 8:1062. doi: 10.3389/fimmu.2017.01062
57. Essandoh K, Li Y, Huo J, Fan GC. MiRNA-Mediated Macrophage Polarization and Its Potential Role in the Regulation of Inflammatory Response. *Shock* (2016) 46(2):122–31. doi: 10.1097/SHK.0000000000000604
58. Liu G, Abraham E. MicroRNAs in Immune Response and Macrophage Polarization. *Arterioscler Thromb Vasc Biol* (2013) 33(2):170–7. doi: 10.1161/ATVBAHA.112.300068
59. Wu XQ, Dai Y, Yang Y, Huang C, Meng XM, Wu BM, et al. Emerging Role of microRNAs in Regulating Macrophage Activation and Polarization in Immune Response and Inflammation. *Immunology* (2016) 148(3):237–48. doi: 10.1111/imm.12608
60. Zhu D, Pan C, Li L, Bian Z, Lv Z, Shi L, et al. MicroRNA-17/20a/106a Modulate Macrophage Inflammatory Responses Through Targeting Signal-Regulatory Protein Alpha. *J Allergy Clin Immunol* (2013) 132(2):426–36 e8. doi: 10.1016/j.jaci.2013.02.005
61. Barna BP, McPeek M, Malur A, Fessler MB, Wingard CJ, Dobbs L, et al. Elevated MicroRNA-33 in Sarcoidosis and a Carbon Nanotube Model of Chronic Granulomatous Disease. *Am J Respir Cell Mol Biol* (2016) 54(6):865–71. doi: 10.1165/rcmb.2015-0332OC
62. Khan MJ, Singh P, Dohare R, Jha R, Rahmani AH, Almatroodi SA, et al. Inhibition of miRNA-34a Promotes M2 Macrophage Polarization and Improves LPS-Induced Lung Injury by Targeting Klf4. *Genes (Basel)* (2020) 11(9):966. doi: 10.3390/genes11090966
63. Eissa MG, Artlett CM. The MicroRNA miR-155 Is Essential in Fibrosis. *Noncoding RNA* (2019) 5(1):23. doi: 10.3390/ncrna5010023
64. Jaiswal A, Maurya M, Maurya P, Barthwal MK. Lin28B Regulates Angiotensin II-Mediated Let-7c/miR-99a MicroRNA Formation Consequently Affecting Macrophage Polarization and Allergic Inflammation. *Inflammation* (2020) 43 (5):1846–61. doi: 10.1007/s10753-020-01258-1
65. Arora S, Dev K, Agarwal B, Das P, Syed MA. Macrophages: Their Role, Activation and Polarization in Pulmonary Diseases. *Immunobiology* (2018) 223(4-5):383–96. doi: 10.1016/j.imbio.2017.11.001
66. Liang Y, Xie J, Che D, Zhang C, Lin Y, Feng L, et al. MiR-124-3p Helps to Protect Against Acute Respiratory Distress Syndrome by Targeting P65. *Biosci Rep* (2020) 40(5):BSR20192132. doi: 10.1042/BSR20192132
67. Shi J, Chen M, Ouyang L, Wang Q, Guo Y, Huang L, et al. miR-142-5p and miR-130a-3p Regulate Pulmonary Macrophage Polarization and Asthma Airway Remodeling. *Immunol Cell Biol* (2020) 98(9):715–25. doi: 10.1111/imcb.12369
68. Huang C, Liu XJ, Zhou Q, Xie J, Ma TT, Meng XM, et al. MiR-146a Modulates Macrophage Polarization by Inhibiting Notch1 Pathway in RAW264. *7 Macrophages Int Immunopharmacol* (2016) 32:46–54. doi: 10.1016/j.intimp.2016.01.009
69. Novosadova E, Chabronova A, Kolek V, Petrek M, Navratilova Z. The Serum Expression of Selected miRNAs in Pulmonary Sarcoidosis With/Without Lofgren's Syndrome. *Mediators Inflamm* (2016) 2016:1246129. doi: 10.1155/2016/1246129
70. Pirlog R, Cismaru A, Nutu A, Berindan-Neagoe I. Field Cancerization in NSCLC: A New Perspective on MicroRNAs in Macrophage Polarization. *Int J Mol Sci* (2021) 22(2):746. doi: 10.3390/ijms22020746
71. Banerjee S, Xie N, Cui H, Tan Z, Yang S, Icyuz M, et al. MicroRNA Let-7c Regulates Macrophage Polarization. *J Immunol* (2013) 190(12):6542–9. doi: 10.4049/jimmunol.1202496
72. Duru N, Wolfson B, Zhou Q. Mechanisms of the Alternative Activation of Macrophages and non-Coding RNAs in the Development of Radiation-Induced Lung Fibrosis. *World J Biol Chem* (2016) 7(4):231–9. doi: 10.4331/wjbc.v7.i4.231

73. Su S, Zhao Q, He C, Huang D, Liu J, Chen F, et al. miR-142-5p and miR-130a-3p are Regulated by IL-4 and IL-13 and Control Profibrogenic Macrophage Program. *Nat Commun* (2015) 6:8523. doi: 10.1038/ncomms9523
74. Wang W, Liu Z, Su J, Chen WS, Wang XW, Bai SX, et al. Macrophage Micro-RNA-155 Promotes Lipopolysaccharide-Induced Acute Lung Injury in Mice and Rats. *Am J Physiol Lung Cell Mol Physiol* (2016) 311(2):L494–506. doi: 10.1152/ajplung.00001.2016
75. Kurowska-Stolarska M, Hasoo MK, Welsh DJ, Stewart L, McIntyre D, Morton BE, et al. The Role of microRNA-155/Liver X Receptor Pathway in Experimental and Idiopathic Pulmonary Fibrosis. *J Allergy Clin Immunol* (2017) 139(6):1946–56. doi: 10.1016/j.jaci.2016.09.021
76. Duru N, Zhang Y, Gernapudi R, Wolfson B, Lo PK, Yao Y, et al. Loss of miR-140 Is a Key Risk Factor for Radiation-Induced Lung Fibrosis Through Reprogramming Fibroblasts and Macrophages. *Sci Rep* (2016) 6:39572. doi: 10.1038/srep39572
77. Zhou D, Wu Y, Wang S, Li J, Luan J. Harnessing Noncoding RNA-Based Macrophage Polarization: Emerging Therapeutic Opportunities for Fibrosis. *Immun Inflamm Dis* (2020) 8(4):793–806. doi: 10.1002/iid3.341
78. Yao MY, Zhang WH, Ma WT, Liu QH, Xing LH, Zhao GF. microRNA-328 in Exosomes Derived From M2 Macrophages Exerts a Promotive Effect on the Progression of Pulmonary Fibrosis *via* FAM13A in a Rat Model. *Exp Mol Med* (2019) 51(6):1–16. doi: 10.1038/s12276-019-0255-x
79. Guiot J, Cambier M, Boeckx A, Henket M, Nivelles O, Gester F, et al. Macrophage-Derived Exosomes Attenuate Fibrosis in Airway Epithelial Cells Through Delivery of Antifibrotic miR-142-3p. *Thorax* (2020) 75 (10):870–81. doi: 10.1136/thoraxjnl-2019-214077
80. Lee H, Groot M, Pinilla-Vera M, Fredenburgh LE, Jin Y. Identification of miRNA-Rich Vesicles in Bronchoalveolar Lavage Fluid: Insights Into the Function and Heterogeneity of Extracellular Vesicles. *J Control Release* (2019) 294:43–52. doi: 10.1016/j.jconrel.2018.12.008
81. Huang R, Qin C, Wang J, Hu Y, Zheng G, Qiu G, et al. Differential Effects of Extracellular Vesicles From Aging and Young Mesenchymal Stem Cells in Acute Lung Injury. *Aging (Albany NY)* (2019) 11(18):7996–8014. doi: 10.18632/aging.102314
82. Xiao T, Zou Z, Xue J, Syed BM, Sun J, Dai X, et al. LncRNA H19-Mediated M2 Polarization of Macrophages Promotes Myofibroblast Differentiation in Pulmonary Fibrosis Induced by Arsenic Exposure. *Environ Pollut* (2021) 268(Pt A):115810. doi: 10.1016/j.envpol.2020.115810
83. Wang R, Xu B. TGF-Beta1-Modified MSC-Derived Exosomal miR-135b Attenuates Cartilage Injury *via* Promoting M2 Synovial Macrophage Polarization by Targeting MAPK6. *Cell Tissue Res* (2021) 384(1):113–27. doi: 10.1007/s00441-020-03319-1

6

Diagnosis of Idiopathic Pulmonary Fibrosis "Pragmatic Challenges in Clinical Practice"

*Vasilios Tzilas[1], Argyris Tzouvelekis[1,2], Serafim Chrysikos[3], Spyridon Papiris[4] and Demosthenes Bouros[1]**

[1] First Academic Department of Pneumonology, Hospital for Thoracic Diseases, "Sotiria", Medical School, National and Kapodistrian University of Athens, Athens, Greece, [2] Division of Immunology, Biomedical Sciences Research Center "Alexander Fleming", Athens, Greece, [3] 5th Department of Pneumonology, Hospital for Thoracic Diseases, "Sotiria", Athens, Greece, [4] 2nd Pulmonary Medicine Department, Attikon University Hospital, Medical School, National and Kapodistrian University of Athens, Athens, Greece

***Correspondence:**
Demosthenes Bouros
debouros@med.uoa.gr,
debouros@gmail.com

The past few years have signaled a major breakthrough on the management of idiopathic pulmonary fibrosis (IPF). Finally, we have drugs in our arsenal able to slow down the inexorable disease natural course. On the other hand, the latter evidence has increased the responsibility for a timely and accurate diagnosis. Establishment of IPF diagnosis directly affects the choice of appropriate treatment. The current diagnostic guidelines represent a major step forward providing an evidence-based road map; yet, clinicians are encountering major diagnostic dilemmas that inevitably affect therapeutic decisions. This review article aims to summarize the current state of knowledge on the diagnostic procedure of IPF based on the current guidelines and discuss pragmatic difficulties and challenges encountered by clinicians with regards to their applicability in the everyday clinical practice.

Keywords: idiopathic pulmonary fibrosis, diagnosis, challenges, pragmatic, clinical practice

INTRODUCTION

Idiopathic pulmonary fibrosis (IPF) represents the most common form of idiopathic interstitial pneumonia (IIPs) and is characterized by the gravest prognosis with a median survival of 3–5 years (1), irrespective of treatment. The past 10 years, large multicenter placebo-controlled clinical trials have significantly shifted the therapeutic dial of IPF (2–4) from harmful agents to Ref. (5) to therapies able to slow down the disease progression (2–4). It is important to note that the efficacy of the antifibrotic agents, pirfenidone, and nintedanib has been tested only in the context of IPF; thus, accurate and timely diagnosis seems to be imperative. It is important to note that disease diagnosis does not represent anymore an academic exercise since it directly influences and guides therapeutic decisions.

DIAGNOSIS OF IPF

Histologically, IPF is characterized by the pattern of usual interstitial pneumonia (UIP), which is denoted by spatial and temporal heterogeneity (6). It is of utmost importance to highlight the fact that UIP pathology is not exclusive to IPF, as it may characterize other diseases including chronic hypersensitivity pneumonitis (HP), connective tissue disorders-associated ILDs, asbestosis, or drug toxicity. In other words, all IPF have UIP pathology, but not all UIP are IPF. High-resolution computed tomography (HRCT) revolutionized the diagnosis of IPF. The presence of honeycombing in a predominantly peripheral and bibasilar distribution has a sufficient positive-predictive value (PPV) for underlying UIP pathology obviating the need for tissue confirmation (7–9). Even in that case, exclusion of other causes of UIP is mandatory to finally establish IPF diagnosis. Furthermore, IPF diagnosis represents a dynamic process and, therefore, close monitoring of the patient is mandatory. In particular, therapeutic decisions can be altered based on disease natural course and treatment responsiveness on an individual basis. In addition, disease diagnosis could be revisited in light of emerging symptoms compatible with connective tissue disorder or exposure to potentially harmful environmental agents.

The patient with IPF typically presents with progressive dyspnea on exertion of insidious onset and non-productive cough. The most characteristic clinical finding is the presence of Velcro rales that can be proven an extremely useful diagnostic tool for early disease diagnosis (10). Clubbing is almost found in 30–50% of patients; yet, its prevalence is much higher following disease progression and development of pulmonary hypertension. Multisystemic manifestations in the context of IPF are highly uncommon and should alert the physician toward alternative diagnoses. Median time from onset of symptoms to first evaluation in an ILD center quite often exceeds 1 year and the length of delay has been associated with increased mortality (11, 12).

Pulmonary function tests usually exhibit a restrictive pattern with concomitant reduction in diffusing capacity of carbon monoxide (DLco). However, the absence of restriction does not exclude the diagnosis of IPF, especially in the context of combined pulmonary fibrosis and emphysema, which is characterized by relatively preserved lung volumes with disproportionately reduced DLco (13). There are also cases discovered early and presumably with an initial FVC > 100% that do not fulfill the criteria of a restrictive pattern, nevertheless, fibrosis is evident on HRCT.

According to current diagnostic criteria (1), HRCT plays a pivotal role in the diagnostic procedure. There are three diagnostic categories based on HRCT appearance: UIP pattern, possible UIP pattern, and inconsistent with UIP. The definition of each category is based on morphological as well as distribution characteristics. UIP pattern is characterized by the presence of reticular abnormalities and honeycombing (with or without traction bronchiectasis) with a subpleural and basal predominance in the absence of inconsistent features. The above radiological features in the absence of honeycombing constitute the possible UIP pattern. Inconsistent features can be categorized as those involving distribution (upper or mid lung and peribronchovascular predominance) and those involving morphology (extensive ground glass opacities, consolidation, mosaic attenuation, nodules, discrete cysts).

The presence of honeycombing is not synonymous with IPF, as it can be seen in other diseases as chronic HP, collagen tissue-related interstitial lung diseases, asbestosis, drug-induced lung toxicity, sarcoidosis, postradiation pneumonitis, and post ARDS. Minimal honeycombing can also be encountered in cases of fibrotic NSIP, which represents a major component of the differential list.

The distribution of honeycombing can offer significant information. Typically, in IPF, it has a subpleural and basilar distribution. Chronic HP can be a great mimic of IPF. However, sometimes in chronic HP, honeycombing can be more marked in the upper/mid lung zones giving a hint to the actual diagnosis. The same upper lobe predominance of honeycombing can be seen in sarcoidosis as well. Furthermore, in sarcoidosis, the fibrotic process often follows the expected perilymphatic route, thus creating a "swath" of honeycombing extending from the hilum to the periphery of the lung. In patients who develop fibrosis post ARDS, it has a striking anterior distribution (**Table 1**).

Besides the distribution of honeycombing, there are other findings on HRCT that increase suspicion toward certain diagnoses. Silva et al. (14) studied 66 patients with biopsy proven IPF, HP, and NSIP. The presence of lobular areas with decreased attenuation, centrilobular nodules, and cysts favored the diagnosis of HP. The best predictors of NSIP were the presence of subpleural sparing and the absence of honeycombing.

In the appropriate clinical setting in patients with a UIP pattern, IPF diagnosis can be established without the need for surgical lung biopsy (SLB). In the cases of possible UIP and inconsistent with UIP, a SLB is recommended in order to reach a final diagnosis. When SLB is necessary, close cooperation with the thoracic surgeon is necessary in order to point the optimal sites for biopsy in order to increase the possibility of an accurate diagnosis. Areas of honeycombing should be avoided in lung sampling since they may reveal non-specific end-stage lung damage and absence of spatial and temporal heterogeneity suggestive of UIP. Samples should be obtained from at least two different

TABLE 1 | Differential diagnosis of radiological honeycombing.

Causes of honeycombing	Comments
Idiopathic pulmonary fibrosis	Distribution predominantly bibasilar and subpleural
Collagen tissue disease	Honeycombing mainly seen in rheumatoid arthritis-ILD
Chronic hypersensitivity pneumonitis	Honeycombing can be seen predominantly in the upper/middle zones. Clues to diagnosis: mosaic attenuation, air trapping in expiratory scans
Asbestosis	Distribution predominantly bibasilar and subpleural. Clues to diagnosis: pleural plaques (±calcification), subpleural lines
NSIP	When seen, honeycombing is minimal. Clues to diagnosis: subpleural sparing, central/peribronchovascular predominance of findings
Sarcoidosis	In rare cases, the distribution is bibasilar and subpleural. Typically, honeycombing is seen in upper/middle zones extending from the periphery toward the hilum. Clues to diagnosis: perilymphatic nodules, hilar/mediastinal lymphadenopathy (±calcification), progressive massive fibrosis
Radiation	Confined to radiation port
End-stage ARDS	Usually involves anterior lung (barotrauma)
Drug toxicity	

lobes, because of the possibility of discordant findings (UIP in one lobe and NSIP in another). In such cases, the UIP pattern drives diagnosis and prognosis as well (15, 16).

Regarding histopathology, current guidelines have classified patients into four categories: UIP, probable UIP, possible UIP, and not UIP (1). Specific combinations of HRCT and SLB pattern with the integration of clinical data are evaluated by a multidisciplinary (MDT) team in order to achieve a final diagnosis.

MDT approach is acknowledged as a major advance in IPF diagnosis. It refers to the constructive exchange of views between a respiratory physician, radiologist, and pathologist with expertise in the field of ILDs. The added value of MDT diagnosis is its association with higher levels of diagnostic confidence and better interobserver agreement (17, 18). Walsh et al. (19) were the first to evaluate the agreement between different multidisciplinary teams in diffuse lung diseases after the 2013 ATS/ERS update (20) on the classification of IIPs. Inter-MDT agreement was acceptable for cases of IPF (weighted kappa coefficient, $\kappa w = 0.71$), while it was moderate for NSIP ($\kappa w = 0.42$) and rather disappointing for HP ($\kappa w = 0.29$) reflecting the lack of diagnostic guidelines for the last two clinical entities. This indirectly impacts the accuracy of IPF diagnosis as well, given the fact that NSIP and HP are frequently major components of its differential.

A PRAGMATIC APPLICATION OF GUIDELINES IN EVERY DAY CLINICAL PRACTICE

The 2011 guidelines are a clear step forward considering that they provide clear guidance on an evidence-based approach. The most crucial caveat of these guidelines is that, in a significant percentage of "real-life" patients with IPF, lack clinical practicality regarding diagnosis, prognosis, and therapeutic decisions.

Challenge 1: Interpretation of HRCT

High-resolution computed tomography plays a pivotal role in disease diagnosis and determines the need of SLB to establish a definite diagnosis. However, accurate identification of honeycombing is not straightforward even amongst thoracic radiologists. Interobserver agreement has been proven poor, and this has been validated in recent studies (21–24). This problem is further accentuated on a community level.

Possible UIP Pattern

An increasing number of studies has shown that in patients with a high suspicion of IPF, a possible UIP pattern retains sufficient PPV for underlying UIP pathology in order to obviate the need for tissue based diagnosis. Raghu et al. (25) studied 315 patients with IPF study that had both HRCT and SLB samples. As expected, UIP pattern had a high PPV for UIP pathology (97.3%). This high PPV was retained for patients with a possible UIP pattern (94%). Though a selection bias is quite obvious given that this evidence refers to patients screened for recruitment into clinical trials and thus should not be generalized; yet, this study highlights the importance of pretest clinical probability. Chung et al. (26) studied 201 patients with pulmonary fibrosis that were subjected to lung biopsy within 1 year of chest CT. Patients with possible UIP on CT scan were more likely to have histologic probable/definite UIP comparing to patients with indeterminate UIP on CT scan (82.4 vs 54.2%, $p = 0.01$). Finally, in the INPULSIS trials, a significant proportion of patients (31.9%, $n = 338$) were enrolled based on possible UIP pattern (with traction bronchiectasis) and no confirmation by SLB. This group of patients exhibited the same progression of disease based on the annual decline of FVC compared to patients with honeycombing on HRCT and/or confirmation by SLB as well as similar treatment response to nintedanib (27). This observation adds further to the notion that in the appropriate clinical setting, possible UIP pattern carries sufficient PPV for UIP pathology.

Recently, a study by Brownell et al. offered valuable new information on this topic (28). Avoiding selection bias, they elegantly showed that the PPV of possible UIP for predicting UIP pathology directly depends on the pretest probability of IPF and the prevalence of IPF in the examined population. In the derivation cohort, possible UIP had a specificity of 91.2% and a PPV of 62.5%. By using two key clinical predictors (male sex, increasing age) and a radiographic predictor (total traction bronchiectasis score), the PPV increased above the acceptable threshold of 90%.

Inconsistent with UIP Pattern

According to guidelines, even if histology is that of a typical UIP pattern when the HRCT appearance is inconsistent with UIP, the diagnosis of IPF is deemed only to be possible. However, the term inconsistent seems to be a misnomer. IPF is actually a great mimic. UIP pathology can exhibit a wide variety of radiological expressions ranging from the typical UIP pattern with peripheral, bibasilar honeycombing, to a pattern resembling HP with areas of mosaic attenuation or to a pattern characterized by extensive ground glass opacities (29, 30). Interestingly, NSIP pathology seems to be much more consistent regarding its radiological expression (31). The key point is that an inconsistent with UIP radiological pattern does not rule out the diagnosis of IPF, but mandates histological confirmation regardless the pretest probability of the patient. In the study by Brownell et al., the maximum PPV achieved for the inconsistent UIP pattern regarding IPF diagnosis was just 38% (28). **Figure 1** summarizes a proposed algorithm for IPF diagnosis based on recent findings as described previously.

Challenge 2: Interpretation of SLB

The interpretation of histological findings is subject to the same limitations as HRCT. The pathologic distinction between UIP and fibrotic NSIP can be especially difficult and is the main reason (>50%) for interobserver variation in the evaluation of diffuse parenchymal lung disease (32). In the same study, the median prevalence for diagnoses with low confidence (<70% likelihood) was 18% while diagnoses made with 100% confidence were reached in only 39% of cases. Thus, it is not surprising that the pathological diagnosis can be reconsidered in almost 20% of cases following integration of clinical and HRCT data (17). The variability in interpretation is accentuated

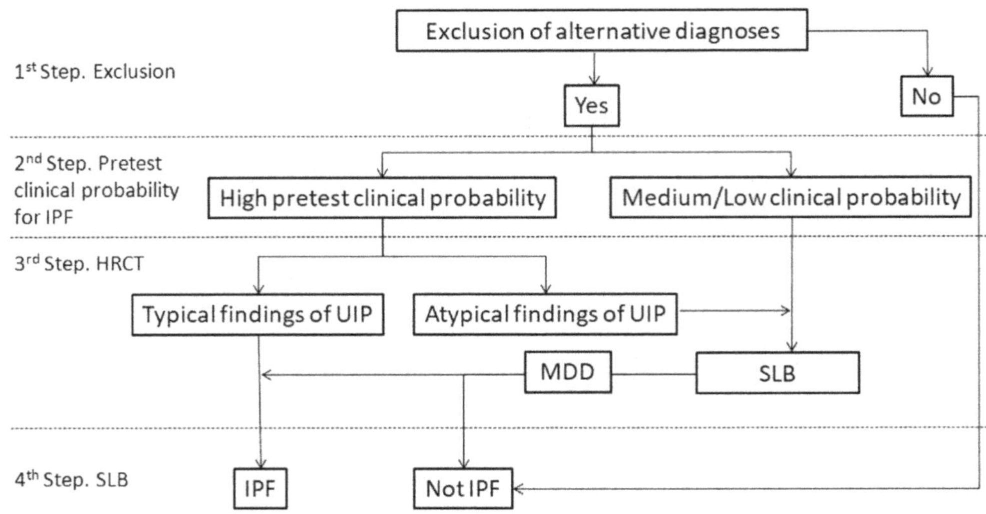

FIGURE 1 | Proposed diagnostic algorithm for idiopathic pulmonary fibrosis (IPF). Typical findings of UIP are radiological signs of lung fibrosis (honeycombing, traction bronchiolectasis, and/or irregular reticular pattern) with a predominantly peripheral/subpleural and bibasilar distribution. Atypical findings of UIP are according to the current definition of inconsistent with UIP pattern. HRCT, high-resolution computed tomography; SLB, surgical lung biopsy.

between thoracic and general pathologists with a poor level of agreement (κ: 0.21), which was shown to have direct clinical implications (33). Also, it is known that biopsies from different sites can produce discordant results, specifically, NSIP vs UIP histology (15, 16). Consequently, sampling error is a possibility and in cases with a definite UIP radiology pattern and NSIP on histology, the radiologic diagnosis actually prevails over histology (34). Finally, histology patterns in interstitial lung diseases are not exclusive to certain diseases. In fact, the same histology can correspond to different diseases and furthermore to the same disease but with strikingly different progression and natural course. SLB is not a gold standard and the risk vs benefit ratio should be carefully examined in each patient.

Challenge 3: Safety of SLB

Surgical lung biopsy in patients with ILDs as it can trigger an acute exacerbation (35, 36), regardless disease severity (37). An alarming observation is that the same parameters that increase the likelihood of IPF (increased age and male sex) (28, 38, 39) represent risk factors that increase mortality following SLB in patients with ILDs (40, 41). Actually, a provisional diagnosis of IPF was identified as a risk factor for increased mortality. Other risk factors are the presence of comorbidities, hypoxemic respiratory failure, severe physiological impairment, pulmonary hypertension, rapidly progressive disease (42).

Two large series (40, 41) reported postoperative hospital mortality rates (1.7%) similar to those reported in patients with lung cancer undergoing lobectomy. The actual postoperative mortality may vary depending on the nature of the procedure (elective vs non-elective) and the risk factors for the individual patient. Thus, the decision to proceed to SLB [*via* video-assisted thoracoscopic surgery (VATS)] should be carefully considered on an individual basis, weighing risks vs diagnostic benefit.

Challenge 4: Current Clinical Practice

By strictly adhering to current guidelines, a large number of patients (almost 50% with a suspicion of IPF) will need to be subjected to SLB. Clinical practice seems to have endorsed the facts that SLB carries a small but significant risk and that the possible UIP pattern in a patient with a high pretest probability of IPF retains sufficient PPV for UIP pathology. It is common practice that in patients with a high clinical probability of IPF (28, 38, 39) (male sex, increased age, and/or extent of fibrosis), we establish a working diagnosis of IPF (43, 44) without resorting to surgical biopsy. Biopsies are reserved for patients in whom establishing a tissue-based diagnosis is clinically meaningful and are fit enough to undergo such a procedure. This is vividly depicted in the study by Hutchinson et al. (40). In a UK study held between 1997 and 2008, only 4.5% of new cases with a provisional diagnosis J84.1 were subjected to SLB (40). Given the fact that the ICD-10 of J84.1 does not accurately describe the IPF population (45, 46), this percentage is likely to be even smaller for actual IPF cases. We eagerly wait to see how the above will be translated in the upcoming guidelines for the diagnosis of IPF.

FUTURE DIRECTIONS

Bronchoscopic Lung Cryobiopsy (BLC)

Bronchoscopic lung cryobiopsy is dynamically emerging during the past few years as an alternative diagnostic tool to SLB, claiming the same diagnostic efficacy and reduced mortality

(47). Cryobiopsies are considerably larger and have minimal crash artifacts as opposed to forceps biopsies when performed by experienced bronchoscopists in appropriate organized centers. Therefore, they allow confident recognition of histological patterns. The vital question that should be addressed is their safety and diagnostic yield against lung biopsies obtained *via* VATS. A recent meta-analysis including 16 studies with BLC (642 patients) and 14 studies with VATS (1,594 patients) (48) reported comparable diagnostic yields for BLC (83.7%) and VATS (92.7%). With regards to safety profile, BLC was associated with severe bleeding in 4.9% of cases and pneumothorax in 9.5% of cases while short-term mortality was similar between BLC (0.7%) and VATS (1.8%). Similar findings have been demonstrated by earlier studies (49, 50). In order to generalize the use of BLC beyond expert centers, it is important to standardize the procedure (e.g., size of cryoprobe, number and site of biopsies, degree of sedation), offer proper training, since it is an operator-dependent procedure (51) and prospectively evaluate safety and diagnostic profile of BLC as opposed to VATS.

Biomarkers

According to the Bayesian diagnostic approach of IPF, it would be very useful to have biomarkers that would increase the pretest probability of IPF. Ideally, these biomarkers would not only have diagnostic value but would also offer clinically relevant prognostic information regarding not only the natural course of the disease but also response to therapy. While for pulmonary embolism, d-dimers are an established diagnostic indicator in a complex disease as IPF, it is unlikely that just one "diagnosticator" will suffice. Considering that IPF diagnosis represent the least critical question for clinicians (given the major improvements of HRCT), in the real-world clinical practice, an ideal biomarker would be the one who could fulfill the unmet need for timely prediction of disease progressiveness and treatment responsiveness. In line with this, most of the studied biomarkers were mostly used as disease prognosticators rather than disease-specific diagnostic tools. Matrix metalloproteinase-(MMP)-7 represents the most extensively studied molecular biomarker that showed promising prognostic value in several independent cohorts of patients with IPF. Despite the fact that elevated MMP-7 levels clearly discriminated patients with IPF from those with HP (52); yet, they showed lack of discriminatory ability between IPF and RA-ILD (53). Further studies using highly standardized sample collection procedures and collection matrices are needed to produce reproducible and reliable diagnostic and prognostic cutoff thresholds (54). The latter observation represents an amenable need for precision medicine approaches (55, 56).

TABLE 2 | Key points for idiopathic pulmonary fibrosis diagnosis.

- Exclusion of other causes is mandatory
- Equally important is to define pretest clinical probability based on age, sex, extend of fibrosis
- Even in the absence of honeycombing, in a patient with a high pretest clinical probability, the presence of other signs of lung fibrosis (traction bronchiolectasis, irregular reticulation) in a predominantly bibasilar/subpleural distribution have sufficient positive-predictive value for usual interstitial pneumonia (UIP) pathology
- Atypical features (inconsistent with UIP) mandates the need for surgical lung biopsy (SLB), regardless pretest clinical probability
- SLB is not a diagnostic panacea, it can be potentially hazardous especially when performed non-electively and should be performed after carefully estimating the clinically meaningful benefit vs risk on an individual basis

Conclusion

The ILD community has made significant progress in understanding IPF. With the development of antifibrotic agents, accurate diagnosis is crucial. Guidance is needed to focus on practical implementation of current guidelines in a real-world clinical setting. An integral first step of the diagnostic process is the exclusion of alternative diagnoses. Equally important is the definition of the pretest probability for every patient with suspected IPF. The diagnostic significance of possible or even definite UIP pattern is completely different when facing a 45-year-old female or a 70-year-old male. Possible UIP pattern seems to carry sufficient PPV in patients with a high pretest probability of IPF. SLB should be considered in patients with inconsistent with UIP pattern after evaluating the individualized benefit risk ratio (**Table 2**). BLC seems an attractive, safer alternative to SLB; yet, standardization and prospective evaluation of the process is required in order to "escape" from expert centers and be embraced by common practice. Finally, biomarkers are sorely needed to fulfill the unmet need of current clinical practice: early prediction of disease progressiveness and treatment responsiveness that will timely guide therapeutic decisions.

AUTHOR CONTRIBUTIONS

VT, AT, and SC wrote the manuscript. SP and DB revised the manuscript for important intellectual content.

REFERENCES

1. Raghu G, Collard HR, Egan JJ, Martinez FJ, Behr J, Brown KK, et al. An official ATS/ERS/JRS/ALAT statement: idiopathic pulmonary fibrosis: evidence-based guidelines for diagnosis and management. *Am J Respir Crit Care Med* (2011) 183:788–824. doi:10.1164/rccm.2009-040GL
2. Noble PW, Albera C, Bradford WZ. Pirfenidone in patients with idiopathic pulmonary fibrosis (CAPACITY): two randomized trials. *Lancet* (2011) 377:1760–9. doi:10.1016/S0140-6736(11)60405-4
3. King TE Jr, Bradford WZ, Castro-Bernardini S, Fagan EA, Glaspole I, Glassberg MK, et al. A phase 3 trial of pirfenidone in patients with idiopathic pulmonary fibrosis. *N Engl J Med* (2014) 370:2083–92. doi:10.1056/NEJMoa1402582
4. Richeldi L, du Bois RM, Raghu G, Azuma A, Brown KK, Costabel U, et al. Efficacy and safety of nintedanib in idiopathic pulmonary fibrosis. *N Engl J Med* (2014) 370:2071–82. doi:10.1056/NEJMoa1402584
5. Idiopathic Pulmonary Fibrosis Clinical Research Network, Raghu G, Anstrom KJ, King TE Jr, Lasky JA, Martinez FJ. Prednisone, azathioprine, and N-acetylcysteine for pulmonary fibrosis. *N Engl J Med* (2012) 366(21):1968–77. doi:10.1056/NEJMoa1113354
6. Smith M, Dalurzo M, Panse P, Parish J, Leslie K. Usual interstitial pneumonia-pattern fibrosis in surgical lung biopsies. Clinical, radiological and histopathological clues to aetiology. *J Clin Pathol* (2013) 66(10):896–903. doi:10.1136/jclinpath-2013-201442
7. Raghu G, Mageto YN, Lockhart D, Schmidt RA, Wood DE, Godwin JD. The accuracy of the clinical diagnosis of new-onset idiopathic pulmonary

fibrosis and other interstitial lung disease: a prospective study. *Chest* (1999) 116:1168–74. doi:10.1378/chest.116.5.1168

8. Hunninghake GW, Zimmerman MB, Schwartz DA, King TE Jr, Lynch J, Hegele R, et al. Utility of a lung biopsy for the diagnosis of idiopathic pulmonary fibrosis. *Am J Respir Crit Care Med* (2001) 164:193–6. doi:10.1164/ajrccm.164.2.2101090
9. Flaherty KR, Thwaite EL, Kazerooni EA, Gross BH, Toews GB, Colby TV, et al. Radiological versus histological diagnosis in UIP and NSIP: survival implications. *Thorax* (2003) 58:143–8. doi:10.1136/thorax.58.2.143
10. Cottin V, Cordier JF. Velcro crackles: the key for early diagnosis of idiopathic pulmonary fibrosis? *Eur Respir J* (2012) 40(3):519–21. doi:10.1183/09031936.00001612
11. Purokivi M, Hodgson U, Myllärniemi M, Salomaa ER, Kaarteenaho R. Are physicians in primary health care able to recognize pulmonary fibrosis? *Eur Clin Respir J* (2017) 4(1):1290339. doi:10.1080/20018525.2017.1290339
12. Lamas DJ, Kawut SM, Bagiella E, Philip N, Arcasoy SM, Lederer DJ. Delayed access and survival in idiopathic pulmonary fibrosis: a cohort study. *Am J Respir Crit Care Med* (2011) 184(7):842–7. doi:10.1164/rccm.201104-0668OC
13. Cottin V, Nunes H, Brillet PY, Delaval P, Devouassoux G, Tillie-Leblond I, et al. Combined pulmonary fibrosis and emphysema: a distinct underrecognised entity. *Eur Respir J* (2005) 26:586–93. doi:10.1183/09031936.05.00021005
14. Silva CI, Müller NL, Lynch DA, Curran-Everett D, Brown KK, Lee KS, et al. Chronic hypersensitivity pneumonitis: differentiation from idiopathic pulmonary fibrosis and nonspecific interstitial pneumonia by using thin-section CT. *Radiology* (2008) 246(1):288–97. doi:10.1148/radiol.2453061881
15. Flaherty KR, Travis WD, Colby TV, Toews GB, Kazerooni EA, Gross BH, et al. Histopathologic variability in usual and nonspecific interstitial pneumonias. *Am J Respir Crit Care Med* (2001) 164:1722–7. doi:10.1164/ajrccm.164.9.2103074
16. Monaghan H, Wells AU, Colby TV, du Bois RM, Hansell DM, Nicholson AG. Prognostic implications of histologic patterns in multiple surgical lung biopsies from patients with idiopathic interstitial pneumonias. *Chest* (2004) 125:522–6. doi:10.1378/chest.125.2.522
17. Flaherty KR, King TE Jr, Raghu G, Lynch JP 3rd, Colby TV, Travis WD, et al. Idiopathic interstitial pneumonia: what is the effect of a multidisciplinary approach to diagnosis? *Am J Respir Crit Care Med* (2004) 170:904–10. doi:10.1164/rccm.200402-147OC
18. Thomeer M, Demedts M, Behr J, Buhl R, Costabel U, Flower CD, et al. Multidisciplinary interobserver agreement in the diagnosis of idiopathic pulmonary fibrosis. *Eur Respir J* (2008) 31:585–91. doi:10.1183/09031936.00063706
19. Walsh SL, Wells AU, Desai SR, Poletti V, Piciucchi S, Dubini A, et al. Multicentre evaluation of multidisciplinary team meeting agreement on diagnosis in diffuse parenchymal lung disease: a case-cohort study. *Lancet Respir Med* (2016) 4(7):557–65. doi:10.1016/S2213-2600(16)30033-9
20. Travis WD, Costabel U, Hansell DM, King TE Jr, Lynch DA, Nicholson AG, et al. An official American Thoracic Society/European Respiratory Society statement: update of the international multidisciplinary classification of the idiopathic interstitial pneumonias. *Am J Respir Crit Care Med* (2013) 188(6):733–48. doi:10.1164/rccm.201308-1483ST
21. Lynch DA, Godwin JD, Safrin S, Starko KM, Hormel P, Brown KK, et al. Idiopathic Pulmonary Fibrosis Study Group. High-resolution computed tomography in idiopathic pulmonary fibrosis: diagnosis and prognosis. *Am J Respir Crit Care Med* (2005) 17:488–93. doi:10.1164/rccm.200412-1756OC
22. Watadani T, Sakai F, Johkoh T, Noma S, Akira M, Fujimoto K, et al. Interobserver variability in the CT assessment of honeycombing in the lungs. *Radiology* (2013) 26:936–44. doi:10.1148/radiol.12112516
23. Sundaram B, Gross BH, Martinez FJ, Oh E, Müller NL, Schipper M, et al. Accuracy of high-resolution CT in the diagnosis of diffuse lung disease: effect of predominance and distribution of findings. *AJR Am J Roentgenol* (2008) 191(4):1032–9. doi:10.2214/AJR.07.3177
24. Walsh SL, Calandriello L, Sverzellati N, Wells AU, Hansell DM; UIP Observer Consort. Interobserver agreement for the ATS/ERS/JRS/ALAT criteria for a UIP pattern on CT. *Thorax* (2016) 7:45–51. doi:10.1136/thoraxjnl-2015-207252
25. Raghu G, Lynch D, Godwin JD, Webb R, Colby TV, Leslie KO, et al. Diagnosis of idiopathic pulmonary fibrosis with high-resolution CT in patients with little or no radiological evidence of honeycombing: secondary analysis of a randomised, controlled trial. *Lancet Respir Med* (2014) 2:277–84. doi:10.1016/S2213-2600(14)70011-6
26. Chung JH, Chawla A, Peljto AL, Cool CD, Groshong SD, Talbert JL, et al. CT scan findings of probable usual interstitial pneumonitis have a high predictive value for histologic usual interstitial pneumonitis. *Chest* (2015) 147:450–9. doi:10.1378/chest.14-0976
27. Raghu G, Wells AU, Nicholson AG, Richeldi L, Flaherty KR, Le Maulf F, et al. Effect of nintedanib in subgroups of idiopathic pulmonary fibrosis by diagnostic criteria. *Am J Respir Crit Care Med* (2017) 195(1):78–85. doi:10.1164/rccm.201602-0402OC
28. Brownell R, Moua T, Henry TS, Elicker BM, White D, Vittinghoff E, et al. The use of pretest probability increases the value of high-resolution CT in diagnosing usual interstitial pneumonia. *Thorax* (2017) 72(5):424–9. doi:10.1136/thoraxjnl-2016-209671
29. Sverzellati N, Wells AU, Tomassetti S, Desai SR, Copley SJ, Aziz ZA, et al. Biopsy-proved idiopathic pulmonary fibrosis: spectrum of nondiagnostic thin-section CT diagnoses. *Radiology* (2010) 254(3):957–64. doi:10.1148/radiol.0990898
30. Yagihashi K, Huckleberry J, Colby TV, Tazelaar HD, Zach J, Sundaram B, et al. Radiologic-pathologic discordance in biopsy-proven usual interstitial pneumonia. *Eur Respir J* (2016) 47(4):1189–97. doi:10.1183/13993003.01680-2015
31. Sumikawa H, Johkoh T, Fujimoto K, Arakawa H, Colby TV, Fukuoka J, et al. Pathologically proved nonspecific interstitial pneumonia: CT pattern analysis as compared with usual interstitial pneumonia CT pattern. *Radiology* (2014) 272(2):549–56. doi:10.1148/radiol.14130853
32. Nicholson AG, Addis BJ, Bharucha H, Clelland CA, Corrin B, Gibbs AR, et al. Interobserver variation between pathologists in diffuse parenchymal lung disease. *Thorax* (2004) 59:500–5. doi:10.1136/thx.2003.011734
33. Lettieri CJ, Veerappan GR, Parker JM, Franks TJ, Hayden D, Travis WD, et al. Discordance between general and pulmonary pathologists in the diagnosis of interstitial lung disease. *Respir Med* (2005) 99(11):1425–30. doi:10.1016/j.rmed.2005.03.008
34. Zander DS. Idiopathic interstitial pneumonias and the concept of the trump card. *Chest* (2004) 125(2):359–60. doi:10.1378/chest.125.2.359
35. Utz JP, Ryu JH, Douglas WW, Hartman TE, Tazelaar HD, Myers JL, et al. High short-term mortality following lung biopsy for usual interstitial pneumonia. *Eur Respir J* (2001) 17:175–9. doi:10.1183/09031936.01.17201750
36. Kreider ME, Hansen-Flaschen J, Ahmad NN, Rossman MD, Kaiser LR, Kucharczuk JC, et al. Complications of video-assisted thoracoscopic lung biopsy in patients with interstitial lung disease. *Ann Thorac Surg* (2007) 83:1140–4. doi:10.1016/j.athoracsur.2006.10.002
37. Chida M, Ono S, Hoshikawa Y, Kondo T. Subclinical idiopathic pulmonary fibrosis is also a risk factor of postoperative acute respiratory distress syndrome following thoracic surgery. *Eur J Cardiothorac Surg* (2008) 34:878–81. doi:10.1016/j.ejcts.2008.07.028
38. Fell CD, Martinez FJ, Liu LX, Murray S, Han MK, Kazerooni EA, et al. Clinical predictors of a diagnosis of idiopathic pulmonary fibrosis. *Am J Respir Crit Care Med* (2010) 181(8):832–7. doi:10.1164/rccm.200906-0959OC
39. Salisbury ML, Xia M, Murray S, Bartholmai BJ, Kazerooni EA, Meldrum CA, et al. Predictors of idiopathic pulmonary fibrosis in absence of radiologic honeycombing: a cross sectional analysis in ILD patients undergoing lung tissue sampling. *Respir Med* (2016) 118:88–95. doi:10.1016/j.rmed.2016.07.016
40. Hutchinson JP, McKeever TM, Fogarty AW, Navaratnam V, Hubbard RB. Surgical lung biopsy for the diagnosis of interstitial lung disease in England: 1997-2008. *Eur Respir J* (2016) 48(5):1453–61. doi:10.1183/13993003.00378-2016
41. Hutchinson JP, Fogarty AW, McKeever TM, Hubbard RB. In-hospital mortality after surgical lung biopsy for interstitial lung disease in the United States 2000 to 2011. *Am J Respir Crit Care Med* (2016) 193:1161–7. doi:10.1164/rccm.201508-1632OC
42. Raj R, Raparia K, Lynch DA, Brown KK. Surgical lung biopsy for interstitial lung diseases. *Chest* (2017) 151(5):1131–40. doi:10.1016/j.chest.2016.06.019
43. Wells AU. Any fool can make a rule and any fool will mind it. *BMC Med* (2016) 14:23. doi:10.1186/s12916-016-0562-1

44. Tzilas V, Bouros D. Usual interstitial pneumonia pattern in the diagnosis of idiopathic pulmonary fibrosis? *Lancet Respir Med* (2016) 4(10):770–2. doi:10.1016/S2213-2600(16)30231-4
45. Tzilas V, Bouros D. Inherent weaknesses of the current ICD coding system regarding idiopathic pulmonary fibrosis. *Eur Respir J* (2015) 45(4):1194–6. doi:10.1183/09031936.00205914
46. Kaunisto J, Kelloniemi K, Sutinen E, Hodgson U, Piilonen A, Kaarteenaho R, et al. Re-evaluation of diagnostic parameters is crucial for obtaining accurate data on idiopathic pulmonary fibrosis. *BMC Pulm Med* (2015) 15:92. doi:10.1186/s12890-015-0074-3
47. Colby TV, Tomassetti S, Cavazza A, Dubini A, Poletti V. Transbronchial cryobiopsy in diffuse lung disease: update for the pathologist. *Arch Pathol Lab Med* (2017) 141(7):891–900. doi:10.5858/arpa.2016-0233-RA
48. Iftikhar IH, Alghothani L, Sardi A, Berkowitz D, Musani AI. Transbronchial lung cryobiopsy and video-assisted thoracoscopic lung biopsy in the diagnosis of diffuse parenchymal lung disease: a meta-analysis of diagnostic test accuracy. *Ann Am Thorac Soc* (2017) 14(7):1197–211. doi:10.1513/AnnalsATS.201701-086SR
49. Ravaglia C, Bonifazi M, Wells AU, Tomassetti S, Gurioli C, Piciucchi S, et al. Safety and diagnostic yield of transbronchial lung cryobiopsy in diffuse parenchymal lung diseases: a comparative study versus video-assisted thoracoscopic lung biopsy and a systematic review of the literature. *Respiration* (2016) 91(3):215–27. doi:10.1159/000444089
50. Johannson KA, Marcoux VS, Ronksley PE, Ryerson CJ. Diagnostic yield and complications of transbronchial lung cryobiopsy for interstitial lung disease. A systematic review and metaanalysis. *Ann Am Thorac Soc* (2016) 13:1828–38. doi:10.1513/AnnalsATS.201606-461SR
51. Poletti V, Hetzel J. Transbronchial cryobiopsy in diffuse parenchymal lung disease: need for procedural standardization. *Respiration* (2015) 90(4): 275–8. doi:10.1159/000439313
52. Rosas IO, Richards TJ, Konishi K, Zhang Y, Gibson K, Lokshin AE, et al. MMP1 and MMP7 as potential peripheral blood biomarkers in idiopathic pulmonary fibrosis. *PLoS Med* (2008) 5(4):e93. doi:10.1371/journal.pmed.0050093
53. White ES, Xia M, Murray S, Dyal R, Flaherty CM, Flaherty KR, et al. Plasma surfactant protein-D, matrix metalloproteinase-7, and osteopontin index distinguishes idiopathic pulmonary fibrosis from other idiopathic interstitial pneumonias. *Am J Respir Crit Care Med* (2016) 194(10):1242–51. doi:10.1164/rccm.201505-0862OC
54. Tzouvelekis A, Herazo-Maya JD, Slade M, Chu JH, Deiuliis G, Ryu C, et al. Validation of the prognostic value of MMP-7 in idiopathic pulmonary fibrosis. *Respirology* (2017) 22(3):486–93. doi:10.1111/resp.12920
55. Tzouvelekis A, Herazo-Maya J, Sakamoto K, Bouros D. Biomarkers in the evaluation and management of idiopathic pulmonary fibrosis. *Curr Top Med Chem* (2016) 16(14):1587–98. doi:10.2174/1568026616666150930120959
56. Tzouvelekis A, Tzilas V, Papiris S, Aidinis V, Bouros D. Diagnostic and prognostic challenges in idiopathic pulmonary fibrosis: a patient's "Q and A" approach. *Pulm Pharmacol Ther* (2017) 42:21–4. doi:10.1016/j.pupt.2016.12.002

7

Targeting Growth Factor and Cytokine Pathways to Treat Idiopathic Pulmonary Fibrosis

Hongbo Ma[1,2†], *Shengming Liu*[1,2†], *Shanrui Li*[1,2†] *and Yong Xia*[1,3]*

[1]Department of Rehabilitation Medicine, West China Hospital, Sichuan University, Chengdu, China, [2]West China School of Pharmacy, Sichuan University, Chengdu, China, [3]Key Laboratory of Rehabilitation Medicine in Sichuan Province/Rehabilitation Medicine Research Institute, Chengdu, China

***Correspondence:**
Yong Xia
yxia4@scu.edu.cn

†These authors have contributed equally to this work and share first authorship

Idiopathic pulmonary fibrosis (IPF) is a chronic interstitial lung disease of unknown origin that usually results in death from secondary respiratory failure within 2–5 years of diagnosis. Recent studies have identified key roles of cytokine and growth factor pathways in the pathogenesis of IPF. Although there have been numerous clinical trials of drugs investigating their efficacy in the treatment of IPF, only Pirfenidone and Nintedanib have been approved by the FDA. However, they have some major limitations, such as insufficient efficacy, undesired side effects and poor pharmacokinetic properties. To give more insights into the discovery of potential targets for the treatment of IPF, this review provides an overview of cytokines, growth factors and their signaling pathways in IPF, which have important implications for fully exploiting the therapeutic potential of targeting cytokine and growth factor pathways. Advances in the field of cytokine and growth factor pathways will help slow disease progression, prolong life, and improve the quality of life for IPF patients in the future.

Keywords: cytokine, growth factor, signaling pathway, clinical trials, idiopathic pulmonary fibrosis, emerging pharmacotherapy

1 INTRODUCTION

Idiopathic pulmonary fibrosis (IPF) is a chronic, progressive fibrotic interstitial lung disease of unknown etiology that usually results in death from secondary respiratory failure within 2–5 years of diagnosis (Meltzer and Noble, 2008). It is a rare familial and sporadic disease. CT imaging of IPF usually shows a typical usual interstitial pneumonia (UIP) pattern, characterized by irregular reticular opacities with obligatory honeycombing, associated with traction bronchiectasis. IPF also exhibits histological features of UIP/IPF pattern characterized by dense fibrosis causing architecture remodeling with frequent honeycombing, patchy lung involvement by fibrosis, subpleural and/or paraseptal distribution, fibroblast foci at the edge of dense scars (Spagnolo et al., 2018; Baratella et al., 2021). With extensive basic and clinical research on the pathogenesis of IPF in recent years, some potential therapeutic targets have been discovered (Wang et al., 2021). A large number of these targets are growth factors, cytokines, and their signaling pathways, including TGF-β, CTGF, IL-13, CCL-2, leukotriene receptor, lipid proinflammatory mediators, and their downstream signaling. In addition, targeting pentraxin 2, galectin-3, oxidative stress, and B cell-mediated autoimmunity showed the potential to treat IPF. Lots of investigational drugs have entered clinical trials to test their efficacies in IPF therapy. However, there are only two currently approved IPF drugs, Pirfenidone and Nintedanib. They both slow the progression of IPF but are not able to reverse lung fibrosis (Chu et al., 2020). Lung transplantation is the only option for patients with end-stage IPF, but the donor organ shortages are an intractable problem worldwide, which means only a minority of patients have the opportunity to undergo lung transplantation (Spagnolo et al., 2018). In addition, lung transplantation is expensive, and the 10-year survival rate after surgery is only 33%–55% (Lederer and Martinez, 2018; Villavicencio et al., 2018). Therefore, there is still an urgent need to develop new drugs to treat IPF.

Although the pathophysiological mechanism of IPF remains unknown, significant progress in understanding the pathogenesis of IPF has been made in the last decade. The current paradigm assumes that recurrent alveolar epithelial cell injury and the crosstalk between dysregulated epithelial cells and mesenchymal, immune, endothelial cells can trigger abnormal wound healing responses and pulmonary fibrosis *via* multiple signaling pathways- (Mei et al., 2021; Moss et al., 2022). The pathogenesis of IPF is believed to be mediated by various cytokines, chemokines, and growth factors (Kelly et al., 2003). Cytokines and growth factors regulate the phenotypic switch of fibroblasts and alveolar epithelial cells (AECs), the recruitment and proliferation of mesenchymal cells, and the deposition and degradation of matrix through multiple mechanisms. Uncoordinated expression of several cytokines may be responsible for the severe matrix remodeling and epithelial-mesenchymal crosstalk in the lung microenvironment of IPF. Although the efficacy of previous anti-inflammatory treatments (e.g., TNF-α neutralization, immunosuppressants) and immunomodulatory treatments (e.g., interferon-γ) in clinical trials for the treatment of IPF has been unsatisfactory, targeting these pathways remains promising. Pirfenidone and Nintedanib, two small-molecule drugs that block multiple cytokine and growth factor signaling pathways, have been approved to slow the progression of pulmonary fibrosis. However, they have obvious defects, such as poor specificity caused by multiple targets and large doses, which lead to undesired side effects. Therefore, it is still necessary to explore the mechanism of the cytokine/growth factor pathway in IPF to find promising targets and develop targeted drugs.

Due to the pivotal role of the cytokine/growth factor pathway in the pathogenesis of IPF, this review comprehensively introduces the association of various growth factors, chemokines, interleukins, lipid proinflammatory mediators and their related signaling pathways with IPF. Related signaling pathways are also attractive therapeutic targets, including RTK and non-RTK pathways, Hedgehog pathway, Wnt pathway and Notch pathway, PI3K/Akt/mTOR pathway, MAPK pathway, and Hippo YAP/TAZ pathway. A large number of drugs, including many small molecules and biologics targeting cytokine/growth factor signaling pathways, have entered clinical trials to determine their efficacy against IPF, as described in this review. Taken together, the aim of this review is to provide an overview of cytokines, growth factors, and the related signaling pathways in IPF, thus providing a basis for the development of novel treatment options to alleviate or even reverse IPF.

2 THE PATHOLOGICAL PROCESS OF IDIOPATHIC PULMONARY FIBROSIS

The complexity of the pathological process of pulmonary fibrosis lies in how crosstalk between epithelial-mesenchymal cells and multiple imbalanced cytokines contribute to the disease. First, alveolar epithelial cells (AECs) are damaged, and the continuity of the basement membrane is interrupted due to a variety of external stimuli, such as radiation, the microbiome, allergens, environmental particles, autoimmunity, antineoplastic drugs (Wilson and Wynn, 2009), and SARS-CoV2 (George et al., 2020). Then, many cytokines and growth factors are released by AECs to recruit and activate inflammatory cells and fibroblasts. Inflammatory cells and some coagulation factors [e.g., tissue factors (TF) and plasminogen activation inhibitors (PAI-1)] are jointly involved in the formation of wound clots (King et al., 2011b; Betensley et al., 2016). Activated AECs and endothelial cells participate in (myo)fibroblast migration, proliferation, and differentiation.

Under normal physiological conditions, the repair process of local lesions is controlled, but in IPF, epithelial-mesenchymal transition (EMT) and differentiation of fibroblasts into myofibroblasts occur, promoting the expansion of myofibroblast population which is the main source of extracellular matrix (ECM) (Yagihashi et al., 2016; Skibba et al., 2020). Notably, EMT may be an indirect mechanism of IPF, because it does not directly contribute to the expansion of the myofibroblast population *via* the epithelial-to-myofibroblasts transition (Rock et al., 2011; Salton et al., 2020). In contrast, EMT is indirectly involved in the pathological process of IPF through the paracrine of fibroblast activating factor (Hill et al., 2019). It has also been reported that EMT is the result of aberrant mechanical forces and signaling pathways in IPF (Qian et al., 2020; Saito et al., 2020; Salton et al., 2020; Su et al., 2020; Wu et al., 2020). Due to the presence of excess fibrin in the ECM, the lung elasticity of IPF patients decreases, which manifests as alveolar collapse and the cystic dilation of residual bronchioles/alveoli. This alveolar collapse leads to a decrease in the effective volume of the alveoli used for gas exchange. Moreover, matrix stiffness forms a positive feedback pathway through the mechanosensor transient receptor potential vanilloid 4 (TRPV4) and α6 integrin, which continuously aggravates pulmonary fibrosis (Rahaman et al., 2014; Chen et al., 2016), causing the loss of pulmonary function (respiratory ventilation) in IPF patients. In addition, excessive ECM encapsulates pulmonary capillaries, resulting in a decrease in the diffusion coefficients of oxygen and carbon dioxide and the loss of gas exchange function in the alveoli, eventually leading to the death of IPF patients from respiratory failure or related syndromes. If injury factors persist, AECs are continuously damaged, often manifesting as AEC death, an increase in the proportion of type II AECs (AT II), and impaired reepithelization (Liu et al., 2017). Therefore, different from normal repair, the repair processes involved in IPF are uncontrolled, continuous, and abnormal.

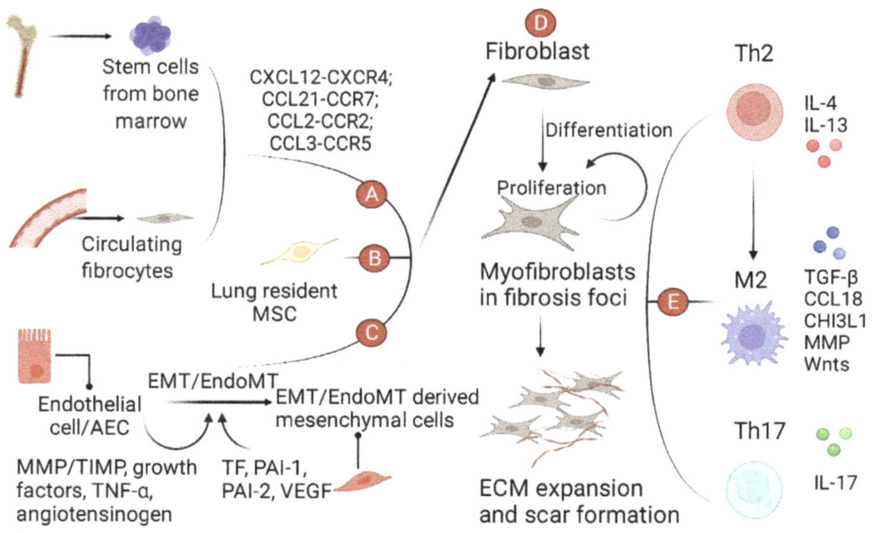

FIGURE 1 | A schematic view of the role of various cells, growth factors and cytokines in IPF. **(A)** Bone marrow-derived mesenchymal progenitor cells and circulating fibrocytes in the peripheral circulation are recruited to the lung by the chemokine-chemokine receptor axis. **(B)** Lung resident MSCs. **(C)** EMT/EndoMT-derived mesenchymal cells. **(D)** Cells from the above three sources aggregate, proliferate, and differentiate into myofibroblasts in the lung, ultimately leading to ECM expansion and scarring. **(E)** Immune cells and cytokines involved in IPF.

A large number of cytokines and their signaling pathways are directly involved in the accumulation of fibroblasts in lung fibrosis foci (**Figure 1**). Fibroblasts are the culprits directly involved in pulmonary fibrosis, and their sources include stem cells recruited from the bone marrow, fibrocytes recruited from the peripheral circulation, mesenchymal stem cells (MSCs) residing in the lung, and EMT/EndoMT-derived interstitial cells. Plasma cells, etc. The CXCL12-CXCR4 axis (Phillips et al., 2004), CCL2-CCR2 axis (Chong et al., 2019), CCL3-CCR5 axis (Ishida et al., 2007; Besnard et al., 2013), and CCL21-CCR7 axis (Ziegenhagen et al., 1998; Habiel and Hogaboam, 2014) are directly involved in the recruitment of fibroblasts. EMT/EndoMT of epithelial and endothelial cells is affected by the coagulation cascade and angiogenesis-related cytokines (TF, PAI-1, and VEGF) and secretion released by AECs (TGF-β, growth factors, TNF-α, MMP/TIMP, and angiotensinogen), which are implicated in multiple signaling pathways (TGF-β, Wnt, SHH, Notch, and ER stress/UPR pathways) (King et al., 2011b; Selman and Pardo, 2014; Betensley et al., 2016).

Growth factors and cytokines are an integral part of the fibrotic microenvironment, which leads to differences in the phenotype of immune cells in the alveoli between patients with pulmonary fibrosis and healthy individuals. Th1/Th2 imbalance and M1-M2 polarization are hallmarks of pulmonary fibrosis. Th2 polarization is characterized by increased secretion of IL-4 and IL-13 and decreased secretion of IFN-γ. M2 polarization can be induced by the microenvironment shaped by Th2 polarization and promotes pulmonary fibrosis through the production of TGF-β, CCL18, chitinase 3-like 1 (CHI3L1), MMPs, and activation of the Wnt/β-catenin pathway (Shenderov et al., 2021). Th17 cells can promote fibroblast proliferation and ECM secretion by secreting IL-17 (Zhang et al., 2019a). In recent years, polymorphisms in immune-related genes have also been reported to be involved in the process of pulmonary fibrosis. For example, an increased risk or severity of IPF is associated with polymorphisms in the TLR3, Toll-interacting protein (TOLLIP), and interleukin-1 receptor antagonist (IL-1RA) genes (Whyte et al., 2000; Korthagen et al., 2012; Noth et al., 2013; O'Dwyer et al., 2013). In addition, activation of TLR2 and TLR9 has been reported to show profibrotic effects, whereas TLR3 has antifibrotic effects (Karampitsakos et al., 2017).

3 THE KEY ROLE OF THE TGF-β SIGNALING PATHWAY IN IDIOPATHIC PULMONARY FIBROSIS

Transforming growth factor-β (TGF-β) is a potent profibrogenic cytokine that plays a central role in the development of pulmonary fibrosis by promoting fibroblast proliferation and phenotype modulation, stimulating the deposition of ECM, and participating in crosstalk with other cytokines and signaling pathways (Ong et al., 2021).

3.1 A Brief Introduction to TGF-β Signalling Pathway

The activation of TGF-β pathway includes five steps, including i) synthesis of TGF-β, ii) activation of latent TGF-β, iii) interaction between TGF-β and TGF-β receptor (TBR), iv) activation of classical and non-classical pathways, and v) regulation of nuclear transcription factors and cell

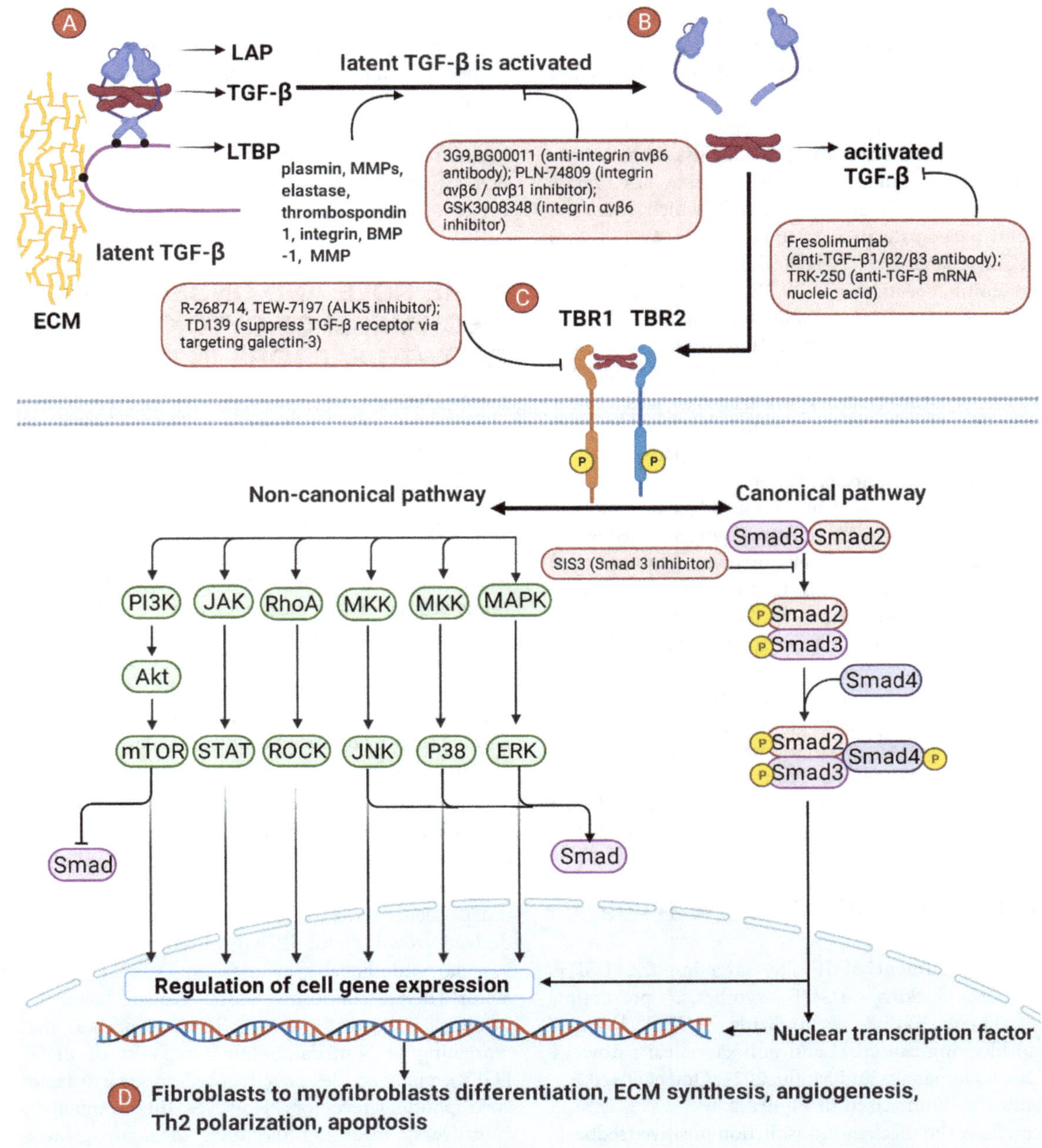

FIGURE 2 | The critical role of the TGF-β pathway and drugs targeting the TGF-β pathway in IPF. **(A)** Latent TGF-β (TGF-β trapped in LAP) binds to ECM through LTBP. **(B)** TGF-β is detached from LAP and activated only in the presence of specific stimuli. **(C)** Activated TGF-β activates the downstream Smad-dependent pathway (canonical pathway) and Smad-independent pathway (non-canonical pathway) by combining with TBR. **(D)** The TGF-β pathway ultimately causes phenotypic reprogramming of AECs, fibroblasts and immune cells and influences fibroblast-to-myofibroblast differentiation, ECM synthesis, angiogenesis, Th2 polarization, and apoptosis.

phenotypes. A brief introduction to the TGF-β pathway is as follows and shown in **Figure 2**.

i) In the endoplasmic reticulum (ER), TGF-β precursors are assembled into dimers wrapped with latency-associated peptides (LAPs). TGF-β-LAPs bind to latent TGF-β binding protein (LTBP) and undergo intracellular proteolytic cleavage by the endopeptidase furin. Then, TGF-β-LAP-LTBPs are secreted into the extracellular medium and eventually bind to ECM (e.g., fibrillin and fibronectin) through LTBP. At this time, latent TGF-β cannot exert its biological function (Derynck and Zhang, 2003).

ii) Latent TGF-β is activated under special conditions [e.g., plasmin (Coutts et al., 2001), thrombospondin 1 (Murphy-Ullrich and Suto, 2018), elastase, integrin, BMP-1 and MMP 2 (Tzavlaki and Moustakas, 2020)] and binds to TGF-β receptor 2 (TBR2).
iii) TBR2 can phosphorylate TGF-β receptor 1 (TBR1) and activate the downstream classical and non-classical pathways.
iv) In classical pathways, Smad2/Smad3 activated by TBR1 binds to Smad4 to form Smad2/Smad3/Smad4, which enter the nucleus and participate in regulating transcription factors (Derynck and Zhang, 2003). Classical pathways also involve Smad7, ubiquitin, coactivator P100, PPAR-γ, Ski/SnoN, and other signal-regulating molecules (Tzavlaki and Moustakas, 2020). In non-classical pathways, TGF-β can activate many signaling pathways, such as the Ras-Raf-Mek1/2-ERK1/2 pathway, TAK1-MKK3/6-P38 pathway, TAK1-MKK4-JNK pathway, and PI3K-Akt-mTOR pathway (Derynck and Zhang, 2003; Ong et al., 2021), and participate in regulating nuclear transcription factors.
v) Some transcription factors of fibroblasts, alveolar epithelial cells, endothelial cells, and Th cells are changed, causing the phenotypic transformation of cells involved in pulmonary fibrosis, which eventually leads to the differentiation of myofibroblasts, the deposition of ECM, the abnormal function of AT II, and an imbalance of immune cells in IPF.

The TGF-β pathway is interrelated with the Wnt/β-catenin pathway, PI3K/Akt pathway, and pathways of other growth factors (Yan et al., 2014). Furthermore, in terms of the pathogenesis of IPF, TGF-β has been implicated in redox imbalance, mitochondrial dysfunction, EMT, MMP/TIMP imbalance, and fibrinolytic system imbalance (Chu et al., 2020).

3.2 Strategies to Treat IPF by Targeting TGF-β Pathway

Strategies for the treatment of IPF by targeting the TGF-β pathway include blocking TGF-β synthesis, preventing activation of latent TGF-β, neutralizing TGF-β ligands/receptors, and blocking canonical and non-canonical pathways (Saito et al., 2018; Hamanaka and Mutlu, 2021; Ong et al., 2021). These strategies are summarized in **Figure 2**.

Integrins mediate the mechanotransduction positive feedback to ECM stiffness in a TGF-β-dependent or TGF-β-independent manner, which is an important therapeutic target. TGF-β-dependent fibrosis is activated by integrins releasing TGF-β through tensile forces generated by actin-cytoskeleton interactions. In the TGF-β-independent pathway, after binding specific ECM ligands to the ectodomain of integrins, integrins bind to the cytoskeleton and various signaling proteins through their cytoplasmic tails, translating the mechanical force of cytoskeleton contraction and ECM stiffness into biochemical signals. Then, F-actin activates the downstream Rho/ROCK-YAP/TAZ signaling pathway *via* FAK phosphorylation, ultimately leading to fibroblast phenotype reprogramming.

There are corresponding preclinical candidate drugs for IPF that target different steps of the TGF-β pathways, including the synthesis, receptor binding, and downstream signal transduction (Ong et al., 2021), but no drug specifically for the TGF-β pathway has been approved due to the side effects of anti-TGF-β treatment (systemic autoimmune, cardiac valve problems, and carcinogenesis) (Henderson et al., 2020). Notably, to avoid systemic autoimmune disease induced by persistent systemic inhibition of TGF-β, it may be necessary to choose the correct dose or duration of treatment, coadminister anti-inflammatory drugs, selectively block TGF-β in targeted organs.

4 THE ROLE AND UNDERLYING MECHANISM OF CYTOKINES AND GROWTH FACTORS IN IDIOPATHIC PULMONARY FIBROSIS

As described above, cytokines, growth factors, and related signaling pathways are intensively involved in the pathogenesis of IPF. Therefore, they might be promising targets to develop novel treatment options for IPF. In this section, we describe the roles of growth factors, chemokines, interleukins, lipid pro-inflammatory mediators, and their signaling pathways in IPF. Many drugs targeting these pathways are in development, and we summarize those that have entered clinical trials to treat patients with IPF. In recent years, therapeutics targeting these pathways have shown many limitations in clinical trials. Therefore, we propose possible approaches to overcome these limitations, aiming to provide insights into the development of therapies with fewer side effects and better efficacy.

4.1 Growth Factors

Growth factors can participate in the development and progression of IPF in TGF-β-dependent or TGF-β-independent ways. These growth factors comprise platelet-derived growth factor (PDGF), fibroblast growth factor (FGF), vascular endothelial growth factor (VEGF), epidermal growth factor (EGF), connective tissue growth factor (CTGF), and insulin-like growth factor (IGF). Due to the successful marketing of Nintedanib (an antagonist of PDGFR/VEGFR/FGFR), many studies have focused on growth factors and their corresponding receptors. However, there remains considerable controversy regarding the roles of many growth factors in promoting fibrosis and resisting fibrosis in IPF. One of the possible reasons for the controversy is that there are many subtypes of these growth factors and their receptors, and the functions of different subtypes differ. Although pharmacological analysis of these subtypes of growth factors is difficult, it is a vital step toward precise treatment and personalized treatment, which is of substantial significance. Next, we introduce the crucial growth factors PDGF, FGF, VEGF, EGF, and CTGF in detail.

4.1.1 Platelet-Derived Growth Factor

Platelet-derived growth factor (PDGF) is a key growth factor that stimulates the proliferation and migration of fibroblasts. In a mouse model of bleomycin-induced IPF, RT–PCR (Maeda et al., 1996), PDGF antibody neutralization (Walsh et al., 1993), and Northern blotting (Zhuo et al., 2004) all demonstrated increased protein or mRNA expression of multiple subtypes of PDGF. However, the main subtypes of PDGF found in these experiments differed slightly, and the specific mechanism requires further research. A clinical study also observed that the high expression of PDGF was correlated with a low overall survival rate (Zhu et al., 2017).

Single strands encoded by the PDGF-A, B, C, and D genes can be combined in pairs to form five types of dimers, AA/BB/AB/CC/DD (Heldin and Westermark, 1999; Li and Eriksson, 2003; Günther et al., 2012). PDGFRs (PDGF receptors) are also homo/heterodimerically formed by combinations of single-chain PDGF-α/PDGF-β. After PDGF binds to the PDGF receptor, PDGFR dimerization can be induced; subsequently, the two PDGFRs after autophosphorylation can couple various downstream signal transduction pathways (Heldin and Westermark, 1999), such as Ras-mitogen-activated protein kinase (MAPK) through Grb2 and Shc adaptor proteins and PI3K and phospholipase C-γ (PLCγ) (Nishioka et al., 2013). PDGFR also participates in the migration and chemotaxis of fibroblasts through the integrin-FAK pathway. PDGF, as the main mitogen, can strongly promote the proliferation of fibroblasts and stimulate collagen synthesis (Heldin and Westermark, 1999). PDGF also participates in cell migration through Ca^{2+} influx and cytoskeleton rearrangement (Nishioka et al., 2013).

4.1.2 Fibroblast Growth Factor

FGFs have been divided into seven subgroups encoded by 22 mammalian genomes. Among the 22 FGFs encoded by genomes, 4 FGFs are FGFR-independent, and the remaining 18 extracellular FGFs bind to 7 FGFR subtypes (FGFR1b, FGFR1c, FGFR2b, FGFR2c, FGFR3b, FGFR3c, and FGFRR4). An FGF can bind to multiple FGFRs. FGFs rely on heparan sulfate proteoglycan (HSPG) and Klotho-type coreceptors to improve their binding to FGFRs (Ornitz and Itoh, 2022). After FGF-FGFR binding, through the autophosphorylation of FGFRs, with the help of FGFR substrate 2 and PLCγ, signals are transferred to the RAS-ERK, PI3K/AKT, PKC, and JAK-STAT signaling cascades, which mediate the survival, proliferation, differentiation, or migration of cells (Inomata et al., 2015; Katoh, 2018).

Subtypes of FGFs have functional differences and play different roles in IPF (Yang et al., 2021). FGF1 (acid FGF or aFGF) has an anti-fibrotic function. The serum FGF1 level of patients with IPF was found to be higher than that of the control group (Shimbori et al., 2016). In rat models induced by TGF-β1, FGF1 could relieve IPF by inhibiting the TGF-β1 signaling pathway and promoting the proliferation of AECs (Shimbori et al., 2016). Further research found that "FGF1 + heparin treatment" could reverse EMT through the MAPK/ERK kinase pathway, leading to phosphorylation of ERK-1 and dephosphorylation of Smad2 (Ramos et al., 2010). FGF2 (basic FGF or bFGF) has a proliferative effect on lung fibroblasts (Hetzel et al., 2005; Khalil et al., 2005), and soluble FGFR2c significantly reduces TGF-β-induced IPF in mice (Ju et al., 2012). However, it has also been reported that FGF2 is antifibrotic in part through decreased collagen expression and fibroblast to myofibroblast differentiation (Koo et al., 2018). FGF9 and FGF18 promote the survival and migration of HLFs and inhibit myofibroblast differentiation *in vitro* (Joannes et al., 2016). More FGF9 was expressed in lung tissue myofibroblasts in patients with IPF than in healthy individuals, and it promoted epithelial cell growth and expansion of pulmonary interstitial through the Wnt7B/β-catenin signaling pathway (Yin et al., 2008). FGF10 plays an antifibrotic role *via* autocrine and paracrine signaling. During autocrine signaling, by activating peroxisome proliferator-activated receptor γ (PPAR γ), FGF10 blocks the lipofibroblast-to-myofibroblast transformation induced by TGF-β1 and promotes the transformation from myofibroblasts to lipofibroblasts. In addition, the FGF10 paracrine signal was considered crucial to the differentiation of alveolar epithelial progenitor cells during development and the maintenance of AT II in a steady state (Wu et al., 2018). FGF21 attenuates the TGF-β pathway *via* decreased oxidative stress in bleomycin-induced pulmonary fibrosis in mice (Zhang et al., 2018). Coadministration of FGF23 and its coreceptor α-Klotho led to a significant reduction in fibrosis and inflammation (Barnes et al., 2019).

In summary, FGF1, FGF10, FGF21, and FGF23 are anti-fibrotic, while FGF2, FGF9, and FGF18 exhibit contradictory functions.

4.1.3 Vascular Endothelial Growth Factor

The VEGF family has seven members: VEGF-A, VEGF-B, VEGF-C, VEGF-D, VEGF-E, placental growth factor, and snake venom vascular endothelial growth factors (Inomata et al., 2015). Most studies have focused on the correlation between VEGF-A and IPF; thus, our description mainly focuses on VEGF-A. The most studied and dominant VEGF-A165 can be divided into VEGF-A165a and VEGF-A165b by the splice site. VEGF-A165a can promote angiogenesis, and VEGF-A165b can inhibit angiogenesis.

VEGF-A can bind to VEGFR1 (Flt-1), VEGFR2 (KDR or Flk1), and their coreceptors neuropilin-1 and neuropilin-2. Among them, VEGFR1 binds to circulating VEGF-α and reduces its bioavailability to VEGFR2. The coreceptors neuropilin-1 and neuropilin-2 assist in the signal transduction of VEGFR1 and VEGFR2. After binding to VEGFR2, VEGF-A165 can activate the downstream Akt pathway, Src signaling pathway, NCK and the p38 MAPK pathway, and integrin/FAK pathway (Fruttiger, 2008; Barratt et al., 2018). VEGF can stimulate the growth of alveolar epithelial type II cells and the production of alveolar surfactant, form new blood vessels, and help epithelial cells and endothelial cells resist apoptosis (Gerber et al., 1998a; Gerber et al., 1998b; Brown et al., 2001; Compernolle et al., 2002; Alavi et al., 2003; Mura et al., 2006; Roberts et al., 2007; Kuhn et al., 2010; Varet et al., 2010; Barratt et al., 2018).

Many contradictory effects of VEGF-A on IPF have been observed in animal models and clinical trials. The possible reasons for these differences are as follows: different animal models, different sampling sites, heterogeneity within and between individuals, and different VEGF-A subtypes caused by diverse splice sites. Different subtypes of VEGF-A may have mutually coordinated pathophysiological relationships. In *in vitro* experiments, VEGF-A165a has been proven to promote the proliferation of AT II and fibroblasts, increase the expansion of ECM, and play a role in promoting fibrosis, and VEGF-A165b could counteract this effect (Varet et al., 2010; Barratt et al., 2017). Thus, VEGF-A165b may be a compensatory protective mechanism.

4.1.4 Epidermal Growth Factor

The EGF receptor (EGFR, also known as ErbB1 or HER1) belongs to the ErbB family receptor tyrosine kinases. EGFR has seven corresponding ligands: EGF, transforming growth factor-α (TGF-α), amphiregulin, betacellulin (BTC), epiregulin, epigen, and heparin-binding EGF-like growth factor (HB-EGF). After ligands bind to EGFR, the autophosphorylation of EGFR can activate the downstream MAPK, Akt, and JNK pathways and promote cell proliferation (Iwamoto and Mekada, 2012).

The relationship between the ErbB family (HER) and IPF remains unclear and thus requires further research. After blocking HER *in vivo*, studies have found that collagen deposition decreases and lung morphology improves, which indirectly indicates that the ErbB family plays a role in fibrosis (Rice et al., 1999; Faress et al., 2007). In addition, in patients with IPF, the mRNA level of EGFR was upregulated in proliferative alveolar epithelial cells around fibrosis, and the mRNA level of EGFR was positively correlated with the mRNA level of type I collagen and negatively correlated with the clinical prognosis (Tzouvelekis et al., 2013).

4.1.5 Connective Tissue Growth Factor

CTGF, also known as CNN2, HCS24, or IGFBP8, belongs to the CNN family. CTGF can interact with a wide range of ECM components, but this also means that the biological action of CTGF is highly dependent on the local microenvironment. CTGF directly binds to other growth factors (e.g., TGF-β, BMPs, and VEGF), which influence signal emission/transduction (Choi, 2012). CTGF can be secreted by interstitial cells, such as proliferating AT II and activated fibroblasts (Pan et al., 2001). The peak of CTGF content mainly appears at the early stage of IPF, and the peak of CTGF appears earlier than the deposition of collagen in the lungs (Wang et al., 2011), which indicates that CTGF may be involved in the early-stage repair of lung tissue injury.

As an auxiliary regulator of TGF-β in IPF in the local microenvironment, CTGF can participate in abnormal tissue repair processes, such as ECM generation and the mobilization of fibroblasts, by assisting TGF-β (Wang et al., 2011). There was an interaction between TGF-β and CTGF in IPF animal models induced by TGF-β/bleomycin, and IPF could be alleviated by the CTGF antibody (FG-3019, pamrevlumab) (Wang et al., 2011). CTGF-deficient transgenic mice had the ability to resist IPF induced by bleomycin (Liu et al., 2011). Therefore, a general belief is that CTGF, as a fibrosis-promoting medium, is a possible target for the research and development of anti-IPF drugs. Pamrevlumab, a human recombinant mAb of CTGF, is the only antibody drug that has shown activity in a phase II clinical trial against IPF. In a recent randomized, placebo-controlled phase II trial for patients with IPF, pamrevlumab showed good safety and certain therapeutic effects, such as slowing the decline of pulmonary function and delaying the progression of fibrosis by HR-CT, which is a milestone of single-target therapy (Lipson et al., 2012; Raghu et al., 2016). The phase III clinical trial of pamrevlumab for IPF is at the recruitment stage (NCT04419558/NCT03955146).

4.2 Chemokines and Chemokine Receptors

Chemokines are small molecule proteins with chemotactic effects on specific cells, and there are four conserved cysteine residues. According to the differences in cysteine residues, chemokines have been divided into four main subfamilies: CXC, CC, CX3C, and XC. Although the role of some chemokines in IPF remains unknown, many studies have demonstrated that chemokines can promote fibrosis or resist fibrosis. It has been reported that pulmonary fibrosis in animal models can be attenuated by knocking out genes encoding chemokines or neutralizing chemokines with antibodies [CCL2-CCR2 (Moore et al., 2001; Murray et al., 2008; Phan et al., 2021), CCL11-CCR3 (Huaux et al., 2005), CCL17 (Agostini and Gurrieri, 2006), CCL21-CCR7 (Habiel and Hogaboam, 2014), CCL22 (Strieter, 2005), CXCL6 (Besnard et al., 2013), CXCL12 (Phillips et al., 2004), CXCL14 (Li et al., 2019), CX3CL1-CX3CR1 (Rivas-Fuentes et al., 2020), CCR5 (Ishida et al., 2007)]. The CXCL11-CXCR3 axis has anti-pulmonary fibrosis effects in a mouse model of bleomycin-induced pulmonary fibrosis (Strieter, 2005).

Chemokines play a crucial role in the pathological process of IPF (**Figure 3**). CXCL12-CXCR4 (Phillips et al., 2004), CCL2-CCR2 (Chong et al., 2019) CCL3-CCR5 (Ishida et al., 2007; Besnard et al., 2013), CCL11-CCR3 (Puxeddu et al., 2006), CCL21-CCR7 (Ziegenhagen et al., 1998; Habiel and Hogaboam, 2014), CCL26 (Kohan et al., 2010) promote the migration of fibrocytes to the lung, whereas CXCL10 (Agostini and Gurrieri, 2006) inhibits the migration of fibrocytes to the lung. CCL2-CCR2 (Hambly et al., 2015), CCL11 (Puxeddu et al., 2006), CCL21-CCR7 (Ziegenhagen et al., 1998; Habiel and Hogaboam, 2014), CCL24 (Kohan et al., 2010) promote fibroblast proliferation. CCL18 (Hambly et al., 2015) and CCL21-CCR7 (Ziegenhagen et al., 1998; Habiel and Hogaboam, 2014) participate in the differentiation of fibroblasts to myofibroblasts and stimulate collagen synthesis. CCL21-CCR7 is involved in the survival of fibroblasts (Ziegenhagen et al., 1998; Habiel and Hogaboam, 2014). CCL2-CCR2 (Agostini and Gurrieri, 2006; Besnard et al., 2013; Hambly et al., 2015), CCL3-CCR5 (Ishida et al., 2007), CCL17-CCR4 (Karman et al., 2021), CCL22-CCR4 (Yogo et al., 2009), CX3CL1-CX3CR1 (Rivas-Fuentes et al., 2020) promote migration of monocytes and macrophages. CCL2 (Rose et al., 2003), CCL17 (Besnard et al., 2013), CCL22 (Besnard et al., 2013), CCR3 (Fulkerson et al., 2006), CCR4 (Yoshinouchi et al., 2007) are involved in type 2 immunity, whereas CCR5 (Loetscher et al., 1998) is involved in type 1 immunity. CXCR3 counteracts the profibrotic effect of IL-13 by assisting IL-13 receptor α2 gene expression (Pignatti et al., 2006; Yoshinouchi et al., 2007; Barnes et al., 2015). A phase II clinical trial of CNTO 888 (CCL2 mAb) failed to provide benefit to FVC in IPF patients (NCT00786201).

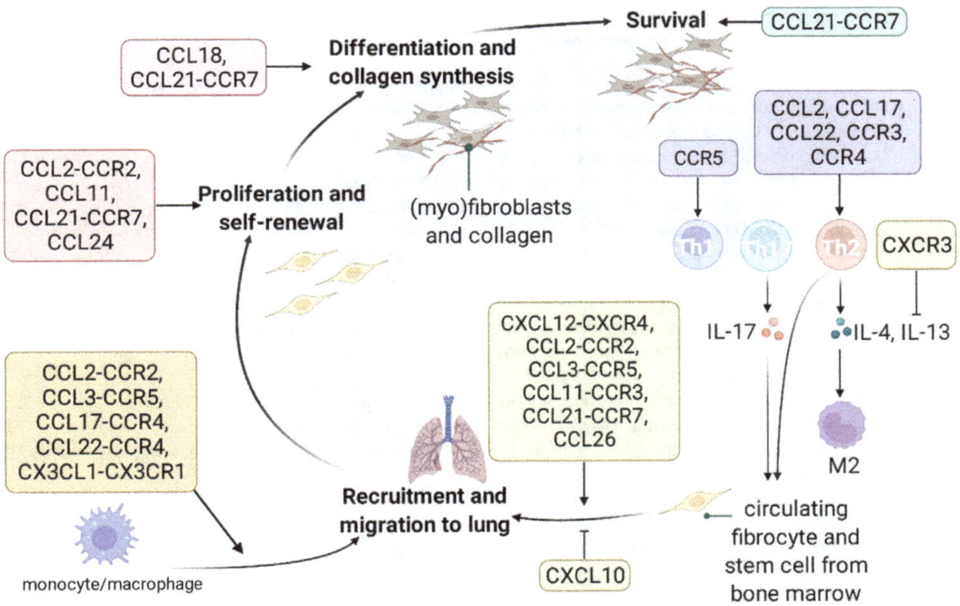

FIGURE 3 | The role and underlying mechanisms of chemokines in IPF. Chemokines are involved in recruitment, proliferation, differentiation, collagen synthesis, survival of fibroblasts, regulation of type 1 and 2 immune balance, and recruitment of monocytes and macrophages.

Nonetheless, the role of chemokines in IPF remains to be further investigated.

4.3 Interleukins

Interleukins are a class of cytokines generated by lymphocytes, monocytes, and other non-monocytes. In addition to affecting fibrosis by modulating the Th1/Th2 balance, many studies have shown that interleukins can also directly affect fibroblasts and epithelial cells (**Table 1**). Thus, interleukins are expected to be developed as drugs and biomarkers for treating IPF.

However, clinical trials of IPF treatments targeting IL-4 and IL-13 have not gone well. Several drugs targeting IL-13 have entered clinical trials for IPF, but none of them have shown protective effects on lung function. Although clinical trials of IPF antibody drugs have mostly failed in phase II, there is still hope for interleukin therapy. Inhibition of IL-11 blocks TGF-β1, PDGF, FGF2, IL-13, OSM (Oncostatin M), and endothelin 1-mediated fibroblast activation (Ng et al., 2019).

Notably, interleukin supplementation alone may not reverse the profibrotic phenotype of cells, and the regulation of cell–cell interactions or phenotypic transformation may be more promising. In addition, anti-inflammatory interleukins should be used with caution in clinical trials, and attention should be given to their side effects on patient immune function. In addition, rational design of interleukin dosage forms is very important because the concentration of the drug in the lungs can explain some of the differences in the study results.

4.4 Lipid Proinflammatory Mediators

Various lipids and their metabolic derivatives play vital roles in IPF. Although glucocorticoids (PLA2 inhibitor) have not shown positive effects in the treatment of IPF in clinical trials, these findings do not indicate that all lipid metabolism pathways have no significance as therapeutic targets of IPF. In contrast, metabolomic studies on fibroblasts have received increasing attention in recent years.

LT and PG are implicated in the pathogenesis of IPF. In arachidonic acid metabolic pathways, phospholipids produce arachidonic acid under the catalysis of phospholipase A2 (PLA2). Then, arachidonic acid produced leukotriene (LT) and prostaglandin (PG) under the catalysis of 5-lipoxygenase (5-LO) and cyclooxygenase (COX), respectively. Among them, PGF2a and LTs promote fibrosis, and PGE2 resists fibrosis (Suryadevara et al., 2020). A phase II trial (NCT02503657) on the safety and tolerability of Tipelukast/MN-001 (LT receptor inhibitor, 5-LO inhibitor and PDE inhibitor) in patients with IPF is ongoing.

The SPHK1/S1P/S1PR axis is involved in pulmonary fibrosis. In sphingolipid metabolism, sphingosine kinase 1 (SPHK1) phosphorylates sphingosine to produce sphingosine-1-phosphate (S1P). Then, the binding of S1P to the S1P receptor can lead to mitochondrial reactive oxygen species (mtROS) and promote YAP1 entry into cell nuclei, affecting the differentiation of myofibroblasts and matrix remodeling (Huang et al., 2020). Targeting the SPHK1/S1P/S1PR axis, PF543 (SPHK1 inhibitor), Mito TEMPO (mitochondria-targeted superoxide dismutase, which can reduce mtROS) and verteporfin (YAP inhibitor) have been reported, but these drugs have not entered clinical trials on IPF treatment.

TABLE 1 | The role and underlying mechanism of interleukins in IPF.

Interleukins	Pro/anti-fibrotic	Mechanism of action	References
IL-1β	Pro-fibrotic	1) IL-1β-driven pulmonary fibrosis is dependent on IL-17A. 2) Gene polymorphism of IL-1β is associated with risk of IPF	Wilson et al. (2010); Korthagen et al. (2012)
IL-4	Pro-fibrotic	1) IL-4 can promote the synthesis of collagen I/III, fibronectin, and other ECM in fibroblasts. 2) IL-4 is a chemokine for fibroblasts. 3) IL-4-induced macrophage-derived IGF-I protects myofibroblasts from apoptosis	Wynes et al. (2004); Antoniou et al. (2007)
IL-6	Pro-fibrotic	1) The IL-6/STAT3/Smad3 axis has profibrotic effects. 2) IL-6 inhibits apoptosis of IPF-derived fibroblasts and promotes apoptosis of normal fibroblasts. 3) High levels of IL-6 and IL-8 are early features of AE-IPFs and are associated with worse outcome	Moodley et al. (2003); Papiris et al. (2018); Epstein Shochet et al. (2020)
IL-8	Pro-fibrotic	1) IL-8 promotes self-renewal, proliferation, and migration of mesenchymal progenitor cells in an autocrine manner. 2) IL-8 stimulates the recruitment and activation of macrophages in a paracrine manner	Yang et al. (2018)
IL-10	Anti-fibrotic	1) IL-10 has powerful anti-inflammatory effects. 2) IL-10 inhibits collagen I synthesis, although the antifibrotic effect of IL-10 is controversial	Arai et al. (2000); Barbarin et al. (2005); Nakagome et al. (2006); García-Prieto et al. (2010); Li et al. (2011)
IL-11	Pro-fibrotic	IL-11 promotes fibrosis *via* JAK/STAT pathway, Ras/Raf/MEK/ERK1/2 pathway, and PI3K/Akt/mTOR pathway	Ng et al. (2019); Kortekaas et al. (2021)
IL-13	Pro-fibrotic	IL-13 stimulates fibroblast proliferation, and induces TGF-β, PDGF, CTGF, collagen I, and fibronectin production	Murray et al. (2008); Passalacqua et al. (2017)
IL-17	Pro-fibrotic	1) IL-17A promotes cell proliferation, ECM deposition, and myofibroblast differentiation through NF-κb and JAK2 signaling. 2) IL-17B is also involved in dysbiosis of lung microbiota. IL-17 cooperates with TGF-β1-mediated Smad2/3 and ERK1/2 to induce EMT in human pulmonary alveolar epithelial cells	Wilson et al. (2010); Wang et al. (2017); Zhang et al. (2019a); Yang et al. (2019)
IL-18	Pro-fibrotic	IL-18 promotes senescence and SASP in pulmonary fibroblasts by blocking the Klotho pathway	Zhang et al. (2019b)
IL-22	Anti-fibrotic	IL-22 inhibits TGF-β-induced signaling pathways and reduces EMT and myofibroblast differentiation	Gu et al. (2021)
IL-24	Pro-fibrotic	IL-24 cooperates with IL-4 to promote macrophage M2 polarization	Rao et al. (2021)
IL-25	Pro-fibrotic	1) IL-25/IL-33/TSLP$^+$ AECs-IL-25R/IL-33R/TSLPR$^+$ (myo)fibroblasts axis is involved in epithelial-mesenchymal crosstalk. 2) Autocrine IL-25/IL-33/TSLP (thymic stromal lymphopoietin) from alveolar epithelial cells can cause damage and phenotypic changes in alveolar epithelial cells	Xu et al. (2020)
IL-31	Pro-fibrotic	1) IL-31 regulates the transcription of ECM and AECs-related genes. 2) IL-31 can cause collagen deposition and decreased lung function	Yombo et al. (2021)
IL-37	Anti-fibrotic	1) IL-37 resulted in enhanced autophagy and attenuated TGF-β1 of IPF fibroblasts. 2) IL-37 inhibits oxidative stress-induced death of AECs	Kim et al. (2019)

The ATX/LPA/LPAR axis plays a potent role in pulmonary fibrosis. Lysophosphatidic acid (LPA) has been proven to activate G protein-mediated signal transduction pathways by binding to its receptors (LPAR1 and LPAR2), which leads to different reactions from lung cells, including the promotion of the apoptosis of epithelial cells, regulation of endothelial permeability, activation of αvβ6 integrin-mediated TGF-β signaling, secretion of IL-8, and recruitment and survival of fibroblasts (Tager et al., 2008; Ninou et al., 2018). LPA can promote the apoptosis of epithelial cells (Suryadevara et al., 2020). LPA is produced by many metabolic pathways *in vivo*, among which ATX/LPA/LPAR is the main pathway. Phosphatidylcholine (PC) generates LPC (lysophosphatidylcholine) under the action of phospholipase A1/phospholipase A2 (PLA1/PLA2), and LPC is hydrolyzed under the action of autotaxin (ATX)/lysoPLD to generate LPA. LPA exerts biological effects by binding to LPAR (Suryadevara et al., 2020). Drugs targeting different positions of the ATX/LPA/LPAR axis have entered clinical trials. The ATX inhibitors BBT-877 and GLPG1690 entered phase I clinical trials (completed) and phase III clinical trials (terminated) on their anti-IPF treatment, respectively. The LPA1 receptor antagonists BMS-986278 (recruiting) and BMS-986020 (completed) have also entered phase II clinical trials.

5 GROWTH FACTOR AND CYTOKINE SIGNALING CASCADES IN IDIOPATHIC PULMONARY FIBROSIS

5.1 Receptor-Type Tyrosine Kinases and Non-Receptor-Type Tyrosine Kinases Signaling Cascades

Due to the central role of growth factors in IPF, the signaling cascade of growth factor receptors is an indispensable topic. Growth factor receptors (GFRs) are receptor-type tyrosine kinases (RTKs), and their counterparts are non-receptor-type tyrosine kinases (non-RTKs) free in the cytoplasm. Src family kinases (SFKs) are a non-RTK family with eleven members, among which Src, Yes and Fyn are ubiquitously reported (Li et al., 2020). RTK and non-RTK signaling crosstalk with

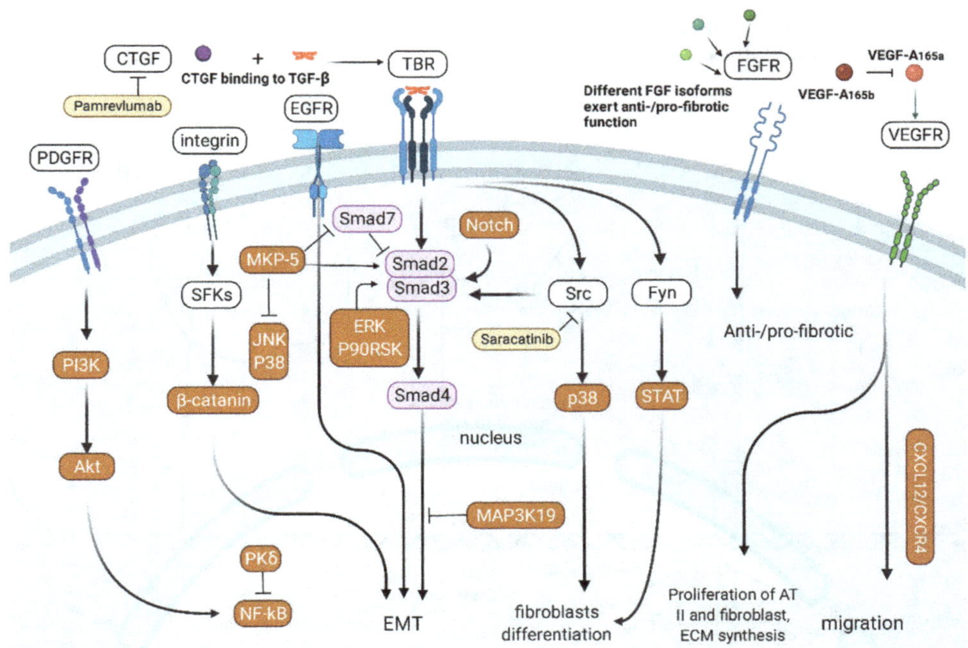

FIGURE 4 | Crosstalk between RTK/non-RTK and other signaling pathways. PDGFR activates NF-κB signaling through the PI3K/Akt pathway. Integrins participate in EMT of epithelial cells through SFK/β-catenin-mediated signaling. TGF-β/Smad signaling interacts with the CTGF, Src, Fyn, and Notch pathways to participate in EMT in epithelial cells. Different subtypes of FGF and VEGF have different pro- or antifibrotic effects.

numerous other pathways and contribute to fibrosis *via* phenotype modulation of fibroblasts and AECs (**Figure 4**).

The combination of TGF-β and TBR can not only initiate the TGF-β/Smad signaling pathway but also indirectly participate in the differentiation of fibroblasts by activating Src/p38 (Pechkovsky et al., 2008) and Fyn/STAT (Xu et al., 2019). Integrins can activate SFKs to activate β-catenin and participate in EMT of epithelial cells (Ulsamer et al., 2012). CTGF participates in abnormal tissue repair by assisting TGF-β. The Notch pathway can also promote TGF-β-mediated fibroblast differentiation through activation of Smads (Aoyagi-Ikeda et al., 2011). MAP3K19 regulates nucleocytoplasmic shuttling of the activated R-Smads, which promotes TGF-β-mediated fibrosis (Boehme et al., 2016). MKP-5, a tyrosine phosphatase negatively regulating the p38 and JNK pathways, inhibits Smad7 activity but promotes Smad3 phosphorylation and the expression of fibrogenic genes (Xylourgidis et al., 2019).

PDGFR activates NF-κB *via* the Src/PI3K/Akt pathway (Cheng et al., 2014). PKCδ attenuates pulmonary fibrosis by enhancing the stability and activity of A20, an inhibitory protein of NF-κB signaling. The PDGFR/mTOR signaling pathway is associated with PINK1/PARP2 dysregulation-induced mitophagy deficiency, leading to myofibroblast differentiation and proliferation (Tsubouchi et al., 2018). Different isoforms of FGF participate in the process of fibrosis through FGFR; for example, FGF1 (Ramos et al., 2010) and FGF10 (Cheng et al., 2014) are anti-fibrotic, while FGF2 is pro-fibrotic (Ju et al., 2012). VEGF-A165a has been proven to promote the proliferation of AT II cells and fibroblasts and ECM expansion, and VEGF-A165b could counteract this effect (Varet et al., 2010; Barratt et al., 2017). VEGFR1 induces pulmonary fibrosis by promoting the migration of VEGFR1+ cells, which is dependent on the SDF-1/CXCR4 axis (Amano et al., 2021). In addition to the above GFR, Gas6/TAM receptor-type tyrosine kinases have also been reported to promote pulmonary fibrosis (Espindola et al., 2018).

5.2 Developmental Pathways: Hedgehog, Wnt, and Notch

Developmental pathways play an important role in the developmental stages of the lung. In adults, some developmental pathways enter a dormant state but are activated again when abnormal lung damage occurs. These signaling pathways include the TGF-β, FGF, Hedgehog, Wnt, and Notch signaling pathways (Chanda et al., 2019) (**Figure 5**). Among them, TGF-β and FGF have been mentioned in the previous section and will not be repeated here.

The Hedgehog pathway starts with the Hedgehog ligand (Hh) and its receptor ptch1 and then activates downstream pathways in a Gli transcription factor-dependent (classical) or independent (non-classical) manner. In the canonical pathway, the binding of Hh to ptch1 relieves the inhibitory effect of ptch1 on Smo. Then, Smo is transferred to the plasma membrane and participates in the regulation of genes in the nucleus by activating full-length Gli to become Gli1/2/3 (active form), thereby inducing AEC

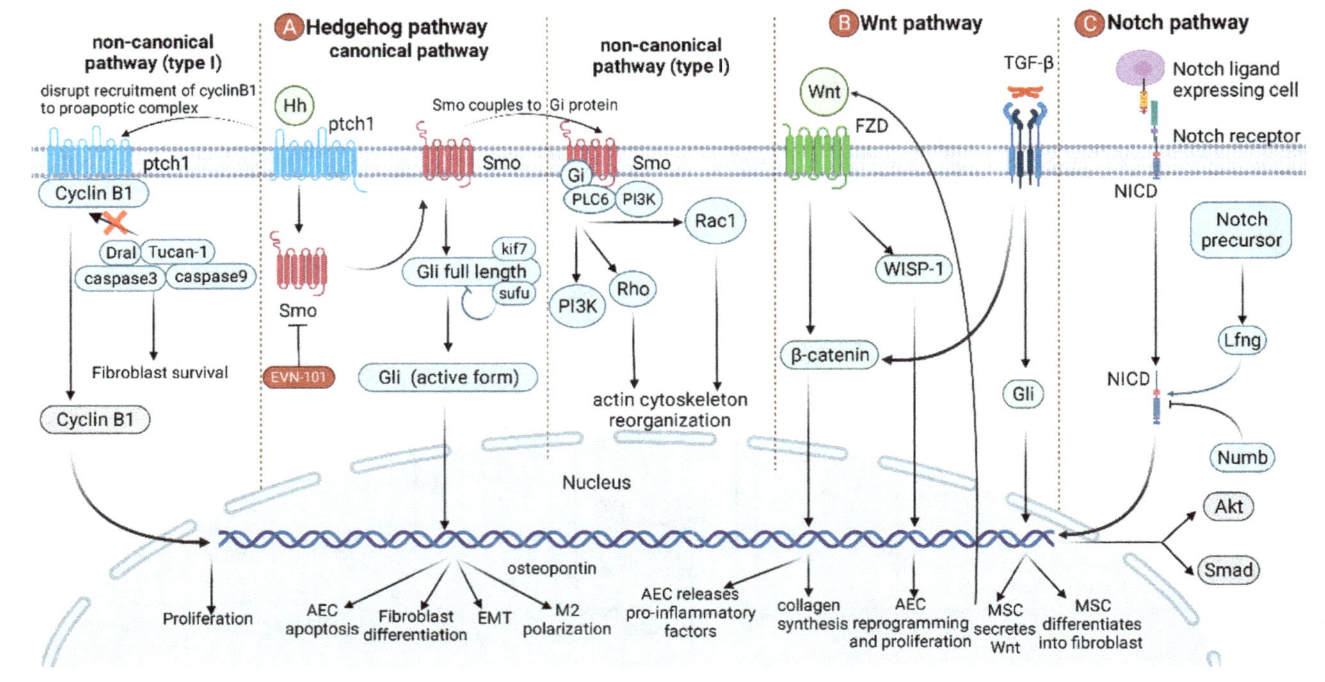

FIGURE 5 | The role of developmental pathways in IPF. **(A)** Canonical hedgehog pathways start from the binding of Hh to ptch1, and Smo then migrates to the plasma membrane, releasing and activating full-length Gli, which leads to AEC apoptosis, fibroblast differentiation, EMT, and M2 polarization. In non-canonical hedgehog pathways (type I), binding of Hh to ptch1 blocks the recruitment of the pro-apoptotic complex by cyclin B1, resulting in anti-apoptosis and promotion of cell proliferation. In non-canonical hedgehog pathways (type II), Smo is coupled to Gi protein, activating downstream PI3K, Rho, and Rac1, resulting in an increase in intracellular calcium concentration and a rearrangement of the cytoskeleton. **(B)** Wnt promotes the accumulation of β-catenin by binding to FZD, thereby stimulating AECs to release proinflammatory factors and promote collagen synthesis in fibroblasts. Wnt also directly induces AEC reprogramming and proliferation *via* WISP-1. TGF-β can induce MSCs to secrete Wnt and promote MSC differentiation. **(C)** The Notch ligand binds to the Notch receptor, causing the Notch intracellular domain (NICD) of the Notch receptor to break and enter the nucleus, leading to gene transcription. Lfng positively regulates this process, while Numb negatively regulates this process. Wnt is also involved in the regulation of Akt and Smad pathways.

apoptosis, fibroblast differentiation, EMT, and M2 polarization (Effendi and Nagano, 2021). In the non-canonical pathway (Type I), the binding of Hh to ptch1 prevents cyclin B1 from recruiting proapoptotic complexes, thereby failing to activate caspase-mediated apoptosis. After entering the nucleus, cyclin B1 can also regulate cell cycle progression by promoting cell proliferation (Robbins et al., 2012; Effendi and Nagano, 2021). In the non-canonical pathway (Type II), the coupling of Smo to Gi protein activates downstream PI3K, Rho, and Rac1, leading to an increase in intracellular calcium concentration and cytoskeleton rearrangement (Robbins et al., 2012; Effendi and Nagano, 2021).

The Wnt signaling pathway is an important signaling pathway in response to postnatal injury and regeneration. Binding of Wnt3a to Frizzled (FZD), followed by β-catenin accumulation, induces AECs to release proinflammatory factors (IL-6, IL-1β) and promotes fibroblast collagen synthesis. In addition, Wnt-inducible signaling protein-1 (WISP-1) is also involved in AEC reprogramming and proliferation (Königshoff et al., 2009). TGF-β promotes the differentiation of mesenchymal stem cells (MSCs) into fibroblasts by activating Gli to secrete Wnt5a, Wnt10a, and Wnt7b, thereby initiating the Wnt pathway (Chen et al., 2018; Martin-Medina et al., 2018). Since Wnt signaling is associated with a large number of normal physiological functions, there are currently no anti-IPF drugs targeting this pathway.

The Notch pathway is a highly conserved signaling pathway that mediates short-range signaling in neighboring cells. The Notch ligand-expressing cell binds to the Notch receptor, causing the Notch intracellular domain (NICD) of the Notch receptor to break and enter the nucleus to lead to gene transcription. Lfng positively regulates this process, while Numb negatively regulates this process (Kiyokawa and Morimoto, 2020). Notch is also involved in the TGF-β/Smad3-mediated transformation of fibroblasts to myofibroblasts (Aoyagi-Ikeda et al., 2011). Notch also induces phosphorylation of Akt by stimulating the expression of insulin-like growth factor-1R (IGF1R), which in turn promotes pulmonary fibrosis by hypoxia-inducible factor-1 (HIF-1) (Eliasz et al., 2010).

5.3 Other Critical Signaling Cascades in Idiopathic Pulmonary Fibrosis: JAK/STAT, PI3K/Akt/mTOR, MAPK, and Hippo-YAP/TAZ

In recent years, research on the molecular mechanism of fibrosis has become increasingly in depth, and the JAK/STAT, PI3K/Akt/

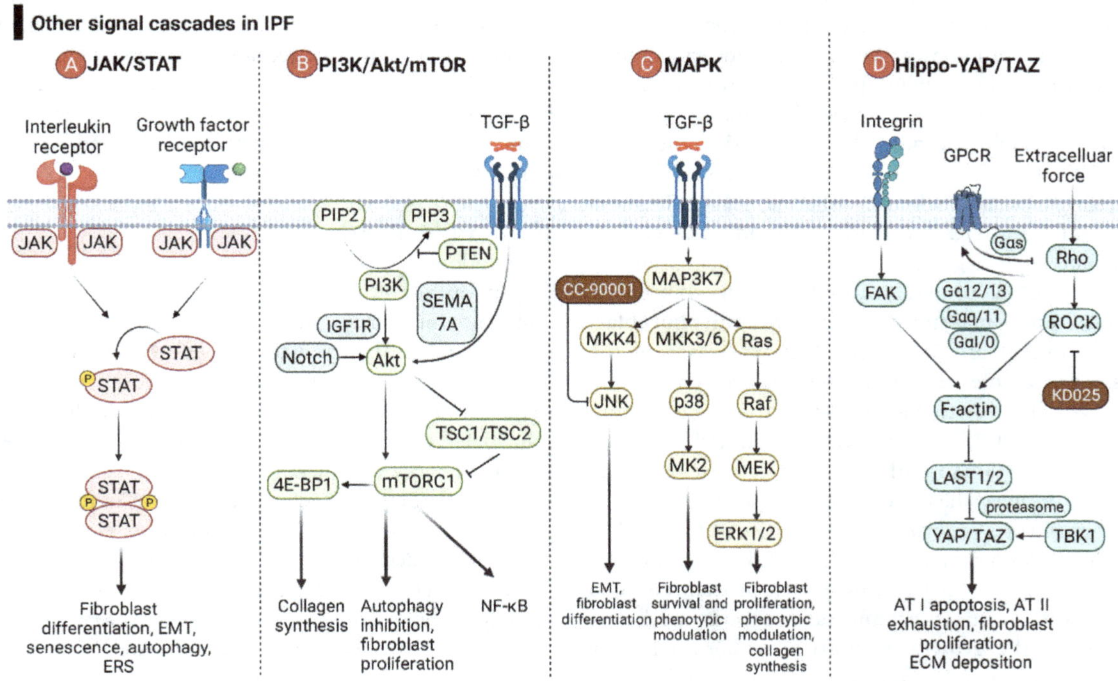

FIGURE 6 | The roles of the JAK/STAT pathway, PI3K/Akt/mTOR pathway, MAPK pathway, and Hippo-YAP/TAZ pathway in IPF. **(A)** After interleukins and growth factors bind to the corresponding receptors, they can activate the JAKs coupled to the receptors, and then JAKs can phosphorylate STAT. Homodimerized STAT enters the nucleus and affects gene transcription. **(B)** Growth factors and cytokines can activate PI3K by binding to receptor-type tyrosine kinases, and then PI3K catalyzes the phosphorylation of PIP2 to PIP3. PIP3 can activate Akt and its downstream mTOR complex (mTORC). PTEN is a negative regulator of the PI3K/Akt/mTOR pathway. TGF-β and Notch are positive regulators of Akt. **(C)** The MAPK pathway consists of three downstream cascades, the JNK, p38, and ERK pathways. JNK and p38 signaling are activated through a pattern of MAP3K-MAP2K-MAPK signaling cascades, while ERK is activated through the MAP3K-Ras-Raf-MEK-ERK cascade. MK2 is a downstream signaling molecule of p38. Growth factors can activate ERK5, and ERK5 and p90RSK can acetylate Smad, thereby promoting the TGF-β/Smad pathway. **(D)** The Hippo-YAP/TAZ pathway is involved in pulmonary fibrosis through the integrin pathway, G protein-coupled receptor pathway, and mechanotransduction pathway. ECM force initiates the Hippo-YAP/TAZ pathway with activation of FAK and Rho/ROCK. FAK and Rho/ROCK relieve the inhibition of the transcription factor YAP/TAZ by large tumor suppressor kinase 1 and 2 (LAST1/2) by promoting the growth, stability, and contractibility of F-actin. Different GPCR signaling pathways regulate LAST1/2 activity through the Rho/ROCK/F-actin pathway.

mTOR, MAPK, and Hippo-YAP/TAZ signaling cascades have received extensive attention (**Figure 6**). Drugs targeting these signaling pathways are already in clinical trials.

Cells respond to inflammatory factors rapidly through JAK/STAT signaling. After interleukins (IL-4, IL-6, IL-11, IL-13, and IL-31) and growth factors (TGF-β, PDGF, VEGF, EGF, and FGF) bind to the corresponding receptors, they can activate and interact with the receptors. Receptor-coupled JAKs (JAK1, JAK2, JAK3, and TYK2) phosphorylate STATs (STAT1, STAT2, STAT3, STAT5, and STAT6) (Montero et al., 2021). Homodimerized STAT enters the nucleus to affect gene transcription, leading to fibroblast differentiation, EMT, senescence, autophagy, and ERS (Montero et al., 2021). Despite numerous isoforms of JAK and STAT, JAK2/STAT3 plays a dominant role in pulmonary fibrosis (Milara et al., 2018). Jaktinib dihydrochloride monohydrate and CC-90001, as JAK1/2 inhibitors, have entered phase II clinical trials (NCT04312594 and NCT03142191, respectively). Since different subtypes of STAT share downstream pathways, blocking only one subtype of STAT may lead to ineffective treatment due to the compensatory effect of other subtypes of STAT. Therefore, no therapeutic drugs targeting STAT have entered clinical trials.

PI3K/Akt/mTOR signaling is involved in autophagy and has caused a huge hit in the field of tumor therapy. A genome-wide association study revealed an association of mTOR with susceptibility to fibrosis (Allen et al., 2020). Growth factors and cytokines activate PI3K by binding to receptor-type tyrosine kinases, which in turn catalyze the phosphorylation of PIP2 to PIP3. PIP3 activates Akt and its downstream mTOR complex (mTORC), which promotes collagen synthesis, proliferation in fibroblasts, and EMT in epithelial cells (Lawrence and Nho, 2018; Fang et al., 2020). PTEN can inhibit the phosphorylation of PIP2, thereby inhibiting the signaling pathway downstream of PI3K and reducing the senescence of AECs (Qiu et al., 2019). Akt relieves the inhibition of mTORC1 by TSC1/TSC2 by phosphorylating TSC2 (Huang and Manning, 2009). mTOR also intersects with NF-κB signaling (Guo et al., 2013). TGF-β signaling can activate Akt in a SEMA 7A-dependent manner, which in turn activates downstream mTOR signaling and promotes lung fibrosis (Reilkoff et al., 2013). mTOR can activate collagen synthesis *via* 4E-BP1 (Woodcock et al., 2019). RPS6KB2 (ribosomal protein S6 kinase B 2) is reported to be involved in the process of aging and IPF due to its activation by growth factors and regulation of the protein kinase mTOR signaling pathway (Hao et al., 2017).

Mitogen-activated protein kinase (MAPK) mainly consists of three downstream cascades, the JNK, p38 and ERK pathways. JNK/p38 is activated *via* a MAP3K-MAP2K-MAPK signaling cascade, whereas ERK is activated *via* a MAP3K-Ras-Raf-MEK-ERK cascade (Woodcock et al., 2019). JNK and p38 signaling participates in apoptosis, necroptosis, and EMT of AEC; fibroblast-to-myofibroblast differentiation; and maintenance of the myofibroblast phenotype (Kasuya et al., 2021). MK2, downstream of the p38 pathway, has a role in fibroblast invasion and fibrosis (Liang et al., 2019). Growth factors can activate ERK5, and then ERK5 and p90RSK can acetylate Smad, thereby promoting the TGF-β/Smad pathway (Kim et al., 2020). The ERK1/2-calpain pathway has been reported to be associated with pulmonary fibrosis *in vivo* and *in vitro* (Zou et al., 2020).

The Hippo-YAP/TAZ pathway is involved in pulmonary fibrosis through the integrin pathway, G protein-coupled receptor pathway, and mechanotransduction pathway. Integrins promote the growth, stability, and contractibility of F-actin by activating FAK, thereby relieving the inhibitory effect of large tumor suppressor kinase 1 and 2 (LAST1/2) on YAP/TAZ. After entering the nucleus, YAP/TAZ regulates AT I apoptosis and AT II exhaustion, fibroblast proliferation and ECM expansion (Sun et al., 2021). The mechanical force of ECM can also activate F-actin *via* Rho/ROCK signaling and promote pulmonary fibrosis (Zhou et al., 2013). Different GPCR signaling pathways (Gαs, Gα12/13, Gαq, and Gαi/o) regulate LAST1/2 activity through the Rho/ROCK/F-actin pathway (Haak et al., 2020). Tank binding kinase 1 (TBK1) activates YAP/TAZ in a proteasomal machinery-dependent but LAST-independent manner (Aravamudhan et al., 2020).

6 ADVANCES IN THE DEVELOPMENT OF ANTI-IPF DRUGS TARGETING CYTOKINE AND GROWTH FACTOR PATHWAYS

6.1 Pirfenidone and Nintedanib, Two FDA-Approved Drugs for Patients With Idiopathic Pulmonary Fibrosis

Antifibrotic therapy provides survival benefit and protection against all-cause and respiratory-related hospitalization for IPF patients (Mooney et al., 2021). FDA approved antifibrotic drugs for treating IPF include Pirfenidone and Nintedanib, and their clinical efficacy is similar though there are no high-quality clinical trials directly comparing the efficacy of the them (Marijic et al., 2021). Regarding their mechanism of action, both of them target multiple growth factor and cytokine-related signaling pathways. Now that the pathogenesis of IPF remains unclear, targeting multiple pathways may be an effective treatment strategy for IPF. In addition, since the mechanisms of Pirfenidone and Nintedanib are not the same, a combination treatment may have synergistic effects. The combination of Pirfenidone and Nintedanib has been shown to be well tolerated and safe, which encourages further research into combination therapy (Flaherty et al., 2018; Vancheri et al., 2018). How to relieve the side effects caused by the off-target effects of Pirfenidone and Nintedanib is also an important topic.

6.1.1 Pirfenidone

Pirfenidone is a pyridine compound approved for marketing in Japan in 2008. It was originally developed as an anti-inflammatory drug. Interestingly, studies in animal models demonstrated that it had the effect of resisting fibrosis of various organs, and it was later approved for IPF treatment. The anti-fibrotic mechanism of Pirfenidone has not been fully elucidated. Published studies indicated that it could inhibit fibrosis mainly by blocking TNF-α and TGF-β/Smad pathways (Oku et al., 2002; Schaefer et al., 2011; Conte et al., 2014).

Three large-scaled RCTs demonstrated that Pirfenidone could delay FVC decline, improve progression-free survival, increase exercise tolerance, and reduce all-cause or IPF related mortality (Taniguchi et al., 2010; Noble et al., 2011; Noble et al., 2012; King et al., 2014). Recently, a systematic review and meta-analysis of RCTs also indicated that Pirfenidone treatment was associated with a longer progression-free-survival and a lower incidence of acute exacerbation (Wu et al., 2021). In the real-world practice, Pirfenidone also provided beneficial effects on survival and pulmonary function decline (Lee et al., 2021). Moreover, A *post hoc* analysis of ASCEND and CAPACITY program suggested a clinically relevant benefit of Pirfenidone in IPF patients with more advanced lung function impairment (Nathan et al., 2019).

However, the use of Pirfenidone has some limitations, such as a short half-life (2.5 h) and a high daily dose (2,403 mg/day). Although generally well tolerated, a minority of patients discontinued treatment due to gastrointestinal and skin-related adverse events. These side effects can be mitigated or prevented by taking it with/after meals, avoiding Sun exposure, wearing protective clothing, and using broad-spectrum sunscreens (Costabel et al., 2014). In addition, caution is recommended prior to Pirfenidone use in IPF patients with severe hepatic and renal insufficiency.

6.1.2 Nintedanib

Nintedanib is a small molecule tyrosinase inhibitor approved for marketing in 2014. Initially, researchers intended to screen drugs that selectively inhibit VEGFR-2 for anticancer treatment. However, in subsequent research, Nintedanib had good antifibrotic and anti-inflammatory effects and was approved for IPF treatment. Nintedanib mainly inhibits tyrosine kinase receptors, such as PDGFR, FGFR, and VEGFR, and non-receptor tyrosine kinases, such as Src and Flt-3 (Hilberg et al., 2008).

The INPULSIS-1 and INPULSIS-2 programs demonstrated that Nintedanib could delay FVC decline and reduce the risk of disease progression (Richeldi et al., 2014; Keating, 2015). However, the parameter of time to first AE and HRQL (Health-related Quality of Life) was inconsistent between

TABLE 2 | Emerging drugs targeting cytokine and growth factor pathways for IPF treatment in clinical trials.

Targets	Drugs	Clinical trial information
TGF-β	GC1008/fresolimumab (TGF-β antibody)	Phase 1 (completed, NCT00125385)
TGF-β	PLN-74809 (integrin αvβ6/αvβ1 inhibitor)	Phase 2 (recruiting, NCT04072315)
		Phase 2 (recruiting, NCT04396756)
TGF-β	TRK-250 (anti-TGF-β mRNA nucleic acid)	Phase 1 (Active, not recruiting, NCT03727802)
TGF-β	TD139 (suppress TGF-β receptor by targeting galectin-3)	Phase 1/2 (completed, NCT02257177)
		Phase 2 (recruiting, NCT03832946)
TGF-β1, CTGF, IL-β23p19, IL-6	PBI-4050 (inhibitor of TGF-β1, CTGF, IL-β23p19, IL-6)	Phase 2 (completed, NCT02538536)
CTGF	Pamrevlumab (CTGF mAb)	Phase 3 (recruiting, NCT03955146); Phase 3 (recruiting, NCT04419558)
IL-13	QAX576 (IL-13 mAb)	Phase 2 (terminated, NCT01266135)
	Tralokinumab (IL-13 mAb)	Phase 2 (terminated, NCT01629667)
	Lebrikizumab (IL-13 mAb)	Phase 2 (completed, NCT01872689)
IL-4, IL-13	SAR156597 (IL-4 and IL-13 Antibody)	Phase 2 (completed, NCT02345070)
CCL-2	CNTO 888 (CCL2 mAb)	Phase 2 (terminated, NCT00786201)
JNK	Jaktinib Dihydrochloride Monohydrate (JNK1/2 inhibitor)	Phase 2 (recruiting, NCT04312594)
	CC-90001 (JNK1/2 inhibitor)	Phase 2 (active, not recruiting, NCT03142191)
Src	Saracatinib (Src kinase inhibitor)	Phase 1/2 (recruiting, NCT04598919)
Hedgehog pathways	taladegib/ENV-101 (Smo receptor inhibitor)	Phase 2 (not yet recruiting, NCT04968574)
ROCK	KD025 (ROCK2 inhibitor)	Phase 2 (completed, NCT02688647)
Leukotrienes	MN-001/Tipelukast (leukotriene receptor antagonist)	Phase 2 (active, not recruiting, NCT02503657)
LPC-ATX-LPA	BMS-986278 (LPA1R antagonist)	Phase 2 (recruiting, NCT04308681)

INPULSIS-1 and INPULSIS-2 (Keating, 2015). Interestingly, despite similar efficacy of Pirfenidone and Nintedanib, there was a higher rate of discontinuation of Nintedanib due to adverse effects (Takehara et al., 2022). Gastrointestinal adverse events (diarrhea, nausea, and vomiting) were reported most commonly (Keating, 2015). Patients treated with Nintedanib who experience diarrhea should maintain hydration and take antidiarrheal therapy as soon as symptoms occur. Dose reduction can also be taken into consideration (Corte et al., 2015).

The timing of antifibrotic therapy may influence the outcome of IPF treatment. A retrospective study indicated that patients who initiated Nintedanib immediately after IPF diagnosis might have reduced hospitalization risk and medical costs compared with those who start treatment later (Singer et al., 2022). A *post hoc* analysis of INPULSIS program suggested that probable UIP with traction bronchiectasis in high-resolution CT might be sufficient for patients to benefit from Nintedanib, implying the importance of early antifibrotic therapy (Lobo, 2016).

Although high-quality clinical trial data are currently lacking to directly demonstrate that Nintedanib is effective in end-stage IPF, the latest *post hoc* analyses of the INPULSIS and INSTAGE programs suggest that it has some effect in IPF patients with more severely impaired gas exchange (Richeldi et al., 2020).

6.1.3 Implications of Pirfenidone and Nintedanib for Anti-Idiopathic Pulmonary Fibrosis Drug Discovery

With the launch of Pirfenidone and Nintedanib in multiple countries, the number of IPF patients not receiving anti-fibrotic therapy will decrease in the future, and it will become increasingly difficult to observe the natural progression of IPF. For ethical reasons and feasibility of patient recruitment, more and more clinical trials of new drugs will use Pirfenidone and Nintedanib as controls. This sets a higher standard for the efficacy of new drugs. In addition, there will be a trend to combine new drugs with existing anti-fibrotic therapies in clinical trials, and whether they can bring additional benefits will be the determining factor. Furthermore, whether a single drug is sufficient to effectively delay the progression of IPF is an important pharmacoeconomic proposition. Since IPF is a rapidly progressive and irreversible disease, whether anti-fibrotic therapy is effective in different stages of IPF, especially in end-stage IPF and suspected IPF, also deserves further study. There are currently no high-quality clinical trials that directly demonstrate the efficacy of antifibrotic therapy in end-stage IPF. In addition, whether patients with suspected IPF on unbiopsied CT images without biopsy require prophylactic antifibrotic therapy remains to be further investigated.

6.2 Anti-Idiopathic Pulmonary Fibrosis Drugs Targeting Cytokine and Growth Factor Pathways in Clinical Trials

With the continuous exploration of the pathophysiological process of IPF and the continuous clarification of the cytokine and growth factor pathways, the targets of IPF treatment have also become diversified. Many targets and drugs developed based on them have entered clinical trials (**Table 2**). Although most of them fail to enter phase III clinical trials, a few drugs show promise in the treatment of IPF. Currently, pamrevlumab (CTGF mAb) and PRM-151 (recombinant pentraxin 2) have successfully entered Phase III clinical trials.

6.3 Information About Clinical Trials That Target Complications and Comorbidities of Idiopathic Pulmonary Fibrosis

Complications and comorbidities are of substantial significance to the disease progression and quality of life in IPF patients.

Cough affects up to 80% of patients with IPF, is frequently disabling, and lacks effective therapy. A 24-week, double-blind, two-treatment, 24 patients enrolled, two-period crossover trial showed that thalidomide improved cough and respiratory quality of life in patients with IPF (Horton et al., 2012).

Patients with IPF are also at risk of developing pulmonary hypertension as the underlying condition worsens (Tanaka et al., 2017). The BUILD-3 program showed no benefit of Bosentan in the life quality of IPF patients (King et al., 2011a). However, a prospective study showed that Bosentan was associated with a trend toward decreased adverse events and improved respiratory status (Tanaka et al., 2017). Sildenafil is an FDA-approved drug for pulmonary arterial hypertension. A double-blind randomized clinical trial showed that the combination of Sildenafil and Nintedanib significantly reduced BNP (B-type natriuretic peptide, an indicator of heart failure) in IPF patients with right ventricular dysfunction compared with Nintedanib alone, but did not improve HRQL (Behr et al., 2019; Suarez-Cuartin and Molina-Molina, 2019). More recently, a systematic review and meta-analysis of RCTs reported that Sildenafil probably reduced all-cause mortality in IPF patients (Pitre et al., 2022), although more studies are needed to confirm this. The 2015 ATS/ERS/JRS/ALAT clinical practice guideline conditionally recommends against the use of Bosentan and Sildenafil, while the 2011 version strongly recommends against the use of them.

Increased bacterial load and loss of microbial diversity have been reported in IPF (Han et al., 2014; Molyneaux et al., 2014), which are associated with disease progression and immune response (Huang et al., 2017; Molyneaux et al., 2017). However, the role of several antibiotics in IPF appears to be controversial. A retrospective study of 85 AE-IPF patients showed that azithromycin may improve survival in patients with AE-IPF compared with a fluoroquinolone-based regimen (Kawamura et al., 2017). On the contrary, a randomized controlled crossover study of 25 IPF patients does not support the use of low-dose azithromycin for chronic cough in IPF (Guler et al., 2021). In addition, a pragmatic randomized unblinded clinical study of 513 IPF patients didn't support the additional use of co-trimoxazole or doxycycline (Martinez et al., 2021). Thus, the selection of antibiotics and the effect of them on immune cells need to be further explored.

Gastroesophageal reflux occurs in a high proportion of IPF patients (Raghu et al., 2015), and chronic microaspiration secondary to gastroesophageal reflux is thought to play a role in disease pathogenesis and progression (Savarino et al., 2013). The 2015 ATS/ERS/JRS/ALAT clinical practice guideline conditionally recommends anti-acid therapy. However, whether anti-acid therapy is effective in IPF patients remains highly controversial (Lee et al., 2011; Lee et al., 2013; Kreuter et al., 2016; Raghu et al., 2018; Tran et al., 2021). In addition, whether anti-acid treatment should choose anti-acid drugs or radical therapy (such as Nissen fundoplication) requires further study (Johannson et al., 2017). Therefore, to investigate the efficacy of anti-acid therapy in slowing the progression of IPF, a phase III, randomized, placebo-controlled, double-blind, multicenter clinical trial using lansoprazole is currently enrolling patients with IPF (NCT04965298).

7 CHALLENGE AND OUTLOOK

Research on the pathogenesis of IPF has made considerable progress. After years of preclinical research and clinical studies, the pathogenesis of IPF has changed from simple inflammation to abnormal epithelial-mesenchymal crosstalk and other pathogenic mechanisms. Based on the emerging pathological mechanism, many studies have systematically studied the key roles of cytokine and growth factor pathways in the pathogenesis of IPF. The approval of Pirfenidone and Nintedanib shows that therapy targeting these pathways is very promising. Although investigational drugs targeting some cytokines such as IFN-γ, TNF-α, and IL-13 have not shown satisfactory efficacy, the development of anti-IPF drugs targeting cytokine and growth factor pathways is still promising. Currently, there are numerous clinical trials investigating the efficacy of these drugs in the treatment of IPF and more drugs may be approved based on the results of these trials.

Advances in the field of cytokine and growth factor pathways would help slow disease progression, prolong lives, and improve the quality of life of IPF patients in the future. Therefore, this review tried to provide an overview of cytokines, growth factors, and their signaling pathways in IPF. Furthermore, key information about emerging drugs targeting these pathways for IPF treatment in clinical trials is provided.

Based on the findings of this review, the following points need to be considered in future studies to make strategies targeting these signaling pathways more promising for the treatment of IPF patients. Although upregulating or antagonizing certain cytokine or growth factor signaling pathways alone may not reverse differentiated cells, promoting fibrotic phenotype transition is more promising. Since cytokine and growth factor signaling pathways also play vital roles in other physiological and pathological processes, including damage repair, defense against infection, autoimmune disease, and antitumor immunity, long-term non-selective targeting of these pathways may lead to undesired side effects. Therefore, the identification of more specific targets and the development of drugs having high selectivity on them, the optimization of drug delivery to increase drug concentrations at the target site, and the identification of biomarkers to help select patients who might benefit more from drugs are all worth exploring. In addition, combination therapy with Pirfenidone and Nintedanib might bring better clinical benefits for IPF patients than single drug administration.

One of the novelties of this review is giving an extensive description of the multiple roles of cytokine and growth factor pathways in pulmonary fibrosis, which provide new insights into therapeutic strategies for IPF. These pathways form a complex network in the pathological process of pulmonary fibrosis, and exploring the crosstalk between different signaling cascades may help discover more potential targets. Clinical trials are a critical stage that all approved drugs must go through. Some of the drugs in clinical trials for the treatment of IPF target cytokines and growth factors. Therefore, we summarize key information from these clinical trials and hope to give insights for the development of more effective drug.

Although IPF is idiopathic by definition, it may become less mysterious with progress in the understanding of the pathogenesis of IPF. This review showed that the number of therapeutic targets from cytokine or growth factor signaling pathways and new targeted drugs entering clinical trials is increasing. These advances show that slowing disease progression, prolonging prognosis, and improving quality of life might be possible in the future for patients with IPF.

In conclusion, cytokine and growth factor signaling pathways are indispensable in the pathogenesis of IPF, and this review hopes to provide theoretical support for the development of novel anti-pulmonary fibrosis drugs targeting cytokine and growth factor pathways.

AUTHOR CONTRIBUTIONS

HBM contributed to the conception of this review and preparation of the manuscript, tables, and figures. SML collected information about the clinical trials. SRL revised the manuscript and helped design the figures; YX contributed to the conception, supervision, and revision of the manuscript. All authors have approved the final article and are included in the disclosure.

REFERENCES

1. Agostini, C., and Gurrieri, C. (2006). Chemokine/cytokine Cocktail in Idiopathic Pulmonary Fibrosis. *Proc. Am. Thorac. Soc.* 3 (4), 357–363. doi:10.1513/pats. 200601-010TK
2. Alavi, A., Hood, J. D., Frausto, R., Stupack, D. G., and Cheresh, D. A. (2003). Role of Raf in Vascular Protection from Distinct Apoptotic Stimuli. *Science* 301 (5629), 94–96. doi:10.1126/science.1082015
3. Allen, R. J., Guillen-Guio, B., Oldham, J. M., Ma, S. F., Dressen, A., Paynton, M. L., et al. (2020). Genome-Wide Association Study of Susceptibility to Idiopathic Pulmonary Fibrosis. *Am. J. Respir. Crit. Care Med.* 201 (5), 564–574. doi:10. 1164/rccm.201905-1017OC
4. Amano, H., Matsui, Y., Hatanaka, K., Hosono, K., and Ito, Y. (2021). VEGFR1-tyrosine Kinase Signaling in Pulmonary Fibrosis. *Inflamm. Regen.* 41 (1), 16. doi:10.1186/s41232-021-00166-7
5. Antoniou, K. M., Pataka, A., Bouros, D., and Siafakas, N. M. (2007). Pathogenetic Pathways and Novel Pharmacotherapeutic Targets in Idiopathic Pulmonary Fibrosis. *Pulm. Pharmacol. Ther.* 20 (5), 453–461. doi:10.1016/j.pupt.2006. 01.002
6. Aoyagi-Ikeda, K., Maeno, T., Matsui, H., Ueno, M., Hara, K., Aoki, Y., et al. (2011). Notch Induces Myofibroblast Differentiation of Alveolar Epithelial Cells via Transforming Growth Factor-{beta}-Smad3 Pathway. *Am. J. Respir. Cell Mol. Biol.* 45 (1), 136–144. doi:10.1165/rcmb.2010-0140oc
7. Arai, T., Abe, K., Matsuoka, H., Yoshida, M., Mori, M., Goya, S., et al. (2000). Introduction of the Interleukin-10 Gene into Mice Inhibited Bleomycin-Induced Lung Injury *In Vivo*. *Am. J. Physiol. Lung Cell Mol. Physiol.* 278 (5), L914–L922. doi:10.1152/ajplung.2000.278.5.L914
8. Aravamudhan, A., Haak, A. J., Choi, K. M., Meridew, J. A., Caporarello, N., Jones, D. L., et al. (2020). TBK1 Regulates YAP/TAZ and Fibrogenic Fibroblast Activation. *Am. J. Physiol. Lung Cell Mol. Physiol.* 318 (5), L852–l863. doi:10.1152/ajplung.00324.2019
9. Baratella, E., Ruaro, B., Giudici, F., Wade, B., Santagiuliana, M., Salton, F., et al. (2021). Evaluation of Correlations between Genetic Variants and High- Resolution Computed Tomography Patterns in Idiopathic Pulmonary Fibrosis. *Diagnostics* 11 (5), 762. doi:10.3390/diagnostics11050762
10. Barbarin, V., Xing, Z., Delos, M., Lison, D., and Huaux, F. (2005). Pulmonary Overexpression of IL-10 Augments Lung Fibrosis and Th2 Responses Induced by Silica Particles. *Am. J. Physiol. Lung Cell Mol. Physiol.* 288 (5), L841–L848. doi:10.1152/ajplung.00329.2004
11. Barnes, J. C., Lumsden, R. V., Worrell, J., Counihan, I. P., O'Beirne, S. L., Belperio, J. A., et al. (2015). CXCR3 Requirement for the Interleukin-13-Mediated Up-Regulation of Interleukin-13Rα2 in Pulmonary Fibroblasts. *Am. J. Respir. Cell Mol. Biol.* 53 (2), 217–225. doi:10.1165/rcmb.2013- 0433OC
12. Barnes, J. W., Duncan, D., Helton, S., Hutcheson, S., Kurundkar, D., Logsdon, N. J., et al. (2019). Role of Fibroblast Growth Factor 23 and Klotho Cross Talk in Idiopathic Pulmonary Fibrosis. *Am. J. Physiol. Lung Cell Mol. Physiol.* 317 (1), L141–l154. doi:10.1152/ajplung.00246.2018
13. Barratt, S. L., Blythe, T., Jarrett, C., Ourradi, K., Shelley-Fraser, G., Day, M. J., et al. (2017). Differential Expression of VEGF-Axxx Isoforms Is Critical for Development of Pulmonary Fibrosis. *Am. J. Respir. Crit. Care Med.* 196 (4), 479–493. doi:10.1164/rccm.201603-0568OC
14. Barratt, S. L., Flower, V. A., Pauling, J. D., and Millar, A. B. (2018). VEGF (Vascular Endothelial Growth Factor) and Fibrotic Lung Disease. *Int. J. Mol. Sci.* 19 (5). doi:10.3390/ijms19051269
15. Behr, J., Kolb, M., Song, J. W., Luppi, F., Schinzel, B., Stowasser, S., et al. (2019). Nintedanib and Sildenafil in Patients with Idiopathic Pulmonary Fibrosis and Right Heart Dysfunction. A Prespecified Subgroup Analysis of a Double-Blind Randomized Clinical Trial (INSTAGE). *Am. J. Respir. Crit. Care Med.* 200 (12), 1505–1512. doi:10.1164/rccm.201903-0488OC
16. Besnard, A. G., Struyf, S., Guabiraba, R., Fauconnier, L., Rouxel, N., Proost, P., et al. (2013). CXCL6 Antibody Neutralization Prevents Lung Inflammation and Fibrosis in Mice in the Bleomycin Model. *J. Leukoc. Biol.* 94 (6), 1317–1323. doi:10.1189/jlb.0313140
17. Betensley, A., Sharif, R., and Karamichos, D. (2016). A Systematic Review of the Role of Dysfunctional Wound Healing in the Pathogenesis and Treatment of Idiopathic Pulmonary Fibrosis. *J. Clin. Med.* 6 (1). doi:10.3390/jcm6010002
18. Boehme, S. A., Franz-Bacon, K., DiTirro, D. N., Ly, T. W., and Bacon, K. B. (2016). MAP3K19 Is a Novel Regulator of TGF-β Signaling that Impacts Bleomycin- Induced Lung Injury and Pulmonary Fibrosis. *PLoS One* 11 (5), e0154874. doi:10.1371/journal.pone.0154874
19. Brown, K. R., England, K. M., Goss, K. L., Snyder, J. M., and Acarregui, M. J. (2001). VEGF Induces Airway Epithelial Cell Proliferation in Human Fetal Lung *In Vitro*. *Am. J. Physiol. Lung Cell Mol. Physiol.* 281 (4), L1001–L1010. doi:10. 1152/ajplung.2001.281.4.L1001
20. Chanda, D., Otoupalova, E., Smith, S. R., Volckaert, T., De Langhe, S. P., and Thannickal, V. J. (2019). Developmental Pathways in the Pathogenesis of Lung Fibrosis. *Mol. Asp. Med.* 65, 56–69. doi:10.1016/j.mam.2018.08.004
21. Chen, H., Qu, J., Huang, X., Kurundkar, A., Zhu, L., Yang, N., et al. (2016). Mechanosensing by the α6-integrin Confers an Invasive Fibroblast Phenotype and Mediates Lung Fibrosis. *Nat. Commun.* 7, 12564. doi:10.1038/ncomms12564
22. Chen, X., Shi, C., Cao, H., Chen, L., Hou, J., Xiang, Z., et al. (2018). The Hedgehog and Wnt/β-Catenin System Machinery Mediate Myofibroblast Differentiation of LR-MSCs in Pulmonary Fibrogenesis. *Cell Death Dis.* 9 (6), 639. doi:10.1038/ s41419-018-0692-9

23. Cheng, S. E., Lee, I. T., Lin, C. C., Hsiao, L. D., and Yang, C. M. (2014). Thrombin Induces ICAM-1 Expression in Human Lung Epithelial Cells via c-Src/PDGFR/ PI3K/Akt-dependent NF-κB/p300 Activation. *Clin. Sci. (Lond)* 127 (3), 171–183. doi:10.1042/cs20130676
24. S. Choi (Editor) (2012). "CCN2 CTGF, FISP12, HCS24, SSig-M2, HBGF-0.8, Ecogenin, IGFBP8, IGFBP-rP2," *Encyclopedia of Signaling Molecules* (New York, NYNew York: Springer), 282. doi:10.1007/978-3-319-67199-4
25. Chong, S. G., Sato, S., Kolb, M., and Gauldie, J. (2019). Fibrocytes and Fibroblasts- Where Are We Now. *Int. J. Biochem. Cell Biol.* 116, 105595. doi:10.1016/j.biocel. 2019.105595
26. Chu, K. A., Yeh, C. C., Kuo, F. H., Lin, W. R., Hsu, C. W., Chen, T. H., et al. (2020). Comparison of Reversal of Rat Pulmonary Fibrosis of Nintedanib, Pirfenidone, and Human Umbilical Mesenchymal Stem Cells from Wharton's Jelly. *Stem Cell Res. Ther.* 11 (1), 513. doi:10.1186/s13287-020-02012-y
27. Compernolle, V., Brusselmans, K., Acker, T., Hoet, P., Tjwa, M., Beck, H., et al. (2002). Loss of HIF-2alpha and Inhibition of VEGF Impair Fetal Lung Maturation, whereas Treatment with VEGF Prevents Fatal Respiratory Distress in Premature Mice. *Nat. Med.* 8 (7), 702–710. doi:10.1038/nm721
28. Conte, E., Gili, E., Fagone, E., Fruciano, M., Iemmolo, M., and Vancheri, C. (2014). Effect of Pirfenidone on Proliferation, TGF-β-Induced Myofibroblast Differentiation and Fibrogenic Activity of Primary Human Lung Fibroblasts. *Eur. J. Pharm. Sci.* 58, 13–19. doi:10.1016/j.ejps.2014.02.014
29. Corte, T., Bonella, F., Crestani, B., Demedts, M. G., Richeldi, L., Coeck, C., et al. (2015). Safety, Tolerability and Appropriate Use of Nintedanib in Idiopathic Pulmonary Fibrosis. *Respir. Res.* 16, 116. doi:10.1186/s12931- 015-0276-5
30. Costabel, U., Bendstrup, E., Cottin, V., Dewint, P., Egan, J. J., Ferguson, J., et al. (2014). Pirfenidone in Idiopathic Pulmonary Fibrosis: Expert Panel Discussion on the Management of Drug-Related Adverse Events. *Adv. Ther.* 31 (4), 375–391. doi:10.1007/s12325-014-0112-1
31. Coutts, A., Chen, G., Stephens, N., Hirst, S., Douglas, D., Eichholtz, T., et al. (2001). Release of Biologically Active TGF-Beta from Airway Smooth Muscle Cells Induces Autocrine Synthesis of Collagen. *Am. J. Physiol. Lung Cell Mol. Physiol.* 280 (5), L999–L1008. doi:10.1152/ajplung.2001.280.5.L999
32. Derynck, R., and Zhang, Y. E. (2003). Smad-dependent and Smad-independent Pathways in TGF-Beta Family Signalling. *Nature* 425 (6958), 577–584. doi:10. 1038/nature02006
33. Effendi, W. I., and Nagano, T. (2021). The Hedgehog Signaling Pathway in Idiopathic Pulmonary Fibrosis: Resurrection Time. *Int. J. Mol. Sci.* 23 (1). doi:10.3390/ijms23010171
34. Eliasz, S., Liang, S., Chen, Y., De Marco, M. A., Machek, O., Skucha, S., et al. (2010). Notch-1 Stimulates Survival of Lung Adenocarcinoma Cells during Hypoxia by Activating the IGF-1R Pathway. *Oncogene* 29 (17), 2488–2498. doi:10.1038/ onc.2010.7
35. Epstein Shochet, G., Brook, E., Bardenstein-Wald, B., and Shitrit, D. (2020). TGF-β Pathway Activation by Idiopathic Pulmonary Fibrosis (IPF) Fibroblast Derived Soluble Factors Is Mediated by IL-6 Trans-signaling. *Respir. Res.* 21 (1), 56. doi:10.1186/s12931-020-1319-0
36. Espindola, M. S., Habiel, D. M., Narayanan, R., Jones, I., Coelho, A. L., Murray, L. A., et al. (2018). Targeting of TAM Receptors Ameliorates Fibrotic Mechanisms in Idiopathic Pulmonary Fibrosis. *Am. J. Respir. Crit. Care Med.* 197 (11), 1443–1456. doi:10.1164/rccm.201707-1519OC
37. Fang, Y., Tian, J., Fan, Y., and Cao, P. (2020). Latest Progress on the Molecular Mechanisms of Idiopathic Pulmonary Fibrosis. *Mol. Biol. Rep.* 47 (12), 9811–9820. doi:10.1007/s11033-020-06000-6
38. Faress, J. A., Nethery, D. E., Kern, E. F., Eisenberg, R., Jacono, F. J., Allen, C. L., et al. (20071985). Bleomycin-induced Pulmonary Fibrosis Is Attenuated by a Monoclonal Antibody Targeting HER2. *J. Appl. Physiol. (1985)* 103 (6), 2077–2083. doi:10.1152/japplphysiol.00239.2007
39. Flaherty, K. R., Fell, C. D., Huggins, J. T., Nunes, H., Sussman, R., Valenzuela, C., et al. (2018). Safety of Nintedanib Added to Pirfenidone Treatment for Idiopathic Pulmonary Fibrosis. *Eur. Respir. J.* 52 (2). doi:10.1183/13993003. 00230-2018
40. Fruttiger, M. (2008). "VEGF Gene Regulation," in *VEGF in Development* (Springer), 30–39.
41. Fulkerson, P. C., Fischetti, C. A., and Rothenberg, M. E. (2006). Eosinophils and CCR3 Regulate Interleukin-13 Transgene-Induced Pulmonary Remodeling. *Am. J. Pathol.* 169 (6), 2117–2126. doi:10.2353/ajpath.2006.060617
42. García-Prieto, E., González-López, A., Cabrera, S., Astudillo, A., Gutiérrez- Fernández, A., Fanjul-Fernandez, M., et al. (2010). Resistance to Bleomycin- Induced Lung Fibrosis in MMP-8 Deficient Mice Is Mediated by Interleukin-10. *PLoS One* 5 (10), e13242. doi:10.1371/journal.pone.0013242
43. George, P. M., Wells, A. U., and Jenkins, R. G. (2020). Pulmonary Fibrosis and COVID-19: the Potential Role for Antifibrotic Therapy. *Lancet Respir. Med.* 8 (8), 807–815. doi:10.1016/s2213-2600(20)30225-3
44. Gerber, H. P., Dixit, V., and Ferrara, N. (1998a). Vascular Endothelial Growth Factor Induces Expression of the Antiapoptotic Proteins Bcl-2 and A1 in Vascular Endothelial Cells. *J. Biol. Chem.* 273 (21), 13313–13316. doi:10.1074/ jbc.273.21.13313
45. Gerber, H. P., McMurtrey, A., Kowalski, J., Yan, M., Keyt, B. A., Dixit, V., et al. (1998b). Vascular Endothelial Growth Factor Regulates Endothelial Cell Survival through the Phosphatidylinositol 3'-kinase/Akt Signal Transduction Pathway. Requirement for Flk-1/KDR Activation. *J. Biol. Chem.* 273 (46), 30336–30343. doi:10.1074/jbc.273.46.30336
46. Gu, P., Wang, D., Zhang, J., Wang, X., Chen, Z., Gu, L., et al. (2021). Protective Function of Interleukin-22 in Pulmonary Fibrosis. *Clin. Transl. Med.* 11 (8), e509. doi:10.1002/ctm2.509
47. Guler, S. A., Clarenbach, C., Brutsche, M., Hostettler, K., Brill, A. K., Schertel, A., et al. (2021). Azithromycin for the Treatment of Chronic Cough in Idiopathic Pulmonary Fibrosis: A Randomized Controlled Crossover Trial. *Ann. Am. Thorac. Soc.* 18 (12), 2018–2026. doi:10.1513/AnnalsATS.202103-266OC
48. Günther, A., Korfei, M., Mahavadi, P., von der Beck, D., Ruppert, C., and Markart, P. (2012). Unravelling the Progressive Pathophysiology of Idiopathic Pulmonary Fibrosis. *Eur. Respir. Rev.* 21 (124), 152–160. doi:10.1183/ 09059180.00001012
49. Guo, F., Li, J., Du, W., Zhang, S., O'Connor, M., Thomas, G., et al. (2013). mTOR Regulates DNA Damage Response through NF-Kb-Mediated FANCD2 Pathway in Hematopoietic Cells. *Leukemia* 27 (10), 2040–2046. doi:10.1038/leu.2013.93
50. Haak, A. J., Ducharme, M. T., Diaz Espinosa, A. M., and Tschumperlin, D. J. (2020). Targeting GPCR Signaling for Idiopathic Pulmonary Fibrosis Therapies. *Trends Pharmacol. Sci.* 41 (3), 172–182. doi:10.1016/j.tips.2019. 12.008
51. Habiel, D. M., and Hogaboam, C. (2014). Heterogeneity in Fibroblast Proliferation and Survival in Idiopathic Pulmonary Fibrosis. *Front. Pharmacol.* 5, 2. doi:10. 3389/fphar.2014.00002
52. Hamanaka, R. B., and Mutlu, G. M. (2021). Metabolic Requirements of Pulmonary Fibrosis: Role of Fibroblast Metabolism. *Febs J.* 288 (22), 6331–6352. doi:10. 1111/febs.15693
53. Hambly, N., Shimbori, C., and Kolb, M. (2015). Molecular Classification of Idiopathic Pulmonary Fibrosis: Personalized Medicine, Genetics and Biomarkers. *Respirology* 20 (7), 1010–1022. doi:10.1111/resp.12569
54. Han, M. K., Zhou, Y., Murray, S., Tayob, N., Noth, I., Lama, V. N., et al. (2014). Lung Microbiome and Disease Progression in Idiopathic Pulmonary Fibrosis: an Analysis of the COMET Study. *Lancet Respir. Med.* 2 (7), 548–556. doi:10. 1016/s2213-2600(14)70069-4
55. Hao, X., Du, Y., Qian, L., Li, D., and Liu, X. (2017). Upregulation of Long Noncoding RNA AP003419.16 Predicts High Risk of Aging-associated I-diopathic P-ulmonary F-ibrosis. *Mol. Med. Rep.* 16 (6), 8085–8091. doi:10. 3892/mmr.2017.7607
56. Heldin, C. H., and Westermark, B. (1999). Mechanism of Action and *In Vivo* Role of Platelet-Derived Growth Factor. *Physiol. Rev.* 79 (4), 1283–1316. doi:10. 1152/physrev.1999.79.4.1283
57. Henderson, N. C., Rieder, F., and Wynn, T. A. (2020). Fibrosis: from Mechanisms to Medicines. *Nature* 587 (7835), 555–566. doi:10.1038/s41586-020-2938-9 Hetzel, M., Bachem, M., Anders, D., Trischler, G., and Faehling, M. (2005).
58. Different Effects of Growth Factors on Proliferation and Matrix Production of Normal and Fibrotic Human Lung Fibroblasts. *Lung* 183 (4), 225–237. doi:10.1007/s00408-004-2534-z

59. Hilberg, F., Roth, G. J., Krssak, M., Kautschitsch, S., Sommergruber, W., Tontsch- Grunt, U., et al. (2008). BIBF 1120: Triple Angiokinase Inhibitor with Sustained Receptor Blockade and Good Antitumor Efficacy. *Cancer Res.* 68 (12), 4774–4782. doi:10.1158/0008-5472.Can-07-6307
60. Hill, C., Jones, M. G., Davies, D. E., and Wang, Y. (2019). Epithelial-mesenchymal Transition Contributes to Pulmonary Fibrosis via Aberrant Epithelial/ fibroblastic Cross-Talk. *J. Lung Health Dis.* 3 (2), 31–35. doi:10.29245/2689- 999x/2019/2.1149
61. Horton, M. R., Santopietro, V., Mathew, L., Horton, K. M., Polito, A. J., Liu, M. C., et al. (2012). Thalidomide for the Treatment of Cough in Idiopathic Pulmonary Fibrosis: a Randomized Trial. *Ann. Intern Med.* 157 (6), 398–406. doi:10.7326/ 0003-4819-157-6-201209180-00003
62. Huang, J., and Manning, B. D. (2009). A Complex Interplay between Akt, TSC2 and the Two mTOR Complexes. *Biochem. Soc. Trans.* 37 (Pt 1), 217–222. doi:10.1042/bst0370217
63. Huang, L. S., Sudhadevi, T., Fu, P., Punathil-Kannan, P. K., Ebenezer, D. L., Ramchandran, R., et al. (2020). Sphingosine Kinase 1/S1P Signaling Contributes to Pulmonary Fibrosis by Activating Hippo/YAP Pathway and Mitochondrial Reactive Oxygen Species in Lung Fibroblasts. *Int. J. Mol. Sci.* 21 (6). doi:10.3390/ijms21062064
64. Huang, Y., Ma, S. F., Espindola, M. S., Vij, R., Oldham, J. M., Huffnagle, G. B., et al. (2017). Microbes Are Associated with Host Innate Immune Response in Idiopathic Pulmonary Fibrosis. *Am. J. Respir. Crit. Care Med.* 196 (2), 208–219. doi:10.1164/rccm.201607-1525OC
65. Huaux, F., Gharaee-Kermani, M., Liu, T., Morel, V., McGarry, B., Ullenbruch, M., et al. (2005). Role of Eotaxin-1 (CCL11) and CC Chemokine Receptor 3 (CCR3) in Bleomycin-Induced Lung Injury and Fibrosis. *Am. J. Pathol.* 167 (6), 1485–1496. doi:10.1016/s0002-9440(10)61235-7
66. Inomata, M., Nishioka, Y., and Azuma, A. (2015). Nintedanib: Evidence for its Therapeutic Potential in Idiopathic Pulmonary Fibrosis. *Core Evid.* 10, 89–98. doi:10.2147/ce.S82905
67. Ishida, Y., Kimura, A., Kondo, T., Hayashi, T., Ueno, M., Takakura, N., et al. (2007). Essential Roles of the CC Chemokine Ligand 3-CC Chemokine Receptor 5 axis in Bleomycin-Induced Pulmonary Fibrosis through Regulation of Macrophage and Fibrocyte Infiltration. *Am. J. Pathol.* 170 (3), 843–854. doi:10.2353/ajpath. 2007.051213
68. Iwamoto, R., Mekada, E., Hofmann, T. G., Krieghoff-Henning, E., Kobayashi, M., Takamatsu, K., et al. (2012). "HB-EGF (Heparin-Binding EGF-like Growth Factor)," in *Encyclopedia of Signaling Molecules*. Editor S. Choi (New York, NY: Springer New York), 849–858. doi:10.1007/978-1-4419-0461-4_127
69. Joannes, A., Brayer, S., Besnard, V., Marchal-Sommé, J., Jaillet, M., Mordant, P., et al. (2016). FGF9 and FGF18 in Idiopathic Pulmonary Fibrosis Promote Survival and Migration and Inhibit Myofibroblast Differentiation of Human Lung Fibroblasts *In Vitro*. *Am. J. Physiol. Lung Cell Mol. Physiol.* 310 (7), L615–L629. doi:10.1152/ajplung.00185.2015
70. Johannson, K. A., Strâmbu, I., Ravaglia, C., Grutters, J. C., Valenzuela, C., Mogulkoc, N., et al. (2017). Antacid Therapy in Idiopathic Pulmonary Fibrosis: More Questions Than Answers? *Lancet Respir. Med.* 5 (7), 591–598. doi:10.1016/s2213-2600(17)30219-9
71. Ju, W., Zhihong, Y., Zhiyou, Z., Qin, H., Dingding, W., Li, S., et al. (2012). Inhibition of α-SMA by the Ectodomain of FGFR2c Attenuates Lung Fibrosis. *Mol. Med.* 18 (1), 992–1002. doi:10.2119/molmed.2011.00425
72. Karampitsakos, T., Woolard, T., Bouros, D., and Tzouvelekis, A. (2017). Toll-like Receptors in the Pathogenesis of Pulmonary Fibrosis. *Eur. J. Pharmacol.* 808, 35–43. doi:10.1016/j.ejphar.2016.06.045
73. Karman, J., Wang, J., Bodea, C., Cao, S., and Levesque, M. C. (2021). Lung Gene Expression and Single Cell Analyses Reveal Two Subsets of Idiopathic Pulmonary Fibrosis (IPF) Patients Associated with Different Pathogenic Mechanisms. *PLoS One* 16 (3), e0248889. doi:10.1371/journal.pone.0248889
74. Kasuya, Y., Kim, J. D., Hatano, M., Tatsumi, K., and Matsuda, S. (2021). Pathophysiological Roles of Stress-Activated Protein Kinases in Pulmonary Fibrosis. *Int. J. Mol. Sci.* 22 (11). doi:10.3390/ijms22116041
75. Katoh, M. (2018). "FGF (Fibroblast Growth Factor)," in *Encyclopedia of Signaling Molecules*. Editor S. Choi (Cham: Springer International Publishing), 1697–1702. doi:10.1007/978-3-319-67199-4_313
76. Kawamura, K., Ichikado, K., Yasuda, Y., Anan, K., and Suga, M. (2017). Azithromycin for Idiopathic Acute Exacerbation of Idiopathic Pulmonary Fibrosis: a Retrospective Single-Center Study. *BMC Pulm. Med.* 17 (1), 94. doi:10.1186/s12890-017-0437-z
77. Keating, G. M. (2015). Nintedanib: A Review of its Use in Patients with Idiopathic Pulmonary Fibrosis. *Drugs* 75 (10), 1131–1140. doi:10.1007/s40265-015-0418-6 Kelly, M., Kolb, M., Bonniaud, P., and Gauldie, J. (2003). Re-evaluation of Fibrogenic Cytokines in Lung Fibrosis. *Curr. Pharm. Des.* 9 (1), 39–49. doi:10.2174/1381612033392341
78. Khalil, N., Xu, Y. D., O'Connor, R., and Duronio, V. (2005). Proliferation of Pulmonary Interstitial Fibroblasts Is Mediated by Transforming Growth Factor-Beta1-Induced Release of Extracellular Fibroblast Growth Factor-2 and Phosphorylation of P38 MAPK and JNK. *J. Biol. Chem.* 280 (52), 43000–43009. doi:10.1074/jbc.M510441200
79. Kim, M. S., Baek, A. R., Lee, J. H., Jang, A. S., Kim, D. J., Chin, S. S., et al. (2019). IL-37 Attenuates Lung Fibrosis by Inducing Autophagy and Regulating TGF-B1 Production in Mice. *J. Immunol.* 203 (8), 2265–2275. doi:10.4049/jimmunol. 1801515
80. Kim, S., Lim, J. H., and Woo, C. H. (2020). Therapeutic Potential of Targeting Kinase Inhibition in Patients with Idiopathic Pulmonary Fibrosis. *Yeungnam Univ. J. Med.* 37 (4), 269–276. doi:10.12701/yujm.2020.00458
81. King, T. E., Jr., Bradford, W. Z., Castro-Bernardini, S., Fagan, E. A., Glaspole, I., Glassberg, M. K., et al. (2014). A Phase 3 Trial of Pirfenidone in Patients with Idiopathic Pulmonary Fibrosis. *N. Engl. J. Med.* 370 (22), 2083–2092. doi:10. 1056/NEJMoa1402582
82. King, T. E., Jr., Brown, K. K., Raghu, G., du Bois, R. M., Lynch, D. A., Martinez, F., et al. (2011a). BUILD-3: a Randomized, Controlled Trial of Bosentan in Idiopathic Pulmonary Fibrosis. *Am. J. Respir. Crit. Care Med.* 184 (1), 92–99. doi:10.1164/rccm.201011-1874OC
83. King, T. E., Jr., Pardo, A., and Selman, M. (2011b). Idiopathic Pulmonary Fibrosis. *Lancet* 378 (9807), 1949–1961. doi:10.1016/s0140-6736(11)60052-4
84. Kiyokawa, H., and Morimoto, M. (2020). Notch Signaling in the Mammalian Respiratory System, Specifically the Trachea and Lungs, in Development, Homeostasis, Regeneration, and Disease. *Dev. Growth Differ.* 62 (1), 67–79. doi:10.1111/dgd.12628
85. Kohan, M., Puxeddu, I., Reich, R., Levi-Schaffer, F., and Berkman, N. (2010). Eotaxin-2/CCL24 and eotaxin-3/CCL26 Exert Differential Profibrogenic Effects on Human Lung Fibroblasts. *Ann. Allergy Asthma Immunol.* 104 (1), 66–72. doi:10.1016/j.anai.2009.11.003
86. Königshoff, M., Kramer, M., Balsara, N., Wilhelm, J., Amarie, O. V., Jahn, A., et al. (2009). WNT1-inducible Signaling Protein-1 Mediates Pulmonary Fibrosis in Mice and Is Upregulated in Humans with Idiopathic Pulmonary Fibrosis. *J. Clin. Invest* 119 (4), 772–787. doi:10.1172/jci33950
87. Koo, H. Y., El-Baz, L. M., House, S., Cilvik, S. N., Dorry, S. J., Shoukry, N. M., et al. (2018). Fibroblast Growth Factor 2 Decreases Bleomycin-Induced Pulmonary Fibrosis and Inhibits Fibroblast Collagen Production and Myofibroblast Differentiation. *J. Pathol.* 246 (1), 54–66. doi:10.1002/path.5106
88. Kortekaas, R. K., Burgess, J. K., van Orsoy, R., Lamb, D., Webster, M., and Gosens, R. (2021). Therapeutic Targeting of IL-11 for Chronic Lung Disease. *Trends Pharmacol. Sci.* 42 (5), 354–366. doi:10.1016/j.tips.2021.01.007
89. Korthagen, N. M., van Moorsel, C. H., Kazemier, K. M., Ruven, H. J., and Grutters, J. C. (2012). IL1RN Genetic Variations and Risk of IPF: a Meta-Analysis and mRNA Expression Study. *Immunogenetics* 64 (5), 371–377. doi:10.1007/ s00251-012-0604-6
90. Kreuter, M., Wuyts, W., Renzoni, E., Koschel, D., Maher, T. M., Kolb, M., et al. (2016). Antacid Therapy and Disease Outcomes in Idiopathic Pulmonary Fibrosis: a Pooled Analysis. *Lancet Respir. Med.* 4 (5), 381–389. doi:10.1016/s2213-2600(16)00067-9
91. Kuhn, H., Krüger, S., Hammerschmidt, S., and Wirtz, H. (2010). High Concentrations of Vascular Endothelial Growth Factor Reduce Stretch-Induced Apoptosis of Alveolar Type II Cells. *Respirology* 15 (2), 343–348. doi:10.1111/j.1440-1843.2009.01701.x
92. Lawrence, J., and Nho, R. (2018). The Role of the Mammalian Target of Rapamycin (mTOR) in Pulmonary Fibrosis. *Int. J. Mol. Sci.* 19 (3). doi:10.3390/ ijms19030778

93. Lederer, D. J., and Martinez, F. J. (2018). Idiopathic Pulmonary Fibrosis. *N. Engl. J. Med.* 378 (19), 1811–1823. doi:10.1056/NEJMra1705751
94. Lee, E. G., Lee, T. H., Hong, Y., Ryoo, J., Heo, J. W., Gil, B. M., et al. (2021). Effects of Low-Dose Pirfenidone on Survival and Lung Function Decline in Patients with Idiopathic Pulmonary Fibrosis (IPF): Results from a Real-World Study. *PLoS One* 16 (12), e0261684. doi:10.1371/journal.pone. 0261684
95. Lee, J. S., Collard, H. R., Anstrom, K. J., Martinez, F. J., Noth, I., Roberts, R. S., et al. (2013). Anti-acid Treatment and Disease Progression in Idiopathic Pulmonary Fibrosis: an Analysis of Data from Three Randomised Controlled Trials. *Lancet Respir. Med.* 1 (5), 369–376. doi:10.1016/ s2213-2600(13)70105-x
96. Lee, J. S., Ryu, J. H., Elicker, B. M., Lydell, C. P., Jones, K. D., Wolters, P. J., et al. (2011). Gastroesophageal Reflux Therapy Is Associated with Longer Survival in Patients with Idiopathic Pulmonary Fibrosis. *Am. J. Respir. Crit. Care Med.* 184 (12), 1390–1394. doi:10.1164/rccm.201101-0138OC
97. Li, H., Zhao, C., Tian, Y., Lu, J., Zhang, G., Liang, S., et al. (2020). Src Family Kinases and Pulmonary Fibrosis: A Review. *Biomed. Pharmacother.* 127, 110183. doi:10.1016/j.biopha.2020.110183
98. Li, L., Li, Q., Wei, L., Wang, Z., Ma, W., Liu, F., et al. (2019). Chemokine (C-X-C Motif) Ligand 14 Contributes to Lipopolysaccharide-Induced Fibrogenesis in Mouse L929 Fibroblasts via Modulating PPM1A. *J. Cell Biochem.* 120 (8), 13372–13381. doi:10.1002/jcb.28612
99. Li, X., and Eriksson, U. (2003). Novel PDGF Family Members: PDGF-C and PDGF-D. *Cytokine Growth Factor Rev.* 14 (2), 91–98. doi:10.1016/s1359-6101(02)00090-4
100. Li, Y., Jiang, D., Liang, J., Meltzer, E. B., Gray, A., Miura, R., et al. (2011). Severe Lung Fibrosis Requires an Invasive Fibroblast Phenotype Regulated by Hyaluronan and CD44. *J. Exp. Med.* 208 (7), 1459–1471. doi:10.1084/jem. 20102510
101. Liang, J., Liu, N., Liu, X., Mena, J. M., Xie, T., Geng, Y., et al. (2019). Mitogen-activated Protein Kinase-Activated Protein Kinase 2 Inhibition Attenuates Fibroblast Invasion and Severe Lung Fibrosis. *Am. J. Respir. Cell Mol. Biol.* 60 (1), 41–48. doi:10.1165/rcmb.2018-0033OC
102. Lipson, K. E., Wong, C., Teng, Y., and Spong, S. (2012). CTGF Is a Central Mediator of Tissue Remodeling and Fibrosis and its Inhibition Can Reverse the Process of Fibrosis. *Fibrogenes. Tissue Repair* 5 (Suppl. 1), S24. doi:10.1186/ 1755-1536-5-s1-s24
103. Liu, S., Shi-wen, X., Abraham, D. J., and Leask, A. (2011). CCN2 Is Required for Bleomycin-Induced Skin Fibrosis in Mice. *Arthritis Rheum.* 63 (1), 239–246. doi:10.1002/art.30074
104. Liu, Y. M., Nepali, K., and Liou, J. P. (2017). Idiopathic Pulmonary Fibrosis: Current Status, Recent Progress, and Emerging Targets. *J. Med. Chem.* 60 (2), 527–553. doi:10.1021/acs.jmedchem.6b00935
105. Lobo, P. (2016). Nintedanib Data Challenge IPF Guidelines. *Lancet Respir. Med.* 4 (8), 610. doi:10.1016/S2213-2600(16)30196-5
106. Loetscher, P., Uguccioni, M., Bordoli, L., Baggiolini, M., Moser, B., Chizzolini, C., et al. (1998). CCR5 Is Characteristic of Th1 Lymphocytes. *Nature* 391 (6665), 344–345. doi:10.1038/34814
107. Maeda, A., Hiyama, K., Yamakido, H., Ishioka, S., and Yamakido, M. (1996). Increased Expression of Platelet-Derived Growth Factor A and Insulin-like Growth Factor-I in BAL Cells during the Development of Bleomycin-Induced Pulmonary Fibrosis in Mice. *Chest* 109 (3), 780–786. doi:10.1378/ chest.109. 3.780
108. Marijic, P., Schwarzkopf, L., Schwettmann, L., Ruhnke, T., Trudzinski, F., and Kreuter, M. (2021). Pirfenidone vs. Nintedanib in Patients with Idiopathic Pulmonary Fibrosis: a Retrospective Cohort Study. *Respir. Res.* 22 (1), 268. doi:10.1186/s12931-021-01857-y
109. Martin-Medina, A., Lehmann, M., Burgy, O., Hermann, S., Baarsma, H. A., Wagner, D. E., et al. (2018). Increased Extracellular Vesicles Mediate WNT5A Signaling in Idiopathic Pulmonary Fibrosis. *Am. J. Respir. Crit. Care Med.* 198 (12), 1527–1538. doi:10.1164/rccm.201708-1580OC
110. Martinez, F. J., Yow, E., Flaherty, K. R., Snyder, L. D., Durheim, M. T., Wisniewski, S. R., et al. (2021). Effect of Antimicrobial Therapy on Respiratory Hospitalization or Death in Adults with Idiopathic Pulmonary Fibrosis: The CleanUP-IPF Randomized Clinical Trial. *Jama* 325 (18), 1841–1851. doi:10. 1001/jama.2021.4956
111. Mei, Q., Liu, Z., Zuo, H., Yang, Z., and Qu, J. (2021). Idiopathic Pulmonary Fibrosis: An Update on Pathogenesis. *Front. Pharmacol.* 12, 797292. doi:10. 3389/fphar.2021.797292
112. Meltzer, E. B., and Noble, P. W. (2008). Idiopathic Pulmonary Fibrosis. *Orphanet J. Rare Dis.* 3, 8. doi:10.1186/1750-1172-3-8
113. Milara, J., Hernandez, G., Ballester, B., Morell, A., Roger, I., Montero, P., et al. (2018). The JAK2 Pathway Is Activated in Idiopathic Pulmonary Fibrosis. *Respir. Res.* 19 (1), 24. doi:10.1186/s12931-018-0728-9
114. Molyneaux, P. L., Cox, M. J., Willis-Owen, S. A., Mallia, P., Russell, K. E., Russell, A. M., et al. (2014). The Role of Bacteria in the Pathogenesis and Progression of Idiopathic Pulmonary Fibrosis. *Am. J. Respir. Crit. Care Med.* 190 (8), 906–913. doi:10.1164/rccm.201403-0541OC
115. Molyneaux, P. L., Willis-Owen, S. A. G., Cox, M. J., James, P., Cowman, S., Loebinger, M., et al. (2017). Host-Microbial Interactions in Idiopathic Pulmonary Fibrosis. *Am. J. Respir. Crit. Care Med.* 195 (12), 1640–1650. doi:10.1164/rccm.201607-1408OC
116. Montero, P., Milara, J., Roger, I., and Cortijo, J. (2021). Role of JAK/STAT in Interstitial Lung Diseases; Molecular and Cellular Mechanisms. *Int. J. Mol. Sci.* 22 (12). doi:10.3390/ijms22126211
117. Moodley, Y. P., Misso, N. L., Scaffidi, A. K., Fogel-Petrovic, M., McAnulty, R. J., Laurent, G. J., et al. (2003). Inverse Effects of Interleukin-6 on Apoptosis of Fibroblasts from Pulmonary Fibrosis and Normal Lungs. *Am. J. Respir. Cell Mol. Biol.* 29 (4), 490–498. doi:10.1165/rcmb.2002-0262OC
118. Mooney, J., Reddy, S. R., Chang, E., Broder, M. S., Gokhale, S., and Corral, M. (2021). Antifibrotic Therapies Reduce Mortality and Hospitalization Among Medicare Beneficiaries with Idiopathic Pulmonary Fibrosis. *J. Manag. Care Spec. Pharm.* 27 (12), 1724–1733. doi:10.18553/jmcp.2021.27.12.1724
119. Moore, B. B., Paine, R., 3rd, Christensen, P. J., Moore, T. A., Sitterding, S., Ngan, R., et al. (2001). Protection from Pulmonary Fibrosis in the Absence of CCR2 Signaling. *J. Immunol.* 167 (8), 4368–4377. doi:10.4049/ jimmunol.167.8.4368 Moss, B. J., Ryter, S. W., and Rosas, I. O. (2022). Pathogenic Mechanisms Underlying Idiopathic Pulmonary Fibrosis. *Annu. Rev. Pathol.* 17, 515–546. doi:10.1146/annurev-pathol-042320-030240
120. Mura, M., Han, B., Andrade, C. F., Seth, R., Hwang, D., Waddell, T. K., et al. (2006). The Early Responses of VEGF and its Receptors during Acute Lung Injury: Implication of VEGF in Alveolar Epithelial Cell Survival. *Crit. Care* 10 (5), R130. doi:10.1186/cc5042
121. Murphy-Ullrich, J. E., and Suto, M. J. (2018). Thrombospondin-1 Regulation of Latent TGF-β Activation: A Therapeutic Target for Fibrotic Disease. *Matrix Biol.* 68-69, 28–43. doi:10.1016/j.matbio.2017.12.009
122. Murray, L. A., Argentieri, R. L., Farrell, F. X., Bracht, M., Sheng, H., Whitaker, B., et al. (2008). Hyper-responsiveness of IPF/UIP Fibroblasts: Interplay between TGFbeta1, IL-13 and CCL2. *Int. J. Biochem. Cell Biol.* 40 (10), 2174–2182. doi:10.1016/j.biocel.2008.02.016
123. Nakagome, K., Dohi, M., Okunishi, K., Tanaka, R., Miyazaki, J., and Yamamoto, K. (2006). *In Vivo* IL-10 Gene Delivery Attenuates Bleomycin Induced Pulmonary Fibrosis by Inhibiting the Production and Activation of TGF-Beta in the Lung. *Thorax* 61 (10), 886–894. doi:10.1136/thx.2005.056317
124. Nathan, S. D., Costabel, U., Albera, C., Behr, J., Wuyts, W. A., Kirchgaessler, K. U., et al. (2019). Pirfenidone in Patients with Idiopathic Pulmonary Fibrosis and More Advanced Lung Function Impairment. *Respir. Med.* 153, 44–51. doi:10. 1016/j.rmed.2019.04.016
125. Ng, B., Dong, J., D'Agostino, G., Viswanathan, S., Widjaja, A. A., Lim, W. W., et al. (2019). Interleukin-11 Is a Therapeutic Target in Idiopathic Pulmonary Fibrosis. *Sci. Transl. Med.* 11 (511). doi:10.1126/scitranslmed.aaw1237
126. Ninou, I., Magkrioti, C., and Aidinis, V. (2018). Autotaxin in Pathophysiology and Pulmonary Fibrosis. *Front. Med. (Lausanne)* 5, 180. doi:10.3389/ fmed.2018. 00180
127. Nishioka, Y., Azuma, M., Kishi, M., and Aono, Y. (2013). Targeting Platelet-Derived Growth Factor as a Therapeutic Approach in Pulmonary Fibrosis. *J. Med. Invest* 60 (3-4), 175–183. doi:10.2152/jmi.60.175
128. Noble, P. W., Albera, C., Bradford, W. Z., Costabel, U., Glassberg, M. K., Kardatzke, D., et al. (2011). Pirfenidone in Patients with Idiopathic Pulmonary Fibrosis (CAPACITY): Two Randomised Trials. *Lancet* 377 (9779), 1760–1769. doi:10. 1016/s0140-6736(11)60405-4

129. Noble, P. W., Barkauskas, C. E., and Jiang, D. (2012). Pulmonary Fibrosis: Patterns and Perpetrators. *J. Clin. Invest* 122 (8), 2756–2762. doi:10.1172/jci60323
130. Noth, I., Zhang, Y., Ma, S. F., Flores, C., Barber, M., Huang, Y., et al. (2013). Genetic Variants Associated with Idiopathic Pulmonary Fibrosis Susceptibility and Mortality: a Genome-wide Association Study. *Lancet Respir. Med.* 1 (4), 309–317. doi:10.1016/s2213-2600(13)70045-6
131. O'Dwyer, D. N., Armstrong, M. E., Trujillo, G., Cooke, G., Keane, M. P., Fallon, P. G., et al. (2013). The Toll-like Receptor 3 L412F Polymorphism and Disease Progression in Idiopathic Pulmonary Fibrosis. *Am. J. Respir. Crit. Care Med.* 188 (12), 1442–1450. doi:10.1164/rccm.201304-0760OC
132. Oku, H., Nakazato, H., Horikawa, T., Tsuruta, Y., and Suzuki, R. (2002). Pirfenidone Suppresses Tumor Necrosis Factor-Alpha, Enhances Interleukin-10 and Protects Mice from Endotoxic Shock. *Eur. J. Pharmacol.* 446 (1-3), 167–176. doi:10.1016/s0014-2999(02)01757-0
133. Ong, C. H., Tham, C. L., Harith, H. H., Firdaus, N., and Israf, D. A. (2021). TGF-β-induced Fibrosis: A Review on the Underlying Mechanism and Potential Therapeutic Strategies. *Eur. J. Pharmacol.* 911, 174510. doi:10.1016/j.ejphar. 2021.174510
134. Ornitz, D. M., and Itoh, N. (2022). New Developments in the Biology of Fibroblast Growth Factors. *WIREs Mech. Dis.* e1549, e1549. doi:10.1002/wsbm.1549
135. Pan, L. H., Yamauchi, K., Uzuki, M., Nakanishi, T., Takigawa, M., Inoue, H., et al. (2001). Type II Alveolar Epithelial Cells and Interstitial Fibroblasts Express Connective Tissue Growth Factor in IPF. *Eur. Respir. J.* 17 (6), 1220–1227. doi:10.1183/09031936.01.00074101
136. Papiris, S. A., Tomos, I. P., Karakatsani, A., Spathis, A., Korbila, I., Analitis, A., et al. (2018). High Levels of IL-6 and IL-8 Characterize Early-On Idiopathic Pulmonary Fibrosis Acute Exacerbations. *Cytokine* 102, 168–172. doi:10.1016/j.cyto.2017.08.019
137. Passalacqua, G., Mincarini, M., Colombo, D., Troisi, G., Ferrari, M., Bagnasco, D., et al. (2017). IL-13 and Idiopathic Pulmonary Fibrosis: Possible Links and New Therapeutic Strategies. *Pulm. Pharmacol. Ther.* 45, 95–100. doi:10.1016/j.pupt. 2017.05.007
138. Pechkovsky, D. V., Scaffidi, A. K., Hackett, T. L., Ballard, J., Shaheen, F., Thompson, P. J., et al. (2008). Transforming Growth Factor Beta1 Induces Alphavbeta3 Integrin Expression in Human Lung Fibroblasts via a Beta3 Integrin-, C-Src-, and P38 MAPK-dependent Pathway. *J. Biol. Chem.* 283 (19), 12898–12908. doi:10.1074/jbc.M708226200
139. Phan, T. H. G., Paliogiannis, P., Nasrallah, G. K., Giordo, R., Eid, A. H., Fois, A. G., et al. (2021). Emerging Cellular and Molecular Determinants of Idiopathic Pulmonary Fibrosis. *Cell Mol. Life Sci.* 78 (5), 2031–2057. doi:10.1007/s00018- 020-03693-7
140. Phillips, R. J., Burdick, M. D., Hong, K., Lutz, M. A., Murray, L. A., Xue, Y. Y., et al. (2004). Circulating Fibrocytes Traffic to the Lungs in Response to CXCL12 and Mediate Fibrosis. *J. Clin. Invest* 114 (3), 438–446. doi:10.1172/jci20997
141. Pignatti, P., Brunetti, G., Moretto, D., Yacoub, M. R., Fiori, M., Balbi, B., et al. (2006). Role of the Chemokine Receptors CXCR3 and CCR4 in Human Pulmonary Fibrosis. *Am. J. Respir. Crit. Care Med.* 173 (3), 310–317. doi:10.1164/rccm.200502-244OC
142. Pitre, T., Khalid, M. F., Cui, S., Zhang, M. C., Husnudinov, R., Mah, J., et al. (2022). Sildenafil for Idiopathic Pulmonary Fibrosis: A Systematic Review and Meta- Analysis. *Pulm. Pharmacol. Ther.* 73-74, 102128. doi:10.1016/j.pupt.2022. 102128
143. Puxeddu, I., Bader, R., Piliponsky, A. M., Reich, R., Levi-Schaffer, F., and Berkman, N. (2006). The CC Chemokine eotaxin/CCL11 Has a Selective Profibrogenic Effect on Human Lung Fibroblasts. *J. Allergy Clin. Immunol.* 117 (1), 103–110. doi:10.1016/j.jaci.2005.08.057
144. Qian, W., Cai, X., Qian, Q., Zhang, W., and Tian, L. (2020). Metastasis-associated Protein 1 Promotes Epithelial-Mesenchymal Transition in Idiopathic Pulmonary Fibrosis by Up-Regulating Snail Expression. *J. Cell Mol. Med.* 24 (11), 5998–6007. doi:10.1111/jcmm.15062
145. Qiu, T., Tian, Y., Gao, Y., Ma, M., Li, H., Liu, X., et al. (2019). PTEN Loss Regulates Alveolar Epithelial Cell Senescence in Pulmonary Fibrosis Depending on Akt Activation. *Aging (Albany NY)* 11 (18), 7492–7509. doi:10.18632/aging.102262
146. Raghu, G., Amatto, V. C., Behr, J., and Stowasser, S. (2015). Comorbidities in Idiopathic Pulmonary Fibrosis Patients: a Systematic Literature Review. *Eur. Respir. J.* 46 (4), 1113–1130. doi:10.1183/13993003.02316-2014
147. Raghu, G., Pellegrini, C. A., Yow, E., Flaherty, K. R., Meyer, K., Noth, I., et al. (2018). Laparoscopic Anti-reflux Surgery for the Treatment of Idiopathic Pulmonary Fibrosis (WRAP-IPF): a Multicentre, Randomised, Controlled Phase 2 Trial. *Lancet Respir. Med.* 6 (9), 707–714. doi:10.1016/s2213-2600(18)30301-1
148. Raghu, G., Scholand, M. B., de Andrade, J., Lancaster, L., Mageto, Y., Goldin, J., et al. (2016). FG-3019 Anti-connective Tissue Growth Factor Monoclonal Antibody: Results of an Open-Label Clinical Trial in Idiopathic Pulmonary Fibrosis. *Eur. Respir. J.* 47 (5), 1481–1491. doi:10.1183/13993003.01030-2015
149. Rahaman, S. O., Grove, L. M., Paruchuri, S., Southern, B. D., Abraham, S., Niese, K. A., et al. (2014). TRPV4 Mediates Myofibroblast Differentiation and Pulmonary Fibrosis in Mice. *J. Clin. Invest* 124 (12), 5225–5238. doi:10.1172/jci75331
150. Ramos, C., Becerril, C., Montaño, M., García-De-Alba, C., Ramírez, R., Checa, M., et al. (2010). FGF-1 Reverts Epithelial-Mesenchymal Transition Induced by TGF-{beta}1 through MAPK/ERK Kinase Pathway. *Am. J. Physiol. Lung Cell Mol. Physiol.* 299 (2), L222–L231. doi:10.1152/ajplung.00070.2010
151. Rao, L. Z., Wang, Y., Zhang, L., Wu, G., Zhang, L., Wang, F. X., et al. (2021). IL-24 Deficiency Protects Mice against Bleomycin-Induced Pulmonary Fibrosis by Repressing IL-4-induced M2 Program in Macrophages. *Cell Death Differ.* 28 (4), 1270–1283. doi:10.1038/s41418-020-00650-6
152. Reilkoff, R. A., Peng, H., Murray, L. A., Peng, X., Russell, T., Montgomery, R., et al. (2013). Semaphorin 7a+ Regulatory T Cells Are Associated with Progressive Idiopathic Pulmonary Fibrosis and Are Implicated in Transforming Growth Factor-B1-Induced Pulmonary Fibrosis. *Am. J. Respir. Crit. Care Med.* 187 (2), 180–188. doi:10.1164/rccm.201206-1109OC
153. Rice, A. B., Moomaw, C. R., Morgan, D. L., and Bonner, J. C. (1999). Specific Inhibitors of Platelet-Derived Growth Factor or Epidermal Growth Factor Receptor Tyrosine Kinase Reduce Pulmonary Fibrosis in Rats. *Am. J. Pathol.* 155 (1), 213–221. doi:10.1016/s0002-9440(10)65115-2
154. Richeldi, L., du Bois, R. M., Raghu, G., Azuma, A., Brown, K. K., Costabel, U., et al. (2014). Efficacy and Safety of Nintedanib in Idiopathic Pulmonary Fibrosis. *N. Engl. J. Med.* 370 (22), 2071–2082. doi:10.1056/NEJMoa1402584
155. Richeldi, L., Kolb, M., Jouneau, S., Wuyts, W. A., Schinzel, B., Stowasser, S., et al. (2020). Efficacy and Safety of Nintedanib in Patients with Advanced Idiopathic Pulmonary Fibrosis. *BMC Pulm. Med.* 20 (1), 3. doi:10.1186/s12890-019-1030-4
156. Rivas-Fuentes, S., Herrera, I., Salgado-Aguayo, A., Buendía-Roldán, I., Becerril, C., and Cisneros, J. (2020). CX3CL1 and CX3CR1 Could Be a Relevant Molecular axis in the Pathophysiology of Idiopathic Pulmonary Fibrosis. *Int. J. Med. Sci.* 17 (15), 2357–2361. doi:10.7150/ijms.43748
157. Robbins, D. J., Fei, D. L., and Riobo, N. A. (2012). The Hedgehog Signal Transduction Network. *Sci. Signal* 5 (246), re6. doi:10.1126/scisignal.2002906 Roberts, J. R., Perkins, G. D., Fujisawa, T., Pettigrew, K. A., Gao, F., Ahmed, A., et al. (2007). Vascular Endothelial Growth Factor Promotes Physical Wound Repair and Is Anti-apoptotic in Primary Distal Lung Epithelial and A549 Cells. *Crit. Care Med.* 35 (9), 2164–2170. doi:10.1097/01.ccm.0000281451.73202.f6
158. Rock, J. R., Barkauskas, C. E., Cronce, M. J., Xue, Y., Harris, J. R., Liang, J., et al. (2011). Multiple Stromal Populations Contribute to Pulmonary Fibrosis without Evidence for Epithelial to Mesenchymal Transition. *Proc. Natl. Acad. Sci. U. S. A.* 108 (52), E1475–E1483. doi:10.1073/pnas.1117988108
159. Rose, C. E., Jr., Sung, S. S., and Fu, S. M. (2003). Significant Involvement of CCL2 (MCP-1) in Inflammatory Disorders of the Lung. *Microcirculation* 10 (3-4), 273–288. doi:10.1038/sj.mn.7800193
160. Saito, A., Horie, M., and Nagase, T. (2018). TGF-β Signaling in Lung Health and Disease. *Int. J. Mol. Sci.* 19 (8). doi:10.3390/ijms19082460
161. Saito, M., Mitani, A., Ishimori, T., Miyashita, N., Isago, H., Mikami, Y., et al. (2020). Active mTOR in Lung Epithelium Promotes Epithelial-Mesenchymal Transition and Enhances Lung Fibrosis. *Am. J. Respir. Cell Mol. Biol.* 62 (6), 699–708. doi:10.1165/rcmb.2019-0255OC

162. Salton, F., Ruaro, B., Confalonieri, P., and Confalonieri, M. (2020). Epithelial-Mesenchymal Transition: A Major Pathogenic Driver in Idiopathic Pulmonary Fibrosis? *Med. Kaunas.* 56 (11). doi:10.3390/medicina56110608
163. Savarino, E., Carbone, R., Marabotto, E., Furnari, M., Sconfienza, L., Ghio, M., et al. (2013). Gastro-oesophageal Reflux and Gastric Aspiration in Idiopathic Pulmonary Fibrosis Patients. *Eur. Respir. J.* 42 (5), 1322–1331. doi:10.1183/ 09031936.00101212
164. Schaefer, C. J., Ruhrmund, D. W., Pan, L., Seiwert, S. D., and Kossen, K. (2011). Antifibrotic Activities of Pirfenidone in Animal Models. *Eur. Respir. Rev.* 20 (120), 85–97. doi:10.1183/09059180.00001111
165. Selman, M., and Pardo, A. (2014). Revealing the Pathogenic and Aging-Related Mechanisms of the Enigmatic Idiopathic Pulmonary Fibrosis. An Integral Model. *Am. J. Respir. Crit. Care Med.* 189 (10), 1161–1172. doi:10.1164/ rccm.201312-2221PP
166. Shenderov, K., Collins, S. L., Powell, J. D., and Horton, M. R. (2021). Immune Dysregulation as a Driver of Idiopathic Pulmonary Fibrosis. *J. Clin. Invest* 131 (2). doi:10.1172/jci143226
167. Shimbori, C., Bellaye, P. S., Xia, J., Gauldie, J., Ask, K., Ramos, C., et al. (2016). Fibroblast Growth Factor-1 Attenuates TGF-B1-Induced Lung Fibrosis. *J. Pathol.* 240 (2), 197–210. doi:10.1002/path.4768
168. Singer, D., Bengtson, L. G. S., Conoscenti, C. S., Anderson, A. J., Brekke, L., Shetty, S. S., et al. (2022). Impact of Timing of Nintedanib Initiation Among Patients Newly Diagnosed with Idiopathic Pulmonary Fibrosis. *J. Med. Econ.* 25, 532–540. doi:10.1080/13696998.2022.2054203
169. Skibba, M., Drelich, A., Poellmann, M., Hong, S., and Brasier, A. R. (2020). Nanoapproaches to Modifying Epigenetics of Epithelial Mesenchymal Transition for Treatment of Pulmonary Fibrosis. *Front. Pharmacol.* 11, 607689. doi:10.3389/fphar.2020.607689
170. Spagnolo, P., Tzouvelekis, A., and Bonella, F. (2018). The Management of Patients with Idiopathic Pulmonary Fibrosis. *Front. Med. (Lausanne)* 5, 148. doi:10. 3389/fmed.2018.00148
171. Strieter, R. M. (2005). Pathogenesis and Natural History of Usual Interstitial Pneumonia: the Whole Story or the Last Chapter of a Long Novel. *Chest* 128 (5 Suppl. 1), 526s–532s. doi:10.1378/chest.128.5_suppl_1.526S
172. Su, J., Morgani, S. M., David, C. J., Wang, Q., Er, E. E., Huang, Y. H., et al. (2020). TGF-β Orchestrates Fibrogenic and Developmental EMTs via the RAS Effector RREB1. *Nature* 577 (7791), 566–571. doi:10.1038/s41586-019-1897-5
173. Suarez-Cuartin, G., and Molina-Molina, M. (2019). Assessing Quality of Life of Idiopathic Pulmonary Fibrosis Patients: the INSTAGE Study. *Breathe (Sheff)* 15 (2), 144–146. doi:10.1183/20734735.0016-2019
174. Sun, M., Sun, Y., Feng, Z., Kang, X., Yang, W., Wang, Y., et al. (2021). New Insights into the Hippo/YAP Pathway in Idiopathic Pulmonary Fibrosis. *Pharmacol. Res.* 169, 105635. doi:10.1016/j.phrs.2021.105635
175. Suryadevara, V., Ramchandran, R., Kamp, D. W., and Natarajan, V. (2020). Lipid Mediators Regulate Pulmonary Fibrosis: Potential Mechanisms and Signaling Pathways. *Int. J. Mol. Sci.* 21 (12). doi:10.3390/ijms21124257
176. Tager, A. M., LaCamera, P., Shea, B. S., Campanella, G. S., Selman, M., Zhao, Z., et al. (2008). The Lysophosphatidic Acid Receptor LPA1 Links Pulmonary Fibrosis to Lung Injury by Mediating Fibroblast Recruitment and Vascular Leak. *Nat. Med.* 14 (1), 45–54. doi:10.1038/nm1685
177. Takehara, K., Koga, Y., Hachisu, Y., Utsugi, M., Sawada, Y., Saito, Y., et al. (2022). Differential Discontinuation Profiles between Pirfenidone and Nintedanib in Patients with Idiopathic Pulmonary Fibrosis. *Cells* 11 (1). doi:10.3390/ cells11010143
178. Tanaka, Y., Hino, M., and Gemma, A. (2017). Potential Benefit of Bosentan Therapy in Borderline or Less Severe Pulmonary Hypertension Secondary to Idiopathic Pulmonary Fibrosis-An Interim Analysis of Results from a Prospective, Single-Center, Randomized, Parallel-Group Study. *BMC Pulm. Med.* 17 (1), 200. doi:10.1186/s12890-017-0523-2
179. Taniguchi, H., Ebina, M., Kondoh, Y., Ogura, T., Azuma, A., Suga, M., et al. (2010). Pirfenidone in Idiopathic Pulmonary Fibrosis. *Eur. Respir. J.* 35 (4), 821–829. doi:10.1183/09031936.00005209
180. Tran, T., Assayag, D., Ernst, P., and Suissa, S. (2021). Effectiveness of Proton Pump Inhibitors in Idiopathic Pulmonary Fibrosis: A Population-Based Cohort Study. *Chest* 159 (2), 673–682. doi:10.1016/j.chest.2020.08.2080
181. Tsubouchi, K., Araya, J., and Kuwano, K. (2018). PINK1-PARK2-mediated Mitophagy in COPD and IPF Pathogeneses. *Inflamm. Regen.* 38, 18. doi:10. 1186/s41232-018-0077-6
182. Tzavlaki, K., and Moustakas, A. (2020). TGF-β Signaling. *Biomolecules* 10 (3). doi:10.3390/biom10030487
183. Tzouvelekis, A., Ntolios, P., Karameris, A., Vilaras, G., Boglou, P., Koulelidis, A., et al. (2013). Increased Expression of Epidermal Growth Factor Receptor (EGF-R) in Patients with Different Forms of Lung Fibrosis. *Biomed. Res. Int.* 2013, 654354. doi:10.1155/2013/654354
184. Ulsamer, A., Wei, Y., Kim, K. K., Tan, K., Wheeler, S., Xi, Y., et al. (2012). Axin Pathway Activity Regulates *In Vivo* pY654-β-Catenin Accumulation and Pulmonary Fibrosis. *J. Biol. Chem.* 287 (7), 5164–5172. doi:10.1074/jbc. M111.322123
185. Vancheri, C., Kreuter, M., Richeldi, L., Ryerson, C. J., Valeyre, D., Grutters, J. C., et al. (2018). Nintedanib with Add-On Pirfenidone in Idiopathic Pulmonary Fibrosis. Results of the INJOURNEY Trial. *Am. J. Respir. Crit. Care Med.* 197 (3), 356–363. doi:10.1164/rccm.201706-1301OC
186. Varet, J., Douglas, S. K., Gilmartin, L., Medford, A. R., Bates, D. O., Harper, S. J., et al. (2010). VEGF in the Lung: a Role for Novel Isoforms. *Am. J. Physiol. Lung Cell Mol. Physiol.* 298 (6), L768–L774. doi:10.1152/ajplung.00353.2009
187. Villavicencio, M. A., Axtell, A. L., Osho, A., Astor, T., Roy, N., Melnitchouk, S., et al. (2018). Single- versus Double-Lung Transplantation in Pulmonary Fibrosis: Impact of Age and Pulmonary Hypertension. *Ann. Thorac. Surg.* 106 (3), 856–863. doi:10.1016/j.athoracsur.2018.04.060
188. Walsh, J., Absher, M., and Kelley, J. (1993). Variable Expression of Platelet-Derived Growth Factor Family Proteins in Acute Lung Injury. *Am. J. Respir. Cell Mol. Biol.* 9 (6), 637–644. doi:10.1165/ajrcmb/9.6.637
189. Wang, Q., Usinger, W., Nichols, B., Gray, J., Xu, L., Seeley, T. W., et al. (2011). Cooperative Interaction of CTGF and TGF-β in Animal Models of Fibrotic Disease. *Fibrogenes. Tissue Repair* 4 (1), 4. doi:10.1186/1755-1536-4-4
190. Wang, Q., Xie, Z. L., Wu, Q., Jin, Z. X., Yang, C., and Feng, J. (2021). Role of Various Imbalances Centered on Alveolar Epithelial Cell/fibroblast Apoptosis Imbalance in the Pathogenesis of Idiopathic Pulmonary Fibrosis. *Chin. Med. J. Engl.* 134 (3), 261–274. doi:10.1097/cm9.0000000000001288
191. Wang, T., Liu, Y., Zou, J. F., and Cheng, Z. S. (2017). Interleukin-17 Induces Human Alveolar Epithelial to Mesenchymal Cell Transition via the TGF-B1 Mediated Smad2/3 and ERK1/2 Activation. *PLoS One* 12 (9), e0183972. doi:10. 1371/journal.pone.0183972
192. Whyte, M., Hubbard, R., Meliconi, R., Whidborne, M., Eaton, V., Bingle, C., et al. (2000). Increased Risk of Fibrosing Alveolitis Associated with Interleukin-1 Receptor Antagonist and Tumor Necrosis Factor-Alpha Gene Polymorphisms. *Am. J. Respir. Crit. Care Med.* 162 (2 Pt 1), 755–758. doi:10.1164/ajrccm.162.2. 9909053
193. Wilson, M. S., Madala, S. K., Ramalingam, T. R., Gochuico, B. R., Rosas, I. O., Cheever, A. W., et al. (2010). Bleomycin and IL-1beta-mediated Pulmonary Fibrosis Is IL-17A Dependent. *J. Exp. Med.* 207 (3), 535–552. doi:10.1084/ jem. 20092121
194. Wilson, M. S., and Wynn, T. A. (2009). Pulmonary Fibrosis: Pathogenesis, Etiology and Regulation. *Mucosal Immunol.* 2 (2), 103–121. doi:10.1038/ mi.2008.85 Woodcock, H. V., Eley, J. D., Guillotin, D., Platé, M., Nanthakumar, C. B., Martufi, M., et al. (2019). The mTORC1/4E-BP1 axis Represents a Critical Signaling Node during Fibrogenesis. *Nat. Commun.* 10 (1), 6. doi:10.1038/s41467-018-07858-8
195. Wu, H., Yu, Y., Huang, H., Hu, Y., Fu, S., Wang, Z., et al. (2020). Progressive Pulmonary Fibrosis Is Caused by Elevated Mechanical Tension on Alveolar Stem Cells. *Cell* 180 (1), 107–e17. e117. doi:10.1016/j.cell. 2019.11.027
196. Wu, J., Chu, X., Chen, C., and Bellusci, S. (2018). Role of Fibroblast Growth Factor 10 in Mesenchymal Cell Differentiation during Lung Development and Disease. *Front. Genet.* 9, 545. doi:10.3389/fgene.2018.00545
197. Wu, W., Qiu, L., Wu, J., Liu, X., and Zhang, G. (2021). Efficacy and Safety of Pirfenidone in the Treatment of Idiopathic Pulmonary Fibrosis Patients: a Systematic Review and Meta-Analysis of Randomised Controlled Trials. *BMJ Open* 11 (12), e050004. doi:10.1136/bmjopen-2021-050004
198. Wynes, M. W., Frankel, S. K., and Riches, D. W. (2004). IL-4-induced Macrophage-Derived IGF-I Protects Myofibroblasts from Apoptosis Following Growth Factor Withdrawal. *J. Leukoc. Biol.* 76 (5), 1019–1027. doi:10.1189/jlb.0504288

199. Xu, Q., Liu, Y., Pan, H., Xu, T., Li, Y., Yuan, J., et al. (2019). Aberrant Expression of miR-125a-3p Promotes Fibroblast Activation via Fyn/STAT3 Pathway during Silica-Induced Pulmonary Fibrosis. *Toxicology* 414, 57–67. doi:10.1016/j.tox. 2019.01.007
200. Xu, X., Zhang, J., and Dai, H. (2020). IL-25/IL-33/TSLP Contributes to Idiopathic Pulmonary Fibrosis: Do Alveolar Epithelial Cells and (Myo) fibroblasts Matter? *Exp. Biol. Med. (Maywood)* 245 (10), 897–901. doi:10. 1177/1535370220915428
201. Xylourgidis, N., Min, K., Ahangari, F., Yu, G., Herazo-Maya, J. D., Karampitsakos, T., et al. (2019). Role of Dual-Specificity Protein Phosphatase DUSP10/MKP-5 in Pulmonary Fibrosis. *Am. J. Physiol. Lung Cell Mol. Physiol.* 317 (5), L678–l689. doi:10.1152/ajplung.00264.2018
202. Yagihashi, K., Huckleberry, J., Colby, T. V., Tazelaar, H. D., Zach, J., Sundaram, B., et al. (2016). Radiologic-pathologic Discordance in Biopsy-Proven Usual Interstitial Pneumonia. *Eur. Respir. J.* 47 (4), 1189–1197. doi:10.1183/13993003.01680-2015
203. Yan, Z., Kui, Z., and Ping, Z. (2014). Reviews and Prospectives of Signaling Pathway Analysis in Idiopathic Pulmonary Fibrosis. *Autoimmun. Rev.* 13 (10), 1020–1025. doi:10.1016/j.autrev.2014.08.028
204. Yang, D., Chen, X., Wang, J., Lou, Q., Lou, Y., Li, L., et al. (2019). Dysregulated Lung Commensal Bacteria Drive Interleukin-17B Production to Promote Pulmonary Fibrosis through Their Outer Membrane Vesicles. *Immunity* 50 (3), 692–e7. e697. doi:10.1016/j.immuni.2019.02.001
205. Yang, L., Herrera, J., Gilbertsen, A., Xia, H., Smith, K., Benyumov, A., et al. (2018). IL-8 Mediates Idiopathic Pulmonary Fibrosis Mesenchymal Progenitor Cell Fibrogenicity. *Am. J. Physiol. Lung Cell Mol. Physiol.* 314 (1), L127–l136. doi:10. 1152/ajplung.00200.2017
206. Yang, L., Zhou, F., Zheng, D., Wang, D., Li, X., Zhao, C., et al. (2021). FGF/FGFR Signaling: From Lung Development to Respiratory Diseases. *Cytokine Growth Factor Rev.* 62, 94–104. doi:10.1016/j.cytogfr.2021.09.002
207. Yin, Y., White, A. C., Huh, S. H., Hilton, M. J., Kanazawa, H., Long, F., et al. (2008). An FGF-WNT Gene Regulatory Network Controls Lung Mesenchyme Development. *Dev. Biol.* 319 (2), 426–436. doi:10.1016/j. ydbio.2008.04.009
208. Yogo, Y., Fujishima, S., Inoue, T., Saito, F., Shiomi, T., Yamaguchi, K., et al. (2009). Macrophage Derived Chemokine (CCL22), Thymus and Activation-Regulated Chemokine (CCL17), and CCR4 in Idiopathic Pulmonary Fibrosis. *Respir. Res.* 10 (1), 80. doi:10.1186/1465-9921-10-80
209. Yombo, D. J. K., Odayar, V., Gupta, N., Jegga, A. G., and Madala, S. K. (2021). The Protective Effects of IL-31RA Deficiency during Bleomycin-Induced Pulmonary Fibrosis. *Front. Immunol.* 12, 645717. doi:10.3389/fimmu.2021. 645717
210. Yoshinouchi, T., Naniwa, T., Shimizu, S., Ohtsuki, Y., Fujita, J., Sato, S., et al. (2007). Expression of Chemokine Receptors CXCR3 and CCR4 in Lymphocytes of Idiopathic Nonspecific Interstitial Pneumonia. *Respir. Med.* 101 (6), 1258–1264. doi:10.1016/j.rmed.2006.10.019
211. Zhang, J., Wang, D., Wang, L., Wang, S., Roden, A. C., Zhao, H., et al. (2019a). Profibrotic Effect of IL-17A and Elevated IL-17RA in Idiopathic Pulmonary Fibrosis and Rheumatoid Arthritis-Associated Lung Disease Support a Direct Role for IL-17A/ IL-17RA in Human Fibrotic Interstitial Lung Disease. *Am. J. Physiol. Lung Cell Mol. Physiol.* 316 (3), L487–l497. doi:10.1152/ajplung.00301.2018
212. Zhang, L. M., Zhang, J., Zhang, Y., Fei, C., Wang, L., Yi, Z. W., et al. (2019b). Interleukin-18 Promotes Fibroblast Senescence in Pulmonary Fibrosis through Down-Regulating Klotho Expression. *Biomed. Pharmacother.* 113, 108756. doi:10.1016/j.biopha.2019.108756
213. Zhang, S., Yu, D., Wang, M., Huang, T., Wu, H., Zhang, Y., et al. (2018). FGF21 Attenuates Pulmonary Fibrogenesis through Ameliorating Oxidative Stress *In Vivo* and *In Vitro*. *Biomed. Pharmacother.* 103, 1516–1525. doi:10.1016/j. biopha.2018.03.100
214. Zhou, Y., Huang, X., Hecker, L., Kurundkar, D., Kurundkar, A., Liu, H., et al. (2013). Inhibition of Mechanosensitive Signaling in Myofibroblasts Ameliorates Experimental Pulmonary Fibrosis. *J. Clin. Invest* 123 (3), 1096–1108. doi:10.1172/jci66700
215. Zhu, X., Fang, X., Chen, W., Han, F., Huang, Z., Luo, B., et al. (2017). Lower Expression of Platelet Derived Growth Factor Is Associated with Better Overall Survival Rate of Patients with Idiopathic Nonspecific Interstitial Pneumonia. *J. Thorac. Dis.* 9 (3), 519–528. doi:10.21037/jtd.2017.02.50
216. Zhuo, Y., Zhang, J., Laboy, M., and Lasky, J. A. (2004). Modulation of PDGF-C and PDGF-D Expression during Bleomycin-Induced Lung Fibrosis. *Am. J. Physiol. Lung Cell Mol. Physiol.* 286 (1), L182–L188. doi:10.1152/ajplung.00083.2003
217. Ziegenhagen, M. W., Schrum, S., Zissel, G., Zipfel, P. F., Schlaak, M., and Müller- Quernheim, J. (1998). Increased Expression of Proinflammatory Chemokines in Bronchoalveolar Lavage Cells of Patients with Progressing Idiopathic Pulmonary Fibrosis and Sarcoidosis. *J. Investig. Med.* 46 (5), 223–231.
218. Zou, M., Zhang, G., Zou, J., Liu, Y., Liu, B., Hu, X., et al. (2020). Inhibition of the ERK1/2-Ubiquitous Calpains Pathway Attenuates Experimental Pulmonary Fibrosis *In Vivo* and *In Vitro*. *Exp. Cell Res.* 391 (1), 111886. doi:10.1016/j.yexcr. 2020.111886

8

Commonalities Between ARDS, Pulmonary Fibrosis and COVID-19: The Potential of Autotaxin as a Therapeutic Target

Konstantinos Ntatsoulis [1†], Theodoros Karampitsakos [2†], Eliza Tsitoura [3†], Elli-Anna Stylianaki [1], Alexios N. Matralis [1], Argyrios Tzouvelekis [2], Katerina Antoniou [3*] and Vassilis Aidinis [1*]*

[1] Institute of Bio-Innovation, Biomedical Sciences Research Center Alexander Fleming, Athens, Greece, [2] Department of Respiratory Medicine, School of Medicine, University of Patras, Patras, Greece, [3] Laboratory of Molecular & Cellular Pneumonology, Department of Respiratory Medicine, School of Medicine, University of Crete, Heraklion, Greece

***Correspondence:**
Argyrios Tzouvelekis
atzouvelekis@upatras.gr
Katerina Antoniou
kantoniou@med.uoc.gr
Vassilis Aidinis
V.Aidinis@Fleming.gr

†These authors have contributed equally to this work

Severe COVID-19 is characterized by acute respiratory distress syndrome (ARDS)-like hyperinflammation and endothelial dysfunction, that can lead to respiratory and multi organ failure and death. Interstitial lung diseases (ILD) and pulmonary fibrosis confer an increased risk for severe disease, while a subset of COVID-19-related ARDS surviving patients will develop a fibroproliferative response that can persist post hospitalization. Autotaxin (ATX) is a secreted lysophospholipase D, largely responsible for the extracellular production of lysophosphatidic acid (LPA), a pleiotropic signaling lysophospholipid with multiple effects in pulmonary and immune cells. In this review, we discuss the similarities of COVID-19, ARDS and ILDs, and suggest ATX as a possible pathologic link and a potential common therapeutic target.

Keywords: COVID-19, ARDS, pulmonary fibrosis, Autotaxin, lysophosphatidic acid

COVID-19

Severe acute respiratory syndrome coronavirus 2 (SARS-CoV-2) infection leads to the development of Coronavirus Disease 2019 (COVID-19), proclaimed pandemic on March 11, 2020 (1, 2). Upon airborne, mainly, CoV-2 transmission, the viral spike (S) glycoprotein mediates viral entry *via* binding to angiotensin-converting enzyme 2 (ACE2), supported by the transmembrane protease serine protease 2 (TMPRSS2) that proteolytically processes the S protein (3, 4). Infected cells in the lung, as detected with immunocytochemistry, include the upper airway bronchiolar epithelium and submucosal gland epithelium, as well as alveolar epithelial cells and macrophages (1). ACE2 is distributed mainly in the intestine, heart, kidney, as well as the lung, where alveolar epithelial type II cells are the major expressing cells. TMPRSS2 is highly expressed in several tissues; in the lung is co- expressed with ACE2 in nasal epithelial cells and alveolar epithelial type II cells, which might partially explain the tissue tropism of CoV-2 infection (3, 4).

CoV-2 infection is either asymptomatic or causes only mild respiratory diseases (non-pneumonia or mild pneumonia) in most individuals. However, a significant number of elderly individuals, frequently with comorbidities (such as cardiovascular diseases, diabetes, obesity), will develop a more severe form of the disease and will require hospital care (1, 2). COVID-19 most common clinical manifestations include fever, fatigue and dry cough, and dyspnea in severe cases (5). Severe COVID-19 associated histopathological changes are found mainly in the lungs, characterized by diffused alveolar damage (DAD), hyaline membranes and fibrin deposits, as well as severe endothelial injury, capillary microthrombi and exudative inflammation (6–12). A systematic review of published case reports and studies identified three main COVID-19 histological patterns: epithelial (85%), vascular (59%) and fibrotic (22%), with a frequent overlap (60%), whereas the epithelial and vascular patterns were present in all stages of severe COVID-19 (13).

COVID-19, ARDS AND PULMONARY FIBROSIS

The rapid replication of SARS- CoV-2 and the associated epithelial cell death may, depending on the underlying genetic, inflammatory or metabolic context, trigger alveolar macrophages to produce excessive amounts of cytokines (such as TNF, IL-1b, IL-6, MIP1, IFN-γ and VEGF), a "cytokine storm", associated with systemic infections such as sepsis or immunotherapies aftermath (14). The highly divert cytokine profile of COVID-19 hyperinflammation resembles, in some cases, other cytokine release syndromes, such as macrophage activation syndrome (15), although it is more heterogeneous and less robust, both quantitively (levels) and qualitatively (number of elevated cytokines). Noteworthy, IL-6 was found to be the most consistently upregulated cytokine and among the most overall predictive biomarkers (16, 17). In turn, the excessive production of cytokines further induces lung injury and Acute Respiratory Distress syndrome (ARDS), leading frequently to respiratory and multi organ failure and death (18).

ARDS develops most commonly in the setting of bacterial and viral pneumonias, or non-pulmonary sepsis, and is characterized by focal epithelial damage and excessive alveolocapillary permeability, leading to interstitial and alveolar edema and hypoxemia in the acute phase (18). Many severe COVID-19 patients will develop ARDS with impaired gas exchange and characteristic CT findings; however, the combination of multiple pathogenetic stimuli in COVID-19-induced ARDS results in a highly heterogeneous, "atypical" clinical appearance that has stimulated considerable controversy (2, 19–24). Nevertheless, excessive inflammation and endothelial dysfunction are among the top candidate pathologic events linking ARDS and COVID-19 (21, 25, 26) and markers of endothelial dysfunction have been recently correlated with COVID-19 mortality (27). Moreover, endothelial dysfunction is also a major characteristic of the most common comorbidities of COVID-19 that are associated with worse prognosis, hypertension, diabetes and obesity (21, 25).

The initial acute exudative inflammatory phase of ARDS is followed by a proliferative phase characterized by alveolar epithelial cell hyperplasia (18). A subset of acute ARDS survivors will further develop a fibroproliferative response, including fibroblast accumulation, deposition of collagen and other lung extracellular matrix (ECM) components (28), the magnitude of which was associated with ARDS duration (29). Moreover, and although invasive mechanical ventilation has revolutionized the management of ARDS, ventilator associated lung injury is considered as an additional contributor to pulmonary fibrosis in ventilated ARDS patients (30). Accordingly, a literature review of published histopathological analyses of COVID-19 lungs *postmortem* indicated, beyond DAD and hyaline membranes, the frequent presence of pulmonary fibrosis (31), while abnormal pulmonary architecture and functions have been reported in many recovering COVID-19 patients (32–34), suggesting persisting fibrotic abnormalities, pending large-scale and long-term follow up studies. Finally, CoV-2 infection *per se* has been reported to induce the expression of different pro-fibrotic factors including TGFβ (35). On the other hand, patients with interstitial lung diseases (ILD) had increased odds for ARDS development and severe COVID-19 (12, 36–39), while COVID-19-related acute exacerbation of ILDs had worse prognosis than non-COVID ILD acute exacerbations (40), thus suggesting pulmonary fibrosis both as a disease risk and a possible complication of COVID-19.

AUTOTAXIN (ATX; *ENPP2*) AND COVID-19

ATX is a secreted glycoprotein that can be detected in most biological fluids, including blood and bronchoalveolar lavage fluid (BALF) (41). A large percentage (~40%) of serum ATX is thought to originate from the adipose tissue (42), while the damaged liver has been suggested as an additional possible source of serum ATX (43). High ATX expression has been reported from endothelial cells in high endothelial venules (HEVs) (44, 45), however their expected relative contribution to circulating levels should be low. Inflammatory macrophages have been also reported to express ATX upon inflammation (46–48), thus contributing to BALF ATX levels (46).

ATX is a constitutively active lysophospholipase D, that catalyzes the extracellular hydrolysis of lysophosphatidylcholine (LPC) to lysophosphatidic acid (LPA) (49). LPC is synthesized from fatty acids or membrane phosphatidylcholine (PC) by phospholipase A_2 (PLA_2) enzymes and is highly abundant in the plasma, associated with oxidized low-density lipoprotein (oxLDL) and albumin (50, 51). LPA is a growth factor-like signaling phospholipid with numerous effects in most cell types through its G-protein coupled receptors (LPAR1-6) (51–53). ATX has been suggested to bind to cell surface integrins (54–56), thus avoiding clearance, as well as localizing LPA production to its adjacent receptors, that exhibit widespread distribution and overlapping functions (51, 57).

Viral infections have been shown to increase systemic ATX levels, including HCV, HIV and HBV (43, 58, 59), while LPA has been also shown to directly affect HCV viral infection and replication (43, 60). Increased *ENPP2* mRNA expression was detected in nasopharyngeal swabs from COVID-19 patients, likely from immune cells (61), suggesting that ATX/LPA might stimulate viral infections, that could include SARS-CoV-2.

Increased serum/plasma ATX levels have been also reported in different diseases, including different forms of cancer, liver diseases, as well as respiratory diseases such as asthma and idiopathic pulmonary fibrosis (IPF) (**Table 1**) (41, 51). A variety of methods has been utilized, while reported levels exhibit remarkable heterogeneity, with no apparent consensus on healthy levels (**Table 1**). Increased ATX serum levels were recently reported in non-surviving ARDS patients, where ATX serum levels were shown to be an independent prognostic factor for 28 day mortality, outperforming the established SOFA/APACHE scores (62). Plasma ATX levels correlated with mortality also in a cohort of patients with severe sepsis (63), suggesting a role for ATX/LPA in systemic hyperinflammation. ATX serum levels in ARDS correlated with the increased IL-6/IL-8 serum levels (62), further supporting an interplay of ATX/LPA with inflammation, as previously suggested in breast cancer (64). ATX serum levels also correlated with the severity of lung injury (62), while increased ATX BALF levels upon endotoxin-induced acute lung injury (ALI) (65, 66), and ventilator-induced lung injury (VILI) in mice (67) have been reported. Moreover, ATX BALF levels in ARDS patients were positively associated with inflammatory and fibrotic mediators (IL-6, IL-8, TNF-α, MMP-7, fibronectin, OSM, and SPARC), suggesting that ATX may also have a role in the fibrotic component of ARDS (62). In line with the above, increased ATX levels have been detected in IPF patients and fibrotic animal models (46, 68), where results from genetic and pharmacologic studies have established a pro-fibrotic role for ATX (46, 69–72). Increased serum ATX levels were very recently detected also in COVID-19 patients hospitalized in the intensive care unit (ICU) as compared with less severe patients hospitalized in the clinic (61), thus adding ATX expression to the commonalities of COVID-19, ARDS and pulmonary fibrosis, and suggesting ATX as a possible pathologic link.

ATX levels in severe COVID-19 patients correlated with the increased IL-6 serum levels (61), as recently also shown in ARDS (62), as well in acute-on-chronic liver failure (ACLF) patients (73), suggesting interdependent regulation of expression. Accordingly, IL-6 has been reported to stimulate ATX expression from adipocytes (73) and human dermal fibroblasts (74). *Vice versa*, LPA has been reported to stimulate the expression of IL-6 from synovial fibroblasts (75, 76) and dermal fibroblasts (74), suggesting an ATX/LPA/IL-6 expression loop. Among the different components of the cytokine storm, IL-6 is the most predictive biomarker in COVID-19 (16, 17), correlating with respiratory failure and the need for mechanical ventilation (77), as well as with mortality risk (78).

Beyond hyperinflammation, and/or as its consequence, endothelial dysfunction is a major characteristic of COVID-19/ARDS (21, 25, 26). The increased ATX levels that were detected in severe COVID-19 patients correlated with markers of endothelial dysfunction (sP-sel, sICAM) (61) that have been independently correlated in the same samples with COVID-19 mortality (27). Similarly, ATX correlated with angiopoietin-2 levels and mortality in severe septic patients (63). In support for a major role of ATX/LPA on vascular homeostasis, ATX expression and LPA signaling have been shown necessary for the embryonic development of the vascular (and neural) system in mice (79–81). In adult mice, in studies unraveling the molecular mechanisms of SARS-CoV and MERS-CoV pathogenesis in the Collaborative Cross mice, *Enpp2*, the gene encoding ATX, has been reported to be a high priority candidate gene for pulmonary hemorrhage (82, 83). More importantly, LPAR1 null mice were reported to be protected from bleomycin (BLM)-induced pulmonary fibrosis, attributed to fibroblast accumulation and reduced vascular leak (68), as well as from *Candida albicans* water-soluble fraction (CAWS)-induced vasculitis, attributed to reduced CXCL1/IL-8-mediated neutrophil infiltration (84). Noteworthy, the stability of LPAR1 in the context of acute lung injury in mice has been proposed to be regulated by ubiquitination (84).

LPA SIGNALING IN PULMONARY AND IMMUNE CELLS

Overall, any ATX effect will rely on its local levels (locally produced and/or extravasated) and its possible cell surface attachment, the local availability of LPC, the cell-specific expression profile of LPA receptors, as well as of the expression of the transmembrane lipid phosphate phosphatases (PLPP1-3; PPA2 A-C) that catabolize LPA (41, 85, 86). In this context, the possible effects of increased ATX levels can be deduced from the corresponding effects of LPA in the relative cells in the tissue microenvironment in question.

A plethora of LPA effects on pulmonary non-immune cells *in vitro* have been reported, as previously reviewed (87–89) and as summarized at **Table 2**. These include the promotion of apoptosis and the secretion of chemotactic signals (IL-8, MCP-1, CXCL1) from epithelial cells, the integrin-mediated activation of TGFβ on epithelial and smooth muscle cells, the modulation of permeability, leukocyte adhesion and cytokine secretion from endothelial cells, and the chemoattraction and accumulation of myofibroblasts (**Table 2**). LPAR1 has been reported as the main receptor mediating these effects, involving different well-known G-protein mediated pathways (**Table 2**). Moreover, LPA has been reported to transactivate different growth factors including TGFβ, PDGF and EGF that activate similar signal transduction pathways, while LPA was reported to signal also *via* RAGE (**Table 2**), further increasing the pleiotropic complexity of LPA signaling in the lung.

The effects of ATX and LPA signaling on the regulation of immune cells have been previously reviewed in detail (87–92). Briefly, high ATX expression from ECs in HEVs in lymph nodes has been reported (44, 45), where ATX has been suggested to facilitate lymphocyte homing *via* the promotion of the adhesion (44), transmigration and motility of lymphocytes (45, 93, 94). Intriguingly, LPA signaling has been proposed to intersect with sphingosine phosphate (S1P) signaling (95), a closely related

TABLE 1 | Autotaxin serum levels in patients of different inflammatory diseases and cancer.

Disease classification	PMID	Disease	Samples (M/F/M+F)	ATX[1]	Method
	33102751	Chronic hepatitis C	28	1.1 ± 0.8	Two-site enzyme immunoassay
		Non-alcoholic steatohepatitis	19	1.4 ± 0.4 *	
		Alcoholic steatohepatitis	15	1.2 ± 0.4 *	
		vs.	*vs.*	*vs.*	
		Chronic hepatitis B	38	0.9 ± 0.3	
	21419756	Chronic Hepatitis C (histologically proven fibrosis)	74	2.40 ± 0.96	Two-site enzyme immunoassay
		Chronic Hepatitis C (FibroScan proven fibrosis)	134	2.20 ± 1.22	
	27981605	Chronic viral hepatitis	14	0.19 (0.13 - 0.35) *	ELISA
			21	0.17 (0.04 - 0.13)	
		vs.	*vs.*	*vs.*	
		Healthy controls	8	0.13 (0.02 - 0.20)	
			12	0.18 (0.09 - 0.35)	
	28425454	Chronic hepatitis C	292	1.16 (0.85 - 1.68) *, #	Two-site enzyme immunoassay
			301	1.64 (1.19 - 2.20) *	
			593	1.39 (1.01 - 1.99) *	
Viral hepatitis		*vs.*	*vs.*	*vs.*	
		Healthy controls	80	0.76 #	
			80	0.82	
			160	0.76	
	31933517	Liver cirrhosis	240	1.58 ± 0.68 #	Two-site enzyme immunoassay
		(multiple aetiologies)	160	1.99 ± 0.73	
		Chronic hepatitis B	33	1.36 ± 0.62 #, ~	
			17	1.82 ± 0.5	
		Chronic hepatitis C	64	1.62 ± 0.67 #, $	
			66	2.09 ± 0.71	
		Non viral hepatitis	143	1.49 ± 0.71 #	
			77	1.96 ± 0.79	
	29114991	Chronic hepatitis B	62	1.10 (0.85-1.24)	Two-site enzyme immunoassay
			39	1.36 (1.23-1.64)	
			101	1.22 (0.95-1.42)	
	25062038	Liver cirrhosis	181	0.77 ± 0.41 *, #	ELISA
			89	0.86 ± 0.43 *	
			270	0.81 ± 0.42 *	
		vs.	*vs.*	*vs.*	
		Healthy controls	35	0.18 ± 0.04 #	
			50	0.35 ± 0.47	
			85	0.26 ± 0.40	
Non-viral liver disorders	29568204	Non-alcoholic fatty liver disease	186	0.86 *	Two-site enzyme immunoassay
		vs.	*vs.*	*vs.*	
		Healthy controls	160	0.76	
	30905718	Liver cirrhosis	50	0.44 ± 0.22 *	ELISA
		vs.	*vs.*	*vs.*	
		Healthy controls	20	0.19 ± 0.06	
	31144415	Non-alcoholic fatty liver disease	173	0.67 ± 0.21 #	Two-site enzyme immunoassay
			134	0.97 ± 0.36	
			307	0.81 ± 0.32	
	31186435	Primary sclerosing cholangitis	193	6.3 ± 3.0 #, *	Homovanillic acid assay
			59	8.6 ± 4.9 *	
			252	6.8 ± 3.7	
		vs.	*vs.*	*vs.*	
		Healthy controls	57	2.5 ± 0.7 #	
			142	3.2 ± 1.5	
Bile duct disorders	31651244	Primary biliary cholangitis – Severe	25	1.25 (0.72 - 4.31)	Two-site enzyme immunoassay
		vs.	*vs.*	*vs.*	
		Primary biliary cholangitis – Moderate	94	1.08 (0.58 - 3.12)	
	27506882	Primary biliary cholangitis	118	10.2 ± 4.4	Homovanillic acid assay
		Primary sclerosing cholangitis	115	7.3 ± 3.4	
		vs.	*vs.*	*vs.*	
		Healthy controls	Undisclosed	3.1 ± 1.7	

(Continued)

TABLE 1 | Continued

Disease classification	PMID	Disease	Samples (M/F/M+F)	ATX[1]	Method
			Undisclosed	2.5 ± 0.7	
			109	2.8 ± 1.4	
	29802350	Primary biliary cholangitis	20	1.00 (0.82 - 1.13) *,#	Two-site enzyme immunoassay
			108	0.78 (0.66 - 0.98) *	
			128	0.97 (0.79 - 1.11) *	
		vs.	*vs.*	*vs.*	
		Healthy controls	80	0.76 #	
			80	0.82	
			160	0.76	
	25450205	Preeclampsia / HELLP syndrome	17	16.8 ± 8.9	Homovanillic acid assay
		Pruritic disorders of pregnancy	33	16.8 ± 6.7	
		Intrahepatic cholestasis of pregnancy	55	43.5 ± 18.2 *, †	
		vs.	*vs.*	*vs.*	
		Normal pregnancy	44	19.6 ± 5.4 *	
		vs.	*vs.*	*vs.*	
		Healthy controls	57	2.5 ± 0.7 #	
			142	3.2 ± 1.5	
Malignancies	2464234	Hepatocellular carcinoma	105	1.94 ± 1.01 #	Two-site enzyme immunoassay
			43	2.87 ± 0.76	
			148	2.21 ± 1.03	
	18710386	Acute myeloid leukemia	26	0.86 ± 0.29	ELISA
		Chronic lymphocytic leukemia	14	0.93 ± 0.30 *	
		Follicular lymphoma	25	1.47 ± 0.69 *	
		Diffuse large B-cell lymphoma	28	0.94 ± 0.39 *	
		vs.	*vs.*	*vs.*	
		Healthy controls	74	0.66 ± 0.12 #	
			46	0.85 ± 0.18	
			120	0.73 ± 0.18	
	27583415	Hepatocellular carcinoma	58	1.07 (0.84 - 1.37) *	Two-site enzyme immunoassay
		vs.	*vs.*	*vs.*	
		Healthy controls	74	0.68 ± 0.12 #	
			46	0.97 ± 0.17	
			120	0.73 ± 0.18	
	29724718[a]	Non-small cell lung cancer	19	0.124 *	TOOS assay
		vs.	*vs.*	*vs.*	
		Healthy controls	49	0.088	
	30921203	Breast cancer	112	0.29 ± 0.04 *	ELISA
		vs.	*vs.*	*vs.*	
		Healthy controls	50	0.25 ± 0.02	
Metabolic disorders	26727116	Obese – overweight people >60 yo	20	0.17 ± 0.01 #	ELISA
			40	0.29 ± 0.02	
			60	0.25 ± 0.11	
	26831013	Diabetic nephropathy	38	0.75 ± 0.27	ELISA
Autoimmune disorders	22493518[b]	Rheumatoid arthritis	10	0.87 ± 0.83 *	ELISA
			16	1.12 ± 1.08 *	
			26	1.03 ± 0.98 *	
		vs.	*vs.*	*vs.*	
		Osteoarthritis	11	0.27 ± 0.19	
			15	0.32 ± 0.19	
			26	0.30 ± 0.19	
	24984830	Multiple sclerosis	20	12.11 ± 1.42 *	TOOS assay
		vs.	*vs.*	*vs.*	
		Other neurological disorders	20	7.05 ± 1.51	
Various disorders	26083365	Chronic liver diseases	18	1.37 ± 0.77 *	Two-site enzyme immunoassay
			17	1.46 ± 0.67 *	
		Follicular lymphoma	10	0.95 ± 0.27 *	
			15	1.28 ± 0.47 *	
		vs.	*vs.*	*vs.*	
		Healthy controls	76	0.98 ± 0.58 #	
			98	1.49 ± 0.98	

(Continued)

TABLE 1 | Continued

Disease classification	PMID	Disease	Samples (M/F/M+F)	ATX[1]	Method
	32826822	Sepsis	84	443.6 (285.8 - 632.2)	TOOS assay
	33568105	Pancreatic diseases	114	0.39 *	ELISA
		Benign pancreatic diseases	94	0.27	
		vs.	*vs.*	*vs.*	
		Healthy controls	120	0.26	
	34130757	Acute respiratory distress syndrome (survivors)	31	39.01 ± 13.89	Human Magnetic Luminex Assay
		Acute respiratory distress syndrome (non-survivors)	21	44.79 ± 13.38	

Only publications analyzing more than 10 samples are included.
[1]All reported values were converted to mg/L and presented as in the original publication as means ± SD, or as median (interquartile range). Individual values represent medians unless stated otherwise.
**: Compared to the same sex group of the controls; $p < 0.05$.*
#: Compared to within-the-group opposite sex; $p < 0.05$.
†: Compared to females with normal pregnancy.
~: Compared to non-viral hepatitis.
$: Compared to hepatitis B.
a: ATX activity mean values are indicated.
b: ATX concentration in the serum was calculated anew by utilizing the supplementary data of this publication.

phospholipid (96), that has been shown to affect lymphocyte egress from the lymph nodes (97).

Non-withstanding the effects of ATX/LPA on lymphocyte homeostasis, highly pertinent for both ILD/IPF and COVID-19, a role for ATX/LPA on the homeostasis of the monocyte phagocyte system is emerging. Macrophages are central players in the pathogenesis of both IPF (98, 99) and COVID-19 (15, 100, 101), exhibiting remarkable heterogeneity and spatiotemporal plasticity. LPA has been suggested to stimulate the expression of macrophage chemotactic factors from ECs, such as monocyte chemoattractant protein-1 (MCP-1) (102) and CXCL1 (103), thus promoting both monocyte migration as well as adhesion to ECs (102–104). Beyond LPA-induced macrophage chemoattraction and adhesion to ECs, inflammatory macrophages *per se* have been reported to express ATX upon BLM-induced pulmonary inflammation and fibrosis, while IPF macrophages have been shown to stain for ATX (46). scRNAseq analysis of BALF cells from COVID-19 patients indicated a predominance of macrophages (100, 101), where *ENPP2* mRNA expression was detected in monocyte-derived alveolar macrophages (Mo-AMs) (61), that have been shown to drive the development of BLM-induced pulmonary fibrosis in mice (105). In turn, accumulating evidence indicates that LPA co-stimulate macrophage maturation and/or activation (47, 106–109), suggesting an autocrine role of ATX/LPA in macrophage pathologic responses. Moreover, LPA has been suggested to stimulate oxLDL uptake and foam cell formation (110, 111), linking macrophages and ATX/LPA with hyperlipidaemia and cardiovascular diseases (112), major comorbidities of COVID-19.

While LPA promotes bone marrow derived monocyte ($CD11b^+$) activation (F4/80 expression) *in vitro* as potently as M-CSF (106), LPA has been also reported to co-stimulate the

TABLE 2 | Reported Lysophosphatidic acid (LPA) effects on pulmonary, non-immune, cells.

Cell type	LPA effect	Receptor	Pathway	PMID
Epithelial cells				
Human bronchial epithelial cells	induction of anchorage dependent apoptosis	LPAR1	-	22021336
	induction of TSLP & CCL20	–	-	18757306
	activation of TGF-β	LPAR2	integrin $\alpha_v\beta_6$	19147812
	induction of soluble ST2 expression	LPAR1, 3	-	21871564
	transactivation of EGFR & secretion of IL-8	-	-	16687414, 16197369
	induction of IL-13Ra2	–	$G_{\alpha i}$	17287216
	enhancement of epithelial barrier integrity	LPAR1, 3	-	19586906, 17359381
	decrease of EGFR-EGF binding	–	-	17640953
	induction of COX-2 expression & PGE2 secretion		$G_{\alpha i}$	18294142
	transactivation of PDGFR-β	–	–	12890682
	redistribution of c-Met on the membrane	-	-	17689924, 23624790

(Continued)

TABLE 2 | Continued

Cell type	LPA effect	Receptor	Pathway	PMID
Human bronchial epithelial cells (BEAS-2B)	transactivation of EGFR inhibition of IFN/TNF-induced CCL5/RANTES expression decrease of EGFR-EGF binding	LPAR1 LPAR1 –	– G_i/PI3K –	17640953 20861350 17640953
Human alveolar epithelial carcinoma cells (A549)	decrease of p53 abundance increase of cell migration promotion of EMT, proliferation and migration	- LPARs RAGE	- PKCδ, cortactin PKB	18025263 21696367 33109194
Human basal cells	induced signaling by CREB	–	ERK1/2	33794877
Mouse alveolar and bronchial epithelial cells	induction of apoptosis induction of apoptosis	LPAR1 LPAR2	- –	22021336 23808384
Mouse lung epithelial cells (MLE12)	induction of migration induction of KC secretion	LPAR1 LPAR1	TrkA ERK, p38	26597701 27448760
Endothelial cells				
Human microvascular endothelial cells	increase of the endothelial layer permeability	LPAR2, 6	-	23084965
Human pulmonary artery endothelial cels	increased adhesive properties	LPAR1, 3	–	25621161
Human aortic endothelial cells	induction of VCAM, E-selectin induction of E-selectin, MCP-1, monocytic migration and adhesion induction of VCAM, ICAM	- – -	G_i ROCK2, NF-κB ROCK2, NF-κB	10595650 30884801 20164172
Human endothelial cells	CXCL1 secretion, monocyte adhesion	LPAR1, 3	–	21531341
Human airway epithelial cells Mouse endothelial cells Bovine pulmonary artery endothelial cells	inhibition of the attachment to the ECM vascular leak/extravasation migration, chemotaxis	LPAR1 LPAR1 - -	Rho-kinase – ERK, Hic-5 -	27500235 18066075 17337598 15333043
Fibroblasts				
Human fibroblasts	chemoattraction, accumulation proliferation, EGFR ectodomain shedding differentiation, profibrotic gene expression (TGFβ, col1a2, FN, SMA)	LPAR1 - LPAR2	– ERK1/2 ERK1/2, Smad 3, Akt, p38	18066075 21362091 23808384
Mouse lung fibroblasts	lamelipodia formation, motility	LPAR1	-	14744855
Mouse fibroblasts (NIH 3T3)	migration, protection from apoptosis, proliferation protection from apoptosis, proliferation	–	– G_i	16219296 11062066
Rat Rat1/c-Myc fibroblasts Mesenchymal cells derived from fibrotic lung allografts	protection from apoptosis promotion of NFAT1 nuclear translocation	– LPAR1	Rac1 β-catenin	11062066 28240604
Smooth muscle cells				
Human smooth muscle cells	proliferation, stimulation of EGFR signaling activation of TGF-β	- –	- integrin $\alpha_v\beta_5$	9252534, 11741820 22025551
Rabbit smooth muscle cells	contraction	-	-	9338431
Stem cells				
Human mesenchymal stem cells	migration migration, differentiation into myofibroblasts	LPAR1 LPAR1	β-catenin –	22782863 24251962

GM-CSF/IL-4-induced conversion of monocytes to DCs (113, 114). Moreover, LPA has been also reported to modulate the activity of TCF4 (115), a decisive transcription factor in plasmacytoid dendritic cells (pDCs) development and homeostasis (116). Increased *ENPP2* expression was detected in COVID-19 DCs and pDCs, correlating with markers of immature DCs (61), while an anti-inflammatory role of LPA has been previously proposed for DCs *via* LPAR2 (117), suggesting that ATX/LPA could be also involved in suppression of DC responses in COVID-19.

Therefore, increases of ATX levels and LPA local production in ARDS, ILD/IPF and COVID-19 can exacerbate numerous

TABLE 3 | Representative small molecules targeting ATX in late-stage preclinical and clinical development.

Compound (Company)	*In vitro* properties			Pre-clinical data			Clinical trials
	IC50(assay)	**Mode of Binding (Ki)ATX inhibitor type (PDB structure entry)**	**ADMET**	**Pharmacokinetics**	**LPA inhibition**	**Disease targeting (Dose, route)**	
GLPG-1690 Ziritaxestat (Galapagos)	131 ± 12 nM (hATX, TOOS assay)[1] 418 nM (mouse plasma, 18:2 LPA, LC-MS/MS)[1] 542 nM (rat plasma, 18:2 LPA, LC-MS/MS)[1] 242 nM (human plasma, 18:2 LPA, LC-MS/MS)[1]	Competitive (15 nM, hATX), type IV inhibitor1 (5MHP)	hERG IC_{50}: = 15 μM[1] CYP3A4 TDI: negative[1]	**iv clearance (L/h·kg)**: 0.23 (mouse), 0.69 (rat), 0.12 (dog)[1] C_{max} (mouse, 30 mg/kg per os): 21.367 μg/mL[1] t_{max} (mouse, 30 mg/kg per os): 1 h[1] $t_{1/2}$ (mouse, 30 mg/kg per os): 3.8 h[1] per os bioavailability (F%): 29 (mouse), 37 (rat), 63 (dog)[1]	95% (maximum) (30 mg/kg per os)[1]	**Pulmonary fibrosis** (3, 10 or 30mg/kg per os)[1]	Phase I NCT03143712 NCT02179502 IPF Phase II NCT02738801 Phase III NCT03711162 NCT03733444 Scleroderma Phase II NCT03798366 NCT03976648
BLD-0409 Cudetaxestat (Blade Therapeutics)	≤ 0.5 μM (LPC assay)[2]	–	–	–	–	**Metabolic disorders** (15mg/kg)[2]	Phase I NCT04146805 NCT04814472 NCT04814498 NCT04939467
ONO-8430506 (Ono Pharmaceuticals)	5.1 nM (recomb. ATX, FS-3 assay)[3] 10.2 nM (hATX, LPC assay)[3, 4] 6.4 nM (mouse plasma, LPC assay)[3] 19 nM (rat plasma, LPC assay)[3] 5.5 nM (human plasma)[3, 4]	type II inhibitor	Protein plasma binding: rat (95.1%), human (99%)[4] High selectivity to ATX[3]	**iv clearance (mL min-1 kg-1):** 8.2 (mouse), 4.7 (rat), 5.8 (dog)[4] **Vdss (L/kg)**: 1.5 (mouse), 1.9 (rat), 2.3 (dog)[4] **Cmax (1 mg/kg per os)**: 124 ng/mL (mouse), 261 ng/mL (rat), 1670 ng/mL (dog)[4] **t1/2** (1 mg/kg per os): 5.4 h (mouse), 2.5 h (rat), 5.9 h (dog)[4] **per os Bioavailability (F)**: 51.6% (rat), 71.1% (dog), 30.8% (monkey)[4]	96% (18:2 LPA, 3 mg/kg)[3] 93% (20:4 LPA, 3 mg/kg)[3] >99% (18:2 & 20:4 LPA, 30 mg/kg)[3]	**Prostatic hyperplasia** (0.3-10mg/kg, id)[3] **Breast cancer** (10mg/kg, per os)[5] **Thyroid cancer** (2mg/kg, per os)[6]	Preclinical evaluation
PF-8380 (Pfizer)	2.8 nM (hATX, FS-3 substrate)[7] 1.7 nM (hATX, LPC substrate)[7] 1.16 nM (mATX, FS-3 substrate)[7] 1.15 nM (fetal fibroblast cell line, LPC substrate)[7] 101 nM (human whole blood)	Competitive (0.02-0.04 nM), type I inhibitor[7]	Solubility (pH = 6.8) = 0.011 mg/mL[8] Poor solubility at physiological pH (7.4)[8] IC50 hERG (cardiotoxicity) = 2.7 μM[8] Permeability (PAMPA assay) = 81%[8]	**rat iv clearance (mL min-1 kg-1)** = 31[7] **Vdss (L/kg)** = 3.2[7] t1/2 = 1.2 h[7] **Cmax** (10 mg/kg per os) = 2.55 μM[7] **tmax** (10 mg/kg per os) = 0.67 h[7] **rat per os F** (10 mg/kg) = 83%[7]	EC50 = 54.7 nM (16:0 LPA)[7] EC50 = 84.6 nM (18:0 LPA)[7] EC50 = 51.7 nM (20:0 LPA)[7]	**Arthritis Hyperalgesia** (30mg/kg, po)[7] **Glioblastoma** (10mg/kg, ip)[9] **Liver fibrosis** (30mg/kg, ip)[10] **Lung allograft fibrosis** (30mg/kg, per os)[11]	Preclinical evaluation

[1-11] *refer to the following hyperlinked publications (PubMed ID):* ***1**: 28414242,* ***2**: 33342311,* ***3**: 24747415,* ***4**: 32551021,* ***5**: 24599971,* ***6**: 25398768,* ***7**: 20392816,* ***8**: 29798825,* ***9**: 24062988,* ***10**: 27981605,* ***11**: 28240604.*

pathogenic responses in the lung, likely in co-ordination with other pathologic inflammatory and fibrotic factors.

PHARMACOLOGIC TARGETING OF ATX AS AN ADDITIONAL THERAPEUTIC OPTION IN COVID-19

Dexamethasone (Dex), the first line of defense against systemic inflammation, has been proven effective in COVID-19 patients requiring oxygen or ventilation (118, 119), the only approved single therapy against severe COVID-19. Remarkably, Dex treatment of ventilated COVID-19 patients attenuated serum ATX levels, suggesting that the therapeutic effects of Dex include the suppression of ATX expression (61) and that ATX can be druggable.

The exacerbated production of IL-6 and other storm cytokines, where present, is considered among the leading causes of COVID-19/ARDS-related mortality, and therefore many clinical trials have been conducted targeting storm cytokines or their receptors, with inconsistent results, spurring controversial opinions on the use of systemic anti-inflammatory drugs (120). ATX and IL-6 levels were shown to correlate in ACLF (73), ARDS (62) and COVID-19 (61) patients, suggesting that simultaneous inhibition of both IL-6 and ATX may be an effective therapeutic strategy for COVID-19, as previously suggested in systemic sclerosis (74).

The antifibrotic compounds pirfenidone and nintedanib, approved for IPF, have shown efficacy in fibrotic lung diseases other than IPF (121–125). Therefore, since COVID-19 and IPF share disease severity risk factors, such as sex/age and comorbidities, existing and developing anti-fibrotic compounds have been suggested as additional therapeutic options in COVID-19 (126–128). Among them, GLPG1690 (**Table 3** and **Figure 1**) targets ATX and, together with the standard of care treatment (pirfenidone or nintedanib), has entered phase III international clinical trials (ISABELA 1 and 2, NCT03711162 and NCT03733444) (129). Given the above, the same or a similar regime might also prove effective in COVID-19.

The crystal structure of ATX has been solved (55, 130, 131), allowing a deep understanding of its structure and function relationship (132) (**Figure 1**), and thus promoting rational drug design. Given the establishment of ATX as a therapeutic target in IPF, as well as the promising results from the initial clinical trials, a plethora of ATX inhibitors have been developed (133, 134); the ones at late-stage development as shown in **Table 3** and their mode in binding at **Figure 1**.

Inducible genetic deletion of ATX in adult life, resulting in 70-80% decreases in serum ATX levels and mRNA expression levels in different tissues, did not have any appreciable effects in gross pathophysiology of major organs (135), suggesting that the bulk of ATX activity in mice is dispensable for adult life. Moreover, potent (IC50 2 nM), long term (3 weeks) pharmacological

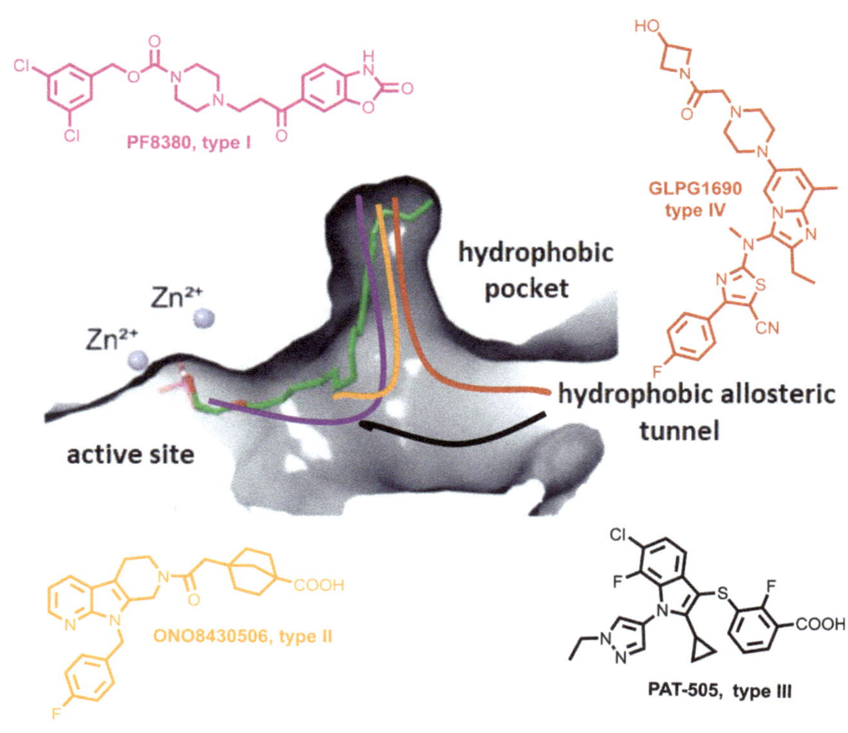

FIGURE 1 | Schematic representation of the mode of binding (color coded) to ATX by the 4 different types of ATX inhibitors (I-IV). The mode of binding of LPA is also displayed (in green).

inhibition of ATX with PF-8380 (120 mg/Kg - 4 times the effective concentration; PO; bid) had no effects in survival or gross pathology of major organs (135), suggesting that ATX pharmaceutical targeting is safe and well tolerated in mice. In humans, GLPG1690 was reported to be well tolerated in a phase 1 randomized clinical trial (NCT02179502), safe and efficacious in a phase 2a randomized placebo-controlled clinical trial (NCT02738801), supporting ATX inhibition as a novel treatment for IPF (136, 137). In addition, administration of BBT-877, another orally available small molecule inhibitor targeting ATX (IC50 ~6.7 nM), to healthy volunteers in a phase I clinical trial (NCT03830125), did not reveal severe adverse events (138, 139). However, the GLPG1690 phase III clinical trial was recently discontinued on account of "low benefit to risk ratio". Likewise, BBT-877's scheduled phase II clinical trial was also postponed due to "toxicity concerns". Since the relative results are not announced yet, it is not known if the toxicity was imposed from the compounds themselves or their target. Nevertheless, several new candidates are emerging, while possible compound toxicity can be eliminated with targeted modifications or bypassed *via* inhaled administration.

CONCLUSIONS

The increased levels of ATX in ILDs/IPF, ARDS and COVID-19 add yet another commonality between them and suggest that LPA signaling is involved in their pathogenesis, including the amplification of vascular damage, the regulation of the immune system and the promotion of fibrosis. Therefore, the therapeutic targeting of ATX in IPF and fibrotic diseases could be also applied in COVID-19, alone or together with approved anti-fibrotic, anti-rheumatic and anti-viral drugs, especially given its predicted short-term administration, as well as the emergency nature and unmet medical need for the treatment of COVID-19 severe cases.

AUTHOR CONTRIBUTIONS

KN, TK, ET, ES and AM drafted the paper. AT and KA critically commented on the draft version. VA finalized the manuscript. All authors contributed to the article and approved the submitted version.

REFERENCES

1. Hu B, Guo H, Zhou P, Shi Z-L. Characteristics of SARS-CoV-2 and COVID-19. *Nat Rev Microbiol* (2020) 19(3):141–54. doi: 10.1038/s41579-020-00459-7
2. Osuchowski MF, Winkler MS, Skirecki T, Cajander S, Shankar-Hari M, Lachmann G, et al. The COVID-19 Puzzle: Deciphering Pathophysiology and Phenotypes of a New Disease Entity. *Lancet Respir Med* (2021) 9 (6):622–42. doi: 10.1016/S2213-2600(21)00218-6
3. Hoffmann M, Kleine-Weber H, Schroeder S, Krüger N, Herrler T, Erichsen S, et al. SARS-CoV-2 Cell Entry Depends on ACE2 and TMPRSS2 and Is Blocked by a Clinically Proven Protease Inhibitor. *Cell* (2020) 181(2):271–80.e8. doi: 10.1016/j.cell.2020.02.052
4. Sungnak W, Huang N, Bécavin C, Berg M, Queen R, Litvinukova M, et al. SARS-CoV-2 Entry Factors Are Highly Expressed in Nasal Epithelial Cells Together With Innate Immune Genes. *Nat Med* (2020) 26(5):681–7. doi: 10.1038/s41591-020-0868-6
5. Wang D, Hu B, Hu C, Zhu F, Liu X, Zhang J, et al. Clinical Characteristics of 138 Hospitalized Patients With 2019 Novel Coronavirus-Infected Pneumonia in Wuhan, China. *Jama* (2020) 323(11):1061–9. doi: 10.1001/jama.2020.1585
6. Guan W-J, Ni Z-Y, Hu Y, Liang W-H, Ou C-Q, He J-X, et al. Clinical Characteristics of Coronavirus Disease 2019 in China. *N Engl J Med* (2020) 382(18):1708–20. doi: 10.1101/2020.02.06.20020974
7. Yang X, Yu Y, Xu J, Shu H, Xia J, Liu H, et al. Clinical Course and Outcomes of Critically Ill Patients With SARS-CoV-2 Pneumonia in Wuhan, China: A Single-Centered, Retrospective, Observational Study. *Lancet Respir Med* (2020) 8(5):475–81. doi: 10.1016/S2213-2600(20)30079-5
8. Chen N, Zhou M, Dong X, Qu J, Gong F, Han Y, et al. Epidemiological and Clinical Characteristics of 99 Cases of 2019 Novel Coronavirus Pneumonia in Wuhan, China: A Descriptive Study. *Lancet* (2020) 395(10223):507–13. doi: 10.1016/S0140-6736(20)30211-7
9. Wu Z, McGoogan JM. Characteristics of and Important Lessons From the Coronavirus Disease 2019 (COVID-19) Outbreak in China: Summary of a Report of 72 314 Cases From the Chinese Center for Disease Control and Prevention. *Jama* (2020) 323(13):1239–42. doi: 10.1001/jama.2020.2648
10. Torres Acosta MA, Singer BD. Pathogenesis of COVID-19-Induced ARDS: Implications for an Ageing Population. *Eur Respir J* (2020) 56(3)10:2002049. doi: 10.1183/13993003.02049-2020
11. Shanmugam C, Mohammed AR, Ravuri S, Luthra V, Rajagopal N, Karre S. COVID-2019 - A Comprehensive Pathology Insight. *Pathol Res Pract* (2020) 216(10):153222. 11. doi: 10.1016/j.prp.2020.153222
12. Bussani R, Schneider E, Zentilin L, Collesi C, Ali H, Braga L, et al. Persistence of Viral RNA, Pneumocyte Syncytia and Thrombosis Are Hallmarks of Advanced COVID-19 Pathology. *EBioMedicine* (2020) 61:103104. doi: 10.1016/j.ebiom.2020.103104
13. Polak SB, Van Gool IC, Cohen D, von der Thüsen JH, van Paassen J. A Systematic Review of Pathological Findings in COVID-19: A Pathophysiological Timeline and Possible Mechanisms of Disease Progression. *Mod Pathol* (2020) 33(11):2128–38. doi: 10.1038/s41379-020-0603-3
14. Fajgenbaum DC, June CH. Cytokine Storm. *N Engl J Med* (2020) 383 (23):2255–73. doi: 10.1056/NEJMra2026131
15. Merad M, Martin JC. Pathological Inflammation in Patients With COVID-19: A Key Role for Monocytes and Macrophages. *Nat Rev Immunol* (2020) 20(6):355–62. doi: 10.1038/s41577-020-0331-4
16. Zhang Z-L, Hou Y-L, Li D-T, Li F-Z. Laboratory Findings of COVID-19: A Systematic Review and Meta-Analysis. *Scand J Clin Lab Invest* (2020) 80 (6):441–7. doi: 10.1080/00365513.2020.1768587
17. Ulhaq ZS, Soraya GV. Interleukin-6 as a Potential Biomarker of COVID-19 Progression. *Med Mal Infect* (2020) 50(4):382–3. doi: 10.1016/j.medmal.2020.04.002

18. Matthay MA, Zemans RL, Zimmerman GA, Arabi YM, Beitler JR, Mercat A, et al. Acute Respiratory Distress Syndrome. *Nat Rev Dis Primers* (2019) 5 (1):18. doi: 10.1038/s41572-019-0069-0
19. Gattinoni L, Coppola S, Cressoni M, Busana M, Rossi S, Chiumello D. COVID-19 Does Not Lead to a "Typical" Acute Respiratory Distress Syndrome. *Am J Respir Crit Care Med* (2020) 201(10):1299–300. doi: 10.1164/rccm.202003-0817LE
20. Ziehr DR, Alladina J, Petri CR, Maley JH, Moskowitz A, Medoff BD, et al. Respiratory Pathophysiology of Mechanically Ventilated Patients With COVID-19: A Cohort Study. *Am J Respir Crit Care Med* (2020) 201 (12):1560–4. doi: 10.1164/rccm.202004-1163LE
21. Mangalmurti NS, Reilly JP, Cines DB, Meyer NJ, Hunter CA, Vaughan AE. COVID-19-Associated Acute Respiratory Distress Syndrome Clarified: A Vascular Endotype? *Am J Respir Crit Care Med* (2020) 202(5):750–3. doi: 10.1164/rccm.202006-2598LE
22. Tobin MJ. Pondering the Atypicality of ARDS in COVID-19 Is a Distraction for the Bedside Doctor. *Intensive Care Med* (2021) 47(3):361–2. doi: 10.1007/s00134-020-06340-8
23. Goligher EC, Ranieri VM, Slutsky AS. Is Severe COVID-19 Pneumonia a Typical or Atypical Form of ARDS? And Does it Matter? *Intensive Care Med* (2021) 47(1):83–5. doi: 10.1007/s00134-020-06320-y
24. Bos LDJ. COVID-19-Related Acute Respiratory Distress Syndrome: Not So Atypical. *Am J Respir Crit Care Med* (2020) 202(4):622–4. doi: 10.1164/rccm.202004-1423LE
25. Huertas A, Montani D, Savale L, Pichon J, Tu L, Parent F, et al. Endothelial Cell Dysfunction: A Major Player in SARS-CoV-2 Infection (COVID-19)? *Eur Respir J* (2020) 56(1):2001634. doi: 10.1183/13993003.01634-2020
26. Vassiliou AG, Kotanidou A, Dimopoulou I, Orfanos SE. Endothelial Damage in Acute Respiratory Distress Syndrome. *Int J Mol Sci* (2020) 21 (22):8793. doi: 10.3390/ijms21228793
27. Vassiliou AG, Keskinidou C, Jahaj E, Gallos P, Dimopoulou I, Kotanidou A, et al. ICU Admission Levels of Endothelial Biomarkers as Predictors of Mortality in Critically Ill COVID-19 Patients. *Cells* (2021) 10(1):186. doi: 10.3390/cells10010186
28. Burnham EL, Janssen WJ, Riches DW, Moss M, Downey GP. The Fibroproliferative Response in Acute Respiratory Distress Syndrome: Mechanisms and Clinical Significance. *Eur Respir J* (2014) 43(1):276–85. doi: 10.1183/09031936.00196412
29. Thille AW, Esteban A, Fernández-Segoviano P, Rodriguez JM, Aramburu JA, Vargas-Errázuriz P, et al. Chronology of Histological Lesions in Acute Respiratory Distress Syndrome With Diffuse Alveolar Damage: A Prospective Cohort Study of Clinical Autopsies. *Lancet Respir Med* (2013) 1(5):395–401. doi: 10.1016/S2213-2600(13)70053-5
30. Cabrera-Benitez NE, Laffey JG, Parotto M, Spieth PM, Villar J, Zhang H, et al. Mechanical Ventilation-Associated Lung Fibrosis in Acute Respiratory Distress Syndrome: A Significant Contributor to Poor Outcome. *Anesthesiology* (2014) 121(1):189–98. doi: 10.1097/ALN.0000000000000264
31. Maiese A, Manetti AC, La Russa R, Di Paolo M, Turillazzi E, Frati P, et al. Autopsy Findings in COVID-19-Related Deaths: A Literature Review. *Forensic Sci Med Pathol* (2020) 17(2):279–96. doi: 10.1007/s12024-020-00310-8
32. Mo X, Jian W, Su Z, Chen M, Peng H, Peng P, et al. Abnormal Pulmonary Function in COVID-19 Patients at Time of Hospital Discharge. *Eur Respir J* (2020) 55(6):2001217. doi: 10.1183/13993003.01217-2020
33. Gassel RJJV, Bels JLM, Raafs A, Bussel BCTV, Poll MCGVD, Simons SO, et al. High Prevalence of Pulmonary Sequelae at 3 Months After Hospital Discharge in Mechanically Ventilated Survivors of COVID-19. *Am J Respir Crit Care Med* (2021) 203(3):371–4. doi: 10.1164/rccm.202010-3823LE
34. Myall KJ, Mukherjee B, Castanheira AM, Lam JL, Benedetti G, Mak SM, et al. Persistent Post-COVID-19 Interstitial Lung Disease. An Observational Study of Corticosteroid Treatment. *Ann Am Thorac Soc* (2021) 18(5):799–806. doi: 10.1513/AnnalsATS.202008-1002OC
35. McDonald LT. Healing After COVID-19: Are Survivors at Risk for Pulmonary Fibrosis? *Am J Physiol Lung Cell Mol Physiol* (2021) 320(2): L257–l65. doi: 10.1152/ajplung.00238.2020
36. Esposito AJ, Menon AA, Ghosh AJ, Putman RK, Fredenburgh LE, El-Chemaly SY, et al. Increased Odds of Death for Patients With Interstitial Lung Disease and COVID-19: A Case-Control Study. *Am J Respir Crit Care Med* (2020) 202(12):1710–3. doi: 10.1164/rccm.202006-2441LE
37. Drake TM, Docherty AB, Harrison EM, Quint JK, Adamali H, Agnew S, et al. Outcome of Hospitalization for COVID-19 in Patients With Interstitial Lung Disease. An International Multicenter Study. *Am J Respir Crit Care Med* (2020) 202(12):1656–65. doi: 10.1164/rccm.202007-2794OC
38. Beltramo G, Cottenet J, Mariet AS, Georges M, Piroth L, Tubert-Bitter P, et al. Chronic Respiratory Diseases Are Predictors of Severe Outcome in COVID-19 Hospitalised Patients: A Nationwide Study. *Eur Respir J* (2021) 2004474. doi: 10.1183/13993003.04474-2020
39. Drake TM, Docherty AB, Harrison EM, Quint JK, Adamali H, Agnew S, et al. Outcome of Hospitalization for COVID-19 in Patients with Interstitial Lung Disease. An International Multicenter Study. *Am J Respir Crit Care Med* (2020) 202(12):1656–65. doi: 10.1164/rccm.202007-2794OC.
40. Kondoh Y, Kataoka K, Ando M, Awaya Y, Ichikado K, Kataoka M, et al. COVID-19 and Acute Exacerbation of Interstitial Lung Disease. *Respir Investig* (2021) 59(5):675–8. doi: 10.1016/j.resinv.2021.06.007
41. Magkrioti C, Galaris A, Kanellopoulou P, Stylianaki EA, Kaffe E, Aidinis V. Autotaxin and Chronic Inflammatory Diseases. *J Autoimmun* (2019) 104:102327. doi: 10.1016/j.jaut.2019.102327
42. Dusaulcy R, Rancoule C, Gres S, Wanecq E, Colom A, Guigne C, et al. Adipose-Specific Disruption of Autotaxin Enhances Nutritional Fattening and Reduces Plasma Lysophosphatidic Acid. *J Lipid Res* (2011) 52(6):1247–55. doi: 10.1194/jlr.M014985
43. Kaffe E, Katsifa A, Xylourgidis N, Ninou I, Zannikou M, Harokopos V, et al. Hepatocyte Autotaxin Expression Promotes Liver Fibrosis and Cancer. *Hepatology* (2017) 65(4):1369–83. doi: 10.1002/hep.28973
44. Kanda H, Newton R, Klein R, Morita Y, Gunn MD, Rosen SD. Autotaxin, an Ectoenzyme That Produces Lysophosphatidic Acid, Promotes the Entry of Lymphocytes Into Secondary Lymphoid Organs. *Nat Immunol* (2008) 9 (4):415–23. doi: 10.1038/ni1573
45. Bai Z, Cai L, Umemoto E, Takeda A, Tohya K, Komai Y, et al. Constitutive Lymphocyte Transmigration Across the Basal Lamina of High Endothelial Venules Is Regulated by the Autotaxin/Lysophosphatidic Acid Axis. *J Immunol* (2013) 190(5):2036–48. doi: 10.4049/jimmunol.1202025
46. Oikonomou N, Mouratis MA, Tzouvelekis A, Kaffe E, Valavanis C, Vilaras G, et al. Pulmonary Autotaxin Expression Contributes to the Pathogenesis of Pulmonary Fibrosis. *Am J Respir Cell Mol Biol* (2012) 47(5):566–74. doi: 10.1165/rcmb.2012-0004OC
47. Ninou I, Sevastou I, Magkrioti C, Kaffe E, Stamatakis G, Thivaios S, et al. Genetic Deletion of Autotaxin From CD11b+ Cells Decreases the Severity of Experimental Autoimmune Encephalomyelitis. *PloS One* (2020) 15(4): e0226050. doi: 10.1371/journal.pone.0226050
48. Kim SJ, Howe C, Mitchell J, Choo J, Powers A, Oikonomopoulos A, et al. Autotaxin Loss Accelerates Intestinal Inflammation by Suppressing TLR4-Mediated Immune Responses. *EMBO Rep* (2020) 21(10):e49332. doi: 10.15252/embr.201949332
49. Umezu-Goto M, Kishi Y, Taira A, Hama K, Dohmae N, Takio K, et al. Autotaxin has Lysophospholipase D Activity Leading to Tumor Cell Growth and Motility by Lysophosphatidic Acid Production. *J Cell Biol* (2002) 158 (2):227–33. doi: 10.1083/jcb.200204026
50. Perrakis A, Moolenaar WH. Autotaxin: Structure-Function and Signaling. *J Lipid Res* (2014) 55(6):1010–18. doi: 10.1194/jlr.R046391
51. Barbayianni E, Kaffe E, Aidinis V, Kokotos G. Autotaxin, A Secreted Lysophospholipase D, as a Promising Therapeutic Target in Chronic Inflammation and Cancer. *Prog Lipid Res* (2015) 58:76–96. doi: 10.1016/j.plipres.2015.02.001
52. Aikawa S, Hashimoto T, Kano K, Aoki J. Lysophosphatidic Acid as a Lipid Mediator With Multiple Biological Actions. *J Biochem* (2015) 157(2):81–9. doi: 10.1093/jb/mvu077
53. Benesch MG, Tang X, Venkatraman G, Bekele RT, Brindley DN. Recent Advances in Targeting the Autotaxin-Lysophosphatidate-Lipid Phosphate Phosphatase Axis *In Vivo*. *J BioMed Res* (2016) 30(4):272–84. doi: 10.7555/JBR.30.20150058
54. Fulkerson Z, Wu T, Sunkara M, Kooi CV, Morris AJ, Smyth SS. Binding of Autotaxin to Integrins Localizes Lysophosphatidic Acid Production to Platelets and Mammalian Cells. *J Biol Chem* (2011) 286(40):34654–63. doi: 10.1074/jbc.M111.276725
55. Hausmann J, Kamtekar S, Christodoulou E, Day JE, Wu T, Fulkerson Z, et al. Structural Basis of Substrate Discrimination and Integrin Binding by

Autotaxin. *Nat Struct Mol Biol* (2011) 18(2):198–204. doi: 10.1038/nsmb.1980

56. Leblanc R, Lee SC, David M, Bordet JC, Norman DD, Patil R, et al. Interaction of Platelet-Derived Autotaxin With Tumor Integrin Alphavbeta3 Controls Metastasis of Breast Cancer Cells to Bone. *Blood* (2014) 124(20):3141–50. doi: 10.1182/blood-2014-04-568683
57. Yung YC, Stoddard NC, Chun J. LPA Receptor Signaling: Pharmacology, Physiology, and Pathophysiology. *J Lipid Res* (2014) 55(7):1192–214. doi: 10.1194/jlr.R046458
58. Kostadinova L, Shive CL, Anthony DD. Elevated Autotaxin and LPA Levels During Chronic Viral Hepatitis and Hepatocellular Carcinoma Associate With Systemic Immune Activation. *Cancers (Basel)* (2019) 11(12):1867. doi: 10.3390/cancers11121867
59. Joshita S, Ichikawa Y, Umemura T, Usami Y, Sugiura A, Shibata S, et al. Serum Autotaxin Is a Useful Liver Fibrosis Marker in Patients With Chronic Hepatitis B Virus Infection. *Hepatol Res* (2018) 48(4):275–85. doi: 10.1111/hepr.12997
60. Farquhar MJ, Humphreys IS, Rudge SA, Wilson GK, Bhattacharya B, Ciaccia M, et al. Autotaxin-Lysophosphatidic Acid Receptor Signalling Regulates Hepatitis C Virus Replication. *J Hepatol* (2017) 66(5):919–29. doi: 10.1016/j.jhep.2017.01.009
61. Nikitopoulou I, Fanidis D, Ntatsoulis K, Moulos P, Mpekoulis G, Evangelidou M, et al. Increased Autotaxin Levels in Severe COVID-19, Correlating With IL-6 Levels, Endothelial Dysfunction Biomarkers, and Impaired Functions of Dendritic Cells. *medRxiv* (2021) 2021.07.30.21261361. doi: 10.1101/2021.07.30.21261361
62. Gao L, Li X, Wang H, Liao Y, Zhou Y, Wang K, et al. Autotaxin Levels in Serum and Bronchoalveolar Lavage Fluid Are Associated With Inflammatory and Fibrotic Biomarkers and the Clinical Outcome in Patients With Acute Respiratory Distress Syndrome. *J Intensive Care* (2021) 9(1):44. doi: 10.1186/s40560-021-00559-3
63. Sexton T, Chalhoub G, Ye S, Morris W, Annabathula R, Dugan A, et al. Autotaxin Activity Predicts 30-Day Mortality in Sepsis Patients and Correlates With Platelet Count and Vascular Dysfunction. *Shock* (2020) 54(6):738–43. doi: 10.1097/SHK.0000000000001569
64. Benesch MG, Tang X, Dewald J, Dong WF, Mackey JR, Hemmings DG, et al. Tumor-Induced Inflammation in Mammary Adipose Tissue Stimulates a Vicious Cycle of Autotaxin Expression and Breast Cancer Progression. *FASEB J* (2015) 29(9):3990–4000. doi: 10.1096/fj.15-274480
65. Mouratis MA, Magkrioti C, Oikonomou N, Katsifa A, Prestwich GD, Kaffe E, et al. Autotaxin and Endotoxin-Induced Acute Lung Injury. *PloS One* (2015) 10(7):e0133619. doi: 10.1371/journal.pone.0133619
66. Zhao J, He D, Su Y, Berdyshev E, Chun J, Natarajan V, et al. Lysophosphatidic Acid Receptor 1 Modulates Lipopolysaccharide-Induced Inflammation in Alveolar Epithelial Cells and Murine Lungs. *Am J Physiol Lung Cell Mol Physiol* (2011) 301(4):L547–56. doi: 10.1152/ajplung.00058.2011
67. Nikitopoulou I, Ninou I, Manitsopoulos N, Dimopoulou I, Orfanos SE, Aidinis V, et al. A Role for Bronchial Epithelial Autotaxin in Ventilator-Induced Lung Injury. *Intensive Care Med Exp* (2021) 9(1):12. doi: 10.1186/s40635-021-00379-7
68. Tager AM, LaCamera P, Shea BS, Campanella GS, Selman M, Zhao Z, et al. The Lysophosphatidic Acid Receptor LPA1 Links Pulmonary Fibrosis to Lung Injury by Mediating Fibroblast Recruitment and Vascular Leak. *Nat Med* (2008) 14(1):45–54. doi: 10.1038/nm1685
69. Ninou I, Kaffe E, Muller S, Budd DC, Stevenson CS, Ullmer C, et al. Pharmacologic Targeting of the ATX/LPA Axis Attenuates Bleomycin-Induced Pulmonary Fibrosis. *Pulm Pharmacol Ther* (2018) 52:32–40. doi: 10.1016/j.pupt.2018.08.003
70. Ninou I, Magkrioti C, Aidinis V. Autotaxin in Pathophysiology and Pulmonary Fibrosis. *Front Med (Lausanne)* (2018) 5:180. doi: 10.3389/fmed.2018.00180
71. Gierse JK, Thorarensen A, Beltey K, Bradshaw-Pierce E, Cortes-Burgos L, Hall T, et al. A Novel Autotaxin Inhibitor Reduces Lysophosphatidic Acid Levels in Plasma and the Site of Inflammation. *J Pharmacol Exp Ther* (2010) 334(1):310–7. doi: 10.1124/jpet.110.165845
72. Tager AM. Autotaxin Emerges as a Therapeutic Target for Idiopathic Pulmonary Fibrosis: Limiting Fibrosis by Limiting Lysophosphatidic Acid Synthesis. *Am J Respir Cell Mol Biol* (2012) 47(5):563–5. doi: 10.1165/rcmb.2012-0235ED
73. Sun S, Wang R, Song J, Guan M, Li N, Zhang X, et al. Blocking Gp130 Signaling Suppresses Autotaxin Expression in Adipocytes and Improves Insulin Sensitivity in Diet-Induced Obesity. *J Lipid Res* (2017) 58: (11):2102–13. doi: 10.1194/jlr.M075655
74. Castelino FV, Bain G, Pace VA, Black KE, George L, Probst CK, et al. An Autotaxin/Lysophosphatidic Acid/Interleukin-6 Amplification Loop Drives Scleroderma Fibrosis. *Arthritis Rheumatol (Hoboken NJ)* (2016) 68 (12):2964–74. doi: 10.1002/art.39797
75. Nikitopoulou I, Oikonomou N, Karouzakis E, Sevastou I, Nikolaidou-Katsaridou N, Zhao Z, et al. Autotaxin Expression From Synovial Fibroblasts Is Essential for the Pathogenesis of Modeled Arthritis. *J Exp Med* (2012) 209(5):925–33. doi: 10.1084/jem.20112012
76. Lei L, Su J, Chen J, Chen W, Chen X, Peng C. The Role of Lysophosphatidic Acid in the Physiology and Pathology of the Skin. *Life Sci* (2019) 220:194–200. doi: 10.1016/j.lfs.2018.12.040
77. Herold T, Jurinovic V, Arnreich C, Lipworth BJ, Hellmuth JC, von Bergwelt-Baildon M, et al. Elevated Levels of IL-6 and CRP Predict the Need for Mechanical Ventilation in COVID-19. *J Allergy Clin Immunol* (2020) 146 (1):128–36.e4. doi: 10.1016/j.jaci.2020.05.008
78. Guirao JJ, Cabrera CM, Jiménez N, Rincón L, Urra JM. High Serum IL-6 Values Increase the Risk of Mortality and the Severity of Pneumonia in Patients Diagnosed With COVID-19. *Mol Immunol* (2020) 128:64–8. doi: 10.1016/j.molimm.2020.10.006
79. Tanaka M, Okudaira S, Kishi Y, Ohkawa R, Iseki S, Ota M, et al. Autotaxin Stabilizes Blood Vessels and Is Required for Embryonic Vasculature by Producing Lysophosphatidic Acid. *J Biol Chem* (2006) 281(35):25822–30. doi: 10.1074/jbc.M605142200
80. van Meeteren LA, Ruurs P, Stortelers C, Bouwman P, van Rooijen MA, Pradere JP, et al. Autotaxin, a Secreted Lysophospholipase D, Is Essential for Blood Vessel Formation During Development. *Mol Cell Biol* (2006) 26 (13):5015–22. doi: 10.1128/MCB.02419-05
81. Fotopoulou S, Oikonomou N, Grigorieva E, Nikitopoulou I, Paparountas T, Thanassopoulou A, et al. ATX Expression and LPA Signalling Are Vital for the Development of the Nervous System. *Dev Biol* (2010) 339(2):451–64. doi: 10.1016/j.ydbio.2010.01.007
82. Gralinski LE, Menachery VD, Morgan AP, Totura AL, Beall A, Kocher J, et al. Allelic Variation in the Toll-Like Receptor Adaptor Protein Ticam2 Contributes to SARS-Coronavirus Pathogenesis in Mice. *G3 (Bethesda)* (2017) 7(6):1653–63. doi: 10.1534/g3.117.041434
83. Gralinski LE, Ferris MT, Aylor DL, Whitmore AC, Green R, Frieman MB, et al. Genome Wide Identification of SARS-CoV Susceptibility Loci Using the Collaborative Cross. *PloS Genet* (2015) 11(10):e1005504. doi: 10.1371/journal.pgen.1005504
84. Zhao J, Wei J, Dong S, Bowser RK, Zhang L, Jacko AM, et al. Destabilization of Lysophosphatidic Acid Receptor 1 Reduces Cytokine Release and Protects Against Lung Injury. *EBioMedicine* (2016) 10:195–203. doi: 10.1016/j.ebiom.2016.07.020
85. Ren H, Panchatcharam M, Mueller P, Escalante-Alcalde D, Morris AJ, Smyth SS. Lipid Phosphate Phosphatase (LPP3) and Vascular Development. *Biochim Biophys Acta* (2013) 1831(1):126–32. doi: 10.1016/j.bbalip.2012.07.012
86. Tang X, Brindley DN. Lipid Phosphate Phosphatases and Cancer. *Biomolecules* (2020) 10(9):1263. doi: 10.3390/biom10091263
87. Magkrioti C, Aidinis V. ATX and LPA Signalling in Lung Pathophysiology. *World J Respirol* (2013) 3(3):77–103. doi: 10.5320/wjr.v3.i3.77
88. Shea BS, Tager AM. Role of the Lysophospholipid Mediators Lysophosphatidic Acid and Sphingosine 1-Phosphate in Lung Fibrosis. *Proc Am Thorac Soc* (2012) 9(3):102–10. doi: 10.1513/pats.201201-005AW
89. Zhao Y, Natarajan V. Lysophosphatidic Acid (LPA) and Its Receptors: Role in Airway Inflammation and Remodeling. *Biochim Biophys Acta* (2013) 1831 (1):86–92. doi: 10.1016/j.bbalip.2012.06.014
90. Kim SJ, Moon HG, Park GY. The Roles of Autotaxin/Lysophosphatidic Acid in Immune Regulation and Asthma. *Biochim Biophys Acta Mol Cell Biol Lipids* (2020) 1865(5):158641. doi: 10.1016/j.bbalip.2020.158641
91. Knowlden S, Georas SN. The Autotaxin-LPA Axis Emerges as a Novel Regulator of Lymphocyte Homing and Inflammation. *J Immunol* (2014) 192 (3):851–7. doi: 10.4049/jimmunol.1302831

92. Lee SC, Dacheux MA, Norman DD, Balazs L, Torres RM, Augelli-Szafran CE, et al. Regulation of Tumor Immunity by Lysophosphatidic Acid. *Cancers (Basel)* (2020) 12(5):1202. doi: 10.3390/cancers12051202
93. Knowlden SA, Capece T, Popovic M, Chapman TJ, Rezaee F, Kim M, et al. Regulation of T Cell Motility *In Vitro* and *In Vivo* by LPA and LPA2. *PloS One* (2014) 9(7):e101655. doi: 10.1371/journal.pone.0101655
94. Katakai T, Kondo N, Ueda Y, Kinashi T. Autotaxin Produced by Stromal Cells Promotes LFA-1-Independent and Rho-Dependent Interstitial T Cell Motility in the Lymph Node Paracortex. *J Immunol* (2014) 193(2):617–26. doi: 10.4049/jimmunol.1400565
95. Hisano Y, Kono M, Cartier A, Engelbrecht E, Kano K, Kawakami K, et al. Lysolipid Receptor Cross-Talk Regulates Lymphatic Endothelial Junctions in Lymph Nodes. *J Exp Med* (2019) 216(7):1582–98. doi: 10.1084/jem.20181895
96. Kunkel GT, Maceyka M, Milstien S, Spiegel S. Targeting the Sphingosine-1-Phosphate Axis in Cancer, Inflammation and Beyond. *Nat Rev Drug Discov* (2013) 12(9):688–702. doi: 10.1038/nrd4099
97. Matloubian M, Lo CG, Cinamon G, Lesneski MJ, Xu Y, Brinkmann V, et al. Lymphocyte Egress From Thymus and Peripheral Lymphoid Organs Is Dependent on S1P Receptor 1. *Nature* (2004) 427(6972):355–60. doi: 10.1038/nature02284
98. Wynn Thomas A, Vannella Kevin M. Macrophages in Tissue Repair, Regeneration, and Fibrosis. *Immunity* (2016) 44(3):450–62. doi: 10.1016/j.immuni.2016.02.015
99. Desai O, Winkler J, Minasyan M, Herzog EL. The Role of Immune and Inflammatory Cells in Idiopathic Pulmonary Fibrosis. *Front Med* (2018) 5:43. doi: 10.3389/fmed.2018.00043
100. Liao M, Liu Y, Yuan J, Wen Y, Xu G, Zhao J, et al. Single-Cell Landscape of Bronchoalveolar Immune Cells in Patients With COVID-19. *Nat Med* (2020) 26(6):842–4. doi: 10.1038/s41591-020-0901-9
101. Grant RA, Morales-Nebreda L, Markov NS, Swaminathan S, Querrey M, Guzman ER, et al. Circuits Between Infected Macrophages and T Cells in SARS-CoV-2 Pneumonia. *Nature* (2021) 590(7847):635–41. doi: 10.1038/s41586-020-03148-w
102. Shimada H, Rajagopalan LE. Rho-Kinase Mediates Lysophosphatidic Acid-Induced IL-8 and MCP-1 Production *via* P38 and JNK Pathways in Human Endothelial Cells. *FEBS Lett* (2010) 584(13):2827–32. doi: 10.1016/j.febslet.2010.04.064
103. Zhou Z, Subramanian P, Sevilmis G, Globke B, Soehnlein O, Karshovska E, et al. Lipoprotein-Derived Lysophosphatidic Acid Promotes Atherosclerosis by Releasing CXCL1 From the Endothelium. *Cell Metab* (2011) 13(5):592–600. doi: 10.1016/j.cmet.2011.02.016
104. Takeda Y, Matoba K, Kawanami D, Nagai Y, Akamine T, Ishizawa S, et al. ROCK2 Regulates Monocyte Migration and Cell to Cell Adhesion in Vascular Endothelial Cells. *Int J Mol Sci* (2019) 20(6):1331. doi: 10.3390/ijms20061331
105. Misharin AV, Morales-Nebreda L, Reyfman PA, Cuda CM, Walter JM, McQuattie-Pimentel AC, et al. Monocyte-Derived Alveolar Macrophages Drive Lung Fibrosis and Persist in the Lung Over the Life Span. *J Exp Med* (2017) 214(8):2387–404. doi: 10.1084/jem.20162152
106. Ray R, Rai V. Lysophosphatidic Acid Converts Monocytes Into Macrophages in Both Mice and Humans. *Blood* (2017) 129(9):1177–83. doi: 10.1182/blood-2016-10-743757
107. Santos-Nogueira E, Lopez-Serrano C, Hernandez J, Lago N, Astudillo AM, Balsinde J, et al. Activation of Lysophosphatidic Acid Receptor Type 1 Contributes to Pathophysiology of Spinal Cord Injury. *J Neurosci* (2015) 35 (28):10224–35. doi: 10.1523/JNEUROSCI.4703-14.2015
108. Kaya B, Doñas C, Wuggenig P, Diaz OE, Morales RA, Melhem H, et al. Lysophosphatidic Acid-Mediated GPR35 Signaling in CX3CR1(+) Macrophages Regulates Intestinal Homeostasis. *Cell Rep* (2020) 32 (5):107979. doi: 10.1016/j.celrep.2020.107979
109. Fransson J, Gómez-Conde AI, Romero-Imbroda J, Fernández O, Leyva L, de Fonseca FR, et al. Activation of Macrophages by Lysophosphatidic Acid Through the Lysophosphatidic Acid Receptor 1 as a Novel Mechanism in Multiple Sclerosis Pathogenesis. *Mol Neurobiol* (2021) 58(2):470–82. doi: 10.1007/s12035-020-02130-x
110. Chang CL, Hsu HY, Lin HY, Chiang W, Lee H. Lysophosphatidic Acid-Induced Oxidized Low-Density Lipoprotein Uptake Is Class A Scavenger Receptor-Dependent in Macrophages. *Prostaglandins Other Lipid Mediat* (2008) 87(1-4):20–5. doi: 10.1016/j.prostaglandins.2008.05.002
111. An D, Hao F, Zhang F, Kong W, Chun J, Xu X, et al. CD14 Is a Key Mediator of Both Lysophosphatidic Acid and Lipopolysaccharide Induction of Foam Cell Formation. *J Biol Chem* (2017) 292(35):14391–400. doi: 10.1074/jbc.M117.781807
112. Schober A, Siess W. Lysophosphatidic Acid in Atherosclerotic Diseases. *Br J Pharmacol* (2012) 167(3):465–82. doi: 10.1111/j.1476-5381.2012.02021.x
113. Martino A, Volpe E, Baldini PM. The Influence of Lysophosphatidic Acid on the Immunophenotypic Differentiation of Human Monocytes Into Dendritic Cells. *Haematologica* (2006) 91(9):1273–4. doi: 10.3324/%x
114. Chen R, Roman J, Guo J, West E, McDyer J, Williams MA, et al. Lysophosphatidic Acid Modulates the Activation of Human Monocyte-Derived Dendritic Cells. *Stem Cells Dev* (2006) 15(6):797–804. doi: 10.1089/scd.2006.15.797
115. Guo L, He P, No YR, Yun CC. Krüppel-Like Factor 5 Incorporates Into the β-Catenin/TCF Complex in Response to LPA in Colon Cancer Cells. *Cell Signal* (2015) 27(5):961–8. doi: 10.1016/j.cellsig.2015.02.005
116. Cisse B, Caton ML, Lehner M, Maeda T, Scheu S, Locksley R, et al. Transcription Factor E2-2 Is an Essential and Specific Regulator of Plasmacytoid Dendritic Cell Development. *Cell* (2008) 135(1):37–48. doi: 10.1016/j.cell.2008.09.016
117. Emo J, Meednu N, Chapman TJ, Rezaee F, Balys M, Randall T, et al. Lpa2 Is a Negative Regulator of Both Dendritic Cell Activation and Murine Models of Allergic Lung Inflammation. *J Immunol* (2012) 188(8):3784–90. doi: 10.4049/jimmunol.1102956
118. Horby P, Lim WS, Emberson JR, Mafham M, Bell JL, Linsell L, et al. Dexamethasone in Hospitalized Patients With Covid-19. *N Engl J Med* (2021) 384(8):693–704. doi: 10.1056/NEJMoa2021436
119. Sterne JAC, Murthy S, Diaz JV, Slutsky AS, Villar J, Angus DC, et al. Association Between Administration of Systemic Corticosteroids and Mortality Among Critically Ill Patients With COVID-19: A Meta-Analysis. *Jama* (2020) 324(13):1330–41. doi: 10.1001/jama.2020.17023
120. Abdin SM, Elgendy SM, Alyammahi SK, Alhamad DW, Omar HA. Tackling the Cytokine Storm in COVID-19, Challenges and Hopes. *Life Sci* (2020) 257:118054. doi: 10.1016/j.lfs.2020.118054
121. Distler O, Highland KB, Gahlemann M, Azuma A, Fischer A, Mayes MD, et al. Nintedanib for Systemic Sclerosis–Associated Interstitial Lung Disease. *N Engl J Med* (2019) 380(26):2518–28. doi: 10.1056/NEJMoa1903076
122. Flaherty KR, Wells AU, Cottin V, Devaraj A, Walsh SLF, Inoue Y, et al. Nintedanib in Progressive Fibrosing Interstitial Lung Diseases. *N Engl J Med* (2019) 381(18):1718–27. doi: 10.1056/NEJMoa1908681
123. Maher TM, Corte TJ, Fischer A, Kreuter M, Lederer DJ, Molina-Molina M, et al. Pirfenidone in Patients With Unclassifiable Progressive Fibrosing Interstitial Lung Disease: A Double-Blind, Randomised, Placebo-Controlled, Phase 2 Trial. *Lancet Respir Med* (2020) 8(2):147–57. doi: 10.1016/S2213-2600(19)30341-8
124. King TEJr., Bradford WZ, Castro-Bernardini S, Fagan EA, Glaspole I, Glassberg MK, et al. A Phase 3 Trial of Pirfenidone in Patients With Idiopathic Pulmonary Fibrosis. *N Engl J Med* (2014) 370(22):2083–92. doi: 10.1056/NEJMoa1402582
125. Richeldi L, du Bois RM, Raghu G, Azuma A, Brown KK, Costabel U, et al. Efficacy and Safety of Nintedanib in Idiopathic Pulmonary Fibrosis. *N Engl J Med* (2014) 370(22):2071–82. doi: 10.1056/NEJMoa1402584
126. Spagnolo P, Balestro E, Aliberti S, Cocconcelli E, Biondini D, Casa GD, et al. Pulmonary Fibrosis Secondary to COVID-19: A Call to Arms? *Lancet Respir Med* (2020) 8(8):750–2. doi: 10.1016/S2213-2600(20)30222-8
127. George PM, Wells AU, Jenkins RG. Pulmonary Fibrosis and COVID-19: The Potential Role for Antifibrotic Therapy. *Lancet Respir Med* (2020) 8(8):807–15. doi: 10.1016/S2213-2600(20)30225-3
128. Vasarmidi E, Tsitoura E, Spandidos DA, Tzanakis N, Antoniou KM. Pulmonary Fibrosis in the Aftermath of the COVID-19 Era (Review). *Exp Ther Med* (2020) 20(3):2557–60. doi: 10.3892/etm.2020.8980
129. Maher TM, Kreuter M, Lederer DJ, Brown KK, Wuyts W, Verbruggen N, et al. Rationale, Design and Objectives of Two Phase III, Randomised, Placebo-Controlled Studies of GLPG1690, a Novel Autotaxin Inhibitor, in Idiopathic Pulmonary Fibrosis (ISABELA 1 and 2). *BMJ Open Respir Res* (2019) 6(1):e000422. doi: 10.1164/ajrccm-conference.2019.199.1_MeetingAbstracts.A4597

130. Nishimasu H, Okudaira S, Hama K, Mihara E, Dohmae N, Inoue A, et al. Crystal Structure of Autotaxin and Insight Into GPCR Activation by Lipid Mediators. *Nat Struct Mol Biol* (2011) 18(2):205–12. doi: 10.1038/nsmb.1998
131. Moolenaar WH, Perrakis A. Insights Into Autotaxin: How to Produce and Present a Lipid Mediator. *Nat Rev Mol Cell Biol* (2011) 12(10):674–9. doi: 10.1038/nrm3188
132. Salgado-Polo F, Perrakis A. The Structural Binding Mode of the Four Autotaxin Inhibitor Types That Differentially Affect Catalytic and Non-Catalytic Functions. *Cancers* (2019) 11(10):1577. doi: 10.3390/cancers11101577
133. Matralis AN, Afantitis A, Aidinis V. Development and Therapeutic Potential of Autotaxin Small Molecule Inhibitors: From Bench to Advanced Clinical Trials. *Med Res Rev* (2018) 39(3):976–1013. doi: 10.1002/med.21551
134. Castagna D, Budd DC, Macdonald SJ, Jamieson C, Watson AJ. Development of Autotaxin Inhibitors: An Overview of the Patent and Primary Literature. *J Med Chem* (2016) 59(12):5604–21. doi: 10.1021/acs.jmedchem.5b01599
135. Katsifa A, Kaffe E, Nikolaidou-Katsaridou N, Economides AN, Newbigging S, McKerlie C, et al. The Bulk of Autotaxin Activity Is Dispensable for Adult Mouse Life. *PloS One* (2015) 10(11):e0143083. doi: 10.1371/journal.pone.0143083
136. van der Aar E, Desrivot J, Dupont S, Heckmann B, Fieuw A, Stutvoet S, et al. Safety, Pharmacokinetics, and Pharmacodynamics of the Autotaxin Inhibitor GLPG1690 in Healthy Subjects: Phase 1 Randomized Trials. *J Clin Pharmacol* (2019) 59(10):1366–78. doi: 10.1002/jcph.1424
137. Maher TM, van der Aar EM, Van de Steen O, Allamassey L, Desrivot J, Dupont S, et al. Safety, Tolerability, Pharmacokinetics, and Pharmacodynamics of GLPG1690, a Novel Autotaxin Inhibitor, to Treat Idiopathic Pulmonary Fibrosis (FLORA): A Phase 2a Randomised Placebo-Controlled Trial. *Lancet Respir Med* (2018) 6(8):627–35. doi: 10.1016/S2213-2600(18)30181-4
138. Lee G, Kang SU, Ryou J-H, Lim J-J, Lee Y-H. Late Breaking Abstract - BBT-877, A Potent Autotaxin Inhibitor in Clinical Development to Treat Idiopathic Pulmonary Fibrosis. *Eur Respir J* (2019) 54(suppl 63):PA1293. doi: 10.1183/13993003.congress-2019.PA1293
139. Lee G, Kang SU, Ryou JH, Lim JJ, Lee DY, Kwon HJ, et al. (2019). BBT-877, a Potent Autotaxin Inhibitor in Clinical Development to Treat Idiopathic Pulmonary Fibrosis. A108 PATHOPHYSIOLOGY IN DIFFUSE PARENCHYMAL LUNG DISEASES, in: *American Thoracic Society International Conference Abstracts*, pp. A2577–A. American Thoracic Society.

9

Idiopathic Pulmonary Fibrosis: Aging, Mitochondrial Dysfunction and Cellular Bioenergetics

Daniel C. Zank[1], Marta Bueno[1,2], Ana L. Mora[1,2] and Mauricio Rojas[1,3,4]**

[1] Division of Pulmonary, Allergy and Critical Care Medicine, University of Pittsburgh School of Medicine, Pittsburgh, PA, United States, [2] Vascular Medicine Institute, University of Pittsburgh School of Medicine, Pittsburgh, PA, United States, [3] McGowan Institute of Regenerative Medicine, University of Pittsburgh School of Medicine, Pittsburgh, PA, United States, [4] Dorothy P. & Richard P. Simmons Center for Interstitial Lung Disease, University of Pittsburgh School of Medicine, Pittsburgh, PA, United States

***Correspondence:**
Ana L. Mora
anamora@pitt.edu;
Mauricio Rojas
rojasm@upmc.edu

At present, the etiology of idiopathic pulmonary fibrosis (IPF) remains elusive. Over the past two decades, however, researchers have identified and described the underlying processes that result in metabolic dysregulation, metabolic reprogramming, and mitochondrial dysfunction observed in the cells of IPF lungs. Metabolic changes and mitochondrial dysfunction in IPF include decreased efficiency of electron transport chain function with increasing production of reactive oxygen species, decreased mitochondrial biogenesis, and impaired mitochondrial macroautophagy, a key pathway for the removal of dysfunctional mitochondria. Metabolic changes in IPF have potential impact on lung cell function, differentiation, and activation of fibrotic responses. These alterations result in activation of TGF-β and predispose to the development of pulmonary fibrosis. IPF is a disease of the aged, and many of these same bioenergetic changes are present to a lesser extent with normal aging, raising the possibility that these anticipated alterations in metabolic processes play important roles in creating susceptibility to the development of IPF. This review explores what is known regarding the cellular metabolic and mitochondrial changes that are found in IPF, and examines this body of literature to identify future research direction and potential points of intervention in the pathogenesis of IPF.

Keywords: aging, mitochondrial dysfunction, lung fibrosis, bioenergetics, mitophagy, senescence

INTRODUCTION

Aging is life's natural destiny. It is biologically defined by a progressive impairment in vital functions coupled with diminished fitness to adapt to environmental stimuli and respond to stress (homeostenosis) (1). Among the predictable cellular alterations that underlie homeostenosis, metabolic dysregulation and alterations in mitochondrial function have been shown to contribute to the aging phenotype. Aging is also associated with increased susceptibility to a wide range of chronic diseases. Lung pathologies are no exception, and the prevalence of several interstitial lung diseases, most notably idiopathic pulmonary fibrosis (IPF), has been found to increase considerably with age. IPF is a progressive and irreversible lung disease, generally diagnosed in the sixth decade of life, whose etiology remains unknown and therapeutic options remain limited (2). Many of the changes in bioenergetics and mitochondrial function seen with aging are also seen in the fibrotic lung and may contribute to IPF (**Table 1**).

TABLE 1 | Mitochondrial changes in the fibrotic lung.

Feature	Change	Model	Reference
Mitochondrial reactive oxygen species	Increased	Bleomycin mouse model Asbestosis mouse model	(44)
Mitochondrial respiration	Decreased ETC complex activity, lower OCR	Human idiopathic pulmonary fibrosis (IPF) lung tissue Human lung fibroblasts Human AECII Alveolar macrophages MHV68 model of lung fibrosis	(5, 15, 42, 43, 63, 66, 69)
ATP production	Decreased	IPF lung fibroblasts IPF lung myofibroblasts IPF total lung	(24, 43, 69)
mtDNA	Increased oxidative damage, insufficient mtDNA repair	IPF total lung Murine AECII Bleomycin mouse model Asbestosis mouse model	(5, 44, 48)
Mitochondrial biogenesis	Decrease	IPF total lung Bleomycin mouse model	(15)
Mitochondrial dynamics	Imbalanced	MHV68 mouse model of fibrosis	(5)
Mitophagy alterations	Reduced levels of mediators of mitochondrial quality control in epithelial cells and fibroblasts Increased mitophagy in macrophages	IPF AECII IPF lung fibroblasts IPF pulmonary macrophages Bleomycin mouse model MHV68 mouse model of fibrosis	(5, 24, 25, 30)
Decreased expression of SIRT3	Acetylation of mitochondrial proteins	IPF total lung Bleomycin mouse model Asbestosis mouse model	(48, 52)

ETC, electron transport chain; OXPHOS, oxidative phosphorylation; AECII, alveolar type II epithelial cells; OCR, oxygen consumption rate.

MITOCHONDRIAL ALTERATIONS WITH AGING AND IPF

Over the past few decades, our understanding of the function and role of mitochondria has moved beyond the initial view of mitochondria as nothing more than a cellular energy generator producing ATP through oxidative phosphorylation (OXPHOS). Mitochondria are now understood to have their own life cycle consisting of biogenesis, fission/fusion dynamics, and recycling through macroautophagy (mitophagy), and to act as an important bidirectional signaling platform, communicating with the nucleus as well as other organelles. Multiple signaling pathways converge and interact to regulate the linked processes of mitochondrial energetics, biogenesis, production of reactive oxygen species (ROS), mitochondrial DNA (mtDNA) preservation and repair, and mitophagy. Dysregulation of many of these regulatory mechanisms that control mitochondrial function have recently been identified in the epithelial cells, fibroblasts, and macrophages in IPF lungs (3). Mitochondrial dysfunction in IPF lung cells contributes to maladaptation to cellular stress, creating vulnerability to injury and promoting the development of pulmonary fibrosis (3–6) (**Figure 1**).

MITOCHONDRIAL BIOGENESIS

Mitochondrial biogenesis, the process of producing additional mitochondria and by extension cellular energy production capacity, is under the control of master regulators PPARγ coactivator-1α (PGC-1α) and PGC-1β, which are nutritional sensors able to induce expression of nuclear respiration factors 1 and 2 (NRF). NRFs upregulate expression of the nuclear and mitochondrial mechanisms necessary for mitochondrial biogenesis (7). With aging, the capacity for mitochondrial biogenesis declines through age-related reduction in upstream activators of PGC-1α and PGC-1β such as AMP-activated protein kinase (AMPK) as well as p53-mediated, senescence-associated repression of these key regulators of mitochondrial biogenesis (8, 9). Moderate exercise, calorie restriction, and resveratrol supplementation have been shown to increase PGC-1α activity and ameliorates aging-related decline in mitochondrial biogenesis (10–12). Expression of PGC1a is reduced in lungs from IPF patients and in fibrotic mouse lungs after bleomycin treatment. Highlighting the critical role of mitochondrial biogenesis in the susceptibility to lung fibrosis, mice deficient in PGC1a are more susceptible to bleomycin-induced lung fibrosis. Thyroid hormone (T4) signaling is known to restore mitochondrial health and function through a PGC-1α-dependent pathway (13, 14). Concordantly, experimental provision of aerosolized T3 and a T4 mimetic attenuated bleomycin- and TGF-β-induced fibrosis in mouse models. T3 supplementation was also associated with reduced alveolar epithelial cell apoptosis, improvement in mitochondrial electron transport chain function, and normalization of swollen mitochondrial morphology. This improvement was

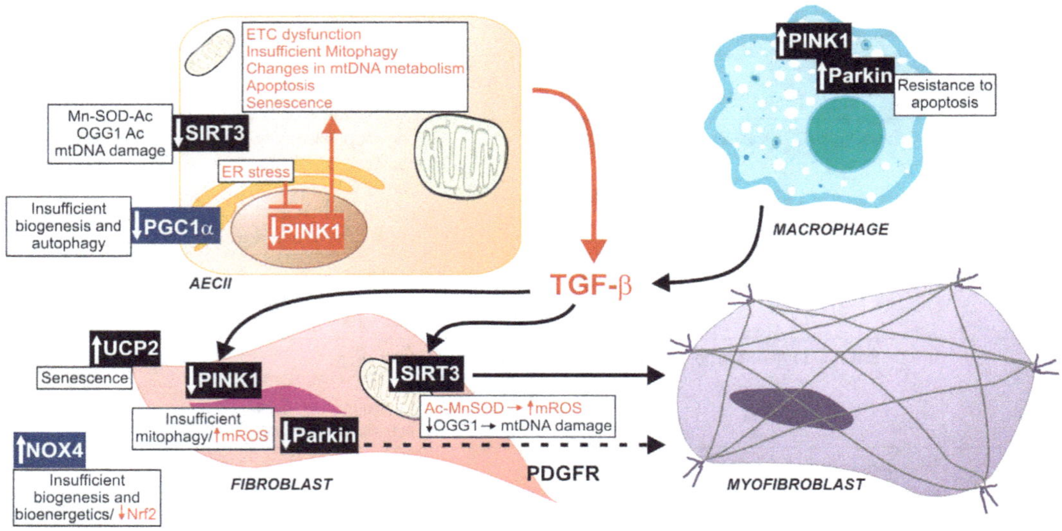

FIGURE 1 | Schematic of profibrotic pathways mediated by mitochondrial dysfunction. Reduced PGC1α in fibrotic lungs has been associated with insufficient biogenesis and diminished autophagy. Similarly, decreased PINK1, a key modulator of mitophagy, and decreased SIRT3 have been found in AECII from fibrotic lungs associated with mitochondrial dysfunction, and increased activation of TGF-β. Profibrotic macrophages exhibit increased rates of mitophagy and resistance to apoptosis resulting in greater release of TGF-β. TGF-β affects mitochondrial function in fibroblasts through decreasing PINK1, Parkin, and SIRT3. Idiopathic pulmonary fibrosis fibroblasts have increased mtDNA damage, mitochondrial dysfunction, impaired mitochondrial biogenesis, and increased rate of senescence. All of these factors contribute to in fibroblast-to-myofibroblast differentiation. Abbreviations: Ac, acetyl group; ETC, type II alveolar epithelial cell electron transport chain, Mn-SOD, manganese super oxide dismutase; mtDNA, mitochondrial DNA, mtROS, mitochondrial reactive oxygen species; NOX4, NADPH oxidase 4; Nrf2, nuclear factor (erythroid-derived 2)-like-2 factor; OGG1, 8-oxoguanine DNA glycosylase 1; PDGFR, platelet-derived growth factor receptor; PINK1, PTEN-induced putative kinase 1; UCP2, uncoupling protein 2; PGC-1α, peroxisome proliferator-activated receptor gamma coactivator 1-alpha.

not seen in PGC-1α knockout mice. These investigations were conducted in response to the finding of increased level and activity of iodothyronine deiodinase 2 in IPF lungs, which is the enzyme responsible for conversion of inactive T4 to the physiologically active T3 form. This is presumed to be an adaptive response to increase the availability of active T3 in fibrotic IPF lung (15).

Idiopathic pulmonary fibrosis and experimental models of pulmonary fibrosis are associated with telomere shortening and DNA damage, which activates the DNA damage sensor poly[ADP-ribose] polymerase 1 (PARP-1) and the checkpoint inhibitor p53. These signaling mechanisms feedback to reduce activation of PPARγ coactivators and reduce mitochondrial biogenesis (9, 16). Impaired mitochondrial biogenesis in IPF potentially creates a mismatch in cellular energy demand and production capacity with resulting mitochondrial dysfunction. Additionally, the ROS-producing enzyme NADPH oxidase-4 (Nox4), which is upregulated in IPF lung fibroblasts, represses mitochondrial biogenesis through direct effect on NRF2 and mitochondrial transcription factor A (TFAM) independent of PGC-1α (17, 18). While these pathways have been demonstrated to play a role in age and disease-related alterations in cellular bioenergetics, and the downstream consequences, such as ROS production, DNA damage, and induction of senescence, are features of lung fibrosis, additional translational investigations in IPF lungs are needed to firmly establish the role of these perturbations in the development of IPF.

MITOPHAGY

Mitophagy is a selective and adaptive response that targets mitochondria for turnover, regulates the number of mitochondria to match cellular energy needs, and removes damaged and dysfunctional mitochondria that can cause cellular stress. Mitophagy and mitochondrial turnover are important processes in maintaining cellular integrity and health. Mitochondrial damage, whether from metabolic alterations, increased ROS production, or an accumulation of mtDNA damage and mutations affecting transcription, results in a reduction of mitochondrial transmembrane potential, reduced ATP production, further increases in ROS, and leakage of mitochondrial contents into the cytosol that, if left unchecked, would eventually lead to cellular injury and apoptosis (19–23).

Selective mitophagy of damaged mitochondria occurs through PTEN-induced putative kinase 1 (PINK1)-Parkin signaling with PINK1 acting as a sensor of mitochondrial membrane depolarization and subsequently activating Parkin, which labels the dysfunctional mitochondrion for trafficking to the autophagosome (19, 24). With aging, a decrease in PINK1 has been observed coupled with a decrease in markers of autophagy and an increase in the size of mitochondria (5, 25). These findings demonstrate that capacity for mitophagy declines as we age.

Deficient mitophagy has been associated with IPF and development of pulmonary fibrosis in response to injury (5, 16, 25–27). Deficiency or dysfunction of multiple mediators of mitophagy has been implicated in the pathobiology of IPF making maintenance or augmentation of mitophagy an attractive avenue of potential intervention. Our work has shown that type II alveolar epithelial cells from IPF lungs are deficient in PINK1 resulting in an accumulation of dysmorphic mitochondria with reduced transmembrane potential, reduced electron transport chain (ETC) activity, increased ROS production, and increased opening of the mitochondrial permeability transition pore. PINK1 knockout was also found to be sufficient to recapitulate this mitochondrial phenotype and confer vulnerability to fibrosis in response to lung injury (5). PINK1 expression has been found to diminish with age and persistent endoplasmic reticulum stress. ER stress has been shown to induce expression of ATF3, a transcriptional repressor of PINK1, in alveolar epithelial cells (28). Interestingly, deficiency of PINK1 in lung epithelial cells was also associated with upregulation of markers of senescence (p16 and p21) and increased levels of TGF-β expression, a key mediator of fibrogenic processes in IPF (5, 28).

As adaptive responses, autophagy and mitophagy are essential to maintaining normal fibroblast function and preventing apoptosis. Impairment of mitophagy, mediated by Parkin deficiency, in IPF lung fibroblasts has been associated with increased deposition of extracellular matrix under profibrotic conditions such as exposure to TGF-β. Defects in mitophagy and autophagy result in increased production of ROS and activation of platelet-derived growth factor receptor (PDGFR)/mammalian target of rapamycin (mTOR) signaling pathways that enhance fibroblast to myofibroblast transformation (24). Supporting these data, Parkin-deficient mice develop more severe lung fibrosis. Induction of autophagy and treatment with antioxidants reduced fibroblast to myofibroblast differentiation, myofibroblast proliferation, and fibrogenesis suggesting that this process is driven by increased mitochondrial ROS (24, 25). Indeed, we now recognize that a subset of surfactant protein C mutations, which causes a familial form of pulmonary fibrosis, acts through mistrafficking of surfactant protein C, accumulation within endosomes, and a late block of macroautophagy and mitophagy within type II alveolar epithelial cells. This results in proteostasis and an accumulation of dysfunctional mitochondria with increased mitochondrial mass but decreased transmembrane potential, which may increase susceptibility to pulmonary fibrosis when an additional "second hit" stressor is present (29).

TGF-β has been shown to variably affect key mediators of mitophagy and promote fibrogenesis. Treatment of alveolar epithelial cells with TGF-β results in initial stabilization of PINK1 on the surface of mitochondria and induction of mitophagy, which appears to be an adaptive response to increased ROS production due to TGF-β's effect on the ETC (30). Longer term exposure to TGF-β results in impaired mitophagy through downregulation of phosphatase and tensin homolog (PTEN), and a subsequent reduction in PINK1 expression (25). Another potential activator of autophagy is T4, which is a well-known activator of AMPK and inhibitor of mTOR (15). Supporting this role of T4 signaling in PINK1-mediated mitochondrial homeostasis and mitophagy, the therapeutic effect of inhaled T3 in mouse models of lung fibrosis required an active PINK1 signaling pathway (15).

On the contrary, pulmonary macrophages isolated from IPF lungs demonstrate increased mitophagy. IPF macrophages are a source of activated TGF-β, and macrophage resistance to apoptosis is necessary for disease progression. IPF macrophages activate TGF-β by producing mitochondrial H_2O_2 through activation of the pro-survival kinase, protein kinase B (Akt1). Increased Akt1 activation and ROS production induce mitophagy as a protective measure and prevent macrophage apoptosis, which stabilizes macrophages to release additional TGF-β and promote local fibroblast activation and proliferation. Blocking mitophagy in alveolar macrophages is protective against bleomycin-induced fibrosis (27). This finding exemplifies the role of mitophagy as an adaptive survival response that, in this case, serves to preserve and promote macrophage signaling.

MITOCHONDRIAL OXPHOS

The processes of mitochondrial respiration and OXPHOS are the highly efficient and preferable means of ATP production, but a natural byproduct of these processes is superoxide and hydrogen peroxide production, which is produced in increasing quantities by dysfunctional mitochondria (31). Mitochondrial ROS (mtROS) serve as a signaling mechanism acting at multiple points throughout the cell that serves to inactivate phosphatases, activate select kinases, and facilitate hypoxia-inducible factor 1-α (HIF-1α), p53, and NF-κB signaling pathways (32–36). Interestingly, mtROS levels have a biphasic effect. At low levels, mtROS stimulate an increase in antioxidant capacity, referred to as mitohormesis, which has a protective effect and has been associated with longevity and resistance to cellular injury. In higher concentrations or with sustained production, ROS propagates free radicals that cause oxidative damage to lipids, proteins, and DNA (37).

Control of OXPHOS and energy production occurs through cooperative signaling mechanisms at mitochondrial, cytosolic, and nuclear levels in order to balance OXPHOS, energetic demands of the cell, and nutrient supply. This complex process limits production of ROS. Additionally, mitochondria have multiple mechanisms for reducing mtROS, but effective regulation of ROS production and mitigation declines with aging and potentiates susceptibility to lung injury and fibrosis (18, 38, 39). Aging is associated with lower ATP production and increased ROS (40). Moreover, older animals have been shown to accumulate higher levels of oxidized proteins in response to lung injury suggesting waning cellular antioxidant defense systems (41).

A profibrotic environment promotes mitochondrial dysfunction in pulmonary epithelial cells. Studies in Mv1Lu cells demonstrate that treatment with TGF-β1 downregulates mitochondrial ETC function, particularly at complex IV, resulting in loss of mitochondrial transmembrane potential and increased mtROS production (42). Increased ROS serves to oxidize and activate latent TGF-β1 creating a self-reinforcing cycle with potential to recruit fibroblasts and promote fibrogenesis (30). This correlates with the findings that type II alveolar epithelial cells from IPF lungs have reduced ETC complex I and IV activity (5), and IPF fibroblasts have reduced ATP content and reduced rate of oxygen consumption indicating poor mitochondrial function (43).

While the effectiveness of antioxidant supplementation in preventing diseases of aging such as IPF has been disappointing and, in some cases, detrimental, overexpression of an antioxidant protective mechanism in mitochondria has shown effectiveness in abrogating the fibrotic response to bleomycin-induced lung injury. Mice that overexpress mitochondria-targeted human catalase predictably show lower levels of mtROS, but also display reduced mtDNA damage and fragmentation with decreased pulmonary fibrosis in response to oxidative injury from asbestos or bleomycin (44). This raises the possibility that mitochondrial-targeted antioxidants may prevent or abrogate the development of IPF by scavenging mtROS at the source.

mtDNA DAMAGE

Mitochondrial DNA is significantly more susceptible to oxidative injury than nuclear DNA, likely due to proximity to the source of ROS, lack of protective histones, and relative paucity of mtDNA repair mechanisms (45). Indeed, oxidative DNA damage is a key mechanism of injury in the commonly used model of bleomycin-induced pulmonary fibrosis (46). In comparison with the nucleus, mitochondria contain fewer and less efficient mechanisms for correcting mutations and repairing DNA damage. Mitochondrial transcription factor A (TFAM) is a key regulator of mtDNA transcription and replication, which also functions to induce *U*-shaped bends in mtDNA. These protective nucleoids can act to sequester damaged DNA and prevent transcription until base excision repair enzymes can correct the damage (47). The base excision repair enzyme, 8-oxoguanine DNA glycosylase 1 (OGG1), plays a critical role in repair of mtDNA oxidative damage, OGG1 deficiency or inactivation predisposes to pulmonary fibrosis (26, 48). The processes of mtROS production and mtDNA damage are intricately linked, and oxidative injury and cellular stress drive apoptotic and senescence pathways that may contribute, at least in part, to both aging and to lung injury and fibrosis. Additional studies in IPF lung-derived cells or tissues are needed to establish the role of mtDNA damage in IPF.

Owing to the evolutionary origin of mitochondria as bacterial endosymbionts, mtDNA contains CpG-rich sequences, which have the potential to act as damage-associated molecular patterns and activate innate immune system mechanisms when they escape the mitochondrial milieu. This pathway may contribute to a pro-fibrotic microenvironment (49). Recently, it has been shown that IPF fibroblasts undergo glycolytic reprogramming associated with release of mtDNA into the cellular interstitium and ultimately into circulation. Furthermore, increased plasma levels of mtDNA were associated with an increase in all-cause mortality suggesting potential use of circulating mtDNA as a biomarker for progression or severity of IPF (50).

SIRTUINS ARE KEY MEDIATORS OF MITOCHONDRIAL HEALTH IMPLICATED IN IPF

Deficiency of the mitochondrial NAD-dependent deacetylase, SIRT3, has been shown to confer susceptibility to epithelial cell apoptosis and fibrosis in both bleomycin and asbestos models of lung injury (48). SIRT3 is an active enzyme in ROS detoxification as well as mtDNA protection and repair pathways, and its dependence on NAD+ as a cofactor directly links SIRT3's function to cellular bioenergetics and TCA cycle activity (51). In the mitochondrion, SIRT3 is implicated in regulation of two redox mechanisms. SIRT3 deacetylates and activates manganese superoxide dismutase (MnSOD) and isocitrate dehydrogenase 2 (IDH2) (52, 53). Low levels of SIRT3 result in increased acetylation and decreased MnSOD activity and an accumulation of mtROS and mtDNA oxidative damage (53). The matrix protein IDH2 is a key provider of the reducing agent, NADPH, necessary for proper functioning of protective antioxidant pathways (52). The mtDNA repair function of OGG1 is also regulated by SIRT3. In the absence of SIRT3, OGG1 is increasingly acetylated and deactivated resulting in unchecked mtDNA damage and lung epithelial cell apoptosis (44, 48).

SIRT3 knockout mice have also been shown to develop increased expression of TGF-β and fibrosis in multiple organs as they age. This has been shown to occur through increased acetylation and deactivation of glycogen synthase kinase-β and stabilization of profibrotic transcription factors, such as smad3 and β-catenin, independent of SIRT3's effect on MnSOD activity (54). Multiple SIRT3-dependent pathways play important roles in preventing mitochondrial damage and vulnerability to fibrosis.

Another sirtuin, SIRT1, has been established to play a role in preventing both aging-related functional decline and age-related diseases such as IPF (55). SIRT1 is a nuclear NAD-dependent deacetylase, but one of its key functions is in modulating mitochondrial biogenesis and function through nuclear-to-mitochondrial signaling pathways (56). These pathways have demonstrated how nuclear DNA damage and telomere shortening can drive mitochondrial dysfunction. Telomerase reverse transcriptase deficiency and shortened telomeres are strongly linked with the development of pulmonary fibrosis, and this chromosomal shortening activates the DNA damage sensor and checkpoint inhibitor p53. Activated p53 represses expression of a key mediator of mitochondrial biogenesis, PPARγ coactivator-1α (PGC-1α) resulting in inefficient OXPHOS and increased ROS production (57). SIRT1 deacetylates and inactivates p53 restoring normal mitochondrial function (9, 56). The nuclear DNA damage sensor, poly[ADP-ribose] polymerase 1 (PARP-1), consumes NAD+ when activated and decreases activity of SIRT1 and PGC-1α. SIRT1 and PGC-1α have also been shown to translocate to the mitochondria and may assist in stabilization of mtDNA (16). Fasting and caloric restriction, long of interest in increasing longevity, and reducing functional decline with aging, increase SIRT1 protein levels and activity (51). SIRT1 translation is inhibited by the microRNA miR-34a, which is highly expressed in models of lung injury. SIRT1 deficiency results in increased acetylation of p53, which acts to induce expression of miR-34a, creating a self-reinforcing cycle and predisposing to development of fibrosis (58). In a bleomycin model of lung injury, upregulation of SIRT1 attenuated fibroblast activation and the development of fibrosis (59). Sirtuins clearly have complex functions in modulating mitochondrial biogenesis, function, ROS production, and mtDNA protection, and this area of investigation has potential to shed new light on the pathogenesis of IPF and other diseases of aging.

METABOLIC REPROGRAMMING IN IPF

Fibrotic lung tissue in IPF has been shown to have increased metabolic activity as demonstrated by increased FDG uptake on PET scan, and increased PET activity correlates with disease progression and mortality (60). Cell-type specific metabolic changes occur in the IPF lung (**Figure 2**). Type II alveolar epithelial cells have downregulation of genes involved in lipid synthesis and metabolism identified through single cell RNA sequencing (61). Fibroblasts have been shown to undergo a metabolic shift away from the highly efficient method of ATP production, OXPHOS, to the less efficient method of glycolysis despite adequate oxygen to continue OxPhos (62–67). Additionally, alveolar macrophages in fibrotic lung tissue increase fatty acid oxidation in response to the shift to glycolysis (66). A similar metabolic shift was initially observed in cancer cells and was eponymously dubbed the Warburg effect after its discoverer (68). The Warburg-like metabolic reprogramming observed in IPF cells results in increased glucose uptake and an accumulation of TCA cycle metabolites and byproducts that act as signaling mechanisms. Kottmann and colleagues demonstrated that glycolytic flux increases lactate production and lowers the local tissue pH resulting in increased activation of TGF-β, stabilization of the transcription factor HIF-1α, and increased transcription of lactate dehydrogenase 5 (LDH5), which synergizes with TGF-β to induce differentiation of fibroblasts to myofibroblasts (62). LDH5 produces lactate, which can be exported by monocarboxylate transporter (MCT)-4 and may be taken up by adjacent cells expressing MCT-1. Shuttled lactate can be oxidized to pyruvate providing additional energy through the TCA cycle and driving OXPHOS. This phenomenon is termed the reverse Warburg effect and promotes fibroblast proliferation and increased levels of mtROS.

Primary myofibroblasts derived from IPF lungs and lung fibroblasts treated with TGF-β demonstrate increased lactate contents. Additionally, IPF myofibroblasts showed increase in expression of glycolytic enzymes including 6-phosphofructo-2-kinase/fructose-2,6-biphosphatase 3 (PFKB3), an enzyme that increases levels of fructose-2,6-bisphosphate and drives glycolysis (63). Glycolytic reprogramming in fibroblasts is, at least partially, driven by TGF-β. Treating normal fibroblasts with TGF-β has been shown to increase transcription of phosphofructokinase (PFK) and hexokinase 2, two key rate-limiting glycolytic enzymes (63). Increased lactate production may be due to shunting of glycolytic products toward anaerobic metabolism due to concurrent mitochondrial dysfunction.

By contrast, a recent study comparing IPF lung tissue to normal human lung using a combined metabolomic and microarray analysis of key metabolic enzymes showed a decrease in the late-stage glycolytic products, fructose 1,6-bisphosphate and phosphoenolpyruvate, and a decrease in PFK and PFKFB3, suggesting an overall reduction in glycolysis in IPF whole lung tissue (69). These findings are in concordance with recent observations in fibroblasts derived from IPF lungs. IPF fibroblasts trended toward having a lower rate of glycolysis, as measured by extracellular acidification rate, and had lesser glycolytic flux in response to TGF-β stimulation compared to normal lung fibroblasts (43). The latter finding may represent a diminished capacity to respond to TGF-β after chronic exposure to this profibrotic cytokine *in vivo*.

Despite these differences, it is known that TGF-β can mediate metabolic reprogramming. TGF-β induces expression of the facultative glucose transporter, glucose transporter 1 (GLUT1),

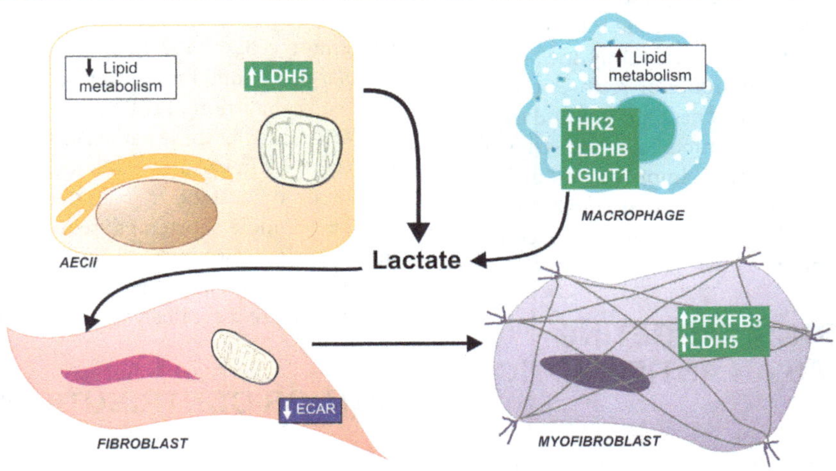

FIGURE 2 | Schematic of metabolic dysfunction in lung fibrosis. Idiopathic pulmonary fibrosis (IPF) lung have a generalized decrease in late stages of glycolysis compared with normal lungs; however, increased levels of lactate were found in IPF lungs suggesting that all products of glycolysis are shuttled toward lactate production. Several studies have been focused in metabolic alterations of specific cell compartments in the IPF lung. IPF lung fibroblasts show decreased glycolytic function determined by extracellular acid production. IPF myofibroblasts have been reported to have higher expression of glycolytic enzymes and lactate content. Single cell RNA sequence data in alveolar epithelial cells show low expression of enzymes necessary for lipid metabolism. By contrast, alveolar macrophages isolated from bleomycin-treated mice show glycolytic reprogramming and increase fatty acid oxidation. Abbreviations: AECII, type II alveolar epithelial cell; GluT1, glucose transporter 1; HK2, hexokinase 2; LDH5, lactate dehydrogenase 5; LDHB, lactate dehydrogenase B; PFKFB3, 6-phosphofructo-2-kinase/fructose-2,6-bisphosphatase 3.

via canonical Smad and PDGFR signaling resulting in increased cellular glucose uptake. Inhibiting GLUT1 upregulation is protective against bleomycin-induced fibrosis (64), and GLUT1 activation of AMPK is integral to fibroblast activation (67). Since metabolic reprogramming appears to be a critical step in promoting fibroblast-to-myofibroblast differentiation, preventing this shift is an intriguing target in attenuating IPF. However, further studies are needed to confirm the metabolic changes in different cell compartments in the IPF lung and determine how these alterations might modify disease progression.

MITOCHONDRIAL DYSFUNCTION AND SENESCENCE

Inducing senescence and apoptosis in fibroblasts are important mechanisms in the wound healing response after injury (70); on the contrary, the aberrant deposition of extracellular matrix seen in IPF is associated with an accumulation of apoptosis-resistant senescent cells (39, 43, 71, 72). Mitochondrial dysfunction has been shown to induce cellular senescence, a process termed mitochondrial dysfunction-associated senescence. In addition, mitophagy defects seem to contribute to a cellular senescence phenotype, which we have observed in the setting of mitochondrial dysfunction induced by PINK1 deficiency *in vivo* (28). Dysfunctional mitochondria are less efficient at oxidizing NADH to NAD+ resulting in a reduced NAD+/NADH ratio, activation of AMPK and p53 resulting in a senescent phenotype (73). Senescent IPF lung epithelial cells, fibroblasts, and myofibroblasts secrete a cell type-specific profile of pro-fibrotic and pro-inflammatory cytokines known as the senescence-associated secretory phenotype (SASP) (72, 74). Senescent fibroblasts exhibit an increased level of the ROS-generating enzyme Nox4 and low levels of the key mediator of cellular antioxidant response pathways, NFE2-related factor 2, and this redox imbalance plays a role in maintaining the senescent phenotype. Treatment with a Nox inhibitor restores the redox balance and results in a decrease in senescent cells and a reduction in fibrosis (18). *In vitro*, mouse model, and *ex vivo* studies in human IPF lung cells have all shown improvement in fibrosis with treatment with a combination of antioxidants (quercetin) and senolytic agents (dasatinib) (72, 74). This approach shows promise as a therapeutic option.

FUTURE DIRECTIONS: TARGETING MITOCHONDRIA AS AN ANTIFIBROTIC THERAPY

Research has extensively shown that both aging and IPF are associated with alterations in cellular bioenergetics and mitochondrial homeostasis. Many of these mitochondrial pathways, especially those involved in maintenance of redox balance, mtDNA protection, and reversal of senescence, have shown promise as therapeutic targets in attenuating or ameliorating fibrosis *in vitro* and in animal models of pulmonary fibrosis. These early investigations of the role of altered bioenergetics in the development of fibrotic lung disease pave the way for translational research to implicate these pathways in human IPF. Other pathways, specifically those involved in maintaining normal mitophagy and turnover of dysfunctional mitochondria and mitochondrial-targeted antioxidants, present potential avenues for altering the natural history of pulmonary fibrosis but require further investigation to identify a point of intervention. Few potential interventions appear ready for human trials to restore mitochondrial biogenesis and mitophagy in alveolar epithelial cells and use of combination senolytic and antioxidant agents to remove senescent cells from injured lung and prevent propagation of SASP signaling (75). These approaches benefit from a history of therapeutic use and safety in treatment of human disease.

There is considerably more to learn about the role of mitochondrial dysfunction in the development and maintenance of the pro-fibrotic conditions that drive IPF, regarding the interplay between mitochondrial and nuclear signaling in overall cellular dysfunction, telomere shortening, and mtDNA damage, and the varying effects of mitochondrial dysfunction in the different cell types (epithelial cells, macrophages, fibroblasts, and myofibroblasts) involved in the development of IPF. Additionally, cellular perturbations seen with normal aging such as decreased macroautophagy and cellular proteostasis have the potential to incite mitochondrial dysfunction and changes in cellular bioenergetics. Development of animal models capable of isolating defects in mitochondrial homeostasis to a particular cell type may be revelatory of the role each cell type plays and shed light on the optimal targets for intervention. Particular attention to the effects of mitochondrial dysfunction on telomere length in the resident progenitor cells of the lungs responsible for regenerating the alveolar epithelium may present novel approaches for preventing stem cell exhaustion in IPF.

While many of these pathways have shown potential as therapeutic targets in isolation, an integrated approach to the bioenergetic and homeostatic changes that are seen with aging and IPF, such as telomere shortening, reduced mitochondrial biogenesis, increased ROS production, and increased nuclear and mtDNA damage, is essential to determining the pathways and therapeutic targets that are most likely to affect the natural history of IPF.

AUTHOR CONTRIBUTIONS

DZ wrote the manuscript along with MB. The manuscript was conceptualized, supervised and modified by ALM and MR. All authors offered intellectual contribution and approved the manuscript.

REFERENCES

1. Khan SS, Singer BD, Vaughan DE. Molecular and physiological manifestations and measurement of aging in humans. *Aging Cell* (2017) 16(4):624–33. doi:10.1111/acel.12601
2. Pardo A, Selman M. Lung fibroblasts, aging, and idiopathic pulmonary fibrosis. *Ann Am Thorac Soc* (2016) 13(Suppl_5):S417–21. doi:10.1513/AnnalsATS.201605-341AW

3. Mora AL, Bueno M, Rojas M. Mitochondria in the spotlight of aging and idiopathic pulmonary fibrosis. *J Clin Invest* (2017) 127(2):405–14. doi:10.1172/JCI87440
4. Okamura DM, Pennathur S. The balance of powers: redox regulation of fibrogenic pathways in kidney injury. *Redox Biol* (2015) 6:495–504. doi:10.1016/j.redox.2015.09.039
5. Bueno M, Lai Y-C, Romero Y, Brands J, St Croix CM, Kamga C, et al. PINK1 deficiency impairs mitochondrial homeostasis and promotes lung fibrosis. *J Clin Invest* (2015) 125(2):521–38. doi:10.1172/JCI74942
6. Schirone L, Forte M, Palmerio S, Yee D, Nocella C, Angelini F, et al. A review of the molecular mechanisms underlying the development and progression of cardiac remodeling. *Oxid Med Cell Longev* (2017) 2017:3920195. doi:10.1155/2017/3920195
7. Lehman JJ, Barger PM, Kovacs A, Saffitz JE, Medeiros DM, Kelly DP. Peroxisome proliferator-activated receptor gamma coactivator-1 promotes cardiac mitochondrial biogenesis. *J Clin Invest* (2000) 106(7):847–56. doi:10.1172/JCI10268
8. Reznick RM, Zong H, Li J, Morino K, Moore IK, Yu HJ, et al. Aging-associated reductions in AMP-activated protein kinase activity and mitochondrial biogenesis. *Cell Metab* (2007) 5(2):151–6. doi:10.1016/j.cmet.2007.01.008
9. Sahin E, Colla S, Liesa M, Moslehi J, Müller FL, Guo M, et al. Telomere dysfunction induces metabolic and mitochondrial compromise. *Nature* (2011) 470(7334):359–65. doi:10.1038/nature09787
10. López-Lluch G, Irusta PM, Navas P, de Cabo R. Mitochondrial biogenesis and healthy aging. *Exp Gerontol* (2008) 43(9):813–9. doi:10.1016/j.exger.2008.06.014
11. Lagouge M, Argmann C, Gerhart-Hines Z, Meziane H, Lerin C, Daussin F, et al. Resveratrol improves mitochondrial function and protects against metabolic disease by activating SIRT1 and PGC-1alpha. *Cell* (2006) 127(6):1109–22. doi:10.1016/j.cell.2006.11.013
12. Short KR, Vittone JL, Bigelow ML, Proctor DN, Rizza RA, Coenen-Schimke JM, et al. Impact of aerobic exercise training on age-related changes in insulin sensitivity and muscle oxidative capacity. *Diabetes* (2003) 52(8):1888–96. doi:10.2337/diabetes.52.8.1888
13. Sinha RA, Singh BK, Zhou J, Wu Y, Farah BL, Ohba K, et al. Thyroid hormone induction of mitochondrial activity is coupled to mitophagy via ROS-AMPK-ULK1 signaling. *Autophagy* (2015) 11(8):1341–57. doi:10.1080/15548627.2015.1061849
14. Lesmana R, Sinha RA, Singh BK, Zhou J, Ohba K, Wu Y, et al. Thyroid hormone stimulation of autophagy is essential for mitochondrial biogenesis and activity in skeletal muscle. *Endocrinology* (2016) 157(1):23–38. doi:10.1210/en.2015-1632
15. Yu G, Tzouvelekis A, Wang R, Herazo-Maya JD, Ibarra GH, Srivastava A, et al. Thyroid hormone inhibits lung fibrosis in mice by improving epithelial mitochondrial function. *Nat Med* (2017) 24(1):39–49. doi:10.1038/nm.4447
16. Fang EF, Scheibye-Knudsen M, Brace LE, Kassahun H, SenGupta T, Nilsen H, et al. Defective mitophagy in XPA via PARP-1 hyperactivation and NAD(+)/SIRT1 reduction. *Cell* (2014) 157(4):882–96. doi:10.1016/j.cell.2014.03.026
17. Amara N, Goven D, Prost F, Muloway R, Crestani B, Boczkowski J. NOX4/NADPH oxidase expression is increased in pulmonary fibroblasts from patients with idiopathic pulmonary fibrosis and mediates TGFbeta1-induced fibroblast differentiation into myofibroblasts. *Thorax* (2010) 65(8):733–8. doi:10.1136/thx.2009.113456
18. Bernard K, Logsdon NJ, Miguel V, Benavides GA, Zhang J, Carter AB, et al. NADPH oxidase 4 (Nox4) suppresses mitochondrial biogenesis and bioenergetics in lung fibroblasts via a nuclear factor erythroid-derived 2-like 2 (Nrf2)-dependent pathway. *J Biol Chem* (2017) 292(7):3029–38. doi:10.1074/jbc.M116.752261
19. Ding W-X, Yin X-M. Mitophagy: mechanisms, pathophysiological roles, and analysis. *Biol Chem* (2012) 393(7):547–64. doi:10.1515/hsz-2012-0119
20. Ashrafi G, Schwarz TL. The pathways of mitophagy for quality control and clearance of mitochondria. *Cell Death Differ* (2013) 20(1):31–42. doi:10.1038/cdd.2012.81
21. Kim I, Rodriguez-Enriquez S, Lemasters JJ. Selective degradation of mitochondria by mitophagy. *Arch Biochem Biophys* (2007) 462(2):245–53. doi:10.1016/j.abb.2007.03.034
22. Kubli DA, Gustafsson ÅB. Mitochondria and mitophagy: the Yin and Yang of cell death control. *Circ Res* (2012) 111(9):1208–21. doi:10.1161/CIRCRESAHA.112.265819
23. Youle RJ, Narendra DP. Mechanisms of mitophagy. *Nat Rev Mol Cell Biol* (2011) 12(1):9–14. doi:10.1038/nrm3028
24. Kobayashi K, Araya J, Minagawa S, Hara H, Saito N, Kadota T, et al. Involvement of PARK2-mediated mitophagy in idiopathic pulmonary fibrosis pathogenesis. *J Immunol* (2016) 197(2):504–16. doi:10.4049/jimmunol.1600265
25. Sosulski ML, Gongora R, Danchuk S, Dong C, Luo F, Sanchez CG. Deregulation of selective autophagy during aging and pulmonary fibrosis: the role of TGFβ1. *Aging Cell* (2015) 14(5):774–83. doi:10.1111/acel.12357
26. Kim S-J, Cheresh P, Jablonski RP, Williams DB, Kamp DW. The role of mitochondrial DNA in mediating alveolar epithelial cell apoptosis and pulmonary fibrosis. *Int J Mol Sci* (2015) 16(9):21486–519. doi:10.3390/ijms160921486
27. Larson-Casey JL, Deshane JS, Ryan AJ, Thannickal VJ, Carter AB. Macrophage Akt1 kinase-mediated mitophagy modulates apoptosis resistance and pulmonary fibrosis. *Immunity* (2016) 44(3):582–96. doi:10.1016/j.immuni.2016.01.001
28. Bueno M, Brands J, Voltz L, Fiedler K, Mays B, St Croix C, et al. ATF3 represses PINK1 gene transcription in lung epithelia to control mitochondrial homeostasis. *Aging Cell* (2018). doi:10.1111/acel.12720
29. Hawkins A, Guttentag SH, Deterding R, Funkhouser WK, Goralski JL, Chatterjee S, et al. A non-BRICHOS SFTPC mutant (SP-CI73T) linked to interstitial lung disease promotes a late block in macroautophagy disrupting cellular proteostasis and mitophagy. *Am J Physiol Lung Cell Mol Physiol* (2015) 308(1):L33–47. doi:10.1152/ajplung.00217.2014
30. Patel AS, Song JW, Chu SG, Mizumura K, Osorio JC, Shi Y, et al. Epithelial cell mitochondrial dysfunction and PINK1 are induced by transforming growth factor-beta1 in pulmonary fibrosis. *PLoS One* (2015) 10(3):e0121246. doi:10.1371/journal.pone.0121246
31. Cui H, Kong Y, Zhang H. Oxidative stress, mitochondrial dysfunction, and aging. *J Signal Transduct* (2012) 2012:646354. doi:10.1155/2012/646354
32. Chandel NS, Maltepe E, Goldwasser E, Mathieu CE, Simon MC, Schumacker PT. Mitochondrial reactive oxygen species trigger hypoxia-induced transcription. *Proc Natl Acad Sci U S A* (1998) 95(20):11715–20. doi:10.1073/pnas.95.20.11715
33. Chandel NS, Vander Heiden MG, Thompson CB, Schumacker PT. Redox regulation of p53 during hypoxia. *Oncogene* (2000) 19(34):3840–8. doi:10.1038/sj.onc.1203727
34. Chandel NS, Trzyna WC, McClintock DS, Schumacker PT. Role of oxidants in NF-B activation and TNF-gene transcription induced by hypoxia and endotoxin. *J Immunol* (2000) 165(2):1013–21. doi:10.4049/jimmunol.165.2.1013
35. Nemoto S, Takeda K, Yu ZX, Ferrans VJ, Finkel T. Role for mitochondrial oxidants as regulators of cellular metabolism. *Mol Cell Biol* (2000) 20(19):7311–8. doi:10.1128/MCB.20.19.7311-7318.2000
36. Rhee SG, Bae YS, Lee SR, Kwon J. Hydrogen peroxide: a key messenger that modulates protein phosphorylation through cysteine oxidation. *Sci STKE* (2000) 2000(53):pe1. doi:10.1126/stke.2000.53.pe1
37. Yun J, Finkel T. Mitohormesis. *Cell Metab* (2014) 19(5):757–66. doi:10.1016/j.cmet.2014.01.011
38. Sundaresan NR, Bindu S, Pillai VB, Samant S, Pan Y, Huang J-Y, et al. SIRT3 blocks aging-associated tissue fibrosis in mice by deacetylating and activating glycogen synthase kinase 3β. *Mol Cell Biol* (2015) 36(5):678–92. doi:10.1128/MCB.00586-15
39. Thannickal VJ. Mechanistic links between aging and lung fibrosis. *Biogerontology* (2013) 14(6):609–15. doi:10.1007/s10522-013-9451-6
40. López-Otín C, Blasco MA, Partridge L, Serrano M, Kroemer G. The hallmarks of aging. *Cell* (2013) 153(6):1194–217. doi:10.1016/j.cell.2013.05.039
41. Friguet B. Oxidized protein degradation and repair in ageing and oxidative stress. *FEBS Lett* (2006) 580(12):2910–6. doi:10.1016/j.febslet.2006.03.028
42. Yoon Y-S, Lee J-H, Hwang S-C, Choi KS, Yoon G. TGF beta1 induces prolonged mitochondrial ROS generation through decreased complex IV activity with senescent arrest in Mv1Lu cells. *Oncogene* (2005) 24(11):1895–903. doi:10.1038/sj.onc.1208262

43. Álvarez D, Cárdenes N, Sellarés J, Bueno M, Corey C, Hanumanthu VS, et al. IPF lung fibroblasts have a senescent phenotype. *Am J Physiol Lung Cell Mol Physiol* (2017) 313(6):L1164–73. doi:10.1152/ajplung.00220.2017
44. Kim S-J, Cheresh P, Jablonski RP, Morales-Nebreda L, Cheng Y, Hogan E, et al. Mitochondrial catalase overexpressed transgenic mice are protected against lung fibrosis in part via preventing alveolar epithelial cell mitochondrial DNA damage. *Free Radic Biol Med* (2016) 101:482–90. doi:10.1016/j.freeradbiomed.2016.11.007
45. Yakes FM, Van Houten B. Mitochondrial DNA damage is more extensive and persists longer than nuclear DNA damage in human cells following oxidative stress. *Proc Natl Acad Sci U S A* (1997) 94(2):514–9. doi:10.1073/pnas.94.2.514
46. Fujita M, Mizuta Y, Ikegame S, Ouchi H, Ye Q, Harada E, et al. Biphasic effects of free radical scavengers against bleomycin-induced pulmonary fibrosis. *Pulm Pharmacol Ther* (2008) 21(5):805–11. doi:10.1016/j.pupt.2008.06.006
47. Hallberg BM, Larsson N-G. TFAM forces mtDNA to make a U-turn. *Nat Struct Mol Biol* (2011) 18(11):1179–81. doi:10.1038/nsmb.2167
48. Jablonski RP, Kim S-J, Cheresh P, Williams DB, Morales-Nebreda L, Cheng Y, et al. SIRT3 deficiency promotes lung fibrosis by augmenting alveolar epithelial cell mitochondrial DNA damage and apoptosis. *FASEB J* (2017) 31(6):2520–32. doi:10.1096/fj.201601077R
49. Zhang Q, Raoof M, Chen Y, Sumi Y, Sursal T, Junger W, et al. Circulating mitochondrial DAMPs cause inflammatory responses to injury. *Nature* (2010) 464(7285):104–7. doi:10.1038/nature08780
50. Ryu C, Sun H, Gulati M, Herazo-Maya JD, Chen Y, Osafo-Addo A, et al. Extracellular mitochondrial DNA is generated by fibroblasts and predicts death in idiopathic pulmonary fibrosis. *Am J Respir Crit Care Med* (2017) 196(12):1571–81. doi:10.1164/rccm.201612-2480OC
51. Kincaid B, Bossy-Wetzel E. Forever young: SIRT3 a shield against mitochondrial meltdown, aging, and neurodegeneration. *Front Aging Neurosci* (2013) 5:48. doi:10.3389/fnagi.2013.00048
52. Yu W, Dittenhafer-Reed KE, Denu JM. SIRT3 protein deacetylates isocitrate dehydrogenase 2 (IDH2) and regulates mitochondrial redox status. *J Biol Chem* (2012) 287(17):14078–86. doi:10.1074/jbc.M112.355206
53. Chen Y, Zhang J, Lin Y, Lei Q, Guan K-L, Zhao S, et al. Tumour suppressor SIRT3 deacetylates and activates manganese superoxide dismutase to scavenge ROS. *EMBO Rep* (2011) 12(6):534–41. doi:10.1038/embor.2011.65
54. Tao R, Vassilopoulos A, Parisiadou L, Yan Y, Gius D. Regulation of MnSOD enzymatic activity by Sirt3 connects the mitochondrial acetylome signaling networks to aging and carcinogenesis. *Antioxid Redox Signal* (2014) 20(10):1646–54. doi:10.1089/ars.2013.5482
55. Tang BL. Sirt1 and the mitochondria. *Mol Cells* (2016) 39(2):87–95. doi:10.14348/molcells.2016.2318
56. Rodgers JT, Lerin C, Haas W, Gygi SP, Spiegelman BM, Puigserver P. Nutrient control of glucose homeostasis through a complex of PGC-1alpha and SIRT1. *Nature* (2005) 434(7029):113–8. doi:10.1038/nature03354
57. Sui B, Hu C, Jin Y. Mitochondrial metabolic failure in telomere attrition-provoked aging of bone marrow mesenchymal stem cells. *Biogerontology* (2016) 17(2):267–79. doi:10.1007/s10522-015-9609-5
58. Shetty SK, Tiwari N, Marudamuthu AS, Puthusseri B, Bhandary YP, Fu J, et al. p53 and miR-34a feedback promotes lung epithelial injury and pulmonary fibrosis. *Am J Pathol* (2017) 187(5):1016–34. doi:10.1016/j.ajpath.2016.12.020
59. Zeng Z, Cheng S, Chen H, Li Q, Hu Y, Wang Q, et al. Activation and overexpression of Sirt1 attenuates lung fibrosis via P300. *Biochem Biophys Res Commun* (2017) 486(4):1021–6. doi:10.1016/j.bbrc.2017.03.155
60. Justet A, Laurent-Bellue A, Thabut G, Dieudonné A, Debray M-P, Borie R, et al. [18F]FDG PET/CT predicts progression-free survival in patients with idiopathic pulmonary fibrosis. *Respir Res* (2017) 18(1):74. doi:10.1186/s12931-017-0556-3
61. Xu Y, Mizuno T, Sridharan A, Du Y, Guo M, Tang J, et al. Single-cell RNA sequencing identifies diverse roles of epithelial cells in idiopathic pulmonary fibrosis. *JCI Insight* (2016) 1(20):e90558. doi:10.1172/jci.insight.90558
62. Kottmann RM, Kulkarni AA, Smolnycki KA, Lyda E, Dahanayake T, Salibi R, et al. Lactic acid is elevated in idiopathic pulmonary fibrosis and induces myofibroblast differentiation via pH-dependent activation of transforming growth factor-β. *Am J Respir Crit Care Med* (2012) 186(8):740–51. doi:10.1164/rccm.201201-0084OC
63. Xie N, Tan Z, Banerjee S, Cui H, Ge J, Liu R-M, et al. Glycolytic reprogramming in myofibroblast differentiation and lung fibrosis. *Am J Respir Crit Care Med* (2015) 192(12):1462–74. doi:10.1164/rccm.201504-0780OC
64. Andrianifahanana M, Hernandez DM, Yin X, Kang J-H, Jung M-Y, Wang Y, et al. Profibrotic up-regulation of glucose transporter 1 by TGF-β involves activation of MEK and mammalian target of rapamycin complex 2 pathways. *FASEB J* (2016) 30(11):3733–44. doi:10.1096/fj.201600428R
65. Xu J, Li J, Yu Z, Rao H, Wang S, Lan H. HMGB1 promotes HLF-1 proliferation and ECM production through activating HIF1-α-regulated aerobic glycolysis. *Pulm Pharmacol Ther* (2017) 45:136–41. doi:10.1016/j.pupt.2017.05.015
66. Xie N, Cui H, Ge J, Banerjee S, Guo S, Dubey S, et al. Metabolic characterization and RNA profiling reveal glycolytic dependence of pro-fibrotic phenotype of alveolar macrophages in lung fibrosis. *Am J Physiol Lung Cell Mol Physiol* (2017) 313(5):L834–44. doi:10.1152/ajplung.00235.2017
67. Cho SJ, Moon J-S, Lee C-M, Choi AMK, Stout-Delgado HW. Glucose transporter 1-dependent glycolysis is increased during aging-related lung fibrosis, and phloretin inhibits lung fibrosis. *Am J Respir Cell Mol Biol* (2017) 56(4):521–31. doi:10.1165/rcmb.2016-0225OC
68. Maher TM. Aerobic glycolysis and the Warburg effect. An unexplored realm in the search for fibrosis therapies? *Am J Respir Crit Care Med* (2015) 192(12):1407–9. doi:10.1164/rccm.201508-1699ED
69. Zhao YD, Yin L, Archer S, Lu C, Zhao G, Yao Y, et al. Metabolic heterogeneity of idiopathic pulmonary fibrosis: a metabolomic study. *BMJ Open Respir Res* (2017) 4(1):e000183. doi:10.1136/bmjresp-2017-000183
70. Demaria M, Ohtani N, Youssef SA, Rodier F, Toussaint W, Mitchell JR, et al. An essential role for senescent cells in optimal wound healing through secretion of PDGF-AA. *Dev Cell* (2014) 31(6):722–33. doi:10.1016/j.devcel.2014.11.012
71. Chilosi M, Poletti V, Rossi A. The pathogenesis of COPD and IPF: distinct horns of the same devil? *Respir Res* (2012) 13:3. doi:10.1186/1465-9921-13-3
72. Schafer MJ, White TA, Iijima K, Haak AJ, Ligresti G, Atkinson EJ, et al. Cellular senescence mediates fibrotic pulmonary disease. *Nat Commun* (2017) 8:14532. doi:10.1038/ncomms14532
73. Wiley CD, Velarde MC, Lecot P, Liu S, Sarnoski EA, Freund A, et al. Mitochondrial dysfunction induces senescence with a distinct secretory phenotype. *Cell Metab* (2016) 23(2):303–14. doi:10.1016/j.cmet.2015.11.011
74. Lehmann M, Korfei M, Mutze K, Klee S, Skronska-Wasek W, Alsafadi HN, et al. Senolytic drugs target alveolar epithelial cell function and attenuate experimental lung fibrosis ex vivo. *Eur Respir J* (2017) 50(2):1602367. doi:10.1183/13993003.02367-2016
75. Mora AL, Rojas M, Pardo A, Selman M. Emerging therapies for idiopathic pulmonary fibrosis, a progressive age-related disease. *Nat Rev Drug Discov* (2017) 16(11):755–72.

10

Catalpol Attenuates Pulmonary Fibrosis by Inhibiting Ang II/AT_1 and TGF-β/Smad-Mediated Epithelial Mesenchymal Transition

Qun Yu[1†], *Dewei Zhu*[1†], *Yang Zou*[1†], *Kai Wang*[2], *Peili Rao*[1] *and Yunhui Shen*[1*]

[1] *School of Pharmacy, Shanghai University of Traditional Chinese Medicine, Shanghai, China,* [2] *Experiment Center for Science and Technology, Shanghai University of Traditional Chinese Medicine, Shanghai, China*

Correspondence:
Yunhui Shen
bravesyh@163.com

[†] *These authors have contributed equally to this work and share first authorship*

Background: Idiopathic pulmonary fibrosis (IPF) is a progressive and devastating chronic lung condition affecting over 3 million people worldwide with a high mortality rate and there are no effective drugs. Angiotensin II (Ang II), as a major effector peptide of the renin angiotensin aldosterone system, has been shown to act in tandem with the transforming growth factor-β (TGF-β) signaling pathway to promote the infiltration of inflammatory cells, production of reactive oxygen species (ROS) and profibrotic factors after lung injury, and to participate in the process of epithelial mesenchymal transition (EMT). Catalpol (CAT) has been shown to have anti-inflammatory and antifibrotic effects. However, the effects and mechanisms of CAT on pulmonary fibrosis are not clear.

Purpose: To assess the effects and mechanisms of catalpol on bleomycin-induced pulmonary fibrosis in mice.

Methods: We used bleomycin-induced mouse model of pulmonary fibrosis to evaluate the alleviation effect of CAT at 7, 14, 28d, respectively. Next, enzyme-linked immunosorbent assay, hematoxylin-eosin staining, immunofluorescence, Masson trichrome staining and western blotting were used to study the underlying mechanism of CAT on bleomycin-induced pulmonary fibrosis.

Results: It's demonstrated that CAT exerted a potent anti-fibrotic function in BLM-induced mice pulmonary fibrosis via alleviating inflammatory, ameliorating collagen deposition, reducing the level of Ang II and HYP and alleviating the degree of EMT. Moreover, CAT attenuate BLM-induced fibrosis by targeting Ang II/AT_1 and TGF-β/Smad signaling *in vivo.*

Conclusion: CAT may serve as a novel therapeutic candidate for the simultaneous blockade of Ang II and TGF-β pathway to attenuate pulmonary fibrosis.

Keywords: idiopathic pulmonary fibrosis, Ang II, TGF-β/Smad signaling pathway, EMT, catalpol

HIGHLIGHTS

- Catalpol significantly ameliorates bleomycin-induced pulmonary fibrosis (PF) in mice.
- Catalpol attenuates pulmonary fibrosis via TGF-β/Smads signaling pathway.
- Catalpol inhibits bleomycin-induced epithelial mesenchymal transition.
- Catalpol decreases the expression of angiotensin II/type 1 receptor (AT_1) in PF mice.

INTRODUCTION

Pulmonary Fibrosis (PF) is a chronic interstitial lung disease characterized by massive proliferation of fibroblasts and accumulation of extracellular matrix (ECM). Pulmonary Fibrosis is accompanied by inflammatory injury, the epithelial-mesenchymal transition (EMT) and destruction of tissue structure (1). Pulmonary Fibrosis will cause lung function damage, scar of lung tissue obstructing the flow of oxygen from lungs into the bloodstream for distribution to other organs and patients will have dry cough, dyspnea and other symptoms. As the condition continues to deteriorate, the integrity of lung tissue structure is destroyed, respiratory function can be further affected, seriously endangering the patient's quality of life and even becoming life-threatening (2). Toxic insults, autoimmune injuries, drug-induced injuries, infectious injuries, traumatic injuries or other unknown factors may cause pulmonary fibrosis. Among them, idiopathic pulmonary fibrosis (IPF) is the most common and prevalent type of pulmonary fibrosis and is associated with risk factors such as genetic alterations, viral infections, lifestyle habits, environmental influences, occupational hazards (3). IPF prevalence has a correlation with age and sex. And the elderly is more prone to IPF and males have a higher incidence rate than females (4, 5). Pulmonary fibrosis is also a sequela in severe patients with the Coronavirus Disease 2019 (COVID-19) and severe acute respiratory syndrome (SARS).

The latest ATS/ERS/JRS/ALAT clinical practice guidelines recommend the conditional use of nintedanib and pirfenidone. In addition, glucocorticoids, immunosuppressive agents, and antioxidants are also used clinically in combination with western medicines to treat pulmonary fibrosis (6–9). The application of angiotensin inhibitor combined with glucocorticoid to treat pulmonary fibrosis also has been reported by many clinicians (10). However, due to the inability of existing drugs in reversing the course of pulmonary fibrosis and the lack of lung organ donors, as well as high treatment costs and so on, the median survival of patients with IPF after diagnosis is only between 3 and 5 years (11, 12). Therefore, the development of affordable and effective anti-fibrotic drugs is urgently needed.

Catalpol (CAT), an iridoid compound, exhibits anti-cancer, neuroprotective, anti-inflammatory, diuretic, hypoglycemic, anti-hepatitis virus effects and anti-fibrosis effect in multiple organs. It has been shown that CAT may inhibit bleomycin-induced pulmonary fibrosis in rats through downregulation of Wnt3a and GSK-3β, β-catenin and phosphorylation of Smad3 (13). CAT has become very popular for clinical medication candidate because of its good safety, fewer toxic side effects and convenient administration. In this context, the research and development of CAT have gradually become hot topics of interest. However, the mechanism by which CAT acts in the treatment of pulmonary fibrosis has not been thoroughly investigated. In this study, a mouse pulmonary fibrosis model was established to further explore the mechanism of action of CAT in the treatment of pulmonary fibrosis, in order to provide a reference basis for the pharmacological research and clinical application of this drug.

MATERIALS AND METHODS

Reagents

Catalpol (CAT, CAS: 2415-24-9, MW: 362.331, purity: 98%, dissolved in normal saline (NS) before use, Chengdu Purifa Technology Co., Ltd., Lot No.: PRF21111722,); Bleomycin for injection (chemical for lung-fibrosis modeling, BLM, Harbin Laibotong Pharmaceutical Co., Ltd., Lot No.: 20120727); Pirfenidone (positive control drug, PFD, Beijing Contini Pharmaceutical Co., Ltd., Lot No.: 20210511); Telmisartan (positive control drug, TEL, Shanghai Xinyi Tianping Pharmaceutical Co., Ltd. Lot No.: 87210302); Haematoxylin and eosin (H&E) (719033, Zhuhai Baso Biotechnology Co., Ltd., China); Masson Staining Kits (C210801, Zhuhai Baso Biotechnology Co., Ltd., China); HYP Kit (Nanjing Jiancheng Bioengineering Institute, Nanjing, China); Ang II Kit (Nanjing Jiancheng Bioengineering Institute, Nanjing, China); RIPA lysis buffer (Beyotime, China); Phosphorylated proteinase inhibitor (Beyotime, China); Phenyl methyl sulfonyl fluoride (PMSF, Beyotime, China); TGF-β1 (ab179695, abcom, USA); Anti-Phospho-Smad2 (18338T, CST, USA); Anti-Phospho-Smad3 (9520T, CST, USA); Anti-Smad2/3 (8685S, CST, USA); Anti-Snail (3879T, CST, USA); Anti-Angiotensin II Type 1 Receptor (ab124734, abcom, United States); Anti-MMP2(ab92536, abcom, USA); Anti-MMP9 (ab283575, abcom, USA); Anti-β-actin (AF7018, Affinity, USA); Horseradish peroxidase (HRP)-linked anti-mouse (A0286, Beyotime, China); Anti-rabbit (A0208, Beyotime, China); α-SMA (19245T, CST, USA); E-cadherin antibody (3195T, CST, USA), N-cadherin antibody (13116T, CST, USA); Goat anti rabbit IgG secondary antibody (A0468/A0423; Beyotime; Biotechnology Co. Ltd., Shanghai, China) and 4', 6-diamidino-2-phenylindole (DAPI; Beyotime; Biotechnology Co. Ltd., Shanghai, China).

Animal Care and Handling

Male C57BL/6 mice (18–20 g), an applicable animal model for BLM-induced PF model, were obtained from Shanghai Jihui Experimental Animal Breeding Co., LTD. The animals were housed in a specific pathogen-free environment and observed under a 12 h light-12 h dark cycle in a well-ventilated room at 23 ± 2°C.They were fed with standard pellet food and tap water *ad libitum*. Being approved by the Animal Care and Use Committee of Shanghai University of Traditional Chinese Medicine, the study was performed in accordance with the guidelines for care and handling of animals of the National Institute of Health (approval number PZSHUTCM220124010).

After a three-day adaptive feeding, the mice were randomized into six groups (n = 20 mice per group): (1) normal saline (NS) + vehicle control group; (2) BLM + vehicle control group, (3) BLM + PFD (300 mg/kg/day) group (14, 15); (4) BLM + TEL (10 mg/kg/day) group (16, 17); (5) BLM + High CAT (200 mg/kg/day) group; (6) BLM + Low CAT (100 mg/kg/day) group (18). On day 0, a single intratracheal instillation of BLM (5 mg/kg) was performed to induce pulmonary fibrosis in C57BL/6 mice (19). Mice in NS group (control group) received an equal volume of NS. One day after BLM induction, mice in PFD groups and TEL group were intragastrically administrated with PFD or TEL, CAT group was intragastrically administrated with high or low dose of CAT, NS group and BLM group were intragastrically administrated with equal volume of NS for 28 days. Body weight was measured every 3 days. On days 7, 14, and 28, 5, 5, and 10 mice were euthanized in each group, respectively, the mice anesthetized with pentobarbital sodium (50 mg/kg) intraperitoneally, lung tissues and blood were collected for subsequent studies.

Histological Examination and Evaluation

Lung tissues from mice were fixed with 4% paraformaldehyde (48 h) and blocked with paraffin, sectioned (5 μM thickness) after deparaffinization in xylene. Haematoxylin and eosin (H&E) and Masson Staining Kits were used for pathological evaluation. The tissues were morphologically analyzed using a StrataFAXS II image analysis system (StrataFAXS II, Vienna, Austria).

Western Blotting Assay

Proteins were extracted from lung tissue using RIPA lysis buffer with 2% phosphorylated proteinase inhibitor, 1% phenyl methyl sulfonyl fluoride, and 2% protease inhibitor, according to the manufacturer's protocol. 30–50 μg of protein from each sample was separated by sodium dodecyl sulfate polyacrylamide gel electrophoresis (10% SDS-PAGE) and transferred to PVDF membranes. After blocking in 5% BSA solution for 2 h at room temperature, the membranes were incubated overnight at 4°C with anti-TGF-β1, anti-Phospho-Smad2, anti-Phospho-Smad3, anti-Smad2/3, anti-Snail, anti-Angiotensin II Type 1 Receptor, United States), anti-MMP2, anti-MMP9 or anti-β-actin.

After washing three times in TBS-T, the membranes were incubated in horseradish peroxidase (HRP)-linked anti-mouse or anti-rabbit for 2 h at room temperature. Detection of protein signal and analysis was performed using Tanon 4600SF (Tiangong Technology Co., Ltd., Shanghai, China) and ImageJ software (National Institute of Mental Health, Bethesda, MD, USA), respectively.

Immunofluorescence Assay

Immunofluorescence was used to verify E-cadherin, N-cadherin and α-SMA expression in lung tissue. Sections were incubated as previously described with anti-α-SMA or anti-E-cadherin antibody, anti-N-cadherin antibody at 4 °C overnight and then incubated with Goat anti rabbit IgG secondary antibody at 37 °C for 1.5 h. After washing, they were counterstained with 4', 6-diamidino-2-phenylindole for 10 min at room temperature in the dark. Images were captured with an immunofluorescence microscope (Leica SP8, Wetzlar, Germany).

Hydroxyproline Assay

Collagen content was assessed by measuring the hydroxyproline (a major component of collagen) content of the tissue as previously described by Woessner (20). After lung tissue was homogenized, a HYP Kit was used to detect the HYP content, following the manufacturer's instructions.

Ang II Assay

Angiotensin II (Ang II), a key vasoactive peptide of the RAAS, mediates pro-inflammatory and pro-fibrotic effects on the lung. After lung tissue was homogenized, an Ang II Kit was used to detect Ang II content following the manufacturer's instructions.

Statistical Analysis

Data are shown as mean ± Standard Error of Mean (SEM). Differences between the groups were evaluated using one-way analysis of variance (ANOVA with Dunnett's *post-hoc* analysis). $P < 0.05$ was considered statistically significant. Statistical analyses and figures were obtained using GraphPad Prism Version 8.0 (GraphPad Software, San Diego, CA, USA).

RESULTS

CAT Attenuates BLM Induced Pulmonary Fibrosis in Mice

Intratracheal instillation of BLM in mice causes destruction of alveolar structure and the formation of fibrosis, and is a widely used model of pulmonary fibrosis. To explore the therapeutic effects of CAT on pulmonary fibrosis (21), we collected lung tissues from mice at 7, 14 and 28d of CAT treatment and performed relevant detection assessments (**Figures 1A,B**). H&E and Masson staining were used to examine the lung histopathological changes, which showed that after BLM modeling, the lung tissue injury was obvious, followed by an obvious interstitial inflammation and inflammatory cell infiltration, increasing with time, interstitial fibrosis was gradually aggravated, and the pathological morphological changes and collagen deposition in lungs were attenuated using CAT (**Figures 1C,D**). Some matrix metalloproteinases (MMPs) are overexpressed in pulmonary fibrosis and may be associated with more severe and advanced pathological stages in the lung (22, 23). In the present study, the protein expression levels of MMP2 and MMP9 in the lungs were evaluated by Western blot analysis at 7, 14, 28d. **Figures 1E–I** showed that compared with the Control group, the BLM-injured lung tissue showed distinct increases in the levels of MMP2 and MMP9 at 14th, 28th time point after modeling ($P < 0.01$), whereas CAT could down-regulate the protein levels of MMP2 and MMP9 in fibrotic lung tissue ($P < 0.05$, $P < 0.01$ or $P < 0.001$). To assess the effect of CAT on lung collagen and ECM, we assessed HYP (a major component of collagen) content in mouse

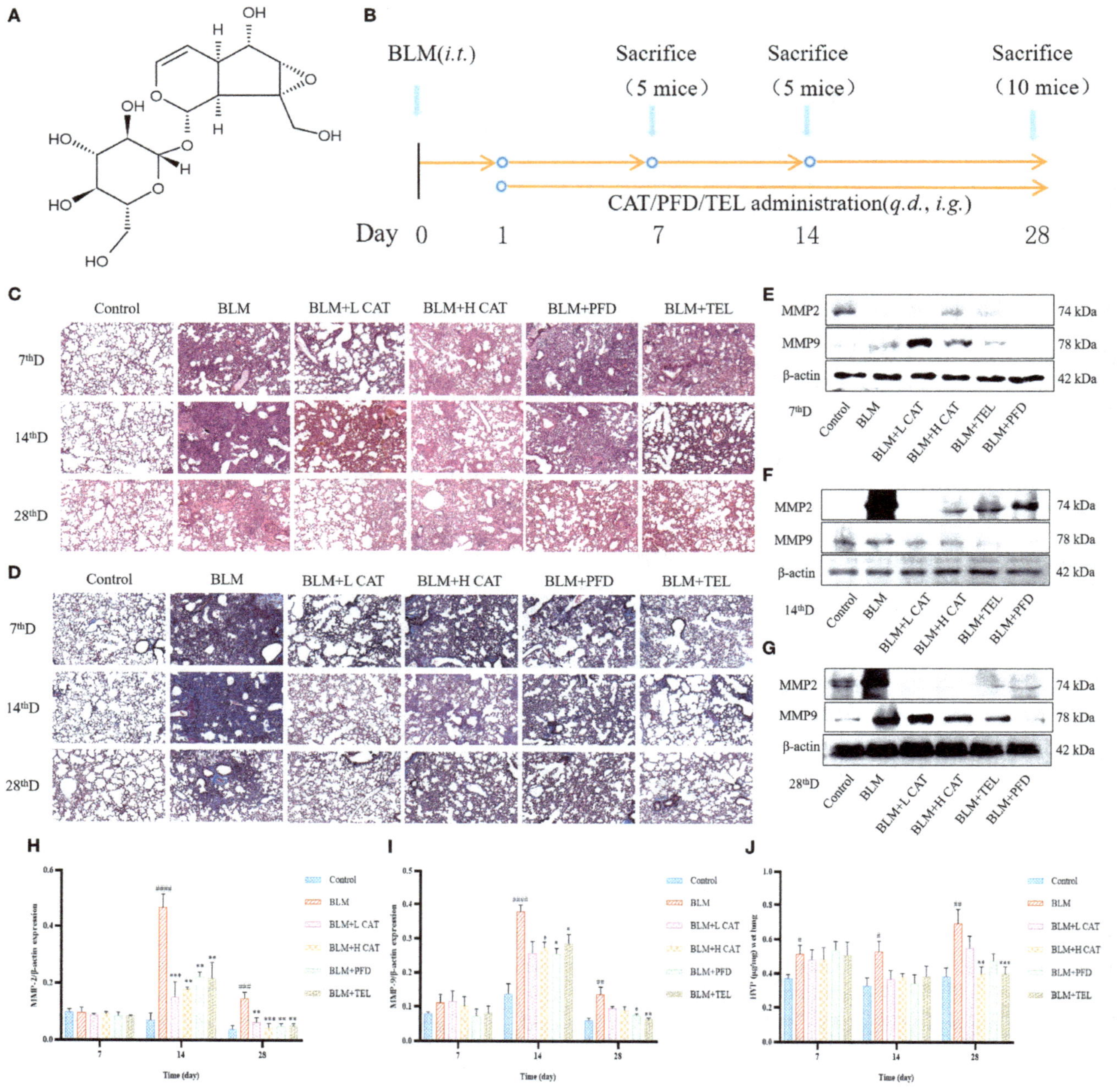

FIGURE 1 | **(A)** Structure of catalpol **(B)** Animal experiment flowchart:C57BL/6 mice were treated by oral gavage with the different doses of CAT (100, 200 mg/kg/day), telmisartan (TEL) (10 mg/kg/day) and pirfenidone (PFD) (300 mg/kg/day) for 28 days followed by intratracheal instillation with BLM (5 mg/kg) or an equal volume of sterile normal saline (NS, Control group), respectively. Control group and BLM group received equal amounts of NS by oral gavage each day (n = 5-10, the number of mice sacrificed per group was 5, 5 and 10 on Day 7, 14 and 28 respectively). From left to right: Samples were collected at 7, 14 and 28th day after BLM administration. **(C)** Representative images of HE staining. Scale bar: 100 μm. **(D)** Representative images of Masson staining. Scale bar: 100 μm. **(E–G)** Expression of MMP2 and MMP9 in the lung tissues at 7, 14, 28d as detected by Western blot. **(H,I)** The MMP2 and MMP9 protein levels at 7, 14, 28d were analyzed by ImageJ software. **(J)** HYP in mouse serum at 7, 14, 28d was measured. $^{\#}P < 0.05$, $^{\#\#}P < 0.01$, $^{\#\#\#}P < 0.001$, $^{\#\#\#\#}P < 0.0001$ compared with the Control group, $^{*}p < 0.05$, $^{**}p < 0.01$, $^{***}p < 0.001$ compared with the BLM group (ANOVA with Dunnett's *post-hoc* analysis).

lungs. As shown in **Figure 1J**, CAT obviously suppressed the expression of HYP compared with BLM group. It is known from the data that CAT could attenuate BLM induced pulmonary fibrosis progression.

CAT Inhibited BLM Induced EMT in Mice

Previous studies have shown that EMT plays an important role in fibrosis in multiple organs, such as promoting epithelial to fibroblast differentiation and participating in the constitution

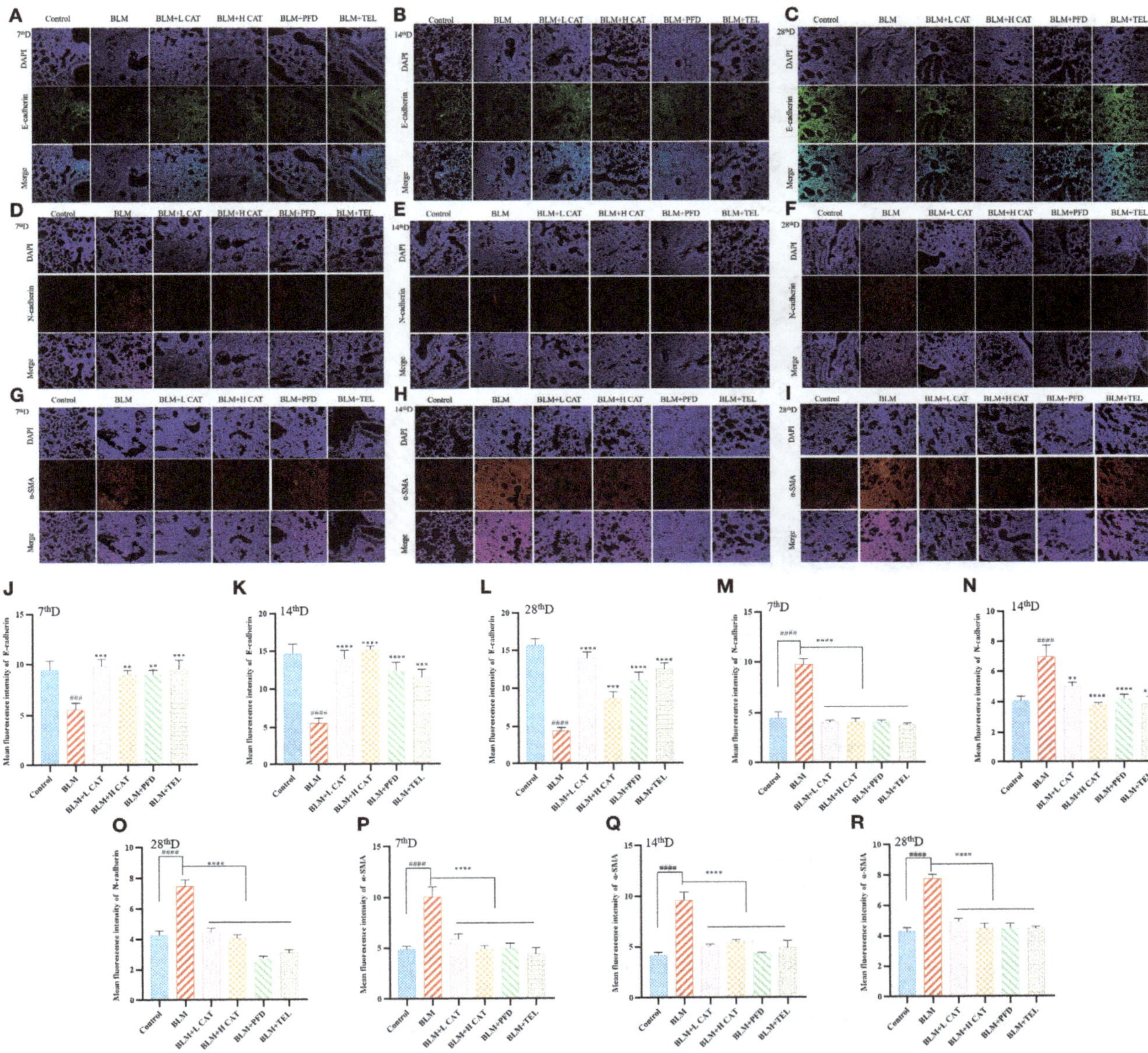

FIGURE 2 | Catalpol inhibits epithelial mesenchymal transition (EMT) in bleomycin induced pulmonary fibrosis. **(A–C,J–L)** Immunofluorescence analysis of E-cadherin in lung sections at 7, 14, 28d, E-cadherin (green), DAPI (blue), the fluorescence intensity of E-cadherin was analyzed by ImageJ software. **(D–F,M–O)** Immunofluorescence analysis of N-cadherin in lung sections at 7, 14, 28d, N-cadherin (red), DAPI (blue), the fluorescence intensity of N-cadherin was analyzed by ImageJ software. **(G–I,P–R)** Immunofluorescence analysis of α-SMA in lung sections at 7, 14, 28d, α-SMA (red), DAPI (blue), the fluorescence intensity of α-SMA was analyzed by ImageJ software. ###$P < 0.001$, ####$P < 0.0001$ compared with the Control group, **$p < 0.01$, ***$p < 0.001$, ****$p < 0.0001$ compared with the BLM group (ANOVA with Dunnett's *post-hoc* analysis).

of fibroblast/myofibroblast foci (24, 25). We further evaluated the role of CAT on EMT progression during BLM induced pulmonary fibrosis in mice. Immunofluorescence analyses revealed that BLM administration in mouse lungs resulted in a significant decrease in E-cadherin expression along with an increase in N-cadherin and α smooth muscle actin (α-SMA), suggesting an epithelial mesenchymal phenotype transition and an increase in myofibroblasts during PF. After CAT administration, the expression of E-cadherin increased, while the expression of N-Cadherin and α-SMA decreased ($P < 0.01$, $P < 0.001$ or $P < 0.0001$) and EMT was inhibited in the lungs of mice compared with that in model group (**Figures 2A–R**).

CAT Attenuates Lung Fibrosis in Mice *via* the Ang II / AT$_1$ Axis

The physiological actions of Ang II are almost all mediated by type 1 angiotensin receptor (AT$_1$) on the cytoplasmic membrane representations, thereby promoting multiple signaling pathways

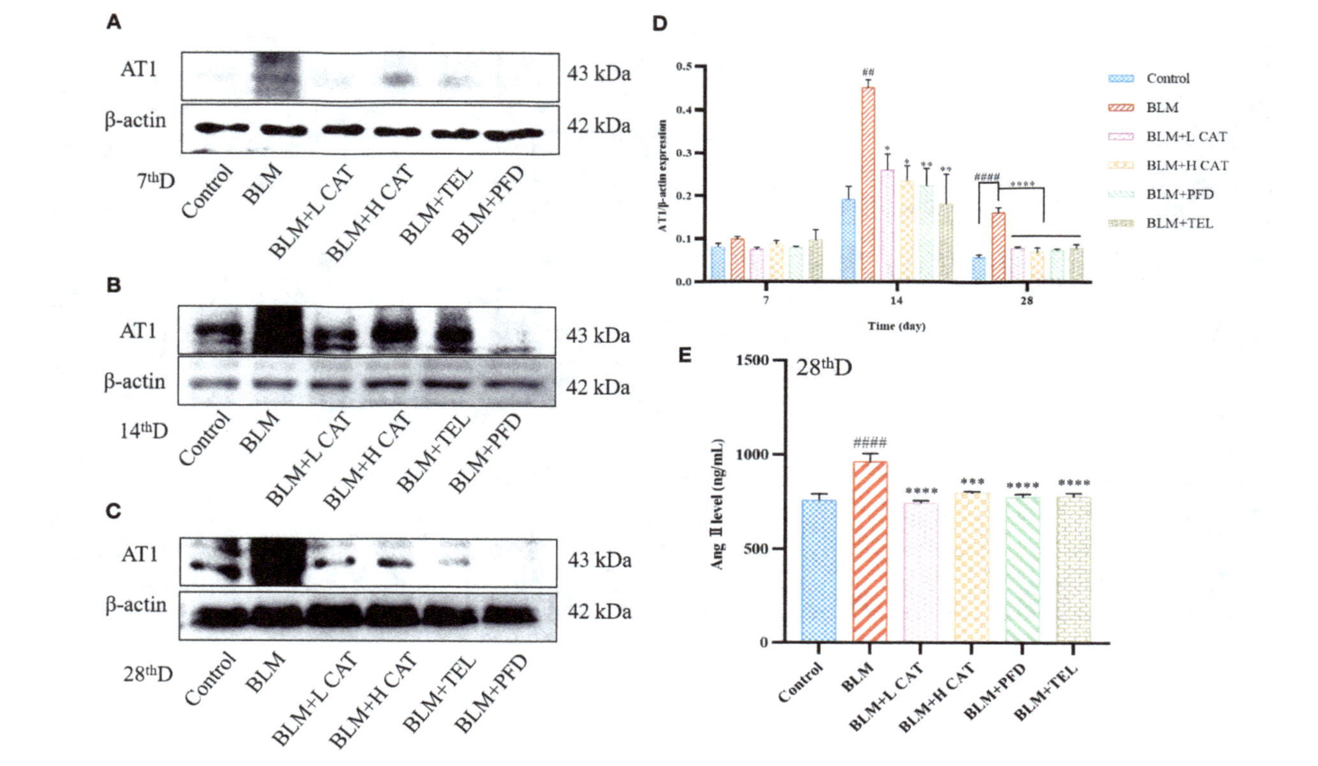

FIGURE 3 | Catalpol inhibits the up-regulation of Ang II and AT_1 in bleomycin-induced pulmonary fibrosis in mice. **(A–D)** Representative Western blots of AT_1 and gray scale quantified data of AT_1-to-β-actin expression ratio at 7, 14, 28d. **(E)** Ang II in mouse serum at 28 day was measured. ##$P < 0.01$, ####$P < 0.0001$ compared with the Control group, *$p < 0.05$, **$p < 0.01$, ***$p < 0.001$ ****$p < 0.0001$ compared with the BLM group (ANOVA with Dunnett's *post-hoc* analysis).

that exert physiological functions. Study has found that not only Ang II has a promoting effect on lung fibroblast proliferation *in vitro*, but also AT_1 as well as TGF-β1 overexpression was found in the model of BLM induced lung fibrosis, accompanied by enhanced collagen synthesis with collagen deposition. Candessartan, an AT_1 receptor antagonist, could reduce TGF-β1 expression and the degree of fibrosis, indicating that Ang II might promote TGF-β1 expression and aggravate the degree of pulmonary fibrosis (26). **Figures 3A–E** showed that treatment with CAT significantly decreased the amount of Ang II in serum ($P < 0.001$ or $P < 0.0001$) and protein of AT_1 in lung tissue.

CAT Attenuates Pulmonary Fibrosis in Mice *via* TGF-β/Smads Signaling Pathway

Small molecules against decapentaplegic homologs (Smad) are classic mediators in the TGF-β signaling pathway and regulate the transcription of a variety of genes, such as AP-1 and snail, which promote pulmonary fibrosis. To determine whether CAT played an important role in the TGF-β signaling pathway in pulmonary fibrosis, we measured the protein expression levels of TGF-β1, Smad2/3, p-Smad2, p-Smad3, Smad7 as well as Snail. As shown in **Figures 4A–H**, TGF-β1, p-Smad2, p-Smad3 and Snail were significantly up-regulated in model group. After CAT treatment, the level of phospho-Smad2 was significantly decreased compared with that of model group ($P < 0.05$). CAT probably acts through TGF-β Signaling pathway to inhibit pulmonary fibrosis development.

Given all the above data, we conclude that catalpol attenuates pulmonary fibrosis by inhibiting Ang II/AT_1 and TGF-β/Smad-mediated epithelial mesenchymal transition (**Figure 5**).

DISCUSSION

Following damage to lung tissue, barrier integrity is generally repaired through the formation of a provisional matrix, transmigration of myofibroblasts and contraction of the wound. Then epithelial cells regenerate and remodel, remove debris and extracellular matrix (ECM) to achieve normal lung healing (27). However, excessive, persistent damage to the alveolar epithelium and/or abnormal wound healing contribute to a dysfunctional, often overexuberant, repair process. The lung develops an inflammatory response in which macrophages and immune cells infiltrate, and produce and release a large number of cytokines and growth factors. Subsequent transformation of alveolar epithelial cells to a mesenchymal phenotype, fibroblast and myofibroblast foci formation, and excessive accumulation of ECM and collagen result in scar formation and destruction of lung architecture, impairing lung function (10, 28).

Renin-angiotensin system (RAS) is the main endocrine regulatory system of the body. Renin (EC 3.4.23.15) is an

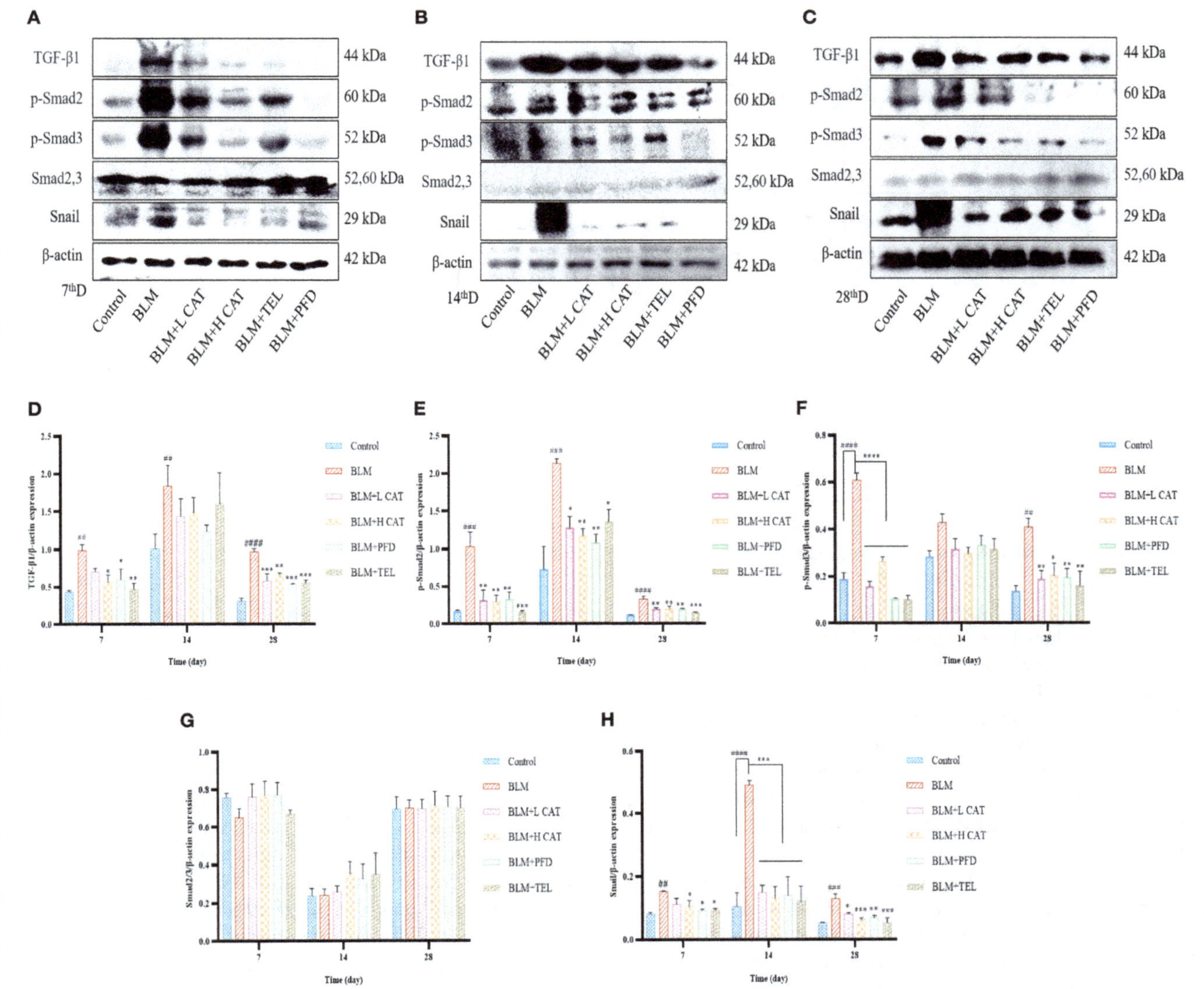

FIGURE 4 | Effect of catalpol on TGF-β/Smad2/3 signaling pathway. **(A–C)** Western blotting was conducted to detect the expression levels of TGF-β1, Smad2,3, p-Smad2, p-Smad3 and Snail in different lung tissue groups at 7, 14, 28d. **(D–H)** Densitometry data of TGF-β1-to-β-actin, p-Smad2-to-β-actin, p-Smad3-to-β-actin, Smad2/3-to-β-actin, Snail-to-β-actin expression ratio at 7, 14, 28d. ##$P < 0.01$, ###$P < 0.001$, ####$P < 0.0001$ compared with the Control group, *$p < 0.05$, **$p < 0.01$, ***$p < 0.001$, ****$p < 0.0001$ compared with the BLM group (ANOVA with Dunnett's *post-hoc* analysis).

aspartyl protease that can catalyze the specific cleavage of angiotensinogen into the decapeptide Ang I. Then, angiotensin converting enzyme (ACE) converts Ang I into the biologically active octapeptide Ang II, and regulate pressure as well as sodium and water homeostasis and so on (29). All major components of the RAS exhibit profibrotic activity, such as Angiotensin converting enzyme (ACE) and angiotensinogen may contribute to increased Ang II production, and Ang II plays important roles in the development of renal, hepatic, as well as pulmonary fibrosis (30, 31). Ang II is hydrolyzed from Ang I under the action of ACE, and the binding of Ang II with AT_1 may be involved in the process of pulmonary fibrosis as a pro-fibrosis mediating factor. Fibroblasts, which make up about 40% of lung cells, are responsible for the deposition of collagen and other ECM proteins. Myofibroblasts expressing α-SMA are extracellular in PF. It has been demonstrated *in vitro* that Ang II can activate the AT_1 to induce human lung fibroblast growth, proliferation, and to mediate the transition of fibroblast phenotype to myofibroblasts as well as procollagen production. And Ang II may also be one of several growth factors that induce and enhance TGF-β and connective tissue growth factor (CTGF) expression at the site of injury (26, 32, 33). Telmisartan, one of the positive controls used in this study, was an Ang II receptor antagonist.

BLM, an agent that induces experimental pulmonary fibrosis, has been described in a variety of experimental animal model

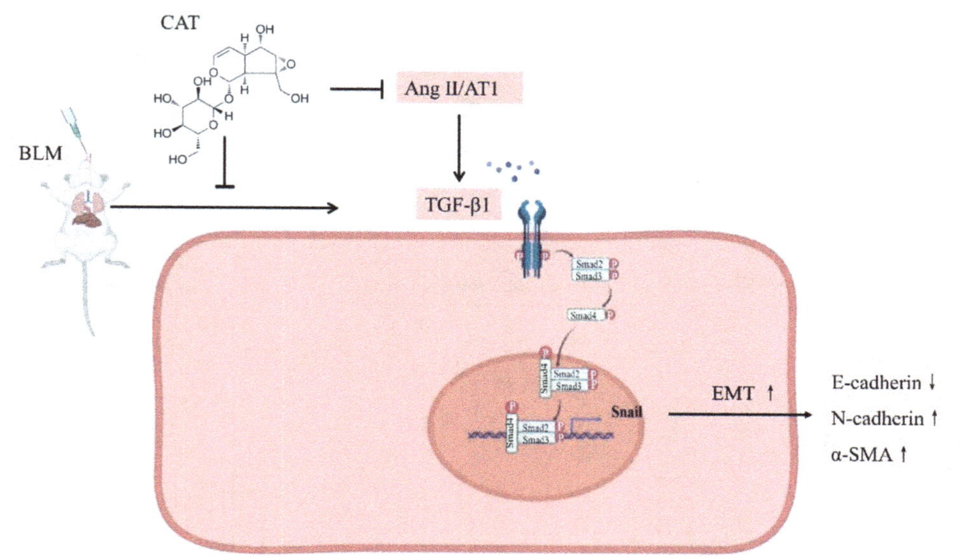

FIGURE 5 | Schematic representation of catalpol regulation of the Ang II/AT_1 and TGF-β/Smad pathway in pulmonary fibrosis.

and this BLM-induced model has the advantages of being simple to perform, widely available and reproducible (21). Intratracheal instillation of BLM in mice causes inflammatory and fibrotic responses within a short period of time. The first 7 days after modeling of BLM induced an inflammatory response characterized by increased levels of proinflammatory cytokines (interleukin-1 β, tumor necrosis factor-α, IL-6, interferon-γ). Inflammation subsequently resolves and fibrosis is detected, in which the expression of profibrotic markers (TGF-β1, Fibronectin, procollagen-1) increased and peaked around day 14. The stage of fibrosis can be maintained for 3–4 weeks after BLM modeling (34). In this experiment, three time points (7, 14, and 28d) were designed to observe the effect of CAT on pulmonary fibrosis at each time point. In this study, Ang II combined with AT_1 was up-regulated in BLM-induced pulmonary fibrosis mice model at 14 and 28 days, and in the CAT treated group, Ang II and AT_1 was down regulated significantly compared with that of the model group. CAT may attenuate pulmonary fibrosis through Ang II/AT_1 axis.

EMT is a crucial step in the process of lung development and many lung diseases (pulmonary fibrosis, chronic obstructive pulmonary disease (COPD), lung cancer). EMT is characterized by epithelial cells losing their characteristics of cell-cell adhesion and apical basal polarity and by gaining some mesenchymal characteristics for migration, invasion, and production of ECM components (35, 36). EMT in organ fibrosis is a major provider of pathogenic mesenchymal cell types with migratory and invasive behavior, such as myofibroblasts (37). Type II EMT is associated with wound healing, tissue regeneration and organ fibrosis, during lung fibrosis, it is generally defined by the detection of several biomarkers that reflect the loss of epithelial phenotype and the gain of mesenchymal phenotype. The changes of these biomarkers include decreased expression of the epithelial cell-cell adhesion molecule CDH1 (E-cadherin) and/or increased expression of mesenchymal markers (CDH2 (N-cadherin), VIM (vimentin), and/or α-SMA), as well as the change of ECM components (fibronectin and collagen) or degrading enzymes (MMP2 and MMP9) (38–40).

TGF-β, a key factor in fibrotic diseases and one of the most studied cytokines, it has various biological effects, such as increasing ECM deposition, recruiting inflammatory cells, contributing to fibrocyte differentiation and epithelial–mesenchymal transition (EMT) (41, 42). TGF-β induces EMT development and progression of lung fibrosis mainly through its canonical Smad dependent pathway. TGF-β family cytokines induce serine/threonine kinase type receptors on the cell membrane to form a functional complex that phosphorylates receptor regulated Smad2 and Smad3, and binds to Smad4, which in turn translocates into the nucleus and participates in transcriptional regulation of target genes (43). Among them, the transcription factors Snail1 and Snail2 downregulate E-cadherin expression and increase the expression of mesenchymal proteins such as N-cadherin, fibronectin and metalloproteinases (27).

The results of pulmonary TGF-β expression in this study may reflect the degree of lung inflammation/EMT in each experimental group. TGF-β and Smad2/3 were significantly upregulated in the model mice, indicating that TGF-β/Smad2/3 pathway is involved in BLM-induced pulmonary fibrosis. After treatment with CAT, the levels of TGF-β, phospho-Smad, as well as the expression of Snail were all decreased. Moreover, CAT can also up-regulate the epithelial cell marker E-cadherin and down-regulate the mesenchymal marker N-cadherin and α-SMA. Our study showed that CAT slowed down EMT progression and reduced myofibroblast proliferation in lung fibrosis. In addition, studies have shown that MMP2 and MMP9 can promote aberrant epithelial repair in fibrotic lungs, degrade ECM and thereby promote aberrant epithelial cell migration as well as promote EMT (22). CAT significantly reduced the MMP2 and MMP9 levels in fibrotic lungs and inhibited the progression of pulmonary fibrosis. CAT may inhibit TGF-β/Smad signaling pathway to attenuate EMT progression of pulmonary fibrosis. Ang II and TGF-β have been proved to promote pulmonary fibrosis. Some studies have shown that there is signal crosstalk between them (44). Ang II binds to AT_1 on the cell membrane and phosphorylates Smad2/3 through the ERK/P38/MAPK pathway. It is then combined with Smad4 and is transferred into the nucleus as a transcription factor to regulate the transcription of TGF-β, procollagen I, procollagen III and fibronectin (33). In addition, Ang II-AT_1 could also directly activate TGF-β signal transduction and induce collagen synthesis in human fetal lung fibroblasts (27). Similarly, Accumulating evidence shows that Ang II stimulates macrophages to release AT_1-enriched exosomes, which promotes fibroblasts activation and lung fibrosis via transforming growth factor-β (TGF-β)/smad2/3 pathway (25, 45–47). In our study, treatment with CAT decreased Ang II and AT_1 as well as TGF-β/Smad2/3, indicating that CAT may attenuate the progression of BLM-induced lung fibrosis in mice partly by inhibiting phosphorylation of Smad2/3 via decreasing Ang II expression.

CONCLUSION

TGF-β1 and Ang II is a critical mediator of tissue fibrosis in disease. These pathways were disease-relevant because the levels of TGF-β and Ang II were increased and positively correlated with Smad2/3 in tissues from patients with idiopathic pulmonary fibrosis or scleroderma-associated interstitial lung disease. Chemicals capable of suppressing TGF-β1-induced production of collagen represent good candidates to treat IPF. Our study points out that the mechanism of CAT protecting against pulmonary fibrosis induced by BLM in mice is related to the regulation of TGF-β1, Smad2, Smad3, Ang II, AT_1, E-cadherin, N-cadherin and α-SMA as well as the phosphorylation of Smad2 and Smad3, also it is given orally which makes it easier to put into clinical practice. In summary, our study points out that catalpol is able to inhibit pulmonary fibrosis, and the mechanism may lie in down-regulating Ang II and AT_1 as well as inhibiting EMT progression through the TGF-β/Smad2/3 signaling pathway.

ETHICS STATEMENT

The animal study was reviewed and approved by Animal Care and Use Committee of Shanghai University of Traditional Chinese Medicine.

AUTHOR CONTRIBUTIONS

Y-HS: conception and design, conceptualization, methodology, data curation, visualization, investigation, supervision, validation, writing-reviewing and editing, project administration, and funding acquisition. QY: software, methodology, data curation, data and image processing, visualization, and validation. D-WZ: investigation, conceptualization, methodology, data curation, visualization, validation, and writing-original draft preparation. YZ: investigation, data curation, data and image processing, and visualization. KW: designed and performed histological experiment. P-LR: carried out a portion of the animal experiments. All authors contributed to and have approved the final manuscript.

REFERENCES

1. Wang J, Li X, Zhong M, Wang Y, Zou L, Wang M, et al. miR-301a suppression within fibroblasts limits the progression of fibrosis through the TSC1/mTOR pathway. *Mol Ther Nucleic Acids.* (2020) 21:217–28. doi: 10.1016/j.omtn.2020.05.027
2. Qiu M, An M, Bian M, Yu S, Liu C, Liu Q. Terrestrosin D from Tribulus terrestris attenuates bleomycin-induced inflammation and suppresses fibrotic changes in the lungs of mice. *Pharm Biol.* (2019) 57:694–700. doi: 10.1080/13880209.2019.1672754
3. Raghu G, Collard HR, Egan JJ, Martinez FJ, Behr J, Brown KK, et al. An official ATS/ERS/JRS/ALAT statement: idiopathic pulmonary fibrosis: evidence-based guidelines for diagnosis and management. *Am J Respir Crit Care Med.* (2011) 183:788–824.
4. Richeldi L, Rubin AS, Avdeev S, Udwadia ZF, Xu ZJ. Idiopathic pulmonary fibrosis in BRIC countries: the cases of Brazil, Russia, India, and China. *BMC Med.* (2015) 13:237. doi: 10.1186/s12916-015-0495-0
5. Olson AL, Gifford AH, Inase N, Fernández Pérez ER, Suda T. The epidemiology of idiopathic pulmonary fibrosis and interstitial lung diseases at risk of a progressive-fibrosing phenotype. *Eur Respir Rev.* (2018) 27:150. doi: 10.1183/16000617.0077-2018
6. Lamb YN. Nintedanib: A review in fibrotic interstitial lung diseases. *Drugs.* (2021) 81:575–86. doi: 10.1007/s40265-021-01487-0
7. Chennakesavulu S, Mishra A, Sudheer A, Sowmya C, Suryaprakash Reddy C, Bhargav E. Pulmonary delivery of liposomal dry powder inhaler formulation for effective treatment of idiopathic pulmonary fibrosis. *Asian J Pharm Sci.* (2018) 13:91–100. doi: 10.1016/j.ajps.2017.08.005
8. Naccache JM, Montil M, Cadranel J, Cachanado M, Cottin V, Crestani B, et al. Study protocol: exploring the efficacy of cyclophosphamide added to corticosteroids for treating acute exacerbation of idiopathic pulmonary fibrosis; a randomized double-blind, placebo-controlled, multi-center phase III trial (EXAFIP). *BMC Pulm Med.* (2019) 19:75. doi: 10.1186/s12890-019-0830-x
9. Fusco R, Cordaro M, Genovese T, Impellizzeri D, Siracusa R, Gugliandolo E, et al. Adelmidrol: a new promising antioxidant and anti-inflammatory therapeutic tool in pulmonary fibrosis. Antioxidants. (2020) 9:601. doi: 10.3390/antiox9070601
10. King TE, Pardo A, Selman M. Idiopathic pulmonary fibrosis. *Lancet.* (2011) 378:1949–61. doi: 10.1016/S0140-6736(11)60052-4
11. Raghu G, Remy-Jardin M, Myers JL, Richeldi L, Ryerson CJ, Lederer DJ, et al. Diagnosis of idiopathic pulmonary fibrosis. an official ATS/ERS/JRS/ALAT clinical practice guideline. *Am J Respir Crit Care Med.* (2018) 198:e44–68. doi: 10.1164/rccm.201807-1255ST
12. Chanda D, Otoupalova E, Smith SR, Volckaert T, De Langhe SP, Thannickal VJ. Developmental pathways in the pathogenesis of lung fibrosis. *Mol Aspects Med.* (2019) 65:56–69. doi: 10.1016/j.mam.2018.08.004
13. Yang F, Hou ZF, Zhu HY, Chen XX, Li WY, Cao RS, et al. Catalpol protects against pulmonary fibrosis through inhibiting TGF-β1/Smad3 and Wnt/β-Catenin signaling pathways. *Front Pharmacol.* (2020) 11:594139. doi: 10.3389/fphar.2020.594139
14. Liu Y, Lu F, Kang L, Wang Z, Wang Y. Pirfenidone attenuates bleomycin-induced pulmonary fibrosis in mice by regulating Nrf2/Bach1 equilibrium. *BMC Pulm Med.* (2017) 17:63. doi: 10.1186/s12890-017-0405-7
15. Qin W, Liu B, Yi M, Li L, Tang Y, Wu B, et al. Antifibrotic agent pirfenidone protects against development of radiation-induced pulmonary fibrosis in a murine model. *Radiat Res.* (2018) 190:396–403. doi: 10.1667/RR15017.1

16. Abdelhamid A, Elsheakh A, Suddek G, Abdelaziz R. Telmisartan alleviates alcohol-induced liver injury by activation of PPAR-γ/ Nrf-2 crosstalk in mice. *Int Immunopharmacol.* (2021) 99:107963. doi: 10.1016/j.intimp.2021.107963
17. Wang W, Song A, Zeng Y, Chen X, Zhang Y, Shi Y, et al. Telmisartan protects chronic intermittent hypoxic mice via modulating cardiac renin-angiotensin system activity. *BMC Cardiovasc Disord.* (2018) 18:133. doi: 10.1186/s12872-018-0875-4
18. Yan J, Wang C, Jin Y, Meng Q, Liu Q, Liu Z, et al. Catalpol ameliorates hepatic insulin resistance in type 2 diabetes through acting on AMPK/NOX4/PI3K/AKT pathway. *Pharmacol Res.* (2018) 130:466–80. doi: 10.1016/j.phrs.2017.12.026
19. Shen YH, Cheng MH, Liu XY, Zhu DW, Gao J. Sodium houttuyfonate inhibits bleomycin induced pulmonary fibrosis in mice. *Front Pharmacol.* (2021) 12:596492. doi: 10.3389/fphar.2021.596492
20. Woessner J. The determination of hydroxyproline in tissue and protein samples containing small proportions of this imino acid. *Arch Biochem Biophys.* (1961) 93:440–7. doi: 10.1016/0003-9861(61)90291-0
21. Moeller A, Ask K, Warburton D, Gauldie J, Kolb M. The bleomycin animal model: a useful tool to investigate treatment options for idiopathic pulmonary fibrosis? *Int J Biochem Cell Biol.* (2008) 40:362–82. doi: 10.1016/j.biocel.2007.08.011
22. Craig VJ, Zhang L, Hagood JS, Owen CA. Matrix metalloproteinases as therapeutic targets for idiopathic pulmonary fibrosis. *Am J Respir Cell Mol Biol.* (2015) 53:585–600. doi: 10.1165/rcmb.2015-0020TR
23. Trombetta A, Soldano S, Contini P, Tomatis V, Ruaro B, Paolino S, et al. A circulating cell population showing both M1 and M2 monocyte/macrophage surface markers characterizes systemic sclerosis patients with lung involvement. *Respir Res.* (2018) 19:186. doi: 10.1186/s12931-018-0891-z
24. Ruaro B, Soldano S, Smith V, Paolino S, Contini P, Montagna P, et al. Correlation between circulating fibrocytes and dermal thickness in limited cutaneous systemic sclerosis patients: a pilot study. *Rheumatol Int.* (2019) 39:1369–76. doi: 10.1007/s00296-019-04315-7
25. Salton F, Ruaro B, Confalonieri P, Confalonieri M. Epithelial-mesenchymal transition: a major pathogenic driver in idiopathic pulmonary fibrosis? *Medicina.* (2020) 56:608. doi: 10.3390/medicina56110608
26. Marshall RP, Gohlke P, Chambers RC, Howell DC, Bottoms SE, Unger T, et al. Angiotensin II and the fibroproliferative response to acute lung injury. *Am J Physiol Lung Cell Mol Physiol.* (2004) 286:L156–64. doi: 10.1152/ajplung.00313.2002
27. Salton F, Volpe MC, Confalonieri M. Epithelial?mesenchymal transition in the pathogenesis of idiopathic pulmonary fibrosis. *Medicina.* (2019) 55:83. doi: 10.3390/medicina55040083
28. Mattoo H, Pillai S. Idiopathic pulmonary fibrosis and systemic sclerosis: pathogenic mechanisms and therapeutic interventions. *Cell Mol Life Sci.* (2021) 78:5527–42. doi: 10.1007/s00018-021-03874-y
29. Takimoto-Ohnishi E, Murakami K. Renin-angiotensin system research: from molecules to the whole body. *J Physiol Sci.* (2019) 69:581–7. doi: 10.1007/s12576-019-00679-4
30. Mezzano SA, Ruiz-Ortega M, Egido J. Angiotensin II and renal fibrosis. *Hypertension.* (2001) 38:635–8. doi: 10.1161/hy09t1.094234
31. Rajapaksha IG, Gunarathne LS, Angus PW, Herath CB. Update on new aspects of the renin-angiotensin system in hepatic fibrosis and portal hypertension: implications for novel therapeutic options. *J Clin Med.* (2021) 10:702. doi: 10.3390/jcm10040702
32. Marshall RP, McAnulty RJ, Laurent GJ. Angiotensin II is mitogenic for human lung fibroblasts via activation of the type 1 receptor. *Am J Respir Crit Care Med.* (2000) 161:1999–2004. doi: 10.1164/ajrccm.161.6.9907004
33. Murphy AM, Wong AL, Bezuhly M. Modulation of angiotensin II signaling in the prevention of fibrosis. *Fibrogenesis Tissue Repair.* (2015) 8:7. doi: 10.1186/s13069-015-0023-z
34. Mouratis MA, Aidinis V. Modeling pulmonary fibrosis with bleomycin. *Curr Opin Pulm Med.* (2011) 17:355–61. doi: 10.1097/MCP.0b013e328349ac2b
35. Jolly MK, Ward C, Eapen MS, Myers S, Hallgren O, Levine H, et al. Epithelial-mesenchymal transition, a spectrum of states: Role in lung development, homeostasis, and disease. *Dev Dyn.* (2018) 247:346–58. doi: 10.1002/dvdy.24541
36. Kalluri R, Weinberg RA. The basics of epithelial-mesenchymal transition. *J Clin Invest.* (2009) 119:1420–8. doi: 10.1172/JCI39104
37. Kyung SY, Kim DY, Yoon JY, Son ES, Kim YJ, Park JW, et al. Sulforaphane attenuates pulmonary fibrosis by inhibiting the epithelial-mesenchymal transition. *BMC Pharmacol Toxicol.* (2018) 19:13. doi: 10.1186/s40360-018-0204-7
38. Jolly MK, Boareto M, Huang B, Jia D, Lu M, Ben-Jacob E, et al. Implications of the hybrid epithelial/mesenchymal phenotype in metastasis. *Front Oncol.* (2015) 5:155. doi: 10.3389/fonc.2015.00155
39. Nieto MA, Huang RY, Jackson RA, Thiery JP. EMT. 2016. *Cell.* (2016) 166:21–45. doi: 10.1016/j.cell.2016.06.028
40. Pain M, Bermudez O, Lacoste P, Royer PJ, Botturi K, Tissot A, et al. Tissue remodelling in chronic bronchial diseases: from the epithelial to mesenchymal phenotype. *Eur Respir Rev.* (2014) 23:118–30. doi: 10.1183/09059180.00004413
41. Li Y, Wang L, Zhang Q, Tian L, Gan C, Liu H, et al. Blueberry juice attenuates pulmonary fibrosis blocking the TGF-β1/Smad signaling pathway. *Front Pharmacol.* (2022) 13:825915. doi: 10.3389/fphar.2022.825915
42. Baratella E, Ruaro B, Giudici F, Wade B, Santagiuliana M, Salton F, et al. Evaluation of correlations between genetic variants and high-resolution computed tomography patterns in idiopathic pulmonary fibrosis. *Diagnostics.* (2021) 11:762. doi: 10.3390/diagnostics11050762
43. Willis BC, Borok Z. TGF-beta-induced EMT: mechanisms and implications for fibrotic lung disease. *Am J Physiol Lung Cell Mol Physiol.* (2007) 293:L525–34. doi: 10.1152/ajplung.00163.2007
44. Uhal BD, Kim JK, Li X, Molina-Molina M. Angiotensin-TGF-beta 1 crosstalk in human idiopathic pulmonary fibrosis: autocrine mechanisms in myofibroblasts and macrophages. *Curr Pharm Des.* (2007) 13:1247–56. doi: 10.2174/138161207780618885
45. Abdul-Hafez A, Shu R, Uhal BD. JunD and HIF-1alpha mediate transcriptional activation of angiotensinogen by TGF-beta1 in human lung fibroblasts. *FASEB J.* (2009) 23:1655–62. doi: 10.1096/fj.08-114611
46. Renzoni EA, Abraham DJ, Howat S, Shi-Wen X, Sestini P, Bou-Gharios G, et al. Gene expression profiling reveals novel TGFbeta targets in adult lung fibroblasts. *Respir Res.* (2004) 5:24. doi: 10.1186/1465-9921-5-24
47. Skibba M, Drelich A, Poellmann M, Hong S, Brasier A. Nanoapproaches to modifying epigenetics of epithelial mesenchymal transition for treatment of pulmonary fibrosis. *Front Pharmacol.* (2020) 11:607689. doi: 10.3389/fphar.2020.607689

11

Enhanced IL-1β Release Following NLRP3 and AIM2 Inflammasome Stimulation is Linked to mtROS in Airway Macrophages in Pulmonary Fibrosis

Athina Trachalaki[1,2,3], Eliza Tsitoura[1], Semeli Mastrodimou[1], Rachele Invernizzi[2], Eirini Vasarmidi[1], Eleni Bibaki[1], Nikolaos Tzanakis[1], Philip L. Molyneaux[2,3], Toby M. Maher[2,3] and Katerina Antoniou[1]*

[1] Laboratory of Molecular and Cellular Pneumonology, Respiratory Medicine Department, School of Medicine, University of Crete, Heraklion, Greece, [2] National Heart and Lung Institute, Imperial College London, London, United Kingdom, [3] Royal Brompton Hospital, London, United Kingdom

***Correspondence:**
Katerina Antoniou
kantoniou@med.uoc.gr

Fibrotic Interstitial lung diseases (ILDs) are complex disorders of variable clinical behaviour. The majority of them cause significant morbidity, whilst Idiopathic Pulmonary Fibrosis (IPF) is recognised as the most relentless. NLRP3, AIM2, and NLRC4 inflammasomes are multiprotein complexes driving IL-1β release; a proinflammatory and profibrotic cytokine. Several pathogenetic factors associated with IPF are identified as inflammasome activators, including increases in mtROS and bacterial burden. Mitochondrial oxidation and alterations in bacterial burden in IPF and other ILDs may lead to augmented inflammasome activity in airway macrophages (AMs). IPF (n=14), non-IPF-ILDs (n=12) patients and healthy subjects (n=12) were prospectively recruited and AMs were isolated from bronchoalveolar lavage. IL-1β release resulting from NLRP3, AIM2 and NLRC4 inflammasomes stimulation in AMs were determined and baseline levels of mitochondrial ROS and microbial burden were also measured. Our results showed that NLRP3 was more inducible in IPF and other ILDs compared to controls. Additionally, following AIM2 activation IL-1β release was significantly higher in IPF compared to controls, whereas similar trends were observed in Non-IPF-ILDs. NLRC4 activation was similar across groups. mtROS was significantly associated with heightened NLRP3 and AIM2 activation, and mitochondrial antioxidant treatment limited inflammasome activation. Importantly, microbial burden was linked to baseline IL-1β release and *AIM2* and *IL-18* relative expression independently of mtROS. In conclusion, the above findings suggested a link between the overactivation of NLRP3 and AIM2 inflammasomes, driven by mitochondrial oxidation, in the pathogenesis of lung fibrosis while changes in the microbiota may prime the inflammasome in the lungs.

Keywords: IPF – idiopathic pulmonary fibrosis, ILD, NLRP3, AIM2, NLRC4, mtROS, mitochondrial reactive oxygen species, microbiome

INTRODUCTION

Interstitial Lung Disease (ILD) is a broad term used to describe multiple complex disorders with different aetiologies and disease behaviours. ILDs are pulmonary fibrotic disorders that affect the lung alveoli causing distraction of the lung parenchyma. The classic paradigm is Idiopathic Pulmonary Fibrosis (IPF), a devastating chronic lung disease of unknown aetiology (1). An interplay of age dependent deregulation of host defence pathways, immune cell homeostasis and microbiome balance is currently speculated to be the underlying cause of the disease (2). Other ILDs are considered to be driven mostly through inflammatory pathways (2).

In the last decade, the landscape of the IPF behaviour has changed with the discovery of two novel antifibrotic drugs (3–5). Of note, the two antifibrotic treatments are similarly effective in other progressive ILDs (6–8). This suggests progressive fibrosis arises from common underlying mechanisms, despite the initial cause, but the exact pathways remain to be identified (9).

Macrophages and monocytes are recognised as drivers of the balance between tissue repair and fibrosis (10). Recent studies in ILD patients have characterised Airway Macrophages (AM) subpopulations which may contribute to different subtypes of pulmonary fibrosis (11). Macrophages, as a source of chemokines and other inflammatory mediators, are responsible for the initial cellular response to injury (12) and can initiate or exacerbate fibrosis (10).

The inflammasome is one central cellular mechanism for chemokine release in macrophages (13). Inflammasomes are cytosolic multiprotein complexes that act as innate immune system sensors. NLRP3, the most studied inflammasome, is activated by a variety of stimuli including ATP, nigericin and ROS (14). Other inflammasomes are more specific and activated by merely one stimulus; NLRC4 by cytosolic Flagellin and AIM2 by cytosolic double stranded DNA (dsDNA) (15). Upon triggering, Inflammasomes cleave pro-IL-1β and pro-IL-18 to their active forms mainly through caspase-1 (15). IL-1β is a potent pro-inflammatory cytokine that can initiate and amplify lung inflammation and has been associated with acute lung injury and fibrosis (16–18). Inflammasome activation has been associated with silicosis, asbestosis and pulmonary fibrosis, mostly in mice models (19–21).

Mitochondria as drivers of metabolic cascades are increasingly recognised as controllers of macrophage activation status (22–25). Mitochondrial reactive oxygen species (mtROS) and oxidised mitochondrial DNA (mtDNA) are both critical for NLRP3 activation (25, 26). It is established that mitochondria homeostasis is defective in aged and IPF individuals (27, 28) and their dysfunction contribute directly to fibrosis in mouse models (29). Our group and others have recently demonstrated that mitochondria in AMs are more oxidised in IPF and other ILDs compared to healthy individuals (30–32).

Microbiota signalling has been shown to alter mitochondrial metabolism and activate the inflammasome (33–35). In IPF, the microbial burden is increased, and its composition is altered (36, 37). Similarly in Chronic Hypersensitivity Pneumonitis (CHP), bacterial burden is higher, albeit at lower levels compared to IPF (38). These alterations have been linked to host immune response transcriptional changes (39) and variable cytokine secretion (40). Of note, streptococcal infection leads to acute exacerbation of lung fibrosis in mice through AIM2 inflammasome activation (41) while inflammasome activation was dysregulated in BAL cells from ILD patients (42).

In this study we hypothesised that alterations in the lung microenvironment including microbiome changes and mitochondrial dysfunction in AMs could drive excessive inflammasome activation with possible implications in the pathogenesis of ILD disease. As such, we sought to determine whether increased mtROS and microbial burden were associated with inflammasome activity in AMs from ILDs, including IPF.

MATERIALS AND METHODS

Patients and Inclusion Criteria

Thirty-six (34) patients were prospectively enrolled at the Respiratory Medicine Department at the University Hospital of Heraklion, Crete, between June 2017 to June 2019.

Twelve (12) healthy controls, and twenty-four (24) ILD patients [fourteen (14) patients with IPF and twelve (12) non-IPF patients] were included. Patients with a recent infection (1 month prior to bronchoscopy) were excluded from the study. ILD patients were treatment naïve. All patients underwent bronchoscopy and Bronchoalveolar Lavage Fluid (BALF) was obtained as part of the diagnostic algorithm.

IPF patients: The diagnosis of IPF was based on either ATS/ERS criteria or the Fleischer Society criteria after Multidisciplinary discussion (22).

Non-IPF patients: Patients with fibrotic Interstitial Lung Diseases as assessed by the presence of reticulation and traction bronchiectasis on High-Resolution Computed Tomography were included. This category included eight (8) patients with fibrotic chronic hypersensitivity pneumonitis (CHP), one (1) with asbestosis related ILD, one (1) with Idiopathic pneumonia with autoimmune features (IPAF) and two (2) with unclassifiable ILD. Any patients with autoimmune diseases treated with immunosuppressive agents were excluded as immunomodulatory treatment could affect inflammatory responses. All patients were evaluated within one month from bronchoscopy, with Pulmonary Lung Function tests.

Control group: Control subjects were either patients undergoing bronchoscopy for the investigation of haemoptysis, without any overt pulmonary comorbidities, with normal bronchoscopy findings and cytology results or healthy volunteers.

Patient demographics, smoking status, and pulmonary function tests (PFTs) were prospectively collected and are summarised in **Table 1**. Since controls were healthy Pulmonary Function Test (PFTs) were not performed.

Abbreviations: AECIIs, alveolar epithelial cells; AIM2, Absent in melanoma 2; AMs, Airway Macrophages; ARDS, Acute Respiratory Distress Syndrome; CHP, chronic hypersensitivity pneumonitis; BALF, Bronchoalveolar Lavage Fluid; dsDNA, double stranded DNA; IPF, Idiopathic Pulmonary Fibrosis; LPS, lipopolysaccharide; NLRC4, NLR Family CARD Domain Containing 4; NLRP3, NOD-, leucine rich region- and pyrin domain-containing-3; NLR, NOD-Like receptor; mtROS, Mitochondrial Reactive Oxygen Species; mtDNA, mitochondrial DNA; ROS, Reactive Oxygen Species.

TABLE 1 | Patient characteristics.

	Control	IPF	Non-IPF	
n	12	14	12	
Age	56.9 ± 14	74.9 ± 6	69 ± 11	P<0001
Male/Female	8/4	12/2	8/4	P ns
Smoking status				P ns
Never smokers	1	2	4	
Smokers	11	13	8	
Pack years	38.1 ± .33.8	40.2 ± 17.4	37.5 ± 19.5	P ns
FVC%		87 ± 21	90 ± 26	P ns
FEV1%		95 ± 19	95 ± 27	P ns
DLCO%		65 ± 21	58 ± 22	P ns
TLC%		81 ± 17	82.8 ± 26	P ns
Macrophages%	93 ± 5	88 ± 5	s89 ± 8	P ns
Lymphocytes%	6 ± 4	6 ± 5	4 ± 3	P ns
Neutrophils%	2 ± 1.5	3 ± 2	4 ± 4	P ns
Eosinophils%	0.4 ± 0.2	1.4 ± 1.3	1.4 ± 1.8	P ns

ns, non significant.

PFTs. Lung volumes (forced expiratory volume in one second – FEV1, forced vital capacity – FVC), and diffusion capacity (DLco, corrected for haemoglobin) were measured using the computerised system (Jaeger 2.12; MasterLab, Würzburg, Germany). Predicted values were obtained from the standardised lung function testing of the European Coal and Steel Community, Luxembourg (1993).

AM Isolation and Culture

Freshly isolated BALF cells were obtained as previously described (30). BALF contains a diverse population of primarily macrophages and variable levels of neutrophils, lymphocytes and eosinophils. To allow macrophage enrichment, BAL cells were cultured for 1 hour prior to experimentation. For each experimental condition $0.5x10^6$ BALF cells were allowed to attach for 1 hour in 24 well plates in DMEM(Biosera) growth media supplemented with 2% FCS (Biosera) and 1x concentration of penicillin-streptomycin (from 100x concentrated solution, Biosera) in a humidified incubator at 37°C containing 5% CO2 at a concentration of 10^6 cells/ml, with subsequent washes to remove non-adherent cells. The remaining attached cell population comprised mainly of macrophages and monocytes from the alveolar space.

Inflammasomes Activation

Human macrophages are known to require a two-step mechanism to activate NLRP3; an evolutionary process preventing uncontrolled NLRP3 activation and IL-1β release. The primary TLR-mediated signal activates NF-kappaB (NF-κB) which results in NLRP3, ASC, pro-IL-1β and pro-IL-18 transcription. The second signal results in proteolytic cleavage of IL-1β and IL-18 by caspase-1 (43).

Here, AMs were primed with 10ng/ml LPS (Liposacccharide E.Coli 0111:B4 strain, Invivogen) to upregulate inflammasome related genes. For NLRP3 activation, cells were primed with LPS for 2 hours and subsequently stimulated with 5 mM ATP(Sigma) for 30 minutes. For the activation of AIM2 and NLRC4 inflammasomes, cells were primed with LPS for 1 hour, followed by transfection with 2 μg/ml dsDNA(naked Poly(dA:dT), InvivoGen) or 0.1ug/ml Ultrapure Flagellin from S. Typhimirium, (InvivoGen) respectively, using Lipofectamine 2000 (Life Technologies) for 4 hours. Inflammasome-specific activation was confirmed using the selective NLRP3 inhibitor MCC950(Cayman) at 1μM, or the caspase-1 inhibitor for the NLRC4 and AIM2 inflammasome (non-selective global inflammasome inhibitor) at 10uM final concentrations, for 1 hour prior to stimulation. The simulation protocol is summarised in **Supplementary Figure 1**.

For the study of mtROS effect on NLRP3 activation, cells were treated with the selective mitochondrial antioxidant agent MitoTempo (Sigma) at a final concentration of 100μM for 1 hour prior to the addition of ATP.

Supernatants and cell lysates were collected after the appropriate stimulation time. ELISA immunoblot was used to quantify IL-1β, as a surrogate marker of inflammasome activation.

Flow Cytometry and mtROS Determination

Mitochondrial ROS was measured by MitoSOX™Red (Invitrogen) staining. $0.5x10^6$ freshly isolated BALF cells resuspended in RPMI-1640, supplemented with 2% FCS, were stained with MitoSOX Red at a final concentration of 5 μM and CD45-FITC for 10 minutes at 37°C. For MitoSOX staining quantification, AMs populations were selected according to high forward and side scatter and CD45 ($FSC^{high}SSC^{high}CD45^{+}$) as previously described (30). Identical cell samples were independently stained with Propidium Iodide (PI) at a final concentration of 1ng/ml, for 5 minutes immediately before flow cytometry analysis, for the detection of necrotic/apoptotic cells. The percentage of MitoSOX positive cells was determined by the percent of cells showing FL-2 fluorescence higher than the unstained control, followed by subtraction of the PI positive percentage of cells. Relative mean fluorescence intensity (MFI) was calculated by normalizing the MFI of the FL-2 channel/MitoSOX positive cells by the MFI of the FL-2 channel of the unstained cells since patient samples displayed wide ranges of autofluorescence. (Data were acquired from Beckman Coulter flow cytometer and analysed with FlowJo 8.7).

Bacterial DNA Extraction and 16S rRNA Gene qPCR

Bacterial DNA extraction and 16S rRNA gene qPCR was performed for quantification of bacterial burden as previously described (36).

Total RNA Extraction and mRNA Expression

1-1.5x10^{6} BALF cells were centrifuged and cell pellets were homogenised in TriReagentTM (MBL) for total RNA extraction, followed by storage at -80°C. Total RNA extraction, cDNA synthesis and real-time PCR were performed as previously described (24). GAPDH levels were used as endogenous control for the normalization of mRNA expression levels in BAL samples. Primer sequences are shown in **Supplementary Table 1**.

Statistical Analysis

Data were analysed using SPSS 25 (IBM) software and graphs were produced using GraphPad Prism 8. Comparisons were made with paired or unpaired student's *t*-test, when appropriate. All data were expressed as means with interquartile range unless stated otherwise. Receiver operating characteristics (ROC) curve analysis was used to select an optimal cut point for mtROS. Spearman's correlation coefficient (*r*) analysis measured the association between two variables. A *p* value less than 0.05 was considered statistically significant (*p<0.05, **p<0.01, ***p<0.001).

Ethics Approval and Patient Consent

The study was approved by the Ethics Committees of the University Hospital of Heraklion (IRB number: 5889). Approval for the study in the UK was obtained from the local research ethics committee (15/SC/0101 and 15-LO-1399). All patients provided written informed consent.

RESULTS

BALF Baseline IL-1β and Inflammasome Components Gene Expression Is Similar in ILDs and Healthy Subjects

Initially, the baseline IL-1β levels were measured in the BAL Fluid (BALF), as a marker of inflammasome pre-activation in the lung microenvironment. Median basal IL-1β concentration in the BALF did not differ significantly between the ILDs and control groups, while some sporadic IL-1β release was detectable in all three groups (**Figure 1A**). IL-1β secretion by unstimulated freshly isolated AMs was also measured and no differences were observed among the groups (**Figure 1B**). Furthermore, we assessed the mRNA expression of genes encoding core inflammasome components *NLRP3*, *NLRC4*, and *AIM2* as well as the gene encoding *IL-18* in BALF cells (**Figures 1C–F**). *NLRP3* relative mRNA expression was significantly elevated in Non-IPF ILDs (p=0.03) and tended to be elevated in IPF as well (p=0.1). *AIM2*, *NLCR4* and *IL-18* expression was similar between groups.

AMs in ILDs Exhibit Enhanced NLRP3 Inflammasome Activation

Typically, monocytes/macrophages require two independent simulation signals to secrete IL-1β *in vitro*; an NF-κB priming step (signal 1), such as LPS or other TLR4 agonists, which leads to the upregulation of inflammasome pathway related genes, followed by a stimulation with a DAMP or PAMP which acts as a second stimulus (signal 2) and leads to robust IL-1β release. Signal 1 alone is known to activate the NLRP3 in a non-canonical way in human myeloid cells (44, 45).

In this study, for NLRP3 inflammasome activation, AMs were primed with LPS followed by ATP stimulation. Treatment with LPS resulted in a significant release of IL-1β by AMs from all groups (**Figure 2A**), although no differences between groups were noted (**Figure 2A**). Upon NLRP3 activation, IPF and non-IPF AMs produced excessive IL-1β compared to controls (p=0.0004 and 0.007 respectively, **Figure 2B**). Between IPF and Non-IPF patients, NLRP3 activity was similar. This effect was NLRP3 specific, as it was abrogated by MCC950 treatment (**Figure 2B**), a novel specific NLRP3 inhibitor (46).

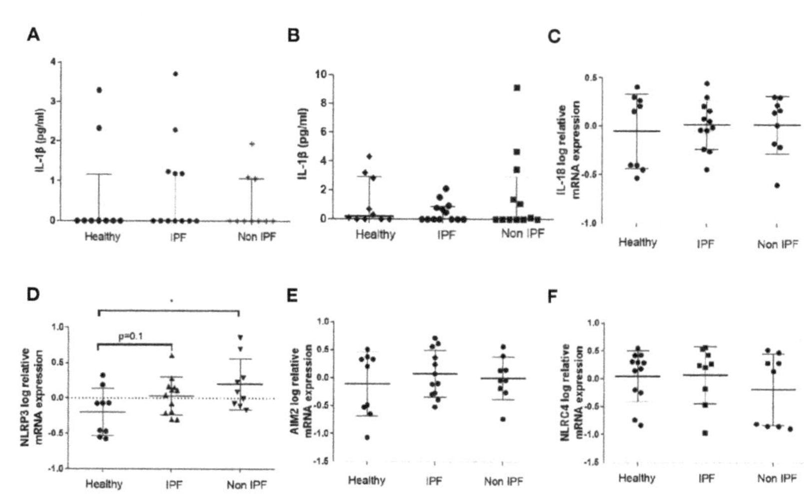

FIGURE 1 | Baseline characterization of the Inflammasome in BALF cells. **(A)** IL-1β protein concentration in BAL fluid as measured by ELISA and **(B)** IL-1β protein release by unstimulated AMs (5-hour culture). Data represented as median with interquartile range Mann-Whitney test. Relative log mRNA expression in unstimulated BALF cells **(C)** *IL18* **(D)** *NLRP3*, **(E)** *AIM2*, **(F)** *NLRC4*. Data represented as mean ± SD, t-test. *p<0.05.

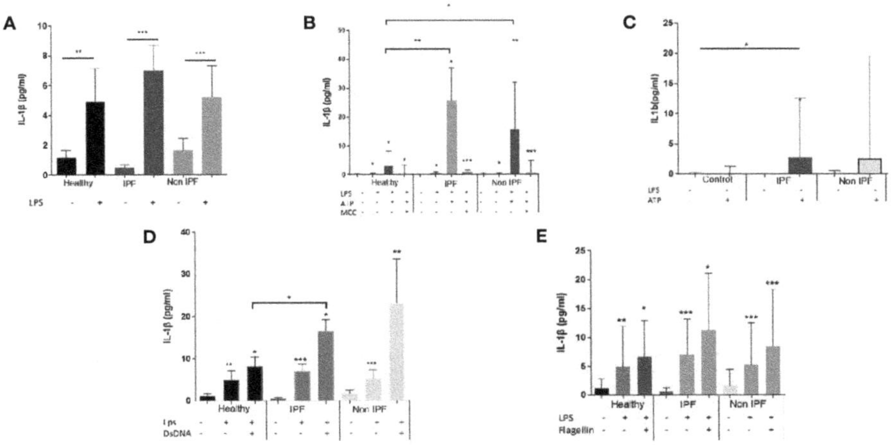

FIGURE 2 | Assay of inflammasomes activation in Airway Macrophages (AMs). **(A)** AMs treated for 5 hours with LPS **(B)** Activation of NLRP3 upon priming with LPS for 2 hours and ATP for 30minutes. Cells were also treated in presence of the Selective NLRP3 inhibitor MCC950 to show specificity of the NLRP3 activation, **(C)** AMs cultured for 2 hours in serum and treated for 30 minutes with ATP without priming with LPS **(D)** AIM2 inflammasome activation: 1 hour of LPS priming followed by 4 hours dsDNA transfection, **(E)** NLRC4 inflammasome activation: 1 hour of LPS priming followed by 4 hours flagellin transfection. For with-in group analysis one-sided paired Wilcoxin test was used. For between group analysis Mann-Whitney test was used. Data presented as median with interquartile range, *$p<0.05$, **$p<0.005$, ***$p<0.0001$.

To determine whether ILD derived AMs were pre-primed by an NF-κB related stimuli in the lungs, we also treated cells with ATP (with no proceeding signal 1). Generally, ATP alone resulted in muted responses compared to LPS/ATP. However, in IPF the addition of ATP was sufficient to generate IL-1β release, compared to healthy controls (p=0.04, **Figure 2C**). Similar trends were noted in non-IPF ILDs (p=0.1, **Figure 2C**). When all ILDs were combined, ATP resulted in increased NLRP3 activation compared to controls (p=0.04).

AIM2 and NLRC4 Activation

For AIM2 activation, cells were primed with LPS followed by transfection with dsDNA. In all three groups the addition of dsDNA resulted in significant IL-1β release (**Figure 2D**). IL-1β production following dsDNA stimulation was significantly elevated in IPF compared to healthy controls (p=0.04) whilst a similar trend was observed for the Non-IPF patients (p=0.09) (**Figure 2D**).

It was recently suggested that in human myeloid cells, in contrast to mice, dsDNA activates the cGAS-STING pathway. This action potentiates lysosomal damage and in turn activates the NLRP3 rather than the AIM2 inflammasome (47). To address this possibility, cells were treated with dsDNA in the presence of MCC950 and a significant inhibition of IL-1β release was observed (**Supplementary Figure 2A**). To test further the above hypothesis of STING-mediated lysosomal damage, cells were treated with chloroquine, a lysosomal acidification inhibitor that blocks lysosomal induced cell death. Chloroquine inhibited dsDNA-mediated inflammasome activation (**Supplementary Figure 1A**).

For the activation of NLRC4, cells were primed with LPS, followed by flagellin transfection. The activation of NLRC4 inflammasome was similar across groups (**Figure 2E**). To confirm the specificity of NLRC4 activation in AMs, both the pan-inflammasome Caspase-1 inhibitor and the NLRP3 specific inhibitor-MCC950 were tested. NLRC4 stimulation resulted in IL-1β release in a caspase-1 dependent and NLRP3-independent manner (**Supplementary Figure 2B**).

NLRP3 and AIM2 Activation Is Associated With Mitochondrial Oxidation and Can Be Inhibited by Antioxidant Treatment

MtROS is widely recognised as an inducer of inflammasome activation and it was previously shown that mtROS is elevated in IPF and Non-IPF AMs (30, 32). It was therefore hypothesised that elevated mtROS could be associated with higher NLRP3 inflammasome activity in ILDs. The levels of mtROS in fresh untreated AMs was measured by flow cytometry using MitoSOX^{TM}red. MtROS was higher in ILD-AMs (IPF and Non-IPF) compared to controls (p=0.03, **Figure 3A**).

Using ROC curves the optimal cut-off value for mtROS level was determined and ILD-AMs samples were stratified according to high or low mtROS. AMs exhibiting high mtROS showed enhanced NLRP3 activation in the absence of LPS priming (p=0.004, **Figure 3B**) and there was also a trend for greater NLRP3 activation in LPS-primed AMs (p=0.08) (**Figure 3C**). AIM2 activation was likewise significantly heightened in AMs with high mtROS (p= 0.02) (**Figure 3D**).

Interestingly, *in vitro* stimulation of AMs with LPS and ATP coincided with a burst of mtROS (**Figures 4A, B**). We subsequently sought to determine whether antioxidant treatment could inhibit IL-1β release by AMs. Treatment with mitoTempo a mitochondria-targeting antioxidant significantly inhibited mtROS accumulation (**Figures 4A, B**) and blocked NLRP3 activation, as assessed by IL-1β release (**Figure 4C**).

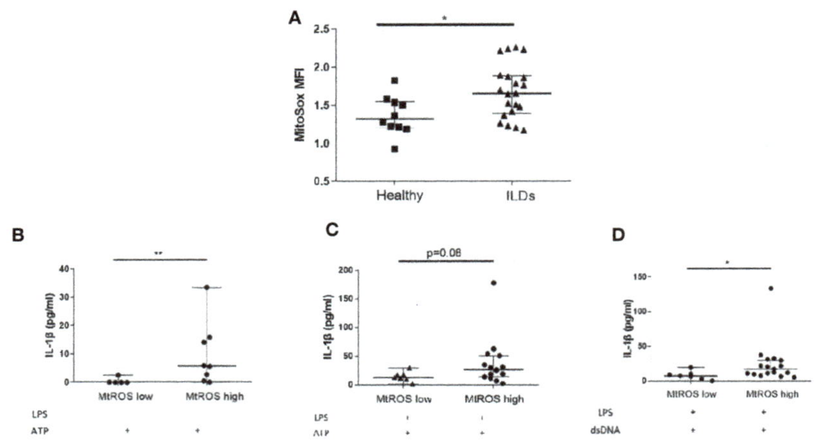

FIGURE 3 | Mitochondrial Oxidation status and the inflammasome. **(A)** MtROS Mean Florescence Intensity Index (MFI) as assessed by flowcytometry in healthy and ILD patients. ILD Patients were categorised according to MtROS MFI using the cut-off value of 1.5(generated by ROC curve). Comparisons on inflammasome activation were made in MtROS high and low groups **(B)** NLRP3 activation without LPS priming, **(C)** NLRP3 activation with LPS priming, **(D)** AIM2 activation (LPS priming followed by dsDNA transfection). Data presented as median with interquartile range, *p<0.05, **p<0.005, Mann-Whitney test.

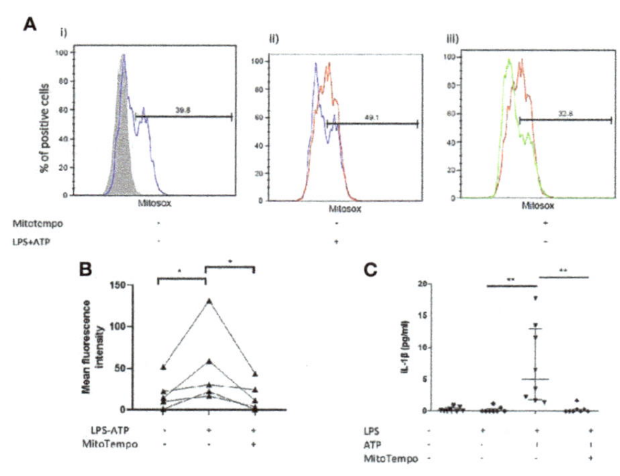

FIGURE 4 | Mitochondrial antioxidant treatment effect on inflammasome activation. AMs were treated with MitoTempo (100μM), a mitochondrial antioxidant for 1 hour prior to the addition of ATP. Cells were subsequently treated with ATP for 30minutes. **(A)** Representative histograms of freshly isolated AMs from ILD subjects, labelled with CD45-FITC and MitoSOX Red analysed by flowcytometry. AMs were selected and percentage of MitoSOX positive cells and mean fluorescence intensities were analysed relative to CD45-FITC labelled populations (grey histograms). AMs were either left untreated(i), treated with (ii) LPS/ATP for NLRP3 activation or (iii) MitoTempo and LPS/ATP. **(B)** MitoSox (assessed by flow-cytometry) and **(C)** IL-1β release measured at baseline, after NLRP3 activation and after NLRP3 activation in the presence of MitoTempo (100μM), Data presented as median with interquartile range, *p<0.05 **p<0.005, Paired Wilcoxon test.

Microbial Burden Is Associated With Baseline *AIM2* and *IL-18* Gene Expression and Il-1β Release

In IPF, it is established that microbial burden is increased and this correlates with disease progression (36, 37). In CHP, microbial burden is also elevated compared to health but at lower levels compared to IPF (38). We hypothesised that microbiota fluctuations in the lung microenvironment could be priming the inflammasomes. BALF microbial burden, as assessed by 16S rRNA gene copies, increased in ILDs relative to healthy individuals (p=0.03) (**Figure 5A**). Furthermore, 16S rRNA gene copies significantly correlated with IL-1β secretion in unstimulated AMs (R^2:0.53; p=0.02)(**Figure 5B**) and *AIM2* (R^2: 0.68 p=0.004, **Figure 5C**) and *IL-18* (R^2: 0.59 p=0.015, **Figure 5D**) relative mRNA expression. There was no association between bacterial burden and mtROS.

DISCUSSION

In this study we demonstrated that AMs in pulmonary fibrosis secrete abundantly IL-1β following stimulation of the NLRP3 and AIM2 inflammasomes compared to healthy subjects. Several factors that could be involved in inflammasomes stimulation have been previously identified in IPF, including increased mtROS and increased microbiome burden. This study showed that higher mtROS was associated with pronounced NLRP3 and AIM2 activation which could be inhibited by antioxidant therapy. Furthermore, BALF microbial burden correlated with baseline IL-1β production, *AIM2* and *IL-18* relative mRNA expression.

The overactivation of the inflammasome has multiple implications in health and disease. Several animal model studies have suggested that NLRP3 activation and subsequent IL-1β release can induce acute lung injury and fibrosis (48–50). In mice models the NLRP3/IL1-b axis is required for the development of bleomycin induced fibrosis (49). In silicosis there is a clear link between NLRP3 and the development of the disease (51). Furthermore, in mice age-dependent mitochondrial dysfunction results in enhanced NLRP3 activation and lung fibrosis (20). In this

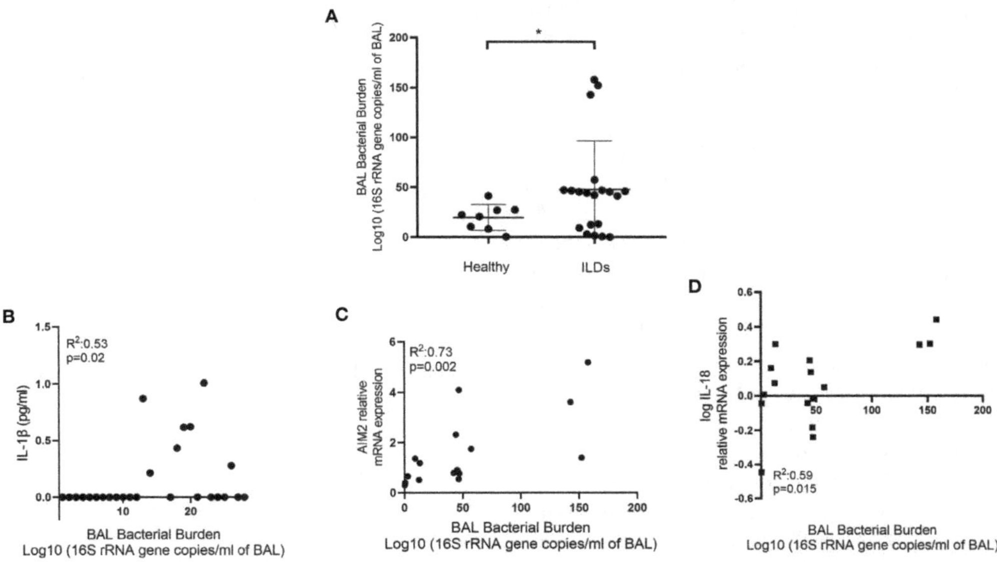

FIGURE 5 | Bacterial burden and the inflammasome. **(A)** Bacterial burden in bronchoalveolar lavage (BAL) of healthy and ILD subjects. Bacterial burden calculated by qPCR and expressed as log10 (16S rRNA gene copies/ml of BAL). Mann-Whitney test. Data are presented as median and interquartile range, *p<0.05. Illustrating correlation between bacterial burden and **(B)** IL-1β release from AMs (Spearman correlation) and **(C)** *AIM2* and **(D)** *IL-18* log relative mRNA expression (Pearson Correlation).

study we provide evidence of an implication of NLRP3 and AIM2 inflammasome in patients with lung fibrosis.

ROS generation by the mitochondria is a well-known trigger of the NLRP3 with mitochondrial death and mitochondrial DNA acting as activators (25). Mitochondrial dysfunction has emerged as a driver of IPF pathogenesis. Mitochondria in IPF AMs have morphological defects and are oxidised (30). Similarly, mtROS is elevated in other ILDs (32). To the best of our knowledge this is the first study to show that in ILD-AMs NLRP3 and AIM2 inflammasome are hyper-inducible and this is associated with mitochondrial oxidation, a hallmark of IPF pathogenesis. In agreement with previous studies (26), we showed that mtROS is crucial for NLRP3 inflammasome activation in patient derived-AMs, since antioxidant treatment inhibits IL-1β release.

It is established that a priming step is required for the activation of the inflammasome which results in the overexpression of several inflammasome components (43). The second signal results in the release of active IL-1β. ROS can act as a direct NLRP3 activator (52), while other studies have suggested that ROS could also exert its role at the priming step (24). Of note, treatment with ATP without LPS pre-stimulation resulted in pronounced IL-1β release in ILDs compared to controls. Furthermore, inflammasome was more inducible in patients with higher mtROS levels, in the absence of LPS priming. This implies that mitochondrial oxidation may be priming the inflammasome in lung fibrosis.

Mitochondria are in the core of metabolic switches in macrophages fighting bacterial infections (53) and a burst of mtROS is crucial for their antibacterial responses (51). By contrast, mitochondrial damage results in deregulated and diminished antioxidant responses to bacteria (54). It is recognised that microbiota are altered in IPF (55, 56). In this study, microbial burden, which is known to be increased in ILDs, was not associated with mtROS, indicating that microbiota changes were not likely the cause of the observed mitochondrial oxidation. The microbial burden was however associated with baseline IL-1β release as well as *AIM2* and *IL-18* mRNA expression in lung fibrosis.

AIM2 inflammasome was recently linked to the pathogenesis of lung fibrosis and progression. Notably, AIM2 is overexpressed in IPF-AMs and this is related to increased Drosha ribonuclease III (DROSHA), a class 2 ribonuclease III enzyme expression (57). Interestingly, a previous study showed that in IPF, peripheral mononuclear cells stimulated to activate the AIM2 released high concentrations of pro-fibrotic mediators and most importantly IL- 1α (58). Of particular interest, GLUT-1 dependent glycolysis promotes exacerbation of lung fibrosis during S. pneumoniae infection *via* AIM2 activation (41) and several studies have suggested a relative abundance of Streptococcus genera in IPF (37, 38, 56). A novel finding of our study is that AIM2 activation is increased in IPF and tended to be higher in other fibrotic ILDs. AIM2 activation was enhanced in patients with higher mtROS and an increase in the bacterial burden was associated with baseline *AIM2* expression

For years, AIM2 was recognised as the central DNA-responding inflammasome. Recent evidence suggests that AIM2 might not be functional in human immune cells in contrast to murine models (47). Researchers showed that cytosolic DNA causes lysosomal damage and activation of the NLRP3 inflammasome through the STING mediated cell death pathway. In our experiments, addition of dsDNA resulted in significant release of IL-1β in all groups. Inhibition of NLRP3 with MCC950, a specific NLRP3 inhibitor, resulted in partial reduction of IL-1β release, as such suggesting that dsDNA activation is to a degree NLRP3-dependent. We also showed that higher mtROS was associated with higher IL-1β production following dsDNA treatment, a result which could be driven by NLRP3 activation rather than AIM2.

In contrast to NLRP3 and AIM2, NLRC4 activation was similar across groups. NLRC4 activation was caspase-1 dependent and NLRP3 independent. A previous transcriptional study in IPF, showed that NLRC4 expression is increased in the peripheral blood and highly associated with increased microbial burden in the lungs (39). Here we focused on AMs and failed to notice overexpression or overactivation of the NLRC4 inflammasome either at baseline or upon stimulation.

Our study sheds light into the pathogenesis of acute exacerbations, a well-recognised complication of IPF and other ILDs (59, 60), characterised by rapid deterioration and death. The pathogenesis of acute exacerbations is not well characterised but is thought to resemble acute lung injury in response to infections or sterile insults (60, 61). Microbiota changes have been implicated in the pathogenesis of IPF exacerbations (37, 56, 62). It is well established that dysregulated NLRP3 inflammasome activity results in uncontrolled inflammation and can cause acute lung injury and fibrosis (18, 50). Intriguingly, a transcriptomic study identified NLRP3 and IL-1β among the top up-regulated genes in AE-IPF (63).

This study indicates that in ILDs NLRP3 and AIM2 can be overactivated. Basal *AIM2* and *IL-18* mRNA expression and IL-1β production was correlated with the bacterial burden in the BALF. Although, it is difficult to prove a direct causal relationship between microbial burden and inflammasome activation, we speculated that microbiota changes prime the inflammasome in the lungs. It is established that microbiota dysbiosis influence systematic immune responses (64) and gut-microbiota changes shape cytokine release from leukocytes (65). More specifically in IPF, disruption of the lung microbiome was associated with variable cytokine production leading to lung inflammation and fibrosis progression (40). Targeting NLRP3, AIM2 or their ultimate effector, IL-1β and IL-18 (66) may prove a novel treatment for ILD exacerbations, which are still considered lethal in most cases.

The main limitation of this study is related to the small number of patients recruited, as differences among different types of lung fibrosis were not established. However, even in this small cohort, we were able to identify changes in lung fibrosis compared to health. Furthermore, different macrophage/monocyte populations exist in the lungs especially following a fibrotic insult (67). It is likely that one or more subpopulations drive the observed excessive inflammasome activation. As such, separation of the different AM populations and subsequent stimulations might be informative of the role of each subpopulation in the disease pathogenesis. One further limitation of our study is the measurement of IL-1β alone and not IL-18 as a marker of inflammasome stimulation. We opted to measure only IL-1β as it is considered a robust marker of inflammasome activation and has generally been associated with initiation and progression of fibrosis. Importantly, IL-1β is not constitutively expressed under homeostasis (68) and has detrimental effects on epithelial cells if over-released (69). Finally, although inflammasome activation in lung fibrosis was increased, we cannot determine whether this plays a causal role in disease progression, nor can we exclude that other factors may relate to the increased inflammasome activation observed here.

In conclusion, this is the first study to show that NLRP3 and AIM2 activation is heightened in ILD-AMs and this is linked to mitochondrial oxidation. Microbial burden is associated to some extent with pre-activation of the inflammasome. Our findings provide evidence of excessive AM-inflammatory response upon activation which could contribute to the progression of fibrosis. Targeting the inflammasome pathway may prove a novel strategy for ILD treatment or a rescue therapy during acute exacerbations of the disease.

ETHICS STATEMENT

The study was approved by the Ethics Committees of the University Hospital of Heraklion (IRB number: 5889). Approval for the study in the UK was obtained from the local research ethics committee (15/SC/0101 and 15-LO-1399). The patients/participants provided their written informed consent to participate in this study.

AUTHOR CONTRIBUTIONS

Conception and design: AT, ET, KA. Analysis interpretation and drafting the manuscript: AT, ET, KA. TM, PM. Technical support and interpretation of the data: AT, ET, SM, RI, EV, EB. All authors critically revised the manuscript and take responsibility for the data presented. All authors contributed to the article and approved the submitted version.

REFERENCES

1. Travis WD, Costabel U, Hansell DM, King TE, Lynch DA, Nicholson AG, et al. An Official American Thoracic Society/European Respiratory Society Statement: Update of the International Multidisciplinary Classification of the Idiopathic Interstitial Pneumonias. *Am J Respir Crit Care Med* (2013) 188 (6):733–48. doi: 10.1164/rccm.201308-1483ST
2. Pardo A, Selman M. Lung Fibroblasts, Aging, and Idiopathic Pulmonary Fibrosis. *Ann Am Thorac Soc* (2016) 13(Suppl 5):S417–s21. doi: 10.1513/AnnalsATS.201605-341AW
3. Margaritopoulos GA, Trachalaki A, Wells AU, Vasarmidi E, Bibaki E, Papastratigakis G, et al. Pirfenidone Improves Survival in IPF: Results From a Real-Life Study. *BMC Pulm Med* (2018) 18(1):177. doi: 10.1186/s12890-018-0736-z
4. Antoniou K, Markopoulou K, Tzouvelekis A, Trachalaki A, Vasarmidi E, Organtzis J, et al. Efficacy and Safety of Nintedanib in a Greek Multicentre Idiopathic Pulmonary Fibrosis Registry: A Retrospective, Observational, Cohort Study. *ERJ Open Res* (2020) 6(1):00172–2019. doi: 10.1183/23120541.00172-2019
5. Trachalaki A, Irfan M, Wells AU. Pharmacological Management of Idiopathic Pulmonary Fibrosis: Current and Emerging Options. *Expert Opin*

Pharmacother (2020) 22(2):191–204. doi: 10.1080/14656566.2020.1822326
6. Brown KK, Martinez FJ, Walsh SLF, Thannickal VJ, Prasse A, Schlenker-Herceg R, et al. The Natural History of Progressive Fibrosing Interstitial Lung Diseases. *Eur Respir J* (2020) 55(6):2000085. doi: 10.1183/13993003.00085-2020
7. Wells AU, Flaherty KR, Brown KK, Inoue Y, Devaraj A, Richeldi L, et al. Nintedanib in Patients With Progressive Fibrosing Interstitial Lung Diseases—subgroup Analyses by Interstitial Lung Disease Diagnosis in the INBUILD Trial: A Randomised, Double-Blind, Placebo-Controlled, Parallel-Group Trial. *Lancet Respir Med* (2020) 8(5):453–60. doi: 10.1016/S2213-2600(20)30036-9
8. Maher TM, Corte TJ, Fischer A, Kreuter M, Lederer DJ, Molina-Molina M, et al. Pirfenidone in Patients With Unclassifiable Progressive Fibrosing Interstitial Lung Disease: A Double-Blind, Randomised, Placebo-Controlled, Phase 2 Trial. *Lancet Respir Med* (2020) 8(2):147–57. doi: 10.1016/S2213-2600(19)30341-8
9. Wollin L, Distler JHW, Redente EF, Riches DWH, Stowasser S, Schlenker-Herceg R, et al. Potential of Nintedanib in Treatment of Progressive Fibrosing Interstitial Lung Diseases. *Eur Respir J* (2019) 54(3):1900161. doi: 10.1183/13993003.00161-2019
10. Wynn TA, Vannella KM. Macrophages in Tissue Repair, Regeneration, and Fibrosis. *Immunity* (2016) 44(3):450–62. doi: 10.1016/j.immuni.2016.02.015
11. Morse C, Tabib T, Sembrat J, Buschur KL, Bittar HT, Valenzi E, et al. Proliferating SPP1/MERTK-Expressing Macrophages in Idiopathic Pulmonary Fibrosis. *Eur Respir J* (2019) 54(2):1802441. doi: 10.1183/13993003.02441-2018
12. Wynn TA, Barron L. Macrophages: Master Regulators of Inflammation and Fibrosis. *Semin Liver Dis* (2010) 30(3):245–57. doi: 10.1055/s-0030-1255354
13. Guermonprez P, Helft J. Inflammasome Activation: A Monocyte Lineage Privilege. *Nat Immunol* (2019) 20(4):383–5. doi: 10.1038/s41590-019-0348-7
14. Stutz A, Kolbe C-C, Stahl R, Horvath GL, Franklin BS, van Ray O, et al. NLRP3 Inflammasome Assembly is Regulated by Phosphorylation of the Pyrin Domain. *J Exp Med* (2017) 214(6):1725–36. doi: 10.1084/jem.20160933
15. Guo H, Callaway JB, Ting JPY. Inflammasomes: Mechanism of Action, Role in Disease, and Therapeutics. *Nat Med* (2015) 21:677. doi: 10.1038/nm.3893
16. Wu J, Yan Z, Schwartz DE, Yu J, Malik AB, Hu G. Activation of NLRP3 Inflammasome in Alveolar Macrophages Contributes to Mechanical Stretch-Induced Lung Inflammation and Injury. *J Immunol* (2013) 190(7):3590–9. doi: 10.4049/jimmunol.1200860
17. Dinarello CA. Biologic Basis for Interleukin-1 in Disease. *Blood* (1996) 87 (6):2095–147. doi: 10.1182/blood.V87.6.2095.bloodjournal8762095
18. Kolb M, Margetts PJ, Anthony DC, Pitossi F, Gauldie J. Transient Expression of IL-1beta Induces Acute Lung Injury and Chronic Repair Leading to Pulmonary Fibrosis. *J Clin Invest* (2001) 107(12):1529–36. doi: 10.1172/JCI12568
19. Dostert C, Pétrilli V, Van Bruggen R, Steele C, Mossman BT, Tschopp J. Innate Immune Activation Through Nalp3 Inflammasome Sensing of Asbestos and Silica. *Science* (2008) 320(5876):674. doi: 10.1126/science.1156995
20. Stout-Delgado HW, Cho SJ, Chu SG, Mitzel DN, Villalba J, El-Chemaly S, et al. Age-Dependent Susceptibility to Pulmonary Fibrosis Is Associated With NLRP3 Inflammasome Activation. *Am J Respir Cell Mol Biol* (2016) 55 (2):252–63. doi: 10.1165/rcmb.2015-0222OC
21. Cassel SL, Eisenbarth SC, Iyer SS, Sadler JJ, Colegio OR, Tephly LA, et al. The Nalp3 Inflammasome is Essential for the Development of Silicosis. *Proc Natl Acad Sci USA* (2008) 105(26):9035–40. doi: 10.1073/pnas.0803933105
22. Ouimet M, Ediriweera HN, Gundra UM, Sheedy FJ, Ramkhelawon B, Hutchison SB, et al. MicroRNA-33-dependent Regulation of Macrophage Metabolism Directs Immune Cell Polarization in Atherosclerosis. *J Clin Invest* (2015) 125(12):4334–48. doi: 10.1172/JCI81676
23. Galván-Peña S, O'Neill LAJ. Metabolic Reprograming in Macrophage Polarization. *Front Immunol* (2014) 5:420. doi: 10.3389/fimmu.2014.00420
24. Zhong Z, Liang S, Sanchez-Lopez E, He F, Shalapour S, X-j L, et al. New Mitochondrial DNA Synthesis Enables NLRP3 Inflammasome Activation. *Nature* (2018) 560(7717):198–203. doi: 10.1038/s41586-018-0372-z
25. Shimada K, Crother TR, Karlin J, Dagvadorj J, Chiba N, Chen S, et al. Oxidized Mitochondrial DNA Activates the NLRP3 Inflammasome During Apoptosis. *Immunity* (2012) 36(3):401–14. doi: 10.1016/j.immuni.2012.01.009
26. Zhou R, Yazdi AS, Menu P, Tschopp J. A Role for Mitochondria in NLRP3 Inflammasome Activation. *Nature* (2011) 469(7329):221–5. doi: 10.1038/nature09663
27. Baumann K. Ageing: The Yin and Yang of Mitochondrial Dysfunction. *Nat Rev Mol Cell Biol* (2016) 17(6):331. doi: 10.1038/nrm.2016.71
28. Rangarajan S, Bernard K, Thannickal VJ. Mitochondrial Dysfunction in Pulmonary Fibrosis. *Ann Am Thorac Soc* (2017) 14(Supplement_5):S383–8. doi: 10.1513/AnnalsATS.201705-370AW
29. Bueno M, Lai Y-C, Romero Y, Brands J, St Croix CM, Kamga C, et al. PINK1 Deficiency Impairs Mitochondrial Homeostasis and Promotes Lung Fibrosis. *J Clin Invest* (2015) 125(2):521–38. doi: 10.1172/JCI74942
30. Tsitoura E, Vasarmidi E, Bibaki E, Trachalaki A, Koutoulaki C, Papastratigakis G, et al. Accumulation of Damaged Mitochondria in Alveolar Macrophages With Reduced OXPHOS Related Gene Expression in IPF. *Respir Res* (2019) 20(1):264. doi: 10.1186/s12931-019-1196-6
31. Larson-Casey JL, Deshane JS, Ryan AJ, Thannickal VJ, Carter AB. Macrophage Akt1 Kinase-Mediated Mitophagy Modulates Apoptosis Resistance and Pulmonary Fibrosis. *Immunity* (2016) 44(3):582–96. doi: 10.1016/j.immuni.2016.01.001
32. Vasarmidi E, Tsitoura E, Mastrodemou S, Trachalaki A, Tzanakis N, Antoniou K. Levels of Oxidised Mitochondria in BAL Macrophages in Fibrotic Ilds. *Eur Respir J* (2020) 56(suppl 64):603. doi: 10.1183/13993003.congress-2020.603
33. Shekhova E. Mitochondrial Reactive Oxygen Species as Major Effectors of Antimicrobial Immunity. *PLoS Pathog* (2020) 16(5):e1008470. doi: 10.1371/journal.ppat.1008470
34. Hirose M, Künstner A, Schilf P, Sünderhauf A, Rupp J, Jöhren O, et al. Mitochondrial Gene Polymorphism Is Associated With Gut Microbial Communities in Mice. *Sci Rep* (2017) 7(1):15293. doi: 10.1038/s41598-017-15377-7
35. Harijith A, Ebenezer DL, Natarajan V. Reactive Oxygen Species At the Crossroads of Inflammasome and Inflammation. *Front Physiol* (2014) 5:352–. doi: 10.3389/fphys.2014.00352
36. Invernizzi R, Barnett J, Rawal B, Nair A, Ghai P, Kingston S, et al. Bacterial Burden n the Lower Airways Predicts Disease Progression in Idiopathic Pulmonary Fibrosis and Is Independent of Radiological Disease Extent. *Eur Respir J* (2020) 55:1901519. doi: 10.1183/13993003.01519-2019
37. Molyneaux PL, Cox MJ, Willis-Owen SA, Mallia P, Russell KE, Russell AM, et al. The Role of Bacteria in the Pathogenesis and Progression of Idiopathic Pulmonary Fibrosis. *Am J Respir Crit Care Med* (2014) 190(8):906–13. doi: 10.1164/rccm.201403-0541OC
38. Invernizzi R, Wu BG, Barnett J, Ghai P, Kingston S, Hewitt RJ, et al. The Respiratory Microbiome in Chronic Hypersensitivity Pneumonitis Is Distinct From That of Idiopathic Pulmonary Fibrosis. *Am J Respir Crit Care Med* (2020) 203(3):339–47. doi: 10.1164/rccm.202002-0460OC
39. Molyneaux PL, Willis-Owen SAG, Cox MJ, James P, Cowman S, Loebinger M, et al. Host-Microbial Interactions in Idiopathic Pulmonary Fibrosis. *Am J Respir Crit Care Med* (2017) 195(12):1640–50. doi: 10.1164/rccm.201607-1408OC
40. O'Dwyer DN, Ashley SL, Gurczynski SJ, Xia M, Wilke C, Falkowski NR, et al. Lung Microbiota Contribute to Pulmonary Inflammation and Disease Progression in Pulmonary Fibrosis. *Am J Respir Crit Care Med* (2019) 199 (9):1127–38. doi: 10.1164/rccm.201809-1650OC
41. Cho SJ, Moon J-S, Nikahira K, Yun HS, Harris R, Hong KS, et al. GLUT1-Dependent Glycolysis Regulates Exacerbation of Fibrosis Via AIM2 Inflammasome Activation. *Thorax* (2020) 75(3):227. doi: 10.1136/thoraxjnl-2019-213571
42. Lasithiotaki I, Giannarakis I, Tsitoura E, Samara KD, Margaritopoulos GA, Choulaki C, et al. NLRP3 Inflammasome Expression in Idiopathic Pulmonary Fibrosis and Rheumatoid Lung. *Eur Respir J* (2016) 47(3):910–8. doi: 10.1183/13993003.00564-2015
43. Bauernfeind FG, Horvath G, Stutz A, Alnemri ES, MacDonald K, Speert D, et al. Cutting Edge: NF-kappaB Activating Pattern Recognition and Cytokine Receptors License NLRP3 Inflammasome Activation by Regulating NLRP3 Expression. *J Immunol (Baltimore Md 1950)* (2009) 183(2):787–91. doi: 10.4049/jimmunol.0901363
44. Gaidt Moritz M, Ebert Thomas S, Chauhan D, Schmidt T, Schmid-Burgk Jonathan L, Rapino F, et al. Human Monocytes Engage an Alternative Inflammasome Pathway. *Immunity* (2016) 44(4):833–46. doi: 10.1016/j.immuni.2016.01.012
45. Netea MG, Nold-Petry CA, Nold MF, Joosten LAB, Opitz B, van der Meer JHM, et al. Differential Requirement for the Activation of the Inflammasome for Processing and Release of IL-1beta in Monocytes and Macrophages. *Blood* (2009) 113(10):2324–35. doi: 10.1182/blood-2008-03-146720

46. Coll RC, Robertson AA, Chae JJ, Higgins SC, Munoz-Planillo R, Inserra MC, et al. A Small-Molecule Inhibitor of the NLRP3 Inflammasome for the Treatment of Inflammatory Diseases. *Nat Med* (2015) 21(3):248–55. doi: 10.1038/nm.3806
47. Gaidt MM, Ebert TS, Chauhan D, Ramshorn K, Pinci F, Zuber S, et al. The DNA Inflammasome in Human Myeloid Cells Is Initiated by a STING-Cell Death Program Upstream of NLRP3. *Cell* (2017) 171(5):1110–24.e18. doi: 10.1016/j.cell.2017.09.039
48. Hoshino T, Okamoto M, Sakazaki Y, Kato S, Young HA, Aizawa H. Role of Proinflammatory Cytokines IL-18 and IL-1beta in Bleomycin-Induced Lung Injury in Humans and Mice. *Am J Respir Cell Mol Biol* (2009) 41(6):661–70. doi: 10.1165/rcmb.2008-0182OC
49. Gasse P, Mary C, Guenon I, Noulin N, Charron S, Schnyder-Candrian S, et al. IL-1r1/MyD88 Signaling and the Inflammasome Are Essential in Pulmonary Inflammation and Fibrosis in Mice. *J Clin Invest* (2007) 117(12):3786–99. doi: 10.1172/JCI32285
50. Grailer JJ, Canning BA, Kalbitz M, Haggadone MD, Dhond RM, Andjelkovic AV, et al. Critical Role for the NLRP3 Inflammasome During Acute Lung Injury. *J Immunol* (2014) 192(12):5974–83. doi: 10.4049/jimmunol.1400368
51. Garaude J, Acín-Pérez R, Martínez-Cano S, Enamorado M, Ugolini M, Nistal-Villán E, et al. Mitochondrial Respiratory-Chain Adaptations in Macrophages Contribute to Antibacterial Host Defense. *Nat Immunol* (2016) 17(9):1037–45. doi: 10.1038/ni.3509
52. Heid ME, Keyel PA, Kamga C, Shiva S, Watkins SC, Salter RD. Mitochondrial Reactive Oxygen Species Induces NLRP3-Dependent Lysosomal Damage and Inflammasome Activation. *J Immunol* (2013) 191(10):5230. doi: 10.4049/jimmunol.1301490
53. Weinberg SE, Sena LA, Chandel NS. Mitochondria in the Regulation of Innate and Adaptive Immunity. *Immunity* (2015) 42(3):406–17. doi: 10.1016/j.immuni.2015.02.002
54. Plataki M, Cho SJ, Harris RM, Huang H-R, Yun HS, Schiffer KT, et al. Mitochondrial Dysfunction in Aged Macrophages and Lung During Primary Streptococcus Pneumoniae Infection is Improved With Pirfenidone. *Sci Rep* (2019) 9(1):971. doi: 10.1038/s41598-018-37438-1
55. Invernizzi R, Molyneaux PL. The Contribution of Infection and The Respiratory Microbiome in Acute Exacerbations of Idiopathic Pulmonary Fibrosis. *Eur Respir Rev* (2019) 28(152):190045. doi: 10.1183/16000617.0045-2019
56. Han MK, Zhou Y, Murray S, Tayob N, Noth I, Lama VN, et al. Lung Microbiome and Disease Progression in Idiopathic Pulmonary Fibrosis: An Analysis of the COMET Study. *Lancet Respir Med* (2014) 2(7):548–56. doi: 10.1016/S2213-2600(14)70069-4
57. Cho SJ, Hong KS, Jeong JH, Lee M, Choi AMK, Stout-Delgado HW, et al. Drosha-Dependent AIM2 Inflammasome Activation Contributes to Lung Inflammation During Idiopathic Pulmonary Fibrosis. *Cells* (2019) 8(8):938. doi: 10.3390/cells8080938
58. Terlizzi M, Molino A, Colarusso C, Donovan C, Imitazione P, Somma P, et al. Activation of the Absent in Melanoma 2 Inflammasome in Peripheral Blood Mononuclear Cells From Idiopathic Pulmonary Fibrosis Patients Leads to the Release of Pro-Fibrotic Mediators. *Front Immunol* (2018) 9:670. doi: 10.3389/fimmu.2018.00670
59. Kolb M, Bondue B, Pesci A, Miyazaki Y, Song JW, Bhatt NY, et al. Acute Exacerbations of Progressive-Fibrosing Interstitial Lung Diseases. *Eur Respir Rev* (2018) 27(150):180071. doi: 10.1183/16000617.0071-2018
60. Miyashita K, Kono M, Saito G, Koyanagi Y, Tsutsumi A, Kobayashi T, et al. Prognosis After Acute Exacerbation in Patients With Interstitial Lung Disease Other Than Idiopathic Pulmonary Fibrosis. *Clin Respir J* (2020) 15(3):336–44. doi: 10.1111/crj.13304
61. Collard HR, Ryerson CJ, Corte TJ, Jenkins G, Kondoh Y, Lederer DJ, et al. Acute Exacerbation of Idiopathic Pulmonary Fibrosis. An International Working Group Report. *Am J Respir Crit Care Med* (2016) 194(3):265–75. doi: 10.1164/rccm.201604-0801CI
62. Molyneaux PL, Cox MJ, Wells AU, Kim HC, Ji W, Cookson WOC, et al. Changes in the Respiratory Microbiome During Acute Exacerbations of Idiopathic Pulmonary Fibrosis. *Respir Res* (2017) 18(1):29. doi: 10.1186/s12931-017-0511-3
63. Carleo A, Deluca D, Bargagli E, Wuyts W, Kaminski N, Prasse A. The Transciptome of BAL Cells At Acute Exacerbation of IPF Reveals New Insights. *Eur Respir J* (2019) 54(suppl 63):PA597. doi: 10.1183/13993003.congress-2019.PA597
64. Zheng D, Liwinski T, Elinav E. Interaction Between Microbiota and Immunity in Health and Disease. *Cell Res* (2020) 30(6):492–506. doi: 10.1038/s41422-020-0332-7
65. Schirmer M, Smeekens SP, Vlamakis H, Jaeger M, Oosting M, Franzosa EA, et al. Linking the Human Gut Microbiome to Inflammatory Cytokine Production Capacity. *Cell* (2016) 167(4):1125–36.e8. doi: 10.1016/j.cell.2016.10.020
66. Mitroulis I, Skendros P, Ritis K. Targeting IL-1beta in Disease; the Expanding Role of NLRP3 Inflammasome. *Eur J Internal Med* (2010) 21(3):157–63. doi: 10.1016/j.ejim.2010.03.005
67. Misharin AV, Morales-Nebreda L, Reyfman PA, Cuda CM, Walter JM, McQuattie-Pimentel AC, et al. Monocyte-Derived Alveolar Macrophages Drive Lung Fibrosis and Persist in the Lung Over the Life Span. *J Exp Med* (2017) 214(8):2387–404. doi: 10.1084/jem.20162152
68. Garlanda C, Dinarello CA, Mantovani A. The Interleukin-1 Family: Back to the Future. *Immunity* (2013) 39(6):1003–18. doi: 10.1016/j.immuni.2013.11.010
69. Choi J, Park J-E, Tsagkogeorga G, Yanagita M, Koo B-K, Han N, et al. Inflammatory Signals Induce AT2 Cell-Derived Damage-Associated Transient Progenitors That Mediate Alveolar Regeneration. *Cell Stem Cell* (2020) 27(3):366–82.e7. doi: 10.1016/j.stem.2020.06.020

12

Acute Exacerbation in Interstitial Lung Disease

Gabriela Leuschner[1] and Jürgen Behr[1,2]*

[1] *Department of Internal Medicine V, Ludwig Maximilians University, Comprehensive Pneumology Center (CPC-M), German Center for Lung Research (DZL), Munich, Germany,* [2] *Asklepios Fachkliniken München-Gauting, Gauting, Germany*

***Correspondence:**
Gabriela Leuschner
gabriela.leuschner@med.uni-muenchen.de

Acute exacerbation of idiopathic pulmonary fibrosis (AE-IPF) has been defined as an acute, clinically significant deterioration that develops within less than 1 month without obvious clinical cause like fluid overload, left heart failure, or pulmonary embolism. Pathophysiologically, damage of the alveoli is the predominant feature of AE-IPF which manifests histopathologically as diffuse alveolar damage and radiologically as diffuse, bilateral ground-glass opacification on high-resolution computed tomography. A growing body of literature now focuses on acute exacerbations of interstitial lung disease (AE-ILD) other than idiopathic pulmonary fibrosis. Based on a shared pathophysiology it is generally accepted that AE-ILD can affect all patients with interstitial lung disease (ILD) but apparently occurs more frequently in patients with an underlying usual interstitial pneumonia pattern. The etiology of AE-ILD is not fully understood, but there are distinct risk factors and triggers like infection, mechanical stress, and microaspiration. In general, AE-ILD has a poor prognosis and is associated with a high mortality within 6–12 months. Although there is a lack of evidence based data, in clinical practice, AE-ILD is often treated with a high dose corticosteroid therapy and antibiotics. This article aims to provide a summary of the clinical features, diagnosis, management, and prognosis of AE-ILD as well as an update on the current developments in the field.

Keywords: acute exacerbation, interstitial lung disease, idiopathic pulmonary fibrosis, definition, diagnosis, management

INTRODUCTION

Interstitial lung diseases (ILD) are a heterogeneous group of diseases. Despite various types of clinical presentation, disease progression, and prognosis, the common feature in most ILDs is a fibrotic destruction of the lung parenchyma. Within the clinical course of ILD, an acute exacerbation [acute exacerbations of interstitial lung disease (AE-ILD)] can occur at any time and is associated with significant morbidity and mortality (1–5). Initially, AE-ILD was described in idiopathic pulmonary

---

Abbreviations: AE-CTD, acute exacerbation of connective tissue disease related interstitial lung disease; AE-HP, acute exacerbation of chronic hypersensitivity pneumonitis; AE-IIP, acute exacerbation of idiopathic interstitial pneumonia; AE-ILD, acute exacerbations of interstitial lung disease; AE-IPF, acute exacerbation of idiopathic pulmonary fibrosis; AE-NSIP, acute exacerbation of non-specific interstitial pneumonia; AE-RA, acute exacerbation of rheumatoid arthritis and interstitial lung disease; ALI, acute lung injury; BAL, bronchoalveolar lavage; CCL, CC-chemokine ligand; CTD-ILD, connective tissue-related interstitial lung disease; DAD, diffuse alveolar damage; DLCO, diffusing capacity of the lung for carbon monoxide; FVC, forced vital capacity; HP, hypersensitivity pneumonitis; HRCT, high-resolution computed tomography; HSP, heat shock protein; IIP, idiopathic interstitial pneumonia; ILD, interstitial lung disease; IPF, idiopathic pulmonary fibrosis; KL-6, Krebs von den Lungen-6; NSIP, non-specific interstitial pneumonia; RA-ILD, interstitial lung disease in patients with rheumatoid arthritis; UIP, usual interstitial pneumonia.

fibrosis (IPF), and according to the official American Thoracic Society/European Respiratory Society/Japanese Respiratory Society/Latin American Thoracic Society IPF guideline, an acute exacerbation of idiopathic pulmonary fibrosis (AE-IPF) has been defined as an acute clinical worsening of dyspnea which develops within less than 1 month without an alternative etiology (6).

Pathophysiologically, AE-ILD resembles an acute lung injury (ALI), which presents histopathologically as diffuse alveolar damage (DAD) in most cases (7). However, DAD is not only found in autopsy studies of patients with IPF but also in patients with connective tissue-related ILD (CTD-ILD), idiopathic fibrotic non-specific interstitial pneumonia (NSIP), and chronic hypersensitivity pneumonitis (HP) (8, 9). Besides the histopathological DAD, AE-ILD and ALI have more clinical features in common, such as an increased oxygen requirement and new bilateral infiltrates on high-resolution computed tomography (HRCT) (e.g., ground-glass opacification/consolidation) (10–12).

While AE-IPF is increasingly recognized better and is perceived as a severe event with high mortality, there is only a limited amount of clinical data on AE-ILD in non-IPF ILD. The aim of this review is to provide a summary of the definition, clinical features, diagnosis, prognosis, and management of AE-ILD. Furthermore, this review will update the current developments in the field of AE-ILD not only in IPF but also in non-IPF ILD.

DEFINITION

Especially in IPF, great efforts have been made to establish a clear definition and diagnosis criteria for AE-IPF (6, 10, 13). In 2007, the IPF Clinical Trials Network (IPFnet) described the clinical presentation, radiological and histopathological findings of AE-IPF and developed diagnostic criteria based on the published literature (13). Just recently, an international working group revised an update on the definition of AE-IPF (**Table 1**) (10). In this document, AE-IPF is defined by a clinically significant respiratory deterioration developing within typically less than 1 month, accompanied by new radiologic abnormalities on HRCT such as diffuse, bilateral ground-glass opacification, and the absence of other obvious clinical causes like fluid overload, left heart failure, or pulmonary embolism (10). In contrast to the previous definition, the authors promote discrimination between a triggered AE-IPF (e.g., infection, post-procedural/postoperative or drug toxicity) and an idiopathic AE-IPF, where no trigger is identified (10). The revised definition aims to be broader and thus allow more inclusion possibilities. In the event of a clinical deterioration with unknown cause, where the criteria for AE-IPF are not met, the term "suspected AE-IPF" can be used (10). This might be the case if there are only unilateral ground glass abnormalities on HRCT or if HRCT data are even missing (13).

CLINCAL FEATURES AND DIAGNOSTIC EVALUATION

Unfortunately, so far, there is no existing official definition of AE-ILD in non-IPF ILD. Since an AE-ILD in non-IPF patients resembles AE-IPF (14–16), in the clinical setting it might be reasonable to apply the definition of AE-IPF to all AE-ILD. Still, it should be pointed out, that the current definition of AE-IPF refers exclusively to IPF and that the authors of the working group report decided against a definition including other ILD (10).

The clinical presentation of AE-ILD is usually a rapid worsening of respiratory symptoms with increased dyspnea within less than 1 month (10, 13). Additional findings can be cough, increased sputum production, fever, and flu-like symptoms (1, 14, 15, 17). Since many patients present with a severe hypoxemia in the arterial blood gas analysis and respiratory failure, admission to the intensive care unit and assisted ventilation is often required (13). Established criteria for a presenting abnormal gas exchange is a Pa_{O2}/Fi_{O2} ratio <225 or a decrease in Pa_{O2} of ≥10 mmHg over time (13).

TABLE 1 | Revised and previous definitions and diagnostic criteria for AE-IPF.

Diagnosis of AE-IPF	Revised diagnosis	Previous diagnosis
Definition		
	An acute, clinically significant, respiratory deterioration characterized by evidence of new widespread alveolar abnormalities	An acute, clinically significant, respiratory deteriorartion of unidentifiable cause
Diagnostic criteria		
– Previous diagnosis	Previous or concurrent diagnosis of IPF	Previous or concurrent diagnosis of IPF
– Clinical presentation	Acute worsening or development of dyspnea typically of less than 1 month	Unexplained worsening or development of dyspnea within 30 days
– Computed tomography findings	New bilateral ground-glass opacity and/or consolidation superimposed on a background pattern consistent with usual interstitial pneumonia (UIP) pattern	New bilateral ground-glass abnormality and/or consolidation superimposed on a background reticular or honeycomb pattern consistent with UIP pattern
– Exclusion of differential diagnosis	Deterioration not fully explained by cardiac failure or fluid overload	Exclusion of alternative causes, including left heart failure, pulmonary embolism and an identifiable cause of acute lung injury
– Concomitant Infection		No evidence of pulmonary infection by endotracheal aspirate or bronchoalveolar lavage

AEIPF, acute exacerbation of idiopathic pulmonary fibrosis; IPF, idiopathic pulmonary fibrosis.

Still, establishing the diagnosis of AE-ILD often comprises a challenge. In order to get to this diagnosis, various diagnostic tests should be performed and differential diagnosis like myocardial infarction, pulmonary embolism, or fluid overload need to be excluded (**Figure 1**). An elementary part of the diagnosis is the HRCT, which should be carried out in all patients who are clinically stable. The important finding in AE-ILD is newly developed, bilateral alveolar infiltrates like ground-glass opacification with or without consolidation on HRCT (**Figure 2**) (6, 14, 16). Three suggested HRCT abnormality patterns are peripheral, multifocal and diffuse ground glass, with the latter two being associated with histologically DAD (13, 18). Several studies have shown that the extent of disease on HRCT seems to be related with the clinical outcome (1, 19–21). If there is no previous HRCT scan available,

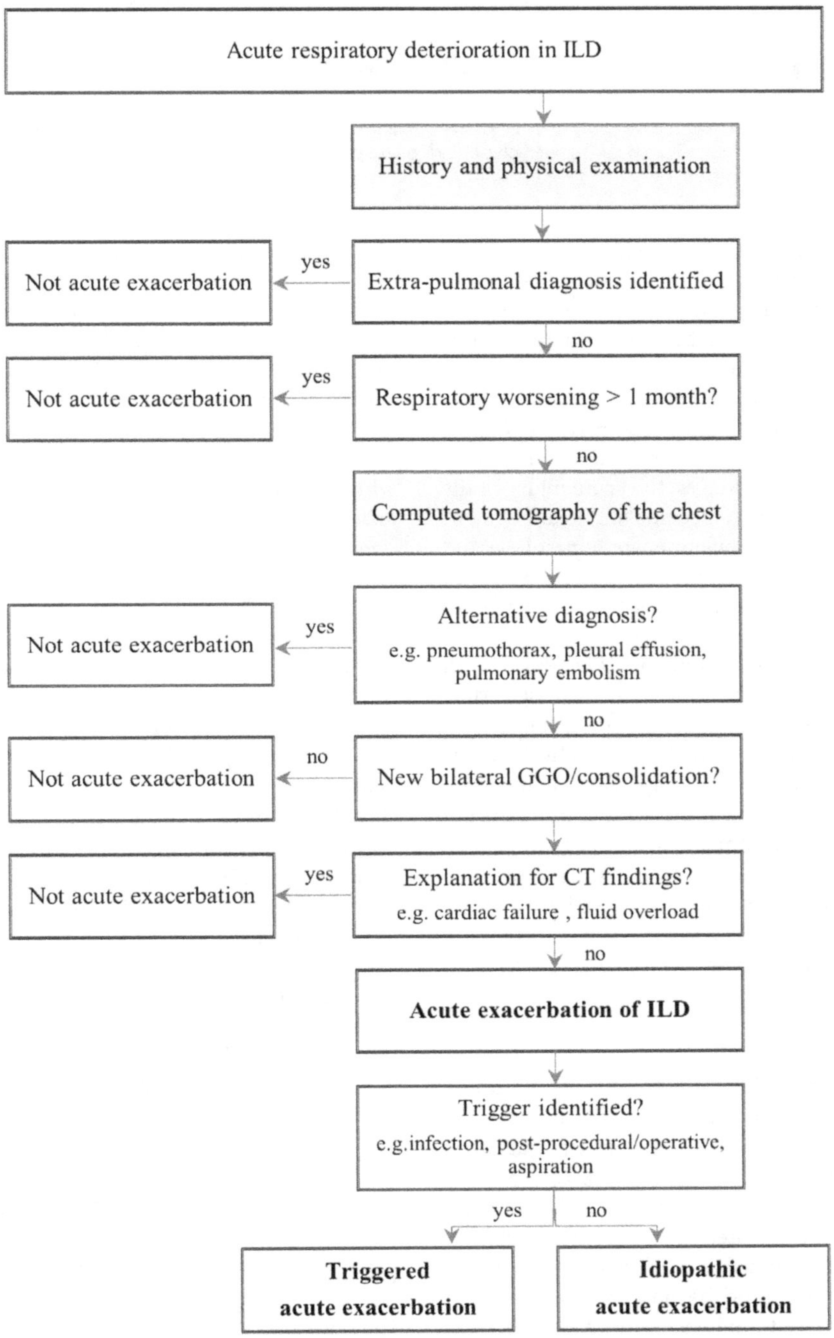

FIGURE 1 | Diagnostic approach to acute exacerbation in interstitial lung disease. Adapted from Ref. (10). Abbreviation: ILD, interstitial lung disease; GGO, ground glass opacity; CT, computed tomography.

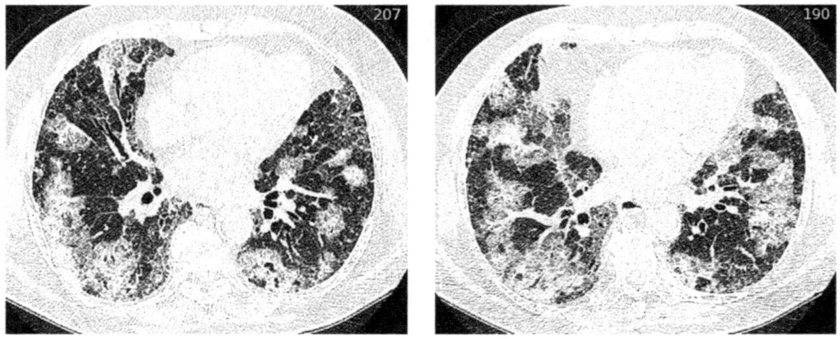

FIGURE 2 | HRCT of an acute exacerbation in IPF. Axial HRCT of a patient with IPF at the time of an acute exacerbation shows extensive bilateral ground-glass opacification. Abbreviation: HRCT, high resolution computed tomography; IPF, idiopathic pulmonary fibrosis.

bilateral ground-glass opacity and/or consolidation on a background of usual interstitial pneumonia (UIP) pattern is sufficient to confirm the radiographic diagnostic criteria of AE-IPF (10). The term "suspected AE-IPF" should be used if there are only unilateral ground glass abnormalities (13).

Histologically, most AE-ILDs are characterized by a DAD, while alternative histological appearances comprise organizing pneumonia, alveolar hemorrhage, and unspecific inflammatory changes (1, 13, 15, 22, 23). In early stages, the acute injury of the lung is characterized by an interstitial edema and hyaline membranes (10). Furthermore, type II pneumocyte hyperplasia and fibroblast foci have been reported in biopsies/autopsies as well as squamous metaplasia and honeycombing with and without hyaline membranes (24).

It has been reported, that patients with AE-ILD present with elevated inflammatory laboratory values such as increased white blood cell count, elevated values of erythrocyte sedimentation rate, and C-reactive protein and increased lactate dehydrogenase (14, 23–25). Although bronchoalveolar lavage (BAL) is not done routinely in AE-ILD, it has also been shown that AE-IPF and AE-HP are associated with an increase in neutrophils in BAL (1, 9, 17, 24–27). Rarely, lymphocytosis has been observed (23, 28), and reactive type II cells hyperplasia has been dectected on BAL (24). Furthermore, BAL is still the subject of research in terms of investigating the pathogenesis of AE and identifying possible prognostic factors.

EPIDEMIOLOGY

Acute exacerbations of interstitial lung disease can occur at any time during the disease, and in some cases it can be the presenting manifestation of an ILD (1, 13, 17). The exact frequency is unknown and the reported incidence rates of AE-ILD broadly vary, most likely due to differences in definition, ILD-entity and disease severity (10, 29). Furthermore, due to incomplete clinical information, definite AE-ILD cannot be confirmed in some cases, although AE-ILD is the suspected and the most probable diagnosis (10). The impact of this relevant difference was investigated in a *post hoc* analysis of the STEP-IPF trail, where a definite AE-IPF occurred in 40 per 1,000 patient-years but combining definite and suspected AE-IPF raised the number to 200 per 1,000 patient-years (30). In a recently published central adjudication on three randomized controlled trials, only 33.2% of the investigator-reported AE-IPF met the criteria (31). A meta-analysis of six randomized-controlled clinical trials identified a weighted average of 41 AE-IPF per 1,000 patient-years (32). In the INPULSIS I and II trial, the 1-year incidence of AE-IPF in the placebo-arm was 7.6% (33).

Compared to clinical trials, retrospective studies report even higher 1-year incidences of AE-IPF, ranging from 7 to 19.1% with highest risk in advanced IPF (1, 2, 34–36). Retrospective analyses of studies from the US and Japan identified the incidences of AE-IPF in approximately 52 per 1,000 patient-years (37, 38). In a registry-based US study, the annual rate of AE in IPF was 133 per 1,000 patient-years (39).

There is much less data on the frequency of AE-ILD in non-IPF ILD compared to AE-IPF. However, the majority of studies indicate that patients with IPF are at a higher risk for developing AE compared to non-IPF ILD (40–43). The estimated 1-year incidence of AE-NSIP is reported to be 4.2%, and the estimated 1-year incidence of AE-CTD ranges from 1.25 to 3.3% (14, 16). Within CTD-ILD, AE seems to be most common in patients with rheumatoid arthritis ILD (RA-ILD) (16). Since the frequency of a UIP pattern is higher in RA-ILD compared to other ILDs, the higher number of AE-RA may be explained by the observation that a UIP pattern *per se* is associated with a higher risk of AE-ILD. Thus, in patients with CTD-ILD and RA-ILD with UIP pattern, a 1-year incidence of 5.6 and 11.1% was found, respectively (14). Furthermore, the 2-year incidence of AE-HP was 11.5% among patients with chronic HP and UIP-like lesions on surgical biopsies (9).

Moreover, ethnicity may play a role, since AE-ILD were initially observed and reported in Japan and Korea, and the literature still is dominated by reports from Asian countries (1, 14, 19, 35). However, two randomized, controlled studies did not support this observation (33, 44, 45).

PATHOGENESIS AND ETIOLOGY

The onset and development of an AE-ILD is unpredictable and until now, it is uncertain, whether an AE-ILD is triggered by an intrinsic factor causing a progression of the underlying disease or a response to an external factor (e.g., infection, aspiration, pulmonary emboli, mechanical stretch) or both (6, 10). Most likely, environmental and genetic factors interact individually leading to AE-IPF in only a subset of patients (13). Concerning the parallels between AE-IPF and acute respiratory distress syndrome, the IPF lung may be generally more vulnerable to intrinsic and extrinsic triggers (10). Still, further research is needed to identify the underlying causes and potential biomarkers for AE-ILD.

Epithelial Injury

During AE-IPF, alveolar injury and loss of epithelial cell integrity may be involved leading to an increased fibrin production and remodeling (13, 46). Morphologically, this leads to neutrophilia in BAL and histopathological DAD (8, 17, 24). Neutrophilic processes are potentially transmitted *via* α-defensins, as they have been shown to be upregulated in patients with AE-IPF (47, 48). α-defensins belong to a family of antimicrobial and cytotoxic peptides contained in mammalian neutrophils (49, 50). Supporting the hypothesis of epithelial injury and proliferation during AE-IPF, a gene expression study of lung tissue detected an increased expression of cyclin A2 and α-defensins together with widespread apoptosis in lungs of patients suffering from AE-IPF in comparison to stable IPF and healthy controls (47). Furthermore, α-defensins were increased in the peripheral blood of patients with AE-IPF, suggesting a potential role as biomarker (47). In a later study including patients with idiopathic interstitial pneumonia (IIP), elevated plasma levels of α-defensins in AE-IIP compared to stable IIP were also seen, but they were not useful as biomarkers due to a lack of specificity (51). Therefore, further studies are needed to clarify the role of α-defensins as biomarker.

Moreover, it could be shown that fibrocytes, which are increased in stable IPF, are even more elevated during AE-IPF (52). Fibrocytes, CD45 and collagen-1 positive cells, are mesenchymal derived progenitor cells which can migrate into injured tissue and can differentiate to fibroblast-like cells playing a role in wound repair, tissue regeneration and pulmonary fibrosis (53, 54). Patients with fibrocytes >5% of total blood leukocytes had a significantly worse survival compared to patients with fibrocytes <5% (52).

Another theory includes the involvement of alternative, so called M2, activation of macrophages in AE-IPF. M2 macrophages play an important role in tumor progression and wound healing (55), and seem to be associated with ILD (56–58). It could be shown that the pro-inflammatory chemokines CXCL1 and Interleukin 8 (produced by classically activated macrophages) and the anti-inflammatory chemokines CC-chemokine ligand (CCL)2, CCL17, CCL18, CCL22, and Interleukin 1ra (produced by alternatively/M2 activated macrophages) were elevated in BAL of patients with AE-IPF in comparison to stable IPF (26). High CCL18 levels in BAL at baseline were further highly predictive for a future AE-IPF (26).

Further markers have been studied, including Krebs von den Lungen-6 (KL-6) and surfactant protein D, which were both identified to be elevated in AE-IPF compared to stable IPF (59) and KL-6 was also increased during the event of AE-HP (60). Furthermore, an elevated serum level of KL-6 at baseline was identified as a predictor for developing AE-ILD in both, IPF and combined pulmonary fibrosis and emphysema (34, 61). KL-6 is a mucin-like glycoprotein, which is mainly expressed in type II penumocytes and bronchial epithelial cells (62). In ILD, a high expression of KL-6 has been detected in regenerating type II cells likely being the primary source of serum KL-6 (63).

Increased levels of Interleukin 6 and Interleukin 8 were also detected in patients with AE-IPF and an increase in either of them was identified to be associated with worse outcome (59, 64). Total protein C, thrombomodulin, plasminogen activator inhibitor 1 (59), and leptin (65) have also been shown to be elevated in the serum of patients with AE-IPF in comparison to stable IPF. In chronic HP, patients with elevated levels of KL-6 and surfactant protein D as well as increased neutrophils in the BAL fluid also have a higher risk for developing AE-HP.

Autoimmunity

Heat shock protein (HSP) 47 is a human collagen-specific molecular chaperone, which is involved in the early stages of biosynthesis and secretion of collagen molecules (66). In AE-IPF, it has been shown that HSP47 serum levels were significantly higher in comparison to stable IPF (67). Furthermore, immunohistochemical analysis detected more HSP47 expression in DAD than in UIP tissues (67). Interestingly, another study identified anti-HSP70 IgG autoantibodies in 25% of patients with IPF and anti-HSP70 positivity was associated with a higher mortality and risk for AE-IPF (68). Mortality among patients with positive anti-HSP70 antibodies was significantly higher compared to patients with negative antibodies (68).

Supporting autoimmune involvement in AE-IPF, one study identified annexin 1 as an autoantigen which increased antibody production and T cell response in AE-IPF with the N-terminus of annexin 1 potentially playing a role in the pathogensis of AE-IPF (69).

Infection

There is an increasing number of findings indicating that infection, both viral and bacterial, might be involved in some cases of AE-ILD. First, in a minority of patients with IIP suffering from AE-IIP, viral ribonucleic acid or a rise in specific immunoglobulins was detected by polymerase chain reaction or pan-viral microarray (70–74). Moreover, changes in the respiratory microbiome were recently identified showing an increased bacterial burden in BAL during an AE-IPF (27). Patients with AE-IPF experienced a markable change in the respiratory microbiome with an increase in *Campylobacter* sp. and *Stenotrophomonas* sp., as well as a significant decrease in *Veillonella* sp. compared to stable IPF (27). The hypothesis of an underlying infection is supported by the fact, that AE-IPF occurs more often between December and May (30, 75) and in the majority of studies an immunosuppressive therapy increases the risk for developing AE-IPF (30, 37, 76).

Microaspiration

Microaspiration might also have a connection to the development of AE-ILD (10). In a *post hoc* analysis of the placebo-treated IPF patients in three clinical trials, none of the patients developing AE-IPF was on an anti-acid therapy (77). Furthermore, patients with AE-IPF had significantly higher levels of pepsin in BAL compared to stable controls, suggesting an involvement of occult aspiration (78).

RISK FACTORS

Several clinical risk factors are discussed playing a potentially crucial role in developing an AE-IPF. First of all, a functionally and clinically advanced stage of disease appears to be an important risk factor. In this context, a low forced vital capacity (FVC) seemed to be the most stable risk factor (2, 26, 30, 34, 35). Other clinical risk factors include a recent decline in FVC (35, 38, 79), a low diffusing capacity of the lung for carbon monoxide (DLCO) (9, 26, 30), a low total lung capacity (9), a low 6-min walking distance (30), an impaired baseline oxygenation (30, 38), an increased dyspnea (30, 35), and a previous AE-IPF (37, 79). However, it should also be considered, that the apparent association between advanced IPF and risk of AE-IPF may be biased by the fact that in advanced disease an AE may have more obvious clinical consequences, while it may even be overlooked in less advanced disease.

In 2007, Selman et al. discriminated IPF patients as rapid or slow progressors based on the duration of symptoms before first presentation (80). Although this study did not analyze AE-IPF, the authors stated that the rapid progression of AE-IPF does not correspond to an AE-IPF (80). Still, some links might be present as the rapid progressors showed a higher rate of fibroblast migration than slow progressors and survival was significantly reduced (80). Until now there is no proof for the theory that rapid progressors and AE-IPF could have a connection but obviously, there is not enough data in this field. Given the association between a recent decline of FVC and an increased risk of AE-IPF (35, 38, 79), it would be further interesting to acknowledge daily variability of FVC. In this context, daily home spirometry is a promising clinical tool to follow the clinical course of IPF patients more closely and potentially detect AE-IPF earlier (81).

Although AE-ILD can occur in different histological forms of ILD, UIP-like lesions were identified to be associated with a higher risk for AE-ILD in patients with chronic HP and CTD-ILD (9, 14). Additional risk factors including male gender (15), a co-existing pulmonary hypertension (36), coronary artery disease (30), a higher body-mass-index (35), and exposure to increased ozone and nitrogen dioxide levels (37) have been reported. Some studies observed a higher risk in former smokers (9, 34), but this finding is inconsistent (2, 26, 82). Similarly, there are different findings concerning age as a potential risk factor: in IPF, younger patients seem to be at a higher risk for AE-IPF (26), whereas a study on CTD-ILD identified higher age as a risk factor for developing AE-CTD (16).

In a retrospective study on patients with ILD and lung cancer undergoing chemotherapy, 21.9% of the patients experienced AE-ILD during the time from diagnosis to the end of the chemotherapy treatment period (83). The authors suggested tegafur-gimeracil–oteracil potassium (S-1) and etoposide as relatively safe options in these patients. Moreover, there is one case-report about a patient with primary lung cancer and subclinical IPF, developing an AE-IPF after hypofractionated stereotactic radiotherapy (84).

A surgical biopsy is another important risk factor triggering AE-ILD. Whereas the incidence rates of developing an AE-ILD after a surgical biopsy for ILD-diagnosis finding are reported to be less than 2.5% (40, 41, 43, 85), AE-ILD after pulmonary resection due to lung cancer can occur in 3–32% (40, 86–88). A decreased FVC and DLCO seemed to be additional risk factors for patients with ILD developing a respiratory deterioration after lung surgery (43, 89). Pulmonary surgery itself seems to be a risk factor, but AE-ILD has also been reported in non-pulmonary surgery and throughout major surgeries the incidences was 3.3% in a study from Korea (90, 91). In IPF, there might be an association between AE-IPF and BAL, as few, individual cases of AE-IPF following BAL exist (92, 93). Furthermore, as this will become increasingly important in the future, the risk of AE-ILD after cryobiopsy needs to be investigated. However, data in this field is still limited and so far, only single cases of AE-ILD following cyrobiopsy have been reported (94, 95).

PROGNOSIS

Acute exacerbations of interstitial lung disease is a life-threatening event and the mortality rate is high. It is assumed that between 35 and 46% of deaths in IPF are caused by AE-IPF (35, 96, 97). In a large number of studies, the in-hospital mortality in AE-IPF is estimated over 50% (1–4, 17, 19, 20, 36, 70, 98) and the median survival after AE-IPF is between 1 and 4 months (2, 36, 75, 82). In IPF, the 1-month mortality ranges between 37 and 53% (37, 99), and the 3-month mortality rate ranges from 63.8 to 73.7% (5, 19, 99). The existing data suggest that patients with IPF have a worse survival compared to ILD patients other than IPF; nonetheless, AE-ILD is also fatal in non-IPF ILD (5, 74). In a study including IPF and non-IPF patients, the overall survival after admission for AE-ILD was 67% at 1 month and 40% at 3 months (4). Similarly to IPF, the highest overall mortality rate of AE-ILD is seen in AE-HP (75–100% mortality) (9, 15). Mortality of AE-ILD in other ILDs ranges from 34 to 83% (5, 16).

Some potential prognostic factors have been identified. First of all, lower baseline pulmonary function parameters (FVC and DLCO) as well as a more impaired oxygenation are associated with a worse outcome in AE-IPF (2, 35, 75). Furthermore, a higher fibrosis score or more extensive disease on HRCT seems to be of prognostic relevance (1, 19–21). A lymphocytosis >15% in the BAL might be another prognostic factor for a favorable outcome in patients with AE-IIP (28). Several markers in the blood could also be potential prognostic markers including lactate dehydrogenase (9, 19, 75), C-reactive protein (2), KL-6 (19, 21), circulating fibrocytes (52), and anti-HSP70 autoantibodies (68). Just recently, Kishaba et al. developed a staging system for AE-IPF, which includes some of these prognostic factors (19).

TREATMENT

So far, there is a lack of evidence based data on effective therapies in AE-ILD. In clinical practice, AE-ILD is often treated with high-dose systemic corticosteroid therapy and antibiotics (9, 14, 16). In AE-IPF, the current international guidelines give a weak recommendation on the treatment with corticosteroids emphasizing that this recommendation is based on anecdotal reports of benefit and the high overall mortality in AE-IPF (6). The authors further point out, that there was a consensus to promote supportive care as an important therapy strategy (6). This includes palliation of symptoms, e.g., with opioids, and supply of oxygen in hypoxemia. Still, there are different opinions on the length of supportive care, and regarding the use of mechanical ventilation (10). Based on an estimated 90% in-hospital mortality, the international guidelines on the management of IPF make a weak recommendation against the use of mechanical ventilation in the case of respiratory failure due to the underlying lung disease (6). The authors point out that this decision has to be made case-by-case together with the physician, the patient, and the family and in accordance with the individual goals of care (6). As a bridge to lung transplantation, mechanical ventilation, or extra-corporal membrane oxygenation may be appropriate and successful in selected patients (6, 100). In a recent retrospective cohort study, the mortality rate in IPF patients undergoing mechanical ventilation significantly decreased from 58.4% in 2006 to 49.3% in 2012 (101). This reminds us to carefully analyze every single patient before a decision for or against mechanical ventilation is taken.

Several studies on different therapy regimens in AE-IPF, other than high-dose intravenous corticosteroids mono, have been published (**Table 2**). In smaller, observational studies, it could be

TABLE 2 | Medical treatment of AE-IPF other than high-dose intravenous corticosteroids mono therapy.

Treatment	Reference	Study design	Number of patients	Treatment/intervention	Clinical outcome
Tacrolimus	Horita et al. (82)	Single-center, retrospective study	15	Steroids mono versus combination steroids plus tacrolimus	Significantly better survival in tacrolimus-group
Cyclosporine	Inase et al. (102)	Single-center, retrospective study	14	Steroids mono versus steroids followed by cyclosporine	Cyclosporine seemed to prevent re-exacerbation and improve survival (no data on significance level)
	Homma et al. (103)	Retrospective study	44	Effect of treatment with steroids mono versus steroids plus cyclosporine before AE-IPF	Significantly better survival in cyclosporine-group
	Sakamoto et al. (104)	Single-center, retrospective study	22	Steroids mono versus combination of steroids plus cyclosporine	Significantly better survival in cyclosporine-group
Rituximab	Donahoe et al. (105)	Pilot- phase I/II-study; historical controls	31	Steroids mono versus combination of steroids plus rituximab/ therapeutic plasma exchanges and IVIG in severely ill IPF	Significantly better 1-year survival in rituximab group
PMX	Seo et al. (99)	Open-label pilot trial	6	Combination of steroids plus PMX	Potential beneficial effect of treatment with PMX
	Abe et al. (106)	Multi-center, retrospective study	160	Combination of steroids plus PMX	PMX improved oxygenation and may improve survival in IP patients with AE
	Abe et al. (107)	Single-center, retrospective study	45	Steroids mono versus combination of steroids plus PMX	PMX treatment significantly improved oxygenation
	Oishi et al. (108)	Single-center, retrospective study	50	Steroids mono versus combination of steroids plus PMX	Significantly better 1-year survival in PMX group
	Oishi et al. (109)	Single-center, retrospective study	26	Stable IPF and healthy controls versus combination of steroids plus PMX in AE-IPF	PMX treatment significantly improved oxygenation
Thrombomodulin i.v.	Isshiki et al. (110)	Single-center, retrospective study	41	Steroids mono versus combination of steroids plus recombinant human soluble thrombomodulin	Thrombomodulin treatment significantly improved 3-month survival
	Kataoka et al. (112)	Single-center, retrospective study	40	Combination of steroids and cyclosporine versus combination of steroids and cyclosporin plus recombinant human soluble thrombomodulin	Thrombomodulin treatment significantly improved 3-month survival
	Tsushima et al. (111)	Single-center, combined prospective and retrospective study	20	Combination of steroids plus recombinant human soluble thrombomodulin	Thrombomodulin treatment significantly improved oxygenation
	Hayakawa et al. (113)	Single arm, non-randomized prospective clinical trial; historical controls	23	Steroids mono versus combination of steroids plus recombinant human soluble thrombomodulin	Thrombomodulin plus steroid pulse therapy improved oxygenation and may improve overall survival
	Abe et al. (114)	Single-center, prospective, non-randomized study	22	Steroids mono versus combination of steroids plus recombinant human soluble thrombomodulin	Thrombomodulin treatment significantly improved 3-month survival
Procalcitonin-guided antibiotic therapy	Ding et al. (115)	Single-center, prospective, randomized study	68	Clinically guided versus procalcitonin-guided antibiotic therapy	Procalcitonin-guided antibiotic therapy had no benefits on survival

(*Continued*)

TABLE 2 | Continued

Treatment	Reference	Study design	Number of patients	Treatment/intervention	Clinical outcome
Cyclophosphamide	Akira et at (20)	Single-center, retrospective study	58	Steroids mono and combination of steroids mono plus cyclophosphamid	No data on treatment-related outcome
	Fujimoto et al. (21)	Multi-institutional, retrospective study	60	Steroids plus cyclophosphamide and steroids plus cyclosporine	No data on treatment-related outcome
	Yokoyama et al. (116)	Single-center, retrospective study	11	Steroids mono and combination of steroids mono plus cyclophosphamide and combination of steroids mono plus cyclosporine	No data on treatment-related outcome

AE-IPF, acute exacerbation of idiopathic pulmonary fibrosis; IPF, idiopathic pulmonary fibrosis; i.v., intravenous; IVIG, intravenous immunoglobulin; PMX, polymyxin B-immobilized fiber column.

shown that the combination of a steroid-pulse therapy with oral tacrolimus (82) or cyclosporine (102–104) was superior to the corticosteroid mono therapy in terms of prognosis in IPF. Other studies identified a positive effect of a treatment with rituximab with plasma exchange and intravenous immunoglobulin (105), polymyxin B-immoblilized fiber column perfusion (99, 106–109), and intra-venous thrombomodulin (110–114). Still, the benefits seen in these studies have to be critically assessed since these were all observational studies with either a historical control or a parallel, untreated control arm, potentially excluding very ill patients from the experimental arm (10). One randomized trial investigated the benefit of a procalcitonin-guided antibiotic therapy compared to a clinical-driven antibiotic therapy but no difference in mechanical ventilation and mortality was seen (115). Several studies reported about a combination therapy of corticosteroids with other immunosuppressant drugs like cyclophosphamide, but it remains unclear whether this is beneficial (20, 21, 116).

Currently, there are indications that an anti-acid therapy could have a protective effect against AE-IPF, as in an analysis of patients from the placebo arm of three large clinical trials, an anti-acid therapy was reported to have a potentially preventive effect on the development of AE-IPF (77). The same potentially preventive effect applies for antifibrotic drugs, although, so far, there is no sufficient data on whether an antifibrotic therapy with nintedanib or pirfenidone should be paused or continued in the event of an AE-IPF. In a phase II trial, patients receiving pirfenidone had a significant reduction in AE-IPF compared to placebo (117). However, a subsequent phase II trial could not reproduce this finding (44). After AE-IPF was not included as an endpoint in the three phase III trials ASCEND and CAPACITY (118, 119), a pooled analysis recently showed that patients receiving pirfenidone had a lower risk for respiratory-related hospitalization compared to healthy controls (120). Interestingly, there is data that the perioperative use of pirfenidone might prevent postoperative AE-IPF (121). In contrast to pirfenidone, AE-IPF was consequently included in the nintedanib clinical study program as a key secondary endpoint; however, the role of nintedanib on AE-IPF needs to be fully understood. Whereas the phase II trial of nintedanib identified a delay in time to the first investigator-reported AE in the nintedanib arm (122), only one of the two INPULSIS phase III twin-trials showed a significant effect of nintedanib on AE-IPF (33). Pooled analysis of the data showed a highly significant prolongation of the time to first AE in IPF due to treatment with nintedanib, thus confirming its preventive effect (45, 123). Still, at this point, more data is needed to validate the effect of pirfenidone and nintedanib in AE-ILD.

Apart from these potentially effective therapeutic approaches, there are a number of drugs that seem to have no preventive effect on AE-IPF, including acetylcystein mono therapy (124), sildenafil (125), bosentan (126), interferon-gamma 1b (127), warfarin (128), ambrisentan (129), and imatinib (130). A combination "triple" therapy (prednisone, azathioprine and acetylcysteine), might even increase the risk for developing AE-IPF (131).

As in AE-IPF, AE-ILD in non-IPF ILD is often treated with a high dose, systemic corticosteroid therapy together with broad-spectrum antibiotics (9, 14, 16). There are some studies additionally using cyclosporine A or cyclophosphamide, but there are no reports on whether there was any benefit in these therapies (9, 16). Similar to IPF, treatment with intra-venous thrombomodulin significantly improved 3-month survival in AE-NSIP (114).

In order to address all therapeutic approaches in this context, one study should be mentioned focusing on a non-steroid approach in AE-IPF: in the event of AE-IPF, prior immunosuppression was immediately stopped and patients were only treated with best supportive care and broad-spectrum antibiotics (132). The median survival of all patients was 1.73 months. Analyzing the single event of AE-IPF, 50% of AE-IPF episodes were survived. Overall, 35.3% of the patients survived AE-IPF and the 1-year survival of the survivors was 83%. Interestingly, patients who had never been treated with immunosuppressant drugs before had a significantly better survival. The 1-year survival in the "never treated" group was 65%, whereas the patients, who had a history of immunosuppression, had a 1-year survival of 17%. Unfortunately, no comparison with a high-dose steroid therapy during AE-IPF was investigated in the study. Nevertheless, this underlines again the lack of evidence based data on therapy strategies in AE-ILD and the necessity for further studies in this field.

FUTURE

Acute exacerbations of interstitial lung diseases are severe events with a high mortality rate. Therefore, it is important to gain further knowledge in this field. As it has been shown that in IPF, an early referral to a specialized center is crucial for survival in general (133), in AE-ILD an early diagnosis and referral might also be important for the patients' prognosis. Therefore, effort should be made to detect early signs of AE-ILD and identify patients who are at a higher risk for developing AE-ILD.

Potential treatment options should be studied in randomized, controlled trials. The currently revised definition of AE-IPF will hopefully allow a more uniform diagnosis, which will help to conduct well designed clinical trials in IPF (10). However, it should be emphasized that, even if it largely follows the framework of AE-IPF guidelines, an official, uniform definition for AE-ILD is needed in the future.

Biomarkers, which can be obtained in an easy and harmless way, are needed to identify patients at a higher risk for developing AE-ILD before symptoms and HRCT features are present. Since biomarkers in BAL might be difficult to obtain in a severely ill patient, serum markers are particularly interesting because of their easier accessibility. Furthermore, daily home spirometry might be a potential tool to understand the clinical course of AE-PF better and even possibly detecting AE-IPF in an early stage (81). There is evidence that home spirometry can potentially improve endpoint efficacy in clinical trials of IPF-therapeutics (134). Therefore, an effort should be made to design studies in that field analyzing the benefit of daily home spirometry in patients with ILD and help establishing home spirometry in clinical, daily routine.

CONCLUSION

Acute exacerbations of interstitial lung disease is a life-threatening event with a high in-hospital mortality rate. The clinical presentation of AE-ILD is similar in non-IPF and IPF, but AE-ILD in non-IPF ILD is less common and the clinical course is less fatal compared to IPF. The new working group report on AE-IPF supports that there are both, idiopathic and triggered AE (e.g., triggered by an infection) (10). So far, there is no evidence as to whether a triggered AE-ILD has a worse prognosis than an idiopathic AE-ILD. Due to the lack of evidence-based therapy options, more studies in this field are urgently needed.

AUTHOR CONTRIBUTIONS

GL and JB wrote the manuscript and have approved the final version of the manuscript for submission.

REFERENCES

1. Kim DS, Park JH, Park BK, Lee JS, Nicholson AG, Colby T. Acute exacerbation of idiopathic pulmonary fibrosis: frequency and clinical features. *Eur Respir J* (2006) 27:143–50. doi:10.1183/09031936.06.00114004
2. Song JW, Hong SB, Lim CM, Koh Y, Kim DS. Acute exacerbation of idiopathic pulmonary fibrosis: incidence, risk factors and outcome. *Eur Respir J* (2011) 37:356–63. doi:10.1183/09031936.00159709
3. Al-Hameed FM, Sharma S. Outcome of patients admitted to the intensive care unit for acute exacerbation of idiopathic pulmonary fibrosis. *Can Respir J* (2004) 11:117–22. doi:10.1155/2004/379723
4. Usui Y, Kaga A, Sakai F, Shiono A, Komiyama K, Hagiwara K, et al. A cohort study of mortality predictors in patients with acute exacerbation of chronic fibrosing interstitial pneumonia. *BMJ Open* (2013) 3:e002971. doi:10.1136/bmjopen-2013-002971
5. Tachikawa R, Tomii K, Ueda H, Nagata K, Nanjo S, Sakurai A, et al. Clinical features and outcome of acute exacerbation of interstitial pneumonia: collagen vascular diseases-related versus idiopathic. *Respiration* (2012) 83:20–7. doi:10.1159/000329893
6. Raghu G, Collard HR, Egan JJ, Martinez FJ, Behr J, Brown KK, et al. An official ATS/ERS/JRS/ALAT statement: idiopathic pulmonary fibrosis: evidence-based guidelines for diagnosis and management. *Am J Respir Crit Care Med* (2011) 183:788–824. doi:10.1164/rccm.2009-040GL
7. Oda K, Ishimoto H, Yamada S, Kushima H, Ishii H, Imanaga T, et al. Autopsy analyses in acute exacerbation of idiopathic pulmonary fibrosis. *Respir Res* (2014) 15:109. doi:10.1186/s12931-014-0109-y
8. Rice AJ, Wells AU, Bouros D, du Bois RM, Hansell DM, Polychronopoulos V, et al. Terminal diffuse alveolar damage in relation to interstitial pneumonias. An autopsy study. *Am J Clin Pathol* (2003) 119:709–14. doi:10.1309/UVARMDY8FE9FJDKU
9. Miyazaki Y, Tateishi T, Akashi T, Ohtani Y, Inase N, Yoshizawa Y. Clinical predictors and histologic appearance of acute exacerbations in chronic hypersensitivity pneumonitis. *Chest* (2008) 134:1265–70. doi:10.1378/chest.08-0866
10. Collard HR, Ryerson CJ, Corte TJ, Jenkins G, Kondoh Y, Lederer DJ, et al. Acute exacerbation of idiopathic pulmonary fibrosis. An international working group report. *Am J Respir Crit Care Med* (2016) 194:265–75. doi:10.1164/rccm.201604-0801CI
11. de Hemptinne Q, Remmelink M, Brimioulle S, Salmon I, Vincent JL. ARDS: a clinicopathological confrontation. *Chest* (2009) 135:944–9. doi:10.1378/chest.08-1741
12. Ferguson ND, Frutos-Vivar F, Esteban A, Fernandez-Segoviano P, Aramburu JA, Najera L, et al. Acute respiratory distress syndrome: underrecognition by clinicians and diagnostic accuracy of three clinical definitions. *Crit Care Med* (2005) 33:2228–34. doi:10.1097/01.CCM.0000181529.08630.49
13. Collard HR, Moore BB, Flaherty KR, Brown KK, Kaner RJ, King TE Jr, et al. Acute exacerbations of idiopathic pulmonary fibrosis. *Am J Respir Crit Care Med* (2007) 176:636–43. doi:10.1164/rccm.200703-463PP
14. Park IN, Kim DS, Shim TS, Lim CM, Lee SD, Koh Y, et al. Acute exacerbation of interstitial pneumonia other than idiopathic pulmonary fibrosis. *Chest* (2007) 132:214–20. doi:10.1378/chest.07-0323
15. Olson AL, Huie TJ, Groshong SD, Cosgrove GP, Janssen WJ, Schwarz MI, et al. Acute exacerbations of fibrotic hypersensitivity pneumonitis: a case series. *Chest* (2008) 134:844–50. doi:10.1378/chest.08-0428
16. Suda T, Kaida Y, Nakamura Y, Enomoto N, Fujisawa T, Imokawa S, et al. Acute exacerbation of interstitial pneumonia associated with collagen vascular diseases. *Respir Med* (2009) 103:846–53. doi:10.1016/j.rmed.2008.12.019
17. Parambil JG, Myers JL, Ryu JH. Histopathologic features and outcome of patients with acute exacerbation of idiopathic pulmonary fibrosis undergoing surgical lung biopsy. *Chest* (2005) 128:3310–5. doi:10.1378/chest.128.5.3310
18. Akira M, Hamada H, Sakatani M, Kobayashi C, Nishioka M, Yamamoto S. CT findings during phase of accelerated deterioration in patients with idiopathic pulmonary fibrosis. *AJR Am J Roentgenol* (1997) 168:79–83. doi:10.2214/ajr.168.1.8976924
19. Kishaba T, Tamaki H, Shimaoka Y, Fukuyama H, Yamashiro S. Staging of acute exacerbation in patients with idiopathic pulmonary fibrosis. *Lung* (2014) 192:141–9. doi:10.1007/s00408-013-9530-0
20. Akira M, Kozuka T, Yamamoto S, Sakatani M. Computed tomography findings in acute exacerbation of idiopathic pulmonary fibrosis. *Am J Respir Crit Care Med* (2008) 178:372–8. doi:10.1164/rccm.200709-1365OC
21. Fujimoto K, Taniguchi H, Johkoh T, Kondoh Y, Ichikado K, Sumikawa H, et al. Acute exacerbation of idiopathic pulmonary fibrosis: high-resolution CT scores predict mortality. *Eur Radiol* (2012) 22:83–92. doi:10.1007/s00330-011-2211-6

22. Churg A, Muller NL, Silva CI, Wright JL. Acute exacerbation (acute lung injury of unknown cause) in UIP and other forms of fibrotic interstitial pneumonias. *Am J Surg Pathol* (2007) 31:277–84. doi:10.1097/01.pas.0000213341.70852.9d
23. Dallari R, Foglia M, Paci M, Cavazza A. Acute exacerbation of idiopathic pulmonary fibrosis. *Eur Respir J* (2004) 23:792. doi:10.1183/09031936.04.00004404
24. Ambrosini V, Cancellieri A, Chilosi M, Zompatori M, Trisolini R, Saragoni L, et al. Acute exacerbation of idiopathic pulmonary fibrosis: report of a series. *Eur Respir J* (2003) 22:821–6. doi:10.1183/09031936.03.00022703
25. Kondoh Y, Taniguchi H, Kawabata Y, Yokoi T, Suzuki K, Takagi K. Acute exacerbation in idiopathic pulmonary fibrosis. Analysis of clinical and pathologic findings in three cases. *Chest* (1993) 103:1808–12. doi:10.1378/chest.103.6.1808
26. Schupp JC, Binder H, Jager B, Cillis G, Zissel G, Muller-Quernheim J, et al. Macrophage activation in acute exacerbation of idiopathic pulmonary fibrosis. *PLoS One* (2015) 10:e0116775. doi:10.1371/journal.pone.0116775
27. Molyneaux PL, Cox MJ, Wells AU, Kim HC, Ji W, Cookson WO, et al. Changes in the respiratory microbiome during acute exacerbations of idiopathic pulmonary fibrosis. *Respir Res* (2017) 18:29. doi:10.1186/s12931-017-0511-3
28. Takei R, Arita M, Kumagai S, Ito Y, Noyama M, Tokioka F, et al. Impact of lymphocyte differential count > 15% in BALF on the mortality of patients with acute exacerbation of chronic fibrosing idiopathic interstitial pneumonia. *BMC Pulm Med* (2017) 17:67. doi:10.1186/s12890-017-0412-8
29. Ryerson CJ, Cottin V, Brown KK, Collard HR. Acute exacerbation of idiopathic pulmonary fibrosis: shifting the paradigm. *Eur Respir J* (2015) 46:512–20. doi:10.1183/13993003.00419-2015
30. Collard HR, Yow E, Richeldi L, Anstrom KJ, Glazer C; IPFnet Investigators. Suspected acute exacerbation of idiopathic pulmonary fibrosis as an outcome measure in clinical trials. *Respir Res* (2013) 14:73. doi:10.1186/1465-9921-14-73
31. de Andrade J, Schwarz M, Collard HR, Gentry-Bumpass T, Colby T, Lynch D, et al. The idiopathic pulmonary fibrosis clinical research network (IPFnet): diagnostic and adjudication processes. *Chest* (2015) 148:1034–42. doi:10.1378/chest.14-2889
32. Atkins CP, Loke YK, Wilson AM. Outcomes in idiopathic pulmonary fibrosis: a meta-analysis from placebo controlled trials. *Respir Med* (2014) 108:376–87. doi:10.1016/j.rmed.2013.11.007
33. Richeldi L, du Bois RM, Raghu G, Azuma A, Brown KK, Costabel U, et al. Efficacy and safety of nintedanib in idiopathic pulmonary fibrosis. *N Engl J Med* (2014) 370:2071–82. doi:10.1056/NEJMoa1402584
34. Ohshimo S, Ishikawa N, Horimasu Y, Hattori N, Hirohashi N, Tanigawa K, et al. Baseline KL-6 predicts increased risk for acute exacerbation of idiopathic pulmonary fibrosis. *Respir Med* (2014) 108:1031–9. doi:10.1016/j.rmed.2014.04.009
35. Kondoh Y, Taniguchi H, Katsuta T, Kataoka K, Kimura T, Nishiyama O, et al. Risk factors of acute exacerbation of idiopathic pulmonary fibrosis. *Sarcoidosis Vasc Diffuse Lung Dis* (2010) 27:103–10.
36. Judge EP, Fabre A, Adamali HI, Egan JJ. Acute exacerbations and pulmonary hypertension in advanced idiopathic pulmonary fibrosis. *Eur Respir J* (2012) 40:93–100. doi:10.1183/09031936.00115511
37. Johannson KA, Vittinghoff E, Lee K, Balmes JR, Ji W, Kaplan GG, et al. Acute exacerbation of idiopathic pulmonary fibrosis associated with air pollution exposure. *Eur Respir J* (2014) 43:1124–31. doi:10.1183/09031936.00122213
38. Kondoh Y, Taniguchi H, Ebina M, Azuma A, Ogura T, Taguchi Y, et al. Risk factors for acute exacerbation of idiopathic pulmonary fibrosis – extended analysis of pirfenidone trial in Japan. *Respir Investig* (2015) 53:271–8. doi:10.1016/j.resinv.2015.04.005
39. Fernandez Perez ER, Daniels CE, Schroeder DR, St Sauver J, Hartman TE, Bartholmai BJ, et al. Incidence, prevalence, and clinical course of idiopathic pulmonary fibrosis: a population-based study. *Chest* (2010) 137:129–37. doi:10.1378/chest.09-1002
40. Sakamoto S, Homma S, Mun M, Fujii T, Kurosaki A, Yoshimura K. Acute exacerbation of idiopathic interstitial pneumonia following lung surgery in 3 of 68 consecutive patients: a retrospective study. *Intern Med* (2011) 50:77–85. doi:10.2169/internalmedicine.50.3390
41. Samejima J, Tajiri M, Ogura T, Baba T, Omori T, Tsuboi M, et al. Thoracoscopic lung biopsy in 285 patients with diffuse pulmonary disease. *Asian Cardiovasc Thorac Ann* (2015) 23:191–7. doi:10.1177/0218492314550724
42. Rotolo N, Imperatori A, Dominioni L, Facchini A, Conti V, Castiglioni M, et al. Efficacy and safety of surgical lung biopsy for interstitial disease. Experience of 161 consecutive patients from a single institution in Italy. *Sarcoidosis Vasc Diffuse Lung Dis* (2015) 32:251–8.
43. Bando M, Ohno S, Hosono T, Yanase K, Sato Y, Sohara Y, et al. Risk of acute exacerbation after video-assisted thoracoscopic lung biopsy for interstitial lung disease. *J Bronchology Interv Pulmonol* (2009) 16:229–35. doi:10.1097/LBR.0b013e3181b767cc
44. Taniguchi H, Ebina M, Kondoh Y, Ogura T, Azuma A, Suga M, et al. Pirfenidone in idiopathic pulmonary fibrosis. *Eur Respir J* (2010) 35:821–9. doi:10.1183/09031936.00005209
45. Costabel U, Inoue Y, Richeldi L, Collard HR, Tschoepe I, Stowasser S, et al. Efficacy of nintedanib in idiopathic pulmonary fibrosis across prespecified subgroups in INPULSIS. *Am J Respir Crit Care Med* (2016) 193:178–85. doi:10.1164/rccm.201503-0562OC
46. Kuhn C III, Boldt J, King TE Jr, Crouch E, Vartio T, McDonald JA. An immunohistochemical study of architectural remodeling and connective tissue synthesis in pulmonary fibrosis. *Am Rev Respir Dis* (1989) 140:1693–703. doi:10.1164/ajrccm/140.6.1693
47. Konishi K, Gibson KF, Lindell KO, Richards TJ, Zhang Y, Dhir R, et al. Gene expression profiles of acute exacerbations of idiopathic pulmonary fibrosis. *Am J Respir Crit Care Med* (2009) 180:167–75. doi:10.1164/rccm.200810-1596OC
48. Mukae H, Iiboshi H, Nakazato M, Hiratsuka T, Tokojima M, Abe K, et al. Raised plasma concentrations of alpha-defensins in patients with idiopathic pulmonary fibrosis. *Thorax* (2002) 57:623–8. doi:10.1136/thorax.57.7.623
49. van Wetering S, Sterk PJ, Rabe KF, Hiemstra PS. Defensins: key players or bystanders in infection, injury, and repair in the lung? *J Allergy Clin Immunol* (1999) 104:1131–8. doi:10.1016/S0091-6749(99)70004-7
50. Ganz T, Lehrer RI. Defensins. *Curr Opin Immunol* (1994) 6:584–9. doi:10.1016/0952-7915(94)90145-7
51. Sakamoto N, Ishimatsu Y, Kakugawa T, Yura H, Tomonaga M, Harada T, et al. Elevated plasma alpha-defensins in patients with acute exacerbation of fibrotic interstitial pneumonia. *Respir Med* (2015) 109:265–71. doi:10.1016/j.rmed.2014.12.015
52. Moeller A, Gilpin SE, Ask K, Cox G, Cook D, Gauldie J, et al. Circulating fibrocytes are an indicator of poor prognosis in idiopathic pulmonary fibrosis. *Am J Respir Crit Care Med* (2009) 179:588–94. doi:10.1164/rccm.200810-1534OC
53. Bucala R, Spiegel LA, Chesney J, Hogan M, Cerami A. Circulating fibrocytes define a new leukocyte subpopulation that mediates tissue repair. *Mol Med* (1994) 1:71–81.
54. Gomperts BN, Strieter RM. Fibrocytes in lung disease. *J Leukoc Biol* (2007) 82:449–56. doi:10.1189/jlb.0906587
55. Mantovani A, Sica A, Sozzani S, Allavena P, Vecchi A, Locati M. The chemokine system in diverse forms of macrophage activation and polarization. *Trends Immunol* (2004) 25:677–86. doi:10.1016/j.it.2004.09.015
56. Mora AL, Torres-Gonzalez E, Rojas M, Corredor C, Ritzenthaler J, Xu J, et al. Activation of alveolar macrophages via the alternative pathway in herpesvirus-induced lung fibrosis. *Am J Respir Cell Mol Biol* (2006) 35:466–73. doi:10.1165/rcmb.2006-0121OC
57. Willems S, Verleden SE, Vanaudenaerde BM, Wynants M, Dooms C, Yserbyt J, et al. Multiplex protein profiling of bronchoalveolar lavage in idiopathic pulmonary fibrosis and hypersensitivity pneumonitis. *Ann Thorac Med* (2013) 8:38–45. doi:10.4103/1817-1737.105718
58. Prasse A, Pechkovsky DV, Toews GB, Jungraithmayr W, Kollert F, Goldmann T, et al. A vicious circle of alveolar macrophages and fibroblasts perpetuates pulmonary fibrosis via CCL18. *Am J Respir Crit Care Med* (2006) 173:781–92. doi:10.1164/rccm.200509-1518OC
59. Collard HR, Calfee CS, Wolters PJ, Song JW, Hong SB, Brady S, et al. Plasma biomarker profiles in acute exacerbation of idiopathic pulmonary fibrosis. *Am J Physiol Lung Cell Mol Physiol* (2010) 299:L3–7. doi:10.1152/ajplung.90637.2008
60. Okamoto T, Fujii M, Furusawa H, Tsuchiya K, Miyazaki Y, Inase N. The usefulness of KL-6 and SP-D for the diagnosis and management of chronic hypersensitivity pneumonitis. *Respir Med* (2015) 109:1576–81. doi:10.1016/j.rmed.2015.10.005
61. Kishaba T, Shimaoka Y, Fukuyama H, Yoshida K, Tanaka M, Yamashiro S, et al. A cohort study of mortality predictors and characteristics of patients with combined pulmonary fibrosis and emphysema. *BMJ Open* (2012) 2:e000988. doi:10.1136/bmjopen-2012-000988

62. Kohno N, Akiyama M, Kyoizumi S, Hakoda M, Kobuke K, Yamakido M. Detection of soluble tumor-associated antigens in sera and effusions using novel monoclonal antibodies, KL-3 and KL-6, against lung adenocarcinoma. *Jpn J Clin Oncol* (1988) 18:203–16.
63. Kohno N, Kyoizumi S, Awaya Y, Fukuhara H, Yamakido M, Akiyama M. New serum indicator of interstitial pneumonitis activity. Sialylated carbohydrate antigen KL-6. *Chest* (1989) 96:68–73. doi:10.1378/chest.96.1.68
64. Papiris SA, Tomos IP, Karakatsani A, Spathis A, Korbila I, Analitis A, et al. High levels of IL-6 and IL-8 characterize early-on idiopathic pulmonary fibrosis acute exacerbations. *Cytokine* (2017). doi:10.1016/j.cyto.2017.08.019
65. Cao M, Swigris JJ, Wang X, Cao M, Qiu Y, Huang M, et al. Plasma leptin is elevated in acute exacerbation of idiopathic pulmonary fibrosis. *Mediators Inflamm* (2016) 2016:6940480. doi:10.1155/2016/6940480
66. Dafforn TR, Della M, Miller AD. The molecular interactions of heat shock protein 47 (Hsp47) and their implications for collagen biosynthesis. *J Biol Chem* (2001) 276:49310–9. doi:10.1074/jbc.M108896200
67. Kakugawa T, Yokota S, Ishimatsu Y, Hayashi T, Nakashima S, Hara S, et al. Serum heat shock protein 47 levels are elevated in acute exacerbation of idiopathic pulmonary fibrosis. *Cell Stress Chaperones* (2013) 18:581–90. doi:10.1007/s12192-013-0411-5
68. Kahloon RA, Xue J, Bhargava A, Csizmadia E, Otterbein L, Kass DJ, et al. Patients with idiopathic pulmonary fibrosis with antibodies to heat shock protein 70 have poor prognoses. *Am J Respir Crit Care Med* (2013) 187:768–75. doi:10.1164/rccm.201203-0506OC
69. Kurosu K, Takiguchi Y, Okada O, Yumoto N, Sakao S, Tada Y, et al. Identification of annexin 1 as a novel autoantigen in acute exacerbation of idiopathic pulmonary fibrosis. *J Immunol* (2008) 181:756–67. doi:10.4049/jimmunol.181.1.756
70. Tomioka H, Sakurai T, Hashimoto K, Iwasaki H. Acute exacerbation of idiopathic pulmonary fibrosis: role of *Chlamydophila pneumoniae* infection. *Respirology* (2007) 12:700–6. doi:10.1111/j.1440-1843.2007.01119.x
71. Ushiki A, Yamazaki Y, Hama M, Yasuo M, Hanaoka M, Kubo K. Viral infections in patients with an acute exacerbation of idiopathic interstitial pneumonia. *Respir Investig* (2014) 52:65–70. doi:10.1016/j.resinv.2013.07.005
72. Wootton SC, Kim DS, Kondoh Y, Chen E, Lee JS, Song JW, et al. Viral infection in acute exacerbation of idiopathic pulmonary fibrosis. *Am J Respir Crit Care Med* (2011) 183:1698–702. doi:10.1164/rccm.201010-1752OC
73. Bando M, Ohno S, Oshikawa K, Takahashi M, Okamoto H, Sugiyama Y. Infection of TT virus in patients with idiopathic pulmonary fibrosis. *Respir Med* (2001) 95:935–42. doi:10.1053/rmed.2001.1151
74. Huie TJ, Olson AL, Cosgrove GP, Janssen WJ, Lara AR, Lynch DA, et al. A detailed evaluation of acute respiratory decline in patients with fibrotic lung disease: aetiology and outcomes. *Respirology* (2010) 15:909–17. doi:10.1111/j.1440-1843.2010.01774.x
75. Simon-Blancal V, Freynet O, Nunes H, Bouvry D, Naggara N, Brillet PY, et al. Acute exacerbation of idiopathic pulmonary fibrosis: outcome and prognostic factors. *Respiration* (2012) 83:28–35. doi:10.1159/000329891
76. Petrosyan F, Culver DA, Reddy AJ. Role of bronchoalveolar lavage in the diagnosis of acute exacerbations of idiopathic pulmonary fibrosis: a retrospective study. *BMC Pulm Med* (2015) 15:70. doi:10.1186/s12890-015-0066-3
77. Lee JS, Collard HR, Anstrom KJ, Martinez FJ, Noth I, Roberts RS, et al. Anti-acid treatment and disease progression in idiopathic pulmonary fibrosis: an analysis of data from three randomised controlled trials. *Lancet Respir Med* (2013) 1:369–76. doi:10.1016/S2213-2600(13)70105-X
78. Lee JS, Song JW, Wolters PJ, Elicker BM, King TE Jr, Kim DS, et al. Bronchoalveolar lavage pepsin in acute exacerbation of idiopathic pulmonary fibrosis. *Eur Respir J* (2012) 39:352–8. doi:10.1183/09031936.00050911
79. Reichmann WM, Yu YF, Macaulay D, Wu EQ, Nathan SD. Change in forced vital capacity and associated subsequent outcomes in patients with newly diagnosed idiopathic pulmonary fibrosis. *BMC Pulm Med* (2015) 15:167. doi:10.1186/s12890-015-0161-5
80. Selman M, Carrillo G, Estrada A, Mejia M, Becerril C, Cisneros J, et al. Accelerated variant of idiopathic pulmonary fibrosis: clinical behavior and gene expression pattern. *PLoS One* (2007) 2:e482. doi:10.1371/journal.pone.0000482
81. Russell AM, Adamali H, Molyneaux PL, Lukey PT, Marshall RP, Renzoni EA, et al. Daily home spirometry: an effective tool for detecting progression in idiopathic pulmonary fibrosis. *Am J Respir Crit Care Med* (2016) 194:989–97. doi:10.1164/rccm.201511-2152OC
82. Horita N, Akahane M, Okada Y, Kobayashi Y, Arai T, Amano I, et al. Tacrolimus and steroid treatment for acute exacerbation of idiopathic pulmonary fibrosis. *Intern Med* (2011) 50:189–95. doi:10.2169/internalmedicine.50.4327
83. Kakiuchi S, Hanibuchi M, Tezuka T, Saijo A, Otsuka K, Sakaguchi S, et al. Analysis of acute exacerbation of interstitial lung disease associated with chemotherapy in patients with lung cancer: a feasibility of S-1. *Respir Investig* (2017) 55:145–52. doi:10.1016/j.resinv.2016.10.008
84. Takeda A, Enomoto T, Sanuki N, Nakajima T, Takeda T, Sayama K, et al. Acute exacerbation of subclinical idiopathic pulmonary fibrosis triggered by hypofractionated stereotactic body radiotherapy in a patient with primary lung cancer and slightly focal honeycombing. *Radiat Med* (2008) 26:504–7. doi:10.1007/s11604-008-0261-8
85. Kondoh Y, Taniguchi H, Kitaichi M, Yokoi T, Johkoh T, Oishi T, et al. Acute exacerbation of interstitial pneumonia following surgical lung biopsy. *Respir Med* (2006) 100:1753–9. doi:10.1016/j.rmed.2006.02.002
86. Mizuno Y, Iwata H, Shirahashi K, Takamochi K, Oh S, Suzuki K, et al. The importance of intraoperative fluid balance for the prevention of postoperative acute exacerbation of idiopathic pulmonary fibrosis after pulmonary resection for primary lung cancer. *Eur J Cardiothorac Surg* (2012) 41:e161–5. doi:10.1093/ejcts/ezs147
87. Suzuki H, Sekine Y, Yoshida S, Suzuki M, Shibuya K, Yonemori Y, et al. Risk of acute exacerbation of interstitial pneumonia after pulmonary resection for lung cancer in patients with idiopathic pulmonary fibrosis based on preoperative high-resolution computed tomography. *Surg Today* (2011) 41:914–21. doi:10.1007/s00595-010-4384-z
88. Watanabe A, Higami T, Ohori S, Koyanagi T, Nakashima S, Mawatari T. Is lung cancer resection indicated in patients with idiopathic pulmonary fibrosis? *J Thorac Cardiovasc Surg* (2008) 136:1357–63, 1363.e1–2. doi:10.1016/j.jtcvs.2008.07.016
89. Park JS, Kim HK, Kim K, Kim J, Shim YM, Choi YS. Prediction of acute pulmonary complications after resection of lung cancer in patients with preexisting interstitial lung disease. *Thorac Cardiovasc Surg* (2011) 59:148–52. doi:10.1055/s-0030-1250644
90. Ghatol A, Ruhl AP, Danoff SK. Exacerbations in idiopathic pulmonary fibrosis triggered by pulmonary and nonpulmonary surgery: a case series and comprehensive review of the literature. *Lung* (2012) 190:373–80. doi:10.1007/s00408-012-9389-5
91. Choi SM, Lee J, Park YS, Cho YJ, Lee CH, Lee SM, et al. Postoperative pulmonary complications after surgery in patients with interstitial lung disease. *Respiration* (2014) 87:287–93. doi:10.1159/000357046
92. Hiwatari N, Shimura S, Takishima T, Shirato K. Bronchoalveolar lavage as a possible cause of acute exacerbation in idiopathic pulmonary fibrosis patients. *Tohoku J Exp Med* (1994) 174:379–86. doi:10.1620/tjem.174.379
93. Sakamoto K, Taniguchi H, Kondoh Y, Wakai K, Kimura T, Kataoka K, et al. Acute exacerbation of IPF following diagnostic bronchoalveolar lavage procedures. *Respir Med* (2012) 106:436–42. doi:10.1016/j.rmed.2011.11.006
94. Tomic R, Cortes-Puentes GA, Murugan P, Joo Kim H, Amin K, Dincer HE. Acute exacerbation of interstitial lung disease after cryobiopsy. *J Bronchology Interv Pulmonol* (2017) 24:319–22. doi:10.1097/LBR.0000000000000369
95. Casoni GL, Tomassetti S, Cavazza A, Colby TV, Dubini A, Ryu JH, et al. Transbronchial lung cryobiopsy in the diagnosis of fibrotic interstitial lung diseases. *PLoS One* (2014) 9:e86716. doi:10.1371/journal.pone.0086716
96. Jeon K, Chung MP, Lee KS, Chung MJ, Han J, Koh WJ, et al. Prognostic factors and causes of death in Korean patients with idiopathic pulmonary fibrosis. *Respir Med* (2006) 100:451–7. doi:10.1016/j.rmed.2005.06.013
97. Natsuizaka M, Chiba H, Kuronuma K, Otsuka M, Kudo K, Mori M, et al. Epidemiologic survey of Japanese patients with idiopathic pulmonary fibrosis and investigation of ethnic differences. *Am J Respir Crit Care Med* (2014) 190:773–9. doi:10.1164/rccm.201403-0566OC
98. Parambil JG, Myers JL, Aubry MC, Ryu JH. Causes and prognosis of diffuse alveolar damage diagnosed on surgical lung biopsy. *Chest* (2007) 132:50–7. doi:10.1378/chest.07-0104
99. Seo Y, Abe S, Kurahara M, Okada D, Saito Y, Usuki J, et al. Beneficial effect of polymyxin B-immobilized fiber column (PMX) hemoperfusion treatment on acute exacerbation of idiopathic pulmonary fibrosis. *Intern Med* (2006) 45:1033–8. doi:10.2169/internalmedicine.45.6018
100. Bozso S, Sidhu S, Garg M, Freed DH, Nagendran J. Canada's longest experience with extracorporeal membrane oxygenation as a bridge to lung

transplantation: a case report. *Transplant Proc* (2015) 47:186–9. doi:10.1016/j.transproceed.2014.10.039
101. Rush B, Wiskar K, Berger L, Griesdale D. The use of mechanical ventilation in patients with idiopathic pulmonary fibrosis in the United States: a nationwide retrospective cohort analysis. *Respir Med* (2016) 111:72–6. doi:10.1016/j.rmed.2015.12.005
102. Inase N, Sawada M, Ohtani Y, Miyake S, Isogai S, Sakashita H, et al. Cyclosporin A followed by the treatment of acute exacerbation of idiopathic pulmonary fibrosis with corticosteroid. *Intern Med* (2003) 42:565–70. doi:10.2169/internalmedicine.42.565
103. Homma S, Sakamoto S, Kawabata M, Kishi K, Tsuboi E, Motoi N, et al. Cyclosporin treatment in steroid-resistant and acutely exacerbated interstitial pneumonia. *Intern Med* (2005) 44:1144–50. doi:10.2169/internalmedicine.44.1144
104. Sakamoto S, Homma S, Miyamoto A, Kurosaki A, Fujii T, Yoshimura K. Cyclosporin A in the treatment of acute exacerbation of idiopathic pulmonary fibrosis. *Intern Med* (2010) 49:109–15. doi:10.2169/internalmedicine.49.2359
105. Donahoe M, Valentine VG, Chien N, Gibson KF, Raval JS, Saul M, et al. Autoantibody-targeted treatments for acute exacerbations of idiopathic pulmonary fibrosis. *PLoS One* (2015) 10:e0127771. doi:10.1371/journal.pone.0127771
106. Abe S, Azuma A, Mukae H, Ogura T, Taniguchi H, Bando M, et al. Polymyxin B-immobilized fiber column (PMX) treatment for idiopathic pulmonary fibrosis with acute exacerbation: a multicenter retrospective analysis. *Intern Med* (2012) 51:1487–91. doi:10.2169/internalmedicine.51.6965
107. Abe S, Hayashi H, Seo Y, Matsuda K, Kamio K, Saito Y, et al. Reduction in serum high mobility group box-1 level by polymyxin B-immobilized fiber column in patients with idiopathic pulmonary fibrosis with acute exacerbation. *Blood Purif* (2011) 32:310–6. doi:10.1159/000330325
108. Oishi K, Aoe K, Mimura Y, Murata Y, Sakamoto K, Koutoku W, et al. Survival from an acute exacerbation of idiopathic pulmonary fibrosis with or without direct hemoperfusion with a polymyxin B-immobilized fiber column: a retrospective analysis. *Intern Med* (2016) 55:3551–9. doi:10.2169/internalmedicine.55.6056
109. Oishi K, Mimura-Kimura Y, Miyasho T, Aoe K, Ogata Y, Katayama H, et al. Association between cytokine removal by polymyxin B hemoperfusion and improved pulmonary oxygenation in patients with acute exacerbation of idiopathic pulmonary fibrosis. *Cytokine* (2013) 61:84–9. doi:10.1016/j.cyto.2012.08.032
110. Isshiki T, Sakamoto S, Kinoshita A, Sugino K, Kurosaki A, Homma S. Recombinant human soluble thrombomodulin treatment for acute exacerbation of idiopathic pulmonary fibrosis: a retrospective study. *Respiration* (2015) 89:201–7. doi:10.1159/000369828
111. Tsushima K, Yamaguchi K, Kono Y, Yokoyama T, Kubo K, Matsumura T, et al. Thrombomodulin for acute exacerbations of idiopathic pulmonary fibrosis: a proof of concept study. *Pulm Pharmacol Ther* (2014) 29:233–40. doi:10.1016/j.pupt.2014.04.008
112. Kataoka K, Taniguchi H, Kondoh Y, Nishiyama O, Kimura T, Matsuda T, et al. Recombinant human thrombomodulin in acute exacerbation of idiopathic pulmonary fibrosis. *Chest* (2015) 148:436–43. doi:10.1378/chest.14-2746
113. Hayakawa S, Matsuzawa Y, Irie T, Rikitake H, Okada N, Suzuki Y. Efficacy of recombinant human soluble thrombomodulin for the treatment of acute exacerbation of idiopathic pulmonary fibrosis: a single arm, non-randomized prospective clinical trial. *Multidiscip Respir Med* (2016) 11:38. doi:10.1186/s40248-016-0074-z
114. Abe M, Tsushima K, Matsumura T, Ishiwata T, Ichimura Y, Ikari J, et al. Efficacy of thrombomodulin for acute exacerbation of idiopathic pulmonary fibrosis and nonspecific interstitial pneumonia: a nonrandomized prospective study. *Drug Des Devel Ther* (2015) 9:5755–62. doi:10.2147/DDDT.S90739
115. Ding J, Chen Z, Feng K. Procalcitonin-guided antibiotic use in acute exacerbations of idiopathic pulmonary fibrosis. *Int J Med Sci* (2013) 10:903–7. doi:10.7150/ijms.4972
116. Yokoyama T, Kondoh Y, Taniguchi H, Kataoka K, Kato K, Nishiyama O, et al. Noninvasive ventilation in acute exacerbation of idiopathic pulmonary fibrosis. *Intern Med* (2010) 49:1509–14. doi:10.2169/internalmedicine.49.3222
117. Azuma A, Nukiwa T, Tsuboi E, Suga M, Abe S, Nakata K, et al. Double-blind, placebo-controlled trial of pirfenidone in patients with idiopathic pulmonary fibrosis. *Am J Respir Crit Care Med* (2005) 171:1040–7. doi:10.1164/rccm.200404-571OC
118. King TE Jr, Bradford WZ, Castro-Bernardini S, Fagan EA, Glaspole I, Glassberg MK, et al. A phase 3 trial of pirfenidone in patients with idiopathic pulmonary fibrosis. *N Engl J Med* (2014) 370:2083–92. doi:10.1056/NEJMoa1402582
119. Noble PW, Albera C, Bradford WZ, Costabel U, Glassberg MK, Kardatzke D, et al. Pirfenidone in patients with idiopathic pulmonary fibrosis (CAPACITY): two randomised trials. *Lancet* (2011) 377:1760–9. doi:10.1016/S0140-6736(11)60405-4
120. Ley B, Swigris J, Day BM, Stauffer JL, Raimundo K, Chou W, et al. Pirfenidone reduces respiratory-related hospitalizations in idiopathic pulmonary fibrosis. *Am J Respir Crit Care Med* (2017) 196(6):756–61. doi:10.1164/rccm.201701-0091OC
121. Iwata T, Yoshida S, Nagato K, Nakajima T, Suzuki H, Tagawa T, et al. Experience with perioperative pirfenidone for lung cancer surgery in patients with idiopathic pulmonary fibrosis. *Surg Today* (2015) 45:1263–70. doi:10.1007/s00595-014-1071-5
122. Richeldi L, Costabel U, Selman M, Kim DS, Hansell DM, Nicholson AG, et al. Efficacy of a tyrosine kinase inhibitor in idiopathic pulmonary fibrosis. *N Engl J Med* (2011) 365:1079–87. doi:10.1056/NEJMoa1103690
123. Kreuter M, Koegler H, Trampisch M, Geier S, Richeldi L. Efficacy of nintedanib on acute exacerbations reported as serious adverse events in the INPULSIS® trials in idiopathic pulmonary fibrosis (IPF). *American Thoracic Society 2016 International Conference.* (Vol. 193), San Francisco: Am J Respir Crit Care Med (2016).
124. Idiopathic Pulmonary Fibrosis Clinical Research Network, Martinez FJ, de Andrade JA, Anstrom KJ, King TE Jr, Raghu G. Randomized trial of acetylcysteine in idiopathic pulmonary fibrosis. *N Engl J Med* (2014) 370:2093–101. doi:10.1056/NEJMoa1401739
125. Idiopathic Pulmonary Fibrosis Clinical Research Network, Zisman DA, Schwarz M, Anstrom KJ, Collard HR, Flaherty KR, et al. A controlled trial of sildenafil in advanced idiopathic pulmonary fibrosis. *N Engl J Med* (2010) 363:620–8. doi:10.1056/NEJMoa1002110
126. King TE Jr, Brown KK, Raghu G, du Bois RM, Lynch DA, Martinez F, et al. BUILD-3: a randomized, controlled trial of bosentan in idiopathic pulmonary fibrosis. *Am J Respir Crit Care Med* (2011) 184:92–9. doi:10.1164/rccm.201011-1874OC
127. King TE Jr, Albera C, Bradford WZ, Costabel U, Hormel P, Lancaster L, et al. Effect of interferon gamma-1b on survival in patients with idiopathic pulmonary fibrosis (INSPIRE): a multicentre, randomised, placebo-controlled trial. *Lancet* (2009) 374:222–8. doi:10.1016/S0140-6736(09)60551-1
128. Noth I, Anstrom KJ, Calvert SB, de Andrade J, Flaherty KR, Glazer C, et al. A placebo-controlled randomized trial of warfarin in idiopathic pulmonary fibrosis. *Am J Respir Crit Care Med* (2012) 186:88–95. doi:10.1164/rccm.201202-0314OC
129. Raghu G, Behr J, Brown KK, Egan JJ, Kawut SM, Flaherty KR, et al. Treatment of idiopathic pulmonary fibrosis with ambrisentan: a parallel, randomized trial. *Ann Intern Med* (2013) 158:641–9. doi:10.7326/0003-4819-158-9-201305070-00003
130. Daniels CE, Lasky JA, Limper AH, Mieras K, Gabor E, Schroeder DR, et al. Imatinib treatment for idiopathic pulmonary fibrosis: randomized placebo-controlled trial results. *Am J Respir Crit Care Med* (2010) 181:604–10. doi:10.1164/rccm.200906-0964OC
131. Idiopathic Pulmonary Fibrosis Clinical Research Network, Raghu G, Anstrom KJ, King TE Jr, Lasky JA, Martinez FJ. Prednisone, azathioprine, and N-acetylcysteine for pulmonary fibrosis. *N Engl J Med* (2012) 366:1968–77. doi:10.1056/NEJMoa1113354
132. Papiris SA, Kagouridis K, Kolilekas L, Papaioannou AI, Roussou A, Triantafillidou C, et al. Survival in idiopathic pulmonary fibrosis acute exacerbations: the non-steroid approach. *BMC Pulm Med* (2015) 15:162. doi:10.1186/s12890-015-0146-4
133. Lamas DJ, Kawut SM, Bagiella E, Philip N, Arcasoy SM, Lederer DJ. Delayed access and survival in idiopathic pulmonary fibrosis: a cohort study. *Am J Respir Crit Care Med* (2011) 184:842–7. doi:10.1164/rccm.201104-0668OC
134. Johannson KA, Vittinghoff E, Morisset J, Lee JS, Balmes JR, Collard HR. Home monitoring improves endpoint efficiency in idiopathic pulmonary fibrosis. *Eur Respir J* (2017) 50:1602406. doi:10.1183/13993003.02406-2016

13

Zoledronic Acid Targeting of the Mevalonate Pathway Causes Reduced Cell Recruitment and Attenuates Pulmonary Fibrosis

Lloyd Tanner[1], Jesper Bergwik[1], Andrew B. Single[1†], Ravi K. V. Bhongir[1], Jonas S. Erjefält[2] and Arne Egesten[1]*

[1]Respiratory Medicine, Allergology, and Palliative Medicine, Department of Clinical Sciences Lund, Lund University and Skåne University Hospital, Lund, Sweden, [2]Unit of Airway Inflammation, Department of Experimental Medical Sciences, Lund University, Lund, Sweden

***Correspondence:**
Lloyd Tanner
lloyd.tanner@med.lu.se

†Present Address:
Andrew B. Single,
Norwegian University of Science and Technology (NTNU), Trondheim, Norway

Background and aim: Idiopathic pulmonary fibrosis (IPF) is a progressive lung disease causing irreparable scarring of lung tissue, with most patients succumbing rapidly after diagnosis. The mevalonate pathway, which is involved in the regulation of cell proliferation, survival, and motility, is targeted by the bisphosphonate zoledronic acid (ZA). The aim of this study was to assess the antifibrotic effects of ZA and to elucidate the mechanisms by which potential IPF treatment occurs.

Methods: A series of *in vitro* and *in vivo* models were employed to identify the therapeutic potential of ZA in treating IPF. *In vitro* transwell assays were used to assess the ability of ZA to reduce fibrotic-related immune cell recruitment. Farnesyl diphosphate synthase (FDPS) was screened as a potential antifibrotic target using a bleomycin mouse model. FDPS-targeting siRNA and ZA were administered to mice following the onset of experimentally-induced lung fibrosis. Downstream analyses were conducted on murine lung tissues and lung fluids including 23-plex cytokine array, flow cytometry, histology, Western blotting, immunofluorescent staining, and PCR analysis.

Results: *In vitro* administration of ZA reduced myofibroblast transition and blocked NF-κB signaling in macrophages leading to impaired immune cell recruitment in a transwell assay. FDPS-targeting siRNA administration significantly attenuated profibrotic cytokine production and lung damage in a murine lung fibrosis model. Furthermore, ZA treatment of mice with bleomycin-induced lung damage displayed decreased cytokine levels in the BALF, plasma, and lung tissue, resulting in less histologically visible fibrotic scarring. Bleomycin-induced upregulation of the ZA target, FDPS, was reduced in lung tissue and fibroblasts upon ZA treatment. Confirmatory increases in FDPS immunoreactivity was seen in human IPF resected lung samples compared to control tissue indicating potential translational value of the approach. Additionally, ZA polarized macrophages towards a less profibrotic phenotype contributing to decreased IPF pathogenesis.

Conclusion: This study highlights ZA as an expedient and efficacious treatment option against IPF in a clinical setting.

Keywords: IPF, Zoledronic Acid, mevalonate, Fibrosis, FDPS, drug repurposing

INTRODUCTION

Idiopathic pulmonary fibrosis (IPF) is a disorder characterized by progressive lung scarring with a median survival time of 3 years postdiagnosis (Raghu et al., 2011, 2019; Chang et al., 2020). IPF is associated with increasing cough and dyspnea, affecting approximately 3 million people worldwide (Martinez et al., 2017; Lederer and Martinez, 2018). Mechanistically, IPF is thought to be driven by chronic and repeated epithelial injury-repair responses leading to epithelial-mesenchymal transition and other resultant changes (Wynn and Vannella, 2016; Skibba et al., 2020; Baratella et al., 2021). Following repeated epithelial damage, fibroblasts and epithelial cells are triggered to transition, migrate, and proliferate resulting in excessive extracellular matrix (ECM) deposition (Hu and Phan, 2013; Cutolo et al., 2018; Piera-Velazquez and Jimenez, 2018; Zhang et al., 2019; Skibba et al., 2020).

Additionally, inflammatory cells such as monocytes and tissue-resident macrophages play crucial roles in tissue injury and wound healing responses, displaying diverse phenotypes to control a multitude of regulatory functions during IPF progression (Vannella and Wynn, 2017; Upagupta et al., 2018; Zhang et al., 2018; Chakarov et al., 2019; Guilliams et al., 2020; Henderson et al., 2020). Current IPF therapies focus on the inhibition of collagen deposition by blocking myofibroblast activation and proliferation, with limited success in achieving overall IPF resolution, necessitating the need for novel therapies (Lederer and Martinez, 2018). Drug repurposing allows for shortened preclinical and clinical trial periods from an estimated 10–12 years to 3–4 years, allowing patients to benefit from cheaper medications (Xue et al., 2018; Fetro and Scherman, 2020).

In this study we repurposed zoledronic acid (ZA), a drug commonly used for the treatment of post-menopausal onset of osteoporosis and hypercalcemia associated with multiple myeloma (Watts and Diab, 2010), in *in vitro* and *in vivo* models of pulmonary fibrosis. In our study, a bleomycin-challenged murine model was used to assess ZA's anti-fibrotic efficacy. Bleomycin-induced fibrosis reproduces several phenotypic features of human IPF, including peripheral alveolar septal thickening, dysregulated cytokine production, and immune cell influx (Tashiro et al., 2017; Tanner and Single, 2019).

The primary target of bisphosphonates is farnesyl diphosphate synthase (FDPS), a key enzyme in the mevalonate pathway (Dunford et al., 2001). Isoprenoid intermediates derived from the mevalonate pathway are utilized in post-translational modifications of several proteins, including Rho GTPases, regulating important cellular functions including modulation of the actin cytoskeleton (Tsou et al., 2014; Larson-Casey et al., 2019). Taken together, increased mevalonate pathway intermediates facilitate the differentiation and movement of pro-fibrotic cell-types and an increased production of reactive oxygen species, potentially leading to IPF onset (Zeng et al., 2003; Chen et al., 2007; Larson-Casey et al., 2016).

We show herein, that FDPS is decreased in control patient lung samples versus IPF lung tissue. Subsequent administration of FDPS-targeting siRNA directly to the lung, reduced bleomycin induced fibrotic lung damage. Similarly, bleomycin administered mice displayed increased *FDPS* expression versus ZA-administered animals. In an IPF context, increased profibrotic macrophage populations have been found in the blood of IPF patients as well as in the lungs of bleomycin-treated mice (Zhou et al., 2014). We show that ZA administration confers beneficial macrophage repolarization and modulation of the fibrotic response, highlighting FDPS as a tractable therapeutic target. ZA is particularly interesting in a clinical context due to its FDA approval and acceptable safety profile, with transient flu-like symptoms and less-commonly occurring osteonecrosis of the jaw the main reported side effects (Rosen et al., 2003).

The aim of this study was to assess the antifibrotic effects of ZA and to delineate any antifibrotic mechanisms associated with FDPS-targeting. The repurposing of bisphosphonates for use in pulmonary fibrosis-related disease is a unique concept that is not currently described in the literature. If successfully applied in the clinic, the novel treatment strategies described in this study would decrease the rate of disease progression associated with IPF.

MATERIALS AND METHODS

Study Design

Further details regarding the materials and methods used can be found in the **Supplementary Material.** *In vivo* murine studies using intratracheally-administered bleomycin were chosen as well-established and relevant models of experimental lung fibrosis (Tashiro et al., 2017; Tanner and Single, 2019). Sample sizes were calculated by power analysis based on previous experience, feasibility, and to conform to the ARRIVE guidelines (arriveguidelines.org). For lung fibrosis experiments testing, $n \geq 8$ to 15 mice per group were used to achieve statistical significance as calculated using G Power Software (ANOVA, with fixed effects, omnibus, one-way). For siRNA experiments, demonstrating FDPS as a target for IPF treatment, $n = 5$ mice per group were used. Mice were randomly assigned to treatment groups. Downstream analyses were conducted with the investigator blinded to the treatment groups, and no animals were excluded as outliers from the reported dataset. All *in vitro* and *in vivo* experiments were performed in 2–4 technical replicates. Macroscopically normal, tumor-free lung tissue samples (control tissue) were obtained during transplantation or resection from patients undergoing cancer surgery or from patients with IPF diagnosed by techniques supplemented by spirometry (**Supplementary Table S2**). Patients undergoing lung biopsies with confirmed distal lung fibrosis (by histological analysis), or high-resolution computerized tomography (HRCT) scans with characteristic IPF features (e. g., opaque fibrosis-like areas and 'honeycombing' in the lung parenchyma) were included in this study (n = 4 per group).

Ethical Approval

All animal experiments in this study were approved by the Malmö-Lund Animal Care Ethics Committee (M17009-18). Lung tissue used for immunoreactivity assays was obtained after written informed consent, approval by the Regional Ethical Review Board in Lund (approval no. LU412-03), and performed in accordance with the Declaration of Helsinki as well as relevant guidelines and regulations.

Fibroblast Transwell Experiment

Human lung fibroblasts (HFL-1; ATCC, Manassas, VA, United States) were cultured until confluent in complete growth medium supplemented with L-glutamine, 100 U/mL penicillin, 100 μg/ml streptomycin, and 10% FBS. Fibroblast chemotaxis was measured using 24-well Nunc (8-μm pore size) Transwell inserts (Thermo Fisher, Waltham, MA, United States). Following confluence, cells were seeded (5×10^5 cells/ml) into the upper chamber in FBS-free medium, whilst the lower chamber contained complete medium with additional 10% FBS as a chemoattractant. Experiments were carried out in experimental triplicate, with each experiment containing 4 biological replicates. Medium containing transforming growth factor beta 1 (TGF-β1; 2 ng/ml) followed by the addition of medium containing zoledronic acid (ZA; 2 μM), medium only, or vehicle only (dimethyl sulfoxide; DMSO 2% and phosphate-buffered saline (PBS) pH 7.4). Following 48 h, medium was removed and cells in the lower chamber were stained (crystal violet) and imaged using a Nikon Eclipse 80i Compound Fluorescent Microscope and analyzed using Nikon NIS Elements F4.60.00.

MTT Assay

Mosmann's MTT [3-(4,5-dimethylthiazol-2-yl)-2,5-diphenyltetrazolium bromide] assay was used to determine cell viability in both RAW264.7 and THP-1 cells. After the addition of the compounds at a starting concentration of 1000 μM (serial diluted to 0.1 μM), and incubation for 48 h, each well received MTT at a concentration of 5 mg/ml in phosphate-buffered saline (PBS), with blank samples receiving only medium and MTT. Each compound concentration tested in this study was completed in triplicate. DMSO was added to each well, followed by plate shaking for 5 min to dissolve the formazan crystals. The absorbance of the formazan salt was measured at 540 nm by a VICTOR 1420 Multilabel plate reader. The following formula **Eq. 1** was used to calculate the cell viability:

$$\begin{aligned} Percentage\ viability &= sample\ absorbance \\ &- blank\ absorbance / control\ absorbance \\ &- blank\ absorbance\ X100 \end{aligned} \tag{1}$$

Nonlinear dose response curves were constructed using GraphPad Prism 4 software (GraphPad Software, San Diego, CA, United States) and Microsoft Excel.

Immunostaining of Embryonic Mouse Fibroblasts

Murine C57BL/6 embryonic fibroblasts (MEFs) were seeded (1×10^4 cells/mL) into 24-well plates containing rounded glass cover slips. TGF-β1 (2 ng/ml) was added to each well, followed by the addition of medium containing ZA or vehicle only. Following 48 h of treatment, cells were washed and fixed with ice cold methanol, containing 0.5% Triton-X100. Slides were blocked using Dako Protein Block (Agilent, Santa Clara, CA, United States) for 1 h at room temperature and then stained with primary antibodies (overnight), rabbit anti-COL1AI, rabbit anti-αSMA, and rabbit anti-fibronectin (Abcam, Cambridge, United Kingdom). Alexa Fluor 488-conjugated goat anti-rabbit antibody (Invitrogen, Carlsbad, CA, United States) was used as secondary antibody (2 h). Glass cover slips were removed and mounted onto glass slides, with nuclei counterstained using DAPI containing fluoroshield (Abcam). Images were visualized using a Nikon Eclipse 80i Compound Fluorescent Microscope and analyzed using Nikon NIS Elements F4.60.00.

Ex vivo Cell Recruitment Assay

BAL was performed on C57BL/6 mice (n = 10) with a total volume of 1 ml PBS containing 100 μM EDTA. BALF was collected in Eppendorf tubes on ice and immediately separated using the Anti-F4/80 MicroBeads UltraPure (mouse; 130-110-443), dead cell removal kit (130-090-101), MS columns (130-042-201), and QuadroMACS™ Separator (130-090-976; Miltenyi Biotec, Bergisch Gladbach, Germany). Purified murine macrophages were counted and run on a BD Accuri C6 flow cytometer to determine cell purity. Concurrently, murine blood was isolated *via* heart puncture and collected in EDTA-containing tubes. Murine PBMCs were isolated using Ficoll-Paque PREMIUM 1.084 (Sigma-Aldrich, Saint Louis, MO, United States) density centrifugation (400 x g for 40 min) and subsequently counted. In the transwell plate, murine macrophages were added to the bottom well (5×10^5 cells/well), with murine PBMCs (6×10^6 cells/well) added to the top chamber. Following 24 h of RANKL (10 ng/ml) macrophage stimulation, cells were harvested and stained for flow cytometry analysis carried out using a BD Accuri C6 (BD, Franklin Lakes, NJ, United States). Samples were separated into 3 aliquots, 1) alveolar macrophages as identified by F4/80 (BM8; 11-4321-42), CD11b (BD553312), and I-A/I-E (BD557000); 2) B and T cells as identified by CD45 (BD553079), CD3 Molecular Complex (BD 555276), CD19 (BD561736); 3) macrophage subtypes and neutrophils as identified by CD11b (BD553312), CD11c (BD558079), Ly-6G (BD551461).

Mouse Macrophage (M1/M2) *Ex Vivo* Assay

BAL was performed on C57BL/6 mice (n = 10) with a total volume of 1 ml PBS containing 100 μM EDTA. BALF was collected in Eppendorf tubes on ice and immediately separated using the Anti-F4/80 MicroBeads UltraPure and QuadroMACS™ Separator as indicated above. Isolated murine macrophages were added to 12-well plates at 5×10^8 cells/well. Cells were stimulated with interleukin-4 (IL-4) and IL-13 (20 ng/ml, PeproTech, NJ, United States) for 48 h followed by flow cytometry analysis (BD Accuri C6) to assess M1/M2 phenotype. Cells were gated using the following antibodies: CD206 (BioLegend, 141705), CD11b (BD553312), CD11c (BD558079), and F4/80 (BD 565635).

Animals

10-12-week-old male C57BL/6 mice (Janvier, Le Genest-Saint-Isle, France) were housed at least 2 weeks in the animal facility at the Biomedical Service Division at Lund University before initiating experiments and were provided with food and water *ad libitum* throughout the study. Mice were randomly allocated into five groups (n = 4-15 animals per group): intratracheally (i.t.)-administered bleomycin (2.5 U/kg) + vehicle (i.p./i.t.), bleomycin (i.t.) +ZA (0.1 mg/kg; i. p./i.t.), saline (i.t.) + vehicle (i.p./i.t.), and saline (i.t.) + ZA (0.1 mg/kg; i. p./i.t.).

siRNA Administration

For lung fibrosis experiments testing the viability of *Fdps* as a drug target in siRNA experiments, $n \geq 4$ to 5 mice per group were used to achieve statistical significance. Mice were randomly assigned to treatment groups. For the siRNA experiments, lung fibrosis was induced by intratracheal introduction of bleomycin (2.5 U/kg) or saline as control. Following 14 days, siRNA targeting mouse *Fdps* (L-059452-01-0020) or nontargeting control (D-001810-01-50) mRNA (Horizon Discovery, Water Beach, United Kingdom) was administered intratracheally at either 25 µg per mouse (*Fdps* siRNA) or 25 µg of nontargeting siRNA. On day 21, mice were euthanized followed by collection of blood, lung tissue, and BALF. Downstream analyses were conducted with the investigator blinded to the treatment groups, and no animals were excluded as outliers from the reported dataset. All *in vitro* and *in vivo* experiments were performed in two to four technical replicates. Human resected lung sections were obtained with informed consent, with a statistically significant n = 4 samples used for disease and control samples.

Blood Collection

Blood was collected in 0.5 M EDTA tubes by cardiac puncture and centrifuged at 1,000 x *g* for 10 min. Plasma supernatant was used for the analysis of inflammatory mediators using a multiplex assay (Bio-plex assay; Bio-Rad, Hercules, CA, United States).

Collection of Lung Tissue

Right lungs were collected in Eppendorf tubes on dry ice and stored at -80°C. The snap-frozen lungs were thawed and homogenized in tissue protein extraction reagent (T-PER) solution (Thermo Fisher Scientific) containing protease inhibitor (Pefabloc SC; Sigma-Aldrich) at a final concentration of 1 mM. Lung homogenates were centrifuged at 9,000 x *g* for 10 min at 4°C, and the supernatants were collected for multiplex analysis. Left lungs were collected in Histofix (Histolab, Göteborg, Sweden) and submerged in 4% buffered paraformaldehyde solution.

Bronchoalveolar Lavage Fluid (BALF) Collection

BAL was performed with a total volume of 1 ml PBS containing 100 µM EDTA. BALF was collected in Eppendorf tubes on ice, with aliquots made for flow cytometry, cytospin differential counts, and an aliquot transferred to -80°C for multiplex cytokine analysis. Cytospin preparations of cells were stained with modified Wright-Giemsa stain (Sigma-Aldrich).

SDS-PAGE and Western Blotting

Lung homogenate lysates were analyzed for total protein concentration (Pierce BCA Protein Assay Kit, Thermoscientific). Samples were run on Mini-PROTEAN® Precast Mini polyacrylamide gel electrophoresis (PAGE) Gels (BioRad). Samples were transferred to Trans-Blot Turbo Mini 0.2 µm; polyvinylidene difluoride (PVDF) Transfer Packs with blots incubated overnight with primary antibodies (1:1000) in blocking buffer, collagen 1A1 (COL1A1; ab88147), arginase 1 (ARG1; ab239731), cluster of differentiation 206 (CD206; ab64693), glyceraldehyde 3-phosphate dehydrogenase (GAPDH; ab8245), farnesyl diphosphate synthase (FDPS; ab153805, Abcam), alpha smooth muscle actin (α-SMA; 19245, cell signaling). Blots were washed with PBS-Tween, before 1 h incubation with Alexa Fluor 488-conjugated goat anti-rabbit/mouse secondary antibodies (Invitrogen, Carlsbad, CA, United States). Blots were imaged using a BioRad ChemiDoc system. Quantification was performed *via* densitometry and normalized using GAPDH.

Flow Cytometry

Flow cytometry was carried out using a BD Accuri C6 (BD). The washed cells were incubated with Fixable Viability Stain 510 (FVS510) (BD564406) to differentiate live and dead cells. Cells were washed with Stain buffer 1x (BD554656) and incubated with Lyse Fix 1x (BD558049 (5x)). Fixed cells were washed with stain buffer and aliquoted into two parts. One was incubated with CD11b (BD553312), CD11c (BD558079), Ly-6G (BD551461) antibodies and the other aliquot was incubated with CD11c, MHC (BD558593), SiglecF (BD562680) antibodies.

Bioplex Cytokine Analysis

For the detection of multiple cytokines in BALF, plasma, and lung homogenate, the Bio-Plex Pro mouse cytokine assay (23-Plex Group I; Bio-Rad) was used on a Luminex-xMAP/Bio-Plex 200 System with Bio-Plex Manager 6.2 software (Bio-Rad). A cytometric magnetic bead-based assay was used to measure cytokine levels, according to the manufacturer's instructions. The detection limits were as follows: Eotaxin (21372.02–1.15 pg/ml), GCSF (124018.4–6.97 pg/ml), GMCSF (1161.99–3.73), IFN-γ (14994.64–0.72 pg/ml), IL-1α (10337.5–0.63 pg/ml), IL-1β (28913.54–1.57 pg/ml), IL-2 (22304.34–1.21 pg/ml), IL-3 (7639.21–0.47 pg/ml), IL-4 (6334.86–0.36 pg/ml), IL-5 (12950.39–0.76 pg/ml), IL-6 (11370.16–0.66 pg/ml), IL-9 (2580.93–2.46 pg/ml), IL-10 (76949.87–4.09 pg/ml), IL-12p40 (323094.58–17.38 pg/ml), IL-12p70 (79308.46–19.51 pg/ml), IL-13 (257172.3–53.85 pg/ml),

IL-17 (8355.61–0.5 pg/ml), KC (23377.88–1.3 pg/ml), MCP-1 (223776.6–45.04 pg/ml), MIP-1α (14038.07–0.58 pg/ml), MIP-1β (928.18–2.39 pg/ml), RANTES (4721.74–4.42 pg/ml), and TNF-α (73020.1–4.61 pg/ml). Cytokine measurements for samples were corrected for protein concentration, measured using a Pierce™ BCA Protein Assay Kit (Thermo Fischer Scientific).

Hydroxyproline Assay

Hydroxyproline levels were determined using the QuickZyme Hydroxyproline Assay kit (Quickzyme Biosciences, Leiden, Netherlands). Hydroxylation of proline groups within the collagen molecule result in the formation of hydroxyproline, with the modified amino acid stabilizing the helical structure in mature collagen (Berg and Prockop, 1973). Hydroxyproline is highly specific for collagen, allowing hydroxyproline measurements to accurately reflect the amount of collagen in fibrotic lung tissue (de Jong et al., 2012). Lung tissues were homogenized as described above. Homogenates were diluted (1:1 vol:vol) with 12 N HCl and hydrolyzed at 95°C for 20 h. After centrifugation at 13,000 × *g* for 10 min, 200 μl from the supernatant was taken and diluted 1:2 with 4 N HCl. Hydroxyproline standard (6.25–300 μM) was prepared in 4 N HCl and transferred to the microtiter plate. Following addition of a chloramine T-containing assay buffer, samples were oxidized for 20 min at RT. Detection reagent containing p-dimethylaminobenzaldehyde was added and after incubation at 60°C for 1 h, absorbance was read at 570 nm with a VICTOR 1420 Multilabel plate reader (PerkinElmer, Waltham, MA, United States). The hydroxyproline content in lung tissue is given as hydroxyproline (μg) per mg lung tissue, corrected using a Pierce™ BCA Protein Assay Kit (Thermo Fisher Scientific).

H&E and Picrosirius Red Staining of Lung Tissue

A segment of the left lung was fixed in Histofix (Histolab) and embedded into paraffin and sectioned (3 μm) with a microtome. The tissue sections were placed on slides (Superfrost Plus; Fisher Scientific) and deparaffinized in serial baths of xylene and ethanol followed by staining using Mayer hematoxylin and 0.2% eosin (Histolab) or picrosirius red staining kit (Abcam, Cambridge, United Kingdom). The stained slides were imaged using an Olympus BX60F microscope with an SC50 camera.

Immunostaining of Murine Lung Sections

Lung tissue sections were fixed as reported above. Lung samples underwent antigen retrieval (pH 9 buffer) using a Dako PT Link pre-treatment module (Agilent). Samples were washed and blocked for 10 min (Dako protein block; Agilent, Santa Clara, CA) before being treated with primary antibodies overnight. Mouse anti-COL1A1, ARG1, and rabbit anti-FDPS, CD206 (Abcam, Cambridge, United Kingdom) antibodies were used. Alexa Fluor 488-conjugated goat/anti-mouse and Alexa Fluor 647 goat/anti-rabbit (Invitrogen, Waltham, CA, United States) were used as secondary antibodies. Glass cover slips were placed onto slides and mounted with DAPI-containing fluoroshield (Abcam). Microscopy was performed on a Widefield Epifluorescence Ti2 microscope equipped with a Nikon DS-Qi2 camera and fluorescence was quantified using ImageJ software.

Real-Time PCR

Extraction of total mRNA from frozen lung tissue and MEF cells was performed using RNeasy Mini Kit (Qiagen, Valencia, CA, United States), in accordance with manufacturer's instructions. RNA concentrations were determined using a NanoDrop ND1000 (Saveen Werner AB, Malmö, Sweden). RNA to cDNA conversion was achieved using an iScript Advanced cDNA Synthesis Kit (Bio-Rad). Gene expression was measured using TaqMan™ Fast Advanced Master Mix together with TaqMan™ probes listed in **Supplementary Table S1**. RT-PCR reactions were analyzed using a QuantStudio™ 7 Flex system (Thermo Fisher Scientific) in 384-well plates. Data was analyzed with QuantStudio™ Real-Time PCR Software v1.3. The obtained Ct-values were normalized to succinate dehydrogenase complex subunit A (*Sdha*) expression, generating ΔCt-values. ΔΔCt-values were obtained by normalizing values to ΔCt-of the PBS only group.

Immunohistochemistry of Human Lung Samples

Macroscopically normal, tumor-free lung tissue samples were obtained during transplantation or resection from patients undergoing cancer surgery, with IPF patients diagnosed/identified by techniques supplemented by spirometry. Patients undergoing lung biopsies with confirmed distal lung fibrosis (by histological analysis), or high-resolution computerized tomography (HRCT) scans with characteristic IPF features (e.g., opaque fibrosis-like areas and "honeycombing" in the lung parenchyma) were included in this study, with clinical data reported in **Supplementary Table S2**. Immediately after collection, samples were placed in 4% buffered formaldehyde. Following dehydration and embedding in paraffin, sections (3 μm) were produced. A single staining protocol (EnVision™ Detection system, K5007, Dako, Glostrup, Denmark) was used for visualization of FDPS. Briefly, after antigen retrieval, FDPS was detected using rabbit anti-FDPS (Abcam) antibody (1:1000) and visualized using secondary goat anti-rabbit antibodies conjugated with peroxidase polymers (Dako). Sections were counter-stained with Mayer's hematoxylin for visualization of background tissue, dehydrated in alcohol/xylene, and mounted on Pertex (Histolab, Göteborg, Sweden). The stained slides were imaged using an Aperio CS2 image capture device. Positive staining was quantified manually (number of cells/area of tissue) or as positivity (positive brown pixels divided by all stained pixels) using computerized image analysis on blinded sections using ImageScope (Aperio, Leica Biosystems, Wetzlar, Germany).

Statistical Analysis

To assess the effects of ZA in murine models, results were compared using one-way analysis of variance (ANOVA) with

Dunnett's post hoc test. In experiments using two groups, results were compared using an unpaired *t*-test with Welch's correction. Results in this study are displayed throughout as mean ± standard error of the mean (SEM). Statistical testing was carried out using GraphPad Prism 9.1.1 with statistical significance defined as $p < 0.05$.

RESULTS

Zoledronic Acid Reduces Fibroblast to Myofibroblast Transition and Production of Fibrotic Proteins

To determine ZA involvement in fibroblast to myofibroblast transition (FMT), human lung fibroblasts (HFL-1) were utilized in a transwell assay (**Figure 1A**). Following stimulation with TGF-β1 for 48 h, cell transition through the transwell membrane was measured. ZA treatment (2 μM) significantly reduced myofibroblast transition ($p < 0.001$). Additionally, staining of mouse embryonic fibroblast cells (MEF) treated with ZA revealed the production of less collagen, fibronectin, and α-smooth muscle actin than in the TGF-β1 control, as measured by immunofluorescence (**Figure 1B**).

Reduced NF-κB Macrophage Signaling Moderates Immune Cell Recruitment

To demonstrate the role of ZA in reducing NF-κB signaling, monocytic (THP1-Blue™ NF-κB) cells were stimulated with RANK ligand (RANKL) for 48 h (**Figure 1C**). ZA significantly reduced RANKL-induced NF-κB signaling at all tested concentrations with ZA not displaying cytotoxicity in either murine macrophages (RAW264.7) or THP1 cells at levels greater than 3 μM (**Figure 1D**). Following reductions in NF-κB, we examined macrophage-mediated immune cell recruitment from murine peripheral blood inhibition by ZA treatment (**Figure 1E**). A wide variety of immune cells were measured using flow cytometry and revealed significant decreases between the RANKL and ZA/RANKL treated samples in recruitment of T cells, neutrophils, inflammatory macrophages, and alveolar macrophages (**Figure 1F**).

Zoledronic Acid Attenuates Murine Weight Loss and Fibrotic Lung Damage

Given the *in vitro* effect of ZA treatment in reducing fibrotic-related damage, a murine model of bleomycin-induced lung damage was employed, with ZA dosed either intratracheally (i.t.) or intraperitoneally (i.p.; 0.1 mg/kg) at day 15 (**Figure 2A**). Murine weight loss was dramatically mitigated following i. p. ZA treatment, whilst i. t. ZA treatment offered less protection (**Figure 2B**). The probability of survival was significantly increased following ZA i. p. administration ($p = 0.0329$), whereas i. t. administration showed no statistically significant difference (**Figure 2C**). Murine lung weight and hydroxyproline levels provide proxies for generalized lung damage and collagen content, with i. p. administration of ZA reducing both lung weight ($p < 0.0001$) and hydroxyproline levels ($p = 0.0143$) compared to vehicle/bleomycin mice (**Figures 2D,E**). Additionally, western blot analysis on lung tissue showed a significantly reduced production of the fibrotic proteins COL1A1 and α-SMA after administration of ZA (**Figure 2F** and **Supplementary Figure S8**). Images of murine lungs revealed decreased areas of fibrosis after i. p. treatment with ZA (**Figure 2G**).

Murine Immune Cell Recruitment to the Lung Is Impaired by Zoledronic Acid

Administration of ZA effectively reduces regulatory T cell involvement in immune cell recruitment in cancer and fibrosis (Ichikawa et al., 2019; Liu et al., 2019), with a large proportion of these recruited cells being macrophages and neutrophils. Investigation of ZA treatment effects on immune cell infiltration into the airways was performed by flow cytometry on BALF obtained from *in vivo* bleomycin studies at day 21. Decreases in neutrophil count and inflammatory macrophages were seen following both i. p. ($p < 0.0001$) and i. t. (neutrophils: $p = 0.0417$; inflammatory macrophages: $p = 0.0213$) ZA administration compared to vehicle/bleomycin samples (**Figures 3A–C**). Giemsa-Wright-stained BALF samples showed bleomycin-treated macrophages were enlarged and present in greater number, a phenomenon not seen in mice treated with ZA (i.p.; **Figure 3D**).

Murine Lung Structure Is Maintained Following Intraperitoneal ZA Administration

To determine whether murine histological damage was reduced more efficaciously by a single route of administration, both i. p. and i. t. lung samples from mice treated with ZA were assessed using H&E and picrosirius red staining (**Figures 4A,B; Supplementary Figure S1 and 2**). ZA administered i. p. quantitatively reduced bleomycin-induced closure of the alveolar structures ($p < 0.0001$), with significant decreases in collagen deposition ($p < 0.0001$) seen in these samples compared to the vehicle/bleomycin samples. Conversely, intratracheally-administered ZA did not confer protection from lung damage as seen in both the H&E ($p = 0.7009$) and picrosirius red staining ($p = 0.0839$).

Cytokine Production Elucidates Decreased Immune Cell Recruitment Following ZA Treatment

The effect of i. p. ZA treatment on inflammatory cytokine levels was investigated in murine samples from the *in vivo* study using a 23-cytokine inflammation multiplex assay (**Supplementary Figures S3–S5**). The majority of cytokines were reduced in the BALF, plasma, and lung tissue following ZA treatment. In particular, lung homogenate decreases were seen for IL-4 ($p = 0.0289$), IL-6 ($p = 0.0007$), GM-CSF ($p < 0.0001$), KC ($p < 0.0001$), and MCP-1 ($p = 0.0389$) compared to the vehicle/bleomycin

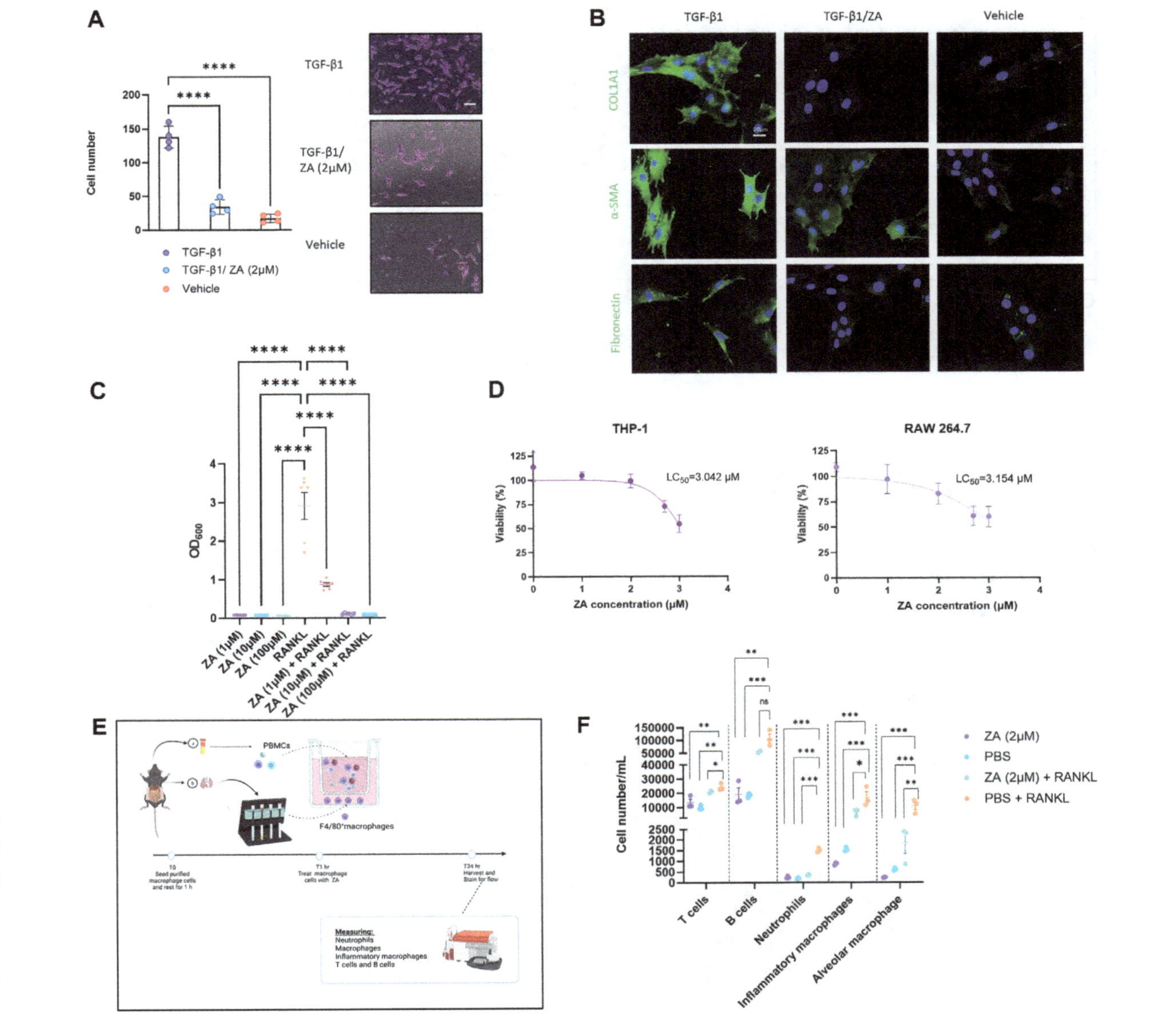

FIGURE 1 | Zoledronic acid (ZA) inhibits *in vitro* transwell migration and fibrotic marker expression, whilst simultaneously reducing nuclear factor kappa-light-chain-enhancer of activated B cells (NF-κB) signaling and immune cell recruitment. **(A)** ZA reduced myofibroblast migration and proliferation in a transwell assay compared to vehicle treatment and no treatment controls (Student's *t*-test, $p < 0.005$ (***) and $p < 0.0001$ (****), with representative myofibroblast cells in lower chamber of transwell insert following 48 h shown. **(B)** Immunostaining of fibroblast cells following 48 h of TGF-β1 treatment, with ZA treatment displaying visually reduced levels of collagen, fibronectin and alpha smooth muscle actin (α-SMA) compared to no treatment control. **(C)** RAW264.7 and THP1-Blue™ NF-κB cells were subjected to receptor activator of nuclear factor kappa beta (RANKL) treatment for 48h, with NF-κB signaling significantly reduced by ZA ($p < 0.0001$) and **(D)** low levels of cytotoxicity reported for ZA against both THP-1 and RAW 264.7 cells. **(E,F)** Isolated murine macrophage cells (bottom well) and peripheral blood mononuclear cells (PBMCs) (top well) were exposed to RANKL in a transwell system, with significant reductions in T cells, neutrophils, and macrophage cells following ZA treatment (drug-treated samples were compared to untreated control samples using a one-way ANOVA followed by a Dunnett's post-hoc test; $N = 3$ technical replicates, from 3 biological replicates per measurement).

group (**Figures 5A–C**). Decreased immune cell recruitment following ZA treatment in murine BALF is supported by reduced murine cytokine levels in murine BALF and plasma. Shared decreases were seen in both fluids for IL-6, GM-CSF, KC, MCP-1, and other cytokines indicative of reduced immune cell recruitment following ZA (i.p.) treatment (**Figures 5A,B; Supplementary Figure S3–S5**).

Bleomycin-Induced FDPS Production in Murine Lung Tissue Is Decreased by Zoledronic Acid Treatment

Increased flux through the mevalonate pathway enhances posttranslational modification of Rac1, promoting macrophage/fibroblast signaling (Larson-Casey et al., 2014,

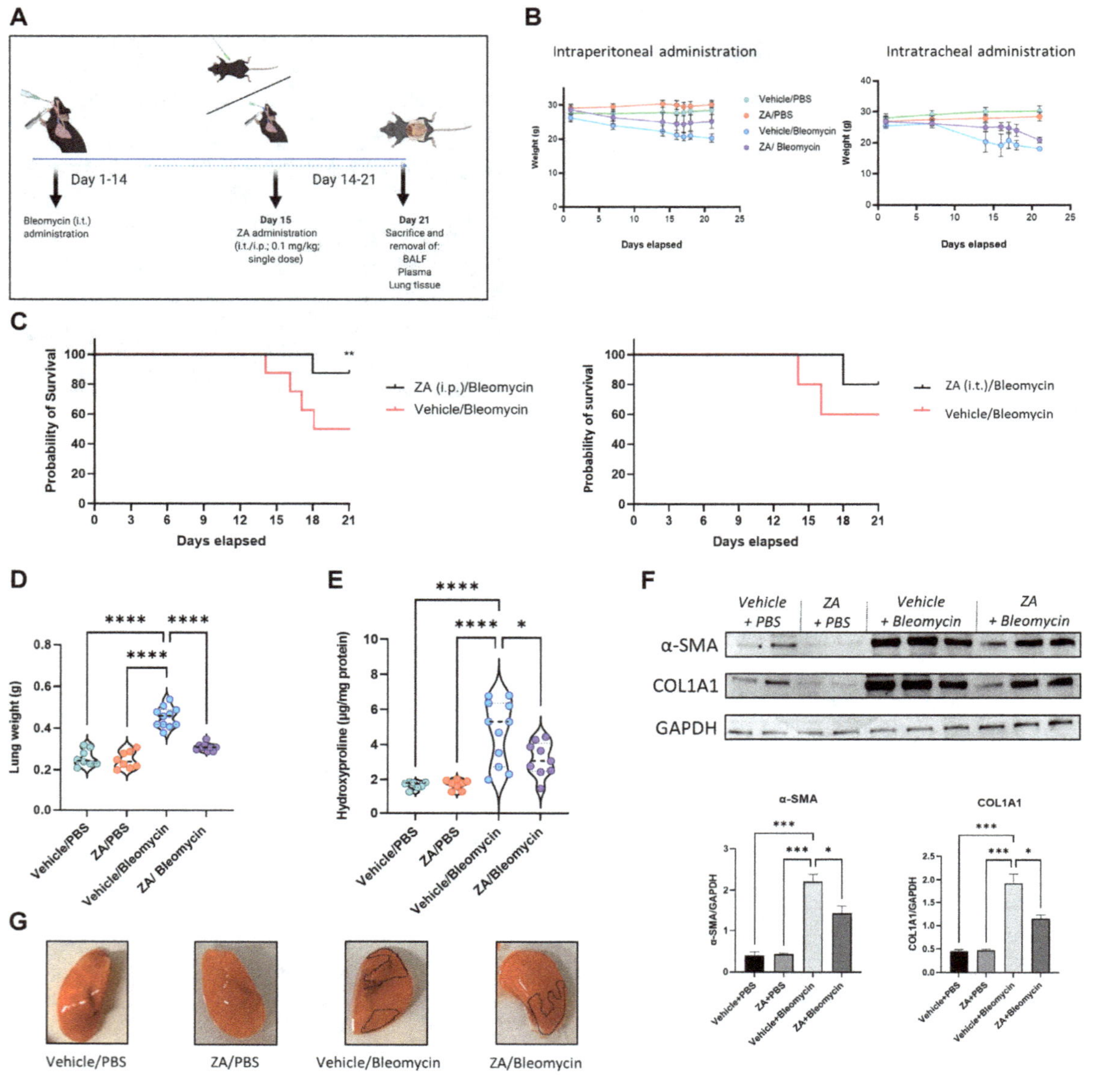

FIGURE 2 | ZA administration, murine weights, survival curve, and lung readouts. **(A)** ZA was administered intraperitoneally (i.p.) and intratracheally (i.t). on day 15 post-bleomycin introduction, with **(B)** murine total weight remaining stable in the ZA (i.p.) group for the duration of 21 days, with both bleomycin groups displaying significant weight loss after 14 days. **(C)** Resultant weight loss in the bleomycin/vehicle group caused significant mortality, with mice in the ZA/Bleo (i.p. and i. t.) groups seemingly protected. **(D)** Murine lung weight showed significant reductions in the ZA treated mice compared to the vehicle/bleomycin group (drug-treated samples were compared to untreated control samples using a one-way ANOVA followed by a Dunnett's post-hoc test: ****$p < 0.0001$). **(E)** Hydroxyproline collagen readout displayed significant reduction following ZA (i.p.) treatment (drug-treated samples were compared to untreated control samples using a one-way ANOVA followed by a Dunnett's post-hoc test: ****$p < 0.0001$). **(F)** Immunoblotting of ZA-treated murine lung lysates displayed significant reductions in both α-SMA and COL1A1 compared to bleomycin only control lysates **(G)** Representative murine images show bleomycin induced lung damage (collagenous deposition highlighted in dotted areas). Mice were allocated into groups as follows: Vehicle (i.p.)/phosphate buffered saline (PBS; i. t.); zoledronic acid (ZA; i. p.)/PBS (i.t.); Vehicle (i.p.)/Bleomycin (i.t.); ZA (i.p.)/ Bleomycin (i.t.).

2016; Politiek and Waterham, 2021). Further elucidation of this mechanism was conducted by probing the downstream signaling pathway (**Figure 6A**) by assessing farnesyl diphosphate synthase (FDPS). Bleomycin-induced FDPS production was significantly decreased following ZA administration, with ZA/bleomycin samples displaying significantly reduced fluorescence ($p = 0.0077$) and immunoreactivity compared to the vehicle/bleomycin group (**Figures 6B,C**). Western blot analysis revealed reduced levels of FDPS in lung homogenates in the ZA/bleomycin group compared to the vehicle/bleomycin group (**Figure 6D**). Furthermore, RT-PCR analysis on lung tissues showed a

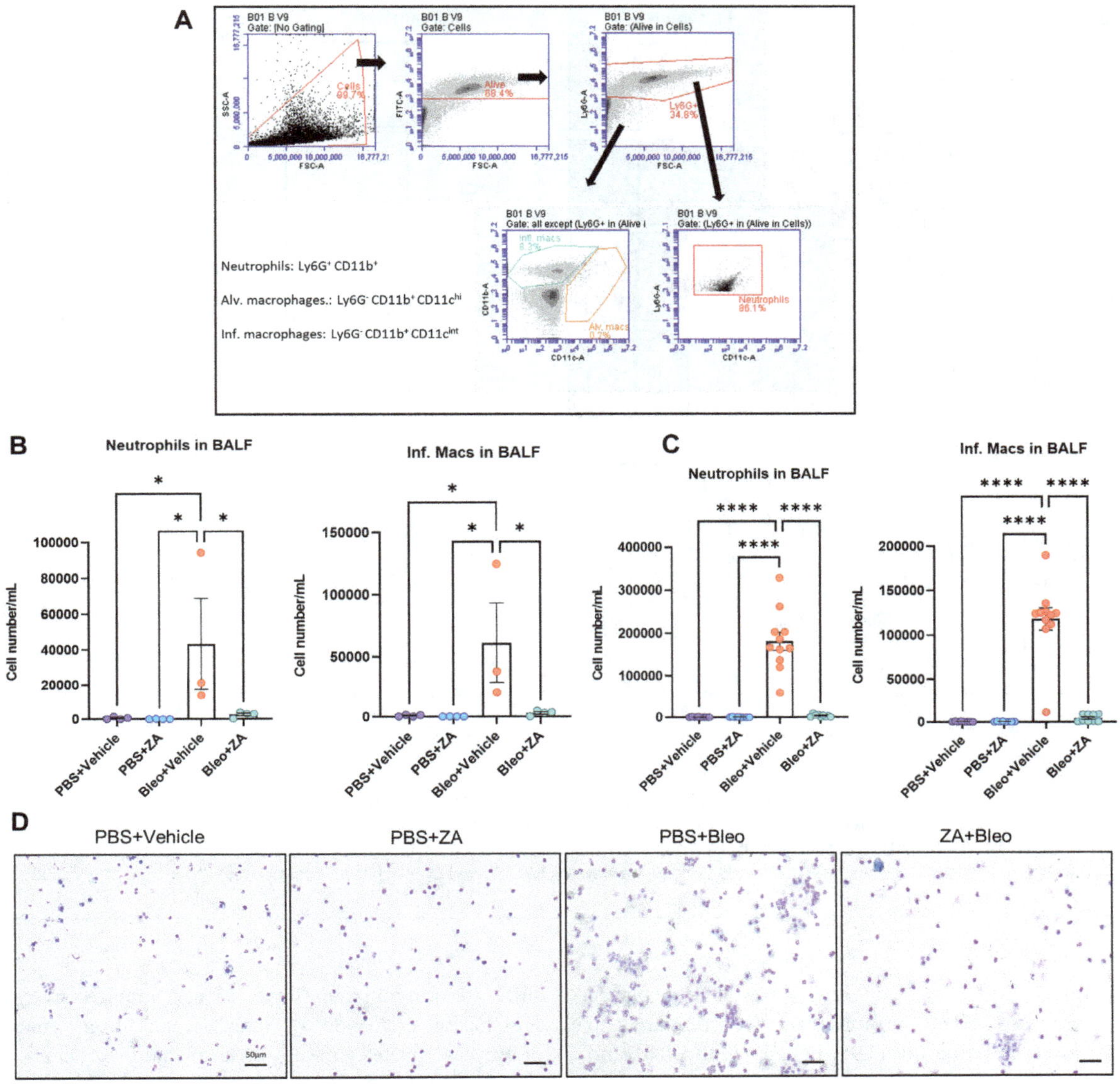

FIGURE 3 | Inflammatory cell influx measured in murine bronchoalveolar lavage fluid (BALF). Murine BALF was assessed for neutrophils and inflammatory macrophages **(B,C)** using flow cytometry, with the representative gating strategy depicted inset **(A)**. Decreased numbers of neutrophils and inflammatory macrophages were detected in response to ZA (i.t.) treatment, with increased significant differences reported between the neutrophils and inflammatory macrophages of mice treated with ZA (i.p.). No significant differences were reported for alveolar macrophage numbers (not shown). Inflammatory cell numbers were compared to the vehicle/bleomycin group using a one-way ANOVA followed by a Dunnett's post-hoc test (*$p < 0.05$; ****$p < 0.0001$). **(D)** Giemsa-Wright stained cytospin slides showing PBS/bleomycin BALF samples containing enlarged inflammatory macrophages, with ZA (i.p.) treatment reducing the presence of inflammatory macrophages. Scale bar = 20 μm.

significantly increased expression of the downstream enzyme *Fdft1* in the vehicle/bleomycin group compared to the ZA/bleomycin group (**Figure 6E**). Trends towards a decreased expression of *Fdps* and the upstream enzyme *Hmgcs1*, after ZA treatment, were also found. No statistical difference in gene expression was seen for the downstream enzyme *Dhdds*, indicative of preferential targeting of the steroid synthesis pathway by ZA. RT-PCR analysis of *Fdps* expression in MEF cells after TGF-β1 exposure showed an increase in FDPS, which was reduced upon ZA treatment (**Figure 6F**). Immunofluorescence staining of the MEF cells revealed a similar trend with enhanced FDPS staining after exposure to TGF-β1, and a decreased staining following ZA treatment (**Figure 6G**).

The role of human IPF and control samples in this study was to demonstrate the potential translational utility of targeting FDPS in IPF patients. Lung samples were stained for FDPS expression using 3,3′-diaminobenzidine (DAB) chromogenic

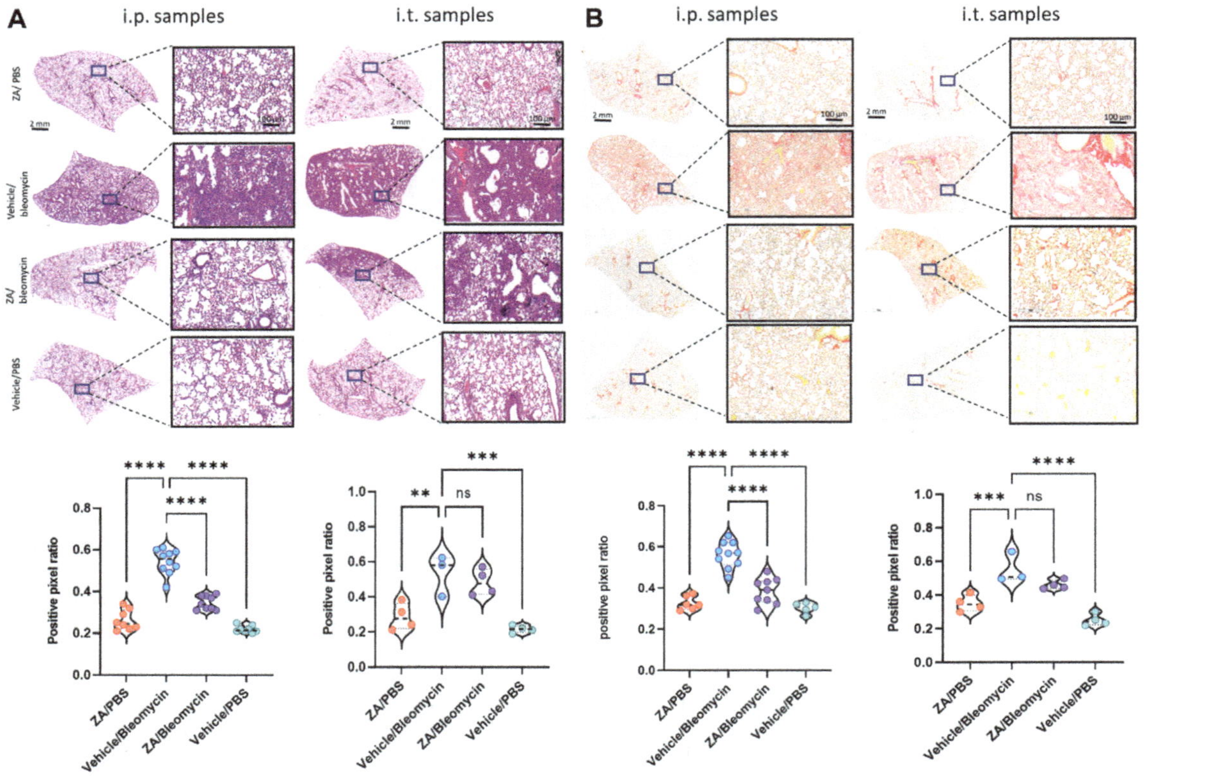

FIGURE 4 | Murine lung staining displays reduced levels of fibrotic-related lung damage following ZA (i.p.) treatment compared to bleomycin/vehicle samples **(A)** ZA (i.p.) significantly decreased lung damage in bleomycin-treated mice (H&E) and **(B)** collagen deposition (picrosirius red) in both macroscopic and microscopic structures compared to vehicle/bleomycin lungs and was confirmed by positive pixel analysis of whole-lung scanned images (scale bar of microscopic image = 100 µm; scale bar of whole lung scan = 2 mm). Statistical analyses were conducted using a one-way ANOVA followed by a Dunnett's post-hoc test ($^{**}p < 0.01$; $^{***}p < 0.005$; $^{*}p < 0.0001$).

staining. Human IPF resected lung samples displayed significantly increased FDPS immunoreactivity compared to controls, indicative of a role for FDPS in IPF (**Figure 6H** and **Supplementary Figure S6**).

Intratracheal Administration of siRNA Confirms FDPS as a Tractable Target for Idiopathic Pulmonary Fibrosis

To verify that reduced FDPS levels in the lungs explains ZA's ability to reduce bleomycin-induced lung damage, intratracheal administration of *FDPS* siRNA was used (**Figure 7A**). Measurement of FDPS protein levels in lung homogenates using western blot confirmed a significant reduction of FDPS levels after siRNA addition (**Figure 7B**). Similar to the ZA treatment, administration of *FDPS*-targeting siRNA resulted in a reduced murine weight loss (**Figure 7C**). Lung weights and hydroxyproline levels were significantly decreased after *FDPS* siRNA administration compared to the control siRNA/bleomycin group (**Figures 7D,E**). Measurements on inflammatory cytokine levels in the BALF after FDPS siRNA administration revealed a very similar pattern to the ZA treatment, whereby a reduction was seen in almost all investigated cytokines compared to the control siRNA/bleomycin group (**Figure 7F** and **Supplementary Figure S7**). Histological evaluation of lung sections from control siRNA/bleomycin treated mice revealed more closure of alveolar structures and increased collagen deposition, whereas lung sections from mice treated with *FDPS*-targeting siRNA were comparable to the control mice (**Figure 7G**). Furthermore, western blot analysis on synthesis of the fibrotic proteins COL1A1 and α-SMA showed a significant decrease in FDPS siRNA treated compared to control siRNA/bleomycin treated mice (**Figure 7H**). Finally, immunofluorescence staining of FDPS in lung sections was amplified in mice treated with control siRNA/bleomycin, which was reduced to control levels upon FDPS siRNA administration (**Figure 7I**).

Farnesyl Diphosphate Synthase Targeting Results in Anti-fibrotic Macrophage Reprogramming

Previous studies have implicated M2 macrophages in IPF pathogenesis, with pro-fibrotic M2 macrophages characterized by expression of CD206 as well as increased metabolism of arginine into ornithine and urea by arginase (Ruaro et al.,

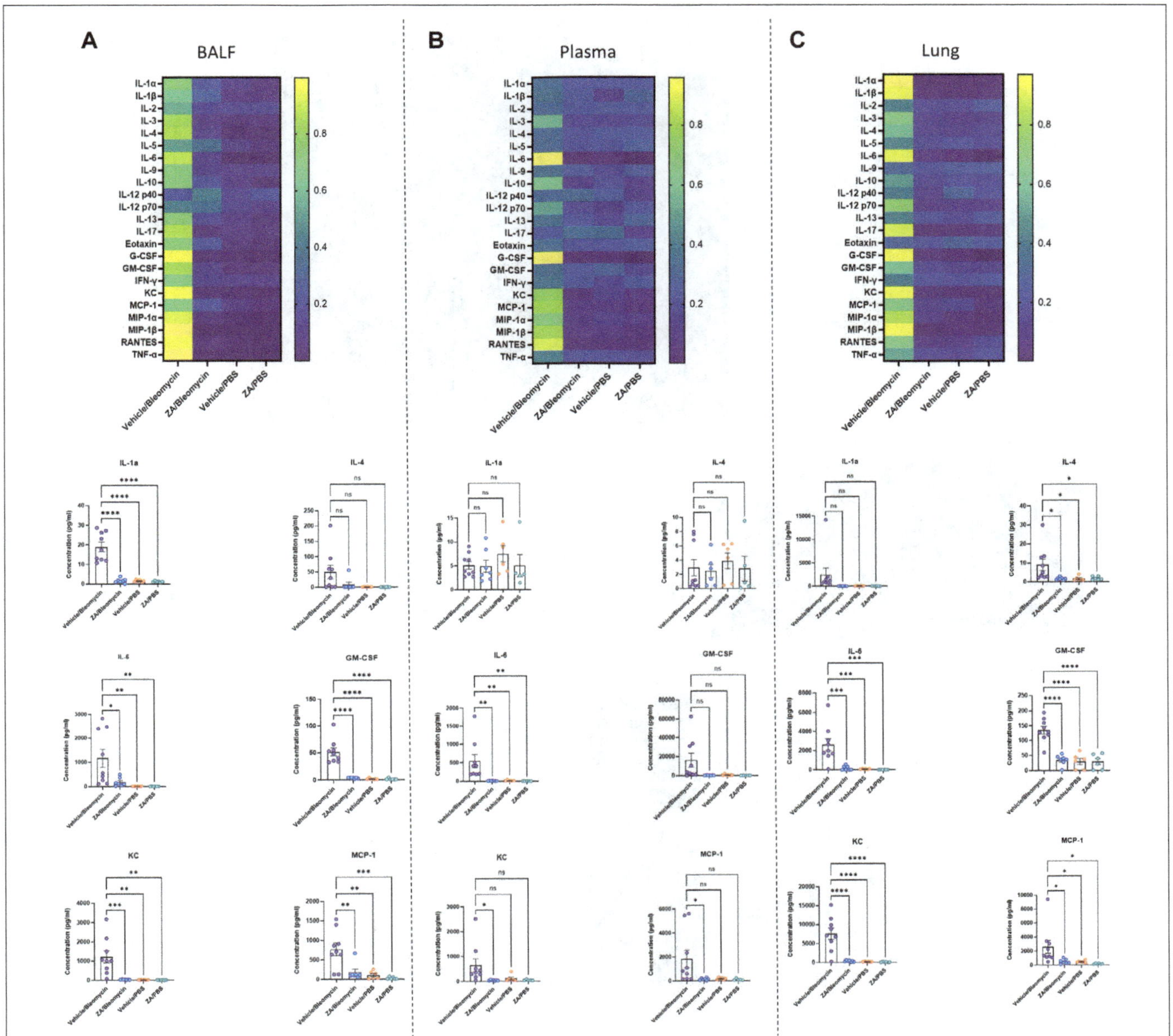

FIGURE 5 | Significantly decreased murine cytokines following intraperitoneal ZA administration. Heatmaps **(A–C)** showing the differences in cytokine levels, as measured by multiplex assay, in murine BALF, plasma, and lung homogenate (yellow indicating high value; blue indicating low value) with selected corresponding significantly decreased or increased cytokine levels below. Cytokine values were compared to the vehicle/bleomycin group using a one-way ANOVA followed by a Dunnett's post-hoc test (*$p < 0.05$; **$p < 0.01$; ***$p < 0.005$; ****$p < 0.001$).

2019; Papadimitriou et al., 2022). Stimulation of macrophages with profibrotic cytokines IL-4 and IL-13 lead to an increased number of M2 macrophages and fewer M1 macrophages indicative of a pro-fibrotic polarization. Addition of ZA to murine *ex vivo* macrophages stimulated with IL-4 and IL-13 resulted in retention of M1 macrophages and a reduction of M2 macrophages (**Figure 8A**). Protein levels of Arg1 and CD206 in the lung, measured by western blot, were found to be significantly increased in the bleomycin/vehicle group, whereas treatment with ZA resulted in a significant decrease of both proteins (**Figure 8B**). This was supported by a trend towards an increased expression of Arg1 seen in the bleomycin/vehicle animals, which was reduced after treatment with ZA (**Figure 8C**). No differences in expression of *CD206* were found between the groups. Immunofluorescence staining of lung sections revealed a bleomycin induced increase in fluorescence from both ARG1 and CD206 compared to the controls. The fluorescent signal for both proteins was almost undetectable in the lung sections from ZA treated mice, and a faint signal was seen in the FDPS siRNA treated mouse lungs (**Figures 8D,E**).

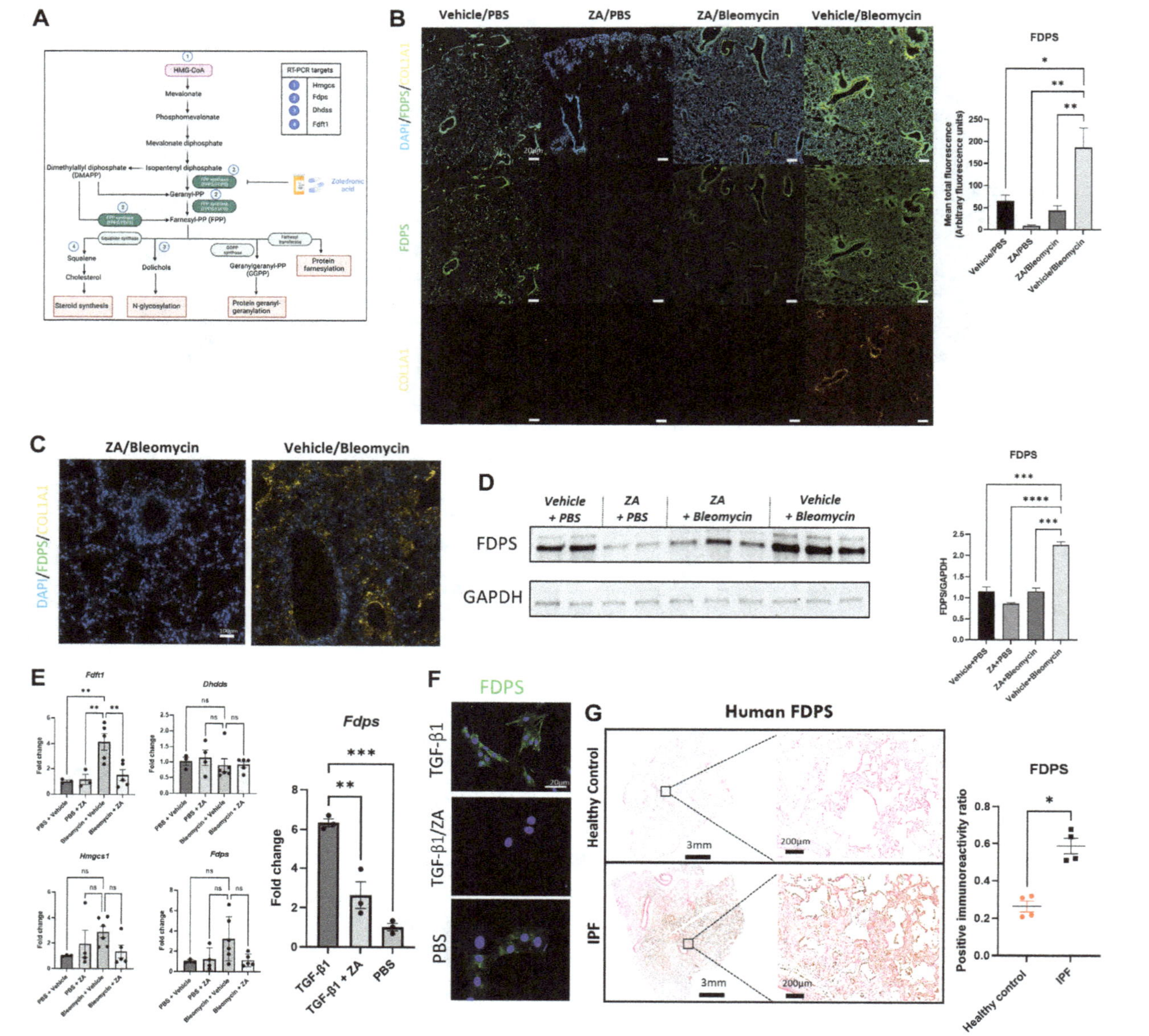

FIGURE 6 | Lower production of FDPS and COL1A1 in murine lungs upon ZA treatment. (A) Mevalonate pathway with key enzymes and intermediates highlighted inset and numbered points indicating PCR measurements (Hmgcs: hydroxymethylglutaryl-CoA synthase; Fdps: farnesyl diphosphate synthase; Dhdds: dehydrodolichol diphosphate synthase; Fdft1: farnesyl-diphosphate farnesyl transferase). **(B)** Murine lung immunofluorescence analysis showed decreased levels of immunoreactivity for FDPS and collagen 1A1 (COL1A1) in ZA (i.p.)-treated mice compared to bleomycin (Bleo) controls (scale bar = 20 μm), with quantification of green fluorescence. ZA-treated and control samples were compared to bleomycin-treated samples using a one-way ANOVA followed by a Dunnett's post-hoc test (**p* < 0.05; ***p* < 0.01) and enlarged images of murine airways displaying co-staining of FDPS and COL1A1 **(C)**. **(D)** Mouse lung homogenate samples analyzed by SDS-PAGE, followed by immunoblotting using rabbit antisera specific to FDPS revealed decreased protein levels within ZA-administered mice. **(E)** RT-PCR analysis of murine lung lysates reveals decreased levels of *Fdft1* and *Fdps* in ZA-treated samples compared to bleomycin controls. Murine embryonic fibroblast cells stimulated with TGF-β1 and treated with ZA/PBS for 48 h displayed significantly reduced *Fdps* levels compared to TGF-β1 control as confirmed by **(F)** immunofluorescent staining of TGF-β1 treated MEF cells (scale bar = 20 μm). **(G)** FDPS immunoreactivity was measured in human IPF and control resected lung tissues, with IPF tissues showing significantly more immunoreactivity than control tissue (**p* = 0.0286) as compared using an unpaired *t* test with Welch's correction. Scale bar = 3 mm and 200 μm for inset images.

DISCUSSION

With current drug targets and therapies predominantly directed toward fibroblast-mediated collagen deposition and fibrotic intercession, our focus turned to indirect intervention into immune cell-mediated inhibitory activities through mevalonate intermediate targeting. The mevalonate pathway has shown utility in multiple diseases, with evidence supporting mevalonate regulation of cell proliferation and energy homeostasis (Clendening et al.,

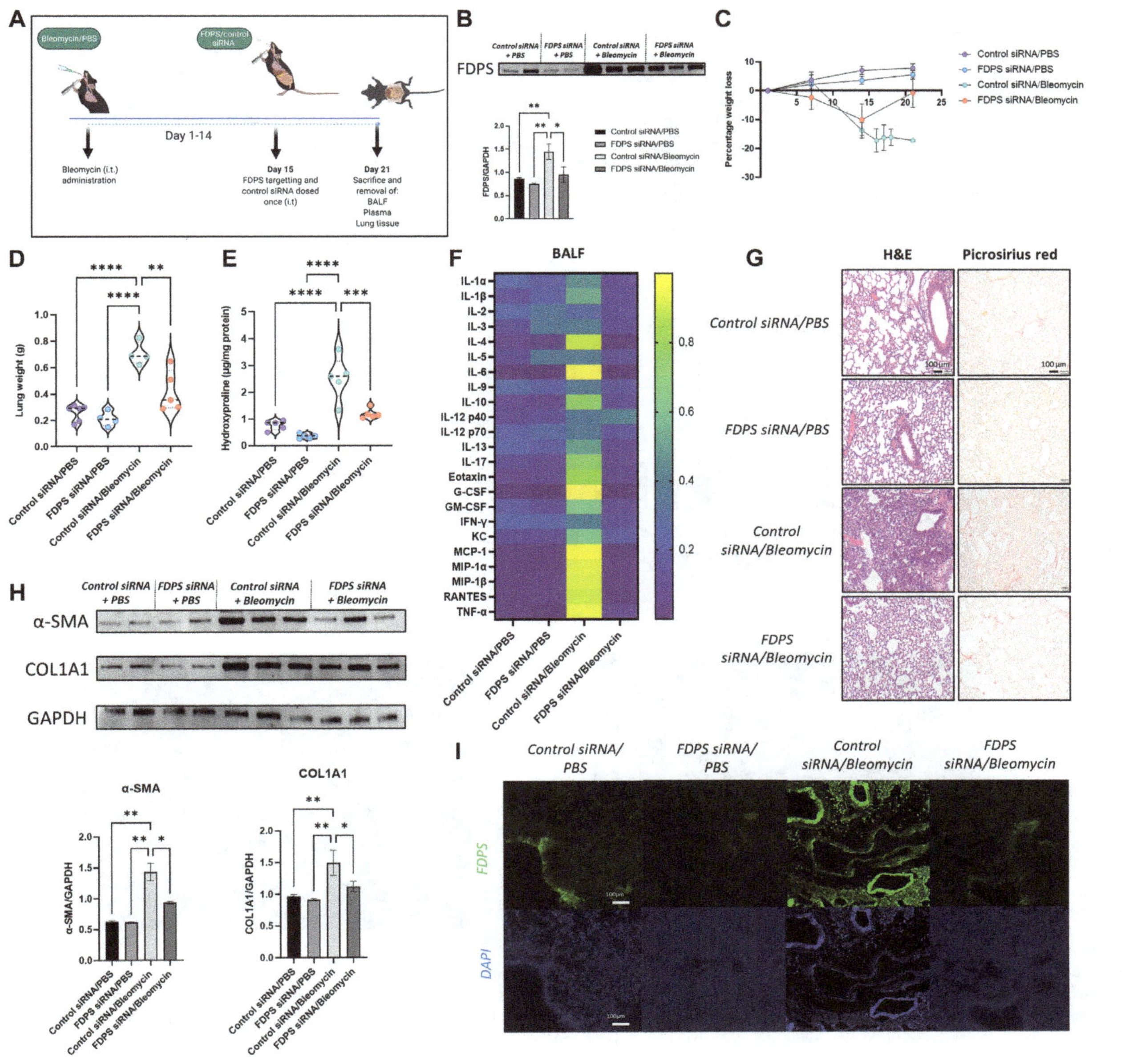

FIGURE 7 | Intratracheal administration of FDPS siRNA confers protection to bleomycin-challenged mice. **(A)** Mice were subjected to bleomycin treatment at day 0, administrated FDPS or control siRNA intratracheally on day 15 and sacrificed on day 21. **(B)** SDS-PAGE followed by western blot analysis using antisera specific for FDPS in mouse lung homogenates confirms significantly decreased levels of FDPS after siRNA administration. Samples were compared using a one-way ANOVA followed by a Dunnett's post-hoc test (*$p < 0.05$, **$p < 0.01$). **(C)** Measurement of murine weight loss following bleomycin exposure shows a protective effect of FDPS siRNA compared to control siRNA. **(D)** Bleomycin induced increases in murine lung weights were significantly reduced after FDPS siRNA treatments compared to control siRNA. Comparison between groups were performed using a one-way ANOVA followed by a Dunnett's post-hoc test (**$p < 0.01$, ****$p < 0.0001$). **(E)** Hydroxyproline levels, which is a measurement of collagen content, was significantly increased in mice treated with bleomycin/control siRNA compared to the FDPS siRNA treated mice. Differences between groups were calculated with a one-way ANOVA followed by a Dunnett's post-hoc test (***$p < 0.001$, ****$p < 0.0001$). **(F)** Heatmap showing the difference in inflammatory cytokine levels in BALF between treatment groups (blue indicating low value; yellow indicating high value). **(G)** Bleomycin/control siRNA mice showed increased lung damage, determined by H&E, and more intense collagen staining (picrosirius red). Lungs from mice receiving FDPS siRNA were resembling lungs from control mice regarding both H&E and collagen. **(H)** Detection and quantification of the fibrotic proteins α-smooth muscle actin (α-SMA) and collagen (COL1A1) using SDS-PAGE followed by western blot revealed a significant increase in both proteins in lungs from bleomycin/control siRNA mice, which was reduced significantly with FDPS siRNA treatment. **(I)** Immunofluorescence staining of lung sections with anti FDPS antibodies displaying an increase immunoreactivity in bleomycin/control siRNA mice, whereas lungs from mice administered FDPS siRNA were similar to lungs from control mice.

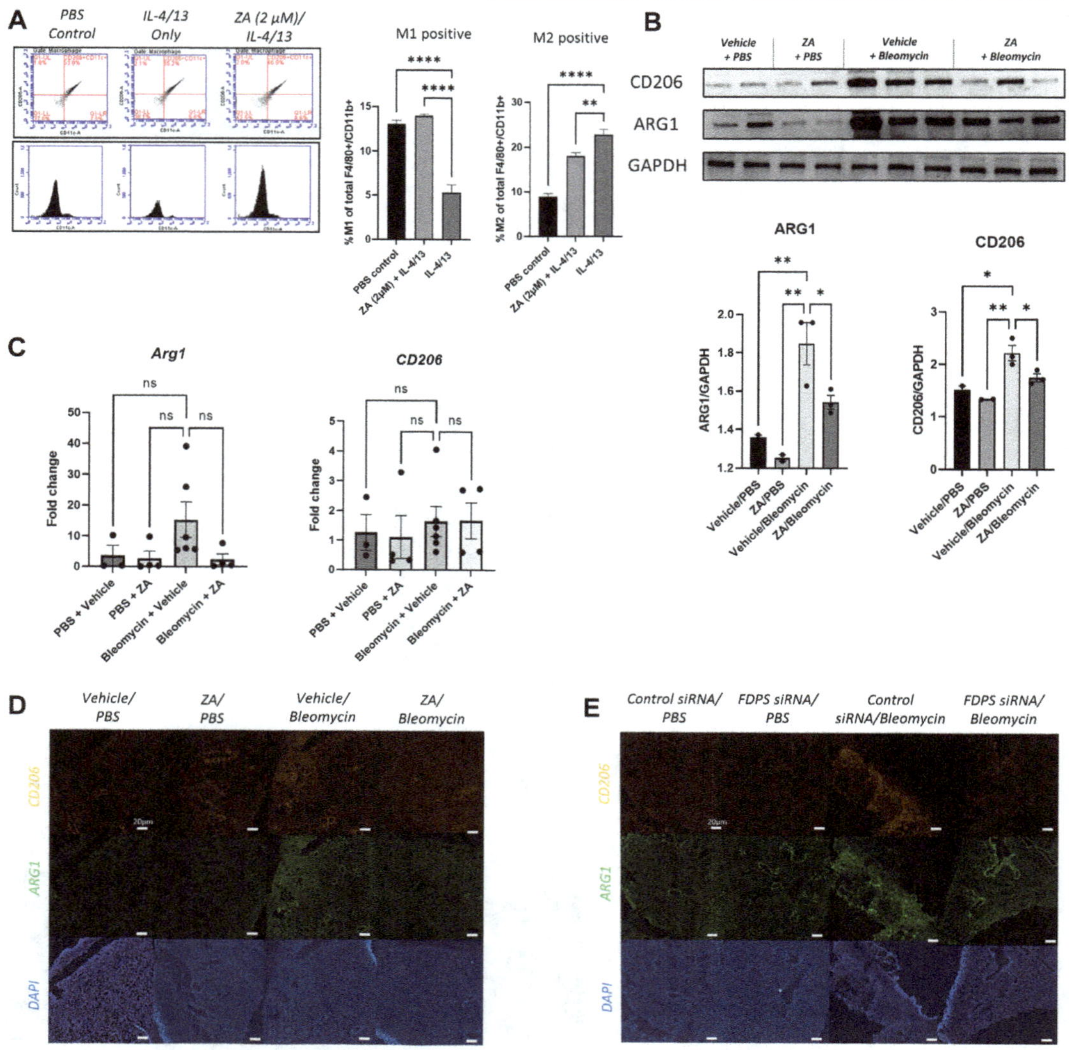

FIGURE 8 | Decreased profibrotic macrophage markers following ZA or FDPS siRNA treatment **(A)** *Ex-vivo* macrophages were analyzed for M1/M2 using flow cytometry, with the gating strategy shown. Stimulation with IL-4/13 for 48 h shifted the macrophages from M1 to M2, which was in part blocked after ZA administration. M1 positive ($CD206^-/CD11c^+/F4/80^+/CD11b^+$) and M2 positive ($CD206^+/CD11c^-/F4/80^+/CD11b^+$) macrophages graphed as percentages. Statistical comparison between groups were performed using a one-way ANOVA with Dunnett's post-hoc test ($^*p < 0.05$; $^{**}p < 0.01$; $^{***}p < 0.001$). **(B)** SDS-PAGE followed by western blot with antibodies for arginase 1 (ARG1) and cluster of differentiation 206 (CD206). Intensity quantification, normalized to Glyceraldehyde 3-phosphate dehydrogenase (GAPDH), of the bands showed decreased protein levels of ARG1 and CD206 after treatment with ZA. Statistical comparison between groups were performed using a one-way ANOVA with Dunnett's post-hoc test ($^*p < 0.05$; $^{**}p < 0.01$; $^{***}p < 0.001$). **(C)** Real-time quantitative PCR (RT-qPCR) analysis of Arg1 and *CD206* in lung after bleomycin exposure and treatment with ZA. The mRNA expression was normalized against succinate dehydrogenase complex subunit A (*Sdha*) and fold change was calculated by difference between all treatment groups compared to PBS/vehicle. Statistical differences between groups were calculated using a one-way ANOVA with Dunnett's post-hoc test **(D,E)** Immunofluorescence staining of ARG1 and CD206 in lung sections revealed an increased signal intensity after bleomycin exposure, which was reduced with administration of ZA **(D)** or FDPS siRNA **(E)**.

2010; Gruenbacher and Thurnher, 2017; Larson-Casey et al., 2019).

HMG-CoA reductase inhibitors such as statins, are reversible competitive inhibitors of HMG-CoA reductase, a molecule that catalyzes the de-acylation of HMG-CoA to mevalonate in cholesterol biosynthesis (Hampton et al., 1996; John R; Burnett and Vasikaran, 2002). Statins have predominantly been used to probe the mevalonate pathway in interstitial lung diseases, offering mixed results. Whilst lung function decline and hospitalizations in IPF patients from the CAPACITY and ASCEND trials was diminished by statin use (Alexeeff et al., 2007; Kreuter et al., 2017), the post-hoc analysis of the INPULSIS trials did not establish beneficial effects of statin use in IPF patients (Kreuter et al., 2018). Furthermore, an FDA report associated statin use with onset of interstitial lung disease (Fernández et al., 2008), with statins shown to increase lung fibrosis in a murine bleomycin model (Xu et al., 2012).

The approach reported in this study utilized a third-generation bisphosphonate, ZA, already employed for the treatment of osteoporosis, through potent effects against the resorptive activity of osteoclasts (Dunstan et al., 2007). This activity is mediated by inhibiting farnesyl diphosphate synthase (FDPS), an enzyme responsible for catalysing the conversion of isopentenyl pyrophosphate and dimethylallyl pyrophosphate to their geranylated and farnesylated states, respectively (Kim et al., 2018). Herein, we report several arguments supporting FDPS targeting by ZA as an appealing and clinically relevant treatment for IPF.

Reported data indicate that increased geranylgeranylation substrates increase Rac1 activity in macrophages, with resultant polarization to a profibrotic phenotype (Larson-Casey et al., 2019). Rac1 also mediates ROS generation (Osborn-Heaford et al., 2012), with IPF-derived fibroblasts and macrophages generating higher levels of ROS (Waghray et al., 2005). Furthermore, IPF-derived BAL cells displayed increased apoptotic resistance and increased TGF-β1 production (Larson-Casey et al., 2016). Our study found that TGF-β1-stimulated HFL-1 cells treated with ZA were less prone to myofibroblast transition and produced decreased levels of fibrotic proteins. RANKL induces phenotypic switching in macrophages from the initial state to M1-like cells, whereas IL-4, IL-10, IL-13, and other cytokines secreted by T helper cells are involved in M2 activation, skewing macrophages toward a profibrotic lineage (Huang et al., 2017). RANK additionally provokes biochemical signaling *via* the recruitment of intracellular TNF receptor-associated factors (TRAFs) after ligand binding and receptor oligomerization. We showed that ZA-treated monocytic cells stimulated with RANKL displayed reduced NF-κB signaling, a key regulator of proinflammatory responses in immune cells. In addition, *ex vivo* macrophage cells from murine BALF exposed to RANKL stimulation and ZA treatment displayed reduced cell recruitment efficiency.

Importantly, uncontrolled lung injury and immune cell recruitment is a hallmark of IPF initiation and progression, resulting in pro-inflammatory and pro-fibrotic cytokine release driving further fibrosis-related immune cell influx and ECM remodeling (Wynn and Ramalingam, 2012; Spagnolo et al., 2018; Upagupta et al., 2018; Baratella et al., 2021). Whilst recent efforts have focused on removal of senescent or damaged fibroblasts (David et al., 2017; Schafer et al., 2017), our approach advantageously suppresses pro-fibrotic mediators and immune cell recruitment with reduced cytotoxicity.

To elucidate the mechanism by which these effects were mediated, we examined murine lung samples. Whilst no direct targeting of FDPS has, to our knowledge, been reported in the airways, FDPS has shown involvement in the progression of cardiac remodelling, with *FDPS*-targeting siRNA attenuating murine cardiac fibrosis (Zhao et al., 2016). This is further supported in our study, with *FDPS*-targeting siRNA reducing fibrotic lung damage. FDPS has displayed involvement in cardiac remodelling, with FDPS-targeting siRNA attenuating murine cardiac fibrosis (Zhao et al., 2016). Furthermore, ZA's ability to decrease FDPS production was demonstrated in human lung tissue, murine lung tissue, and directly in fibroblast cells, correlating with subsequent decreases in collagen deposition. In addition, our study examined the most appropriate route of ZA administration, a key factor in any drug discovery program. Surprisingly, intraperitoneal administration of ZA produced the most effective alleviation of lung fibrosis. We hypothesize that intratracheal administration of ZA to the murine lung may produce cytotoxic damage or result in elimination of the macrophage population entirely [44]. Conversely, intraperitoneal introduction of ZA displayed the ability to repolarize murine macrophages to an anti-fibrotic phenotype, highlighting further advantages of ZA administration (Kaneko et al., 2018).

Important limitations addressed in this study include whether treatment using ZA can display utility in human IPF pathologies. Whilst the translational aspect of this study is suggested using murine lung sections, it is important to demonstrate that ZA treatment successfully reduces FDPS levels and subsequent IPF lung damage in human clinical trials. Transition to such clinical trials is eased by the pre-existing FDA approval of ZA (i.v.) for osteoporosis, multiple myeloma, and bone metastases in cancer.

Together, our findings demonstrate that ZA possesses a mechanism of action targeting FDPS to suppress pulmonary fibrosis, which is distinct from currently employed therapeutic interventions. This study highlights the downstream effects of FDPS inhibition, including decreasing myofibroblast transition, decreasing inflammatory cell recruitment, reducing pro-fibrotic macrophage populations, and eventual inhibition of fibrotic-related lung remodelling. These data support the use of ZA in clinical trials for the treatment of IPF.

ETHICS STATEMENT

The studies involving human participants were reviewed and approved by the Regional Ethical Review Board in Lund (approval no. LU412-03), and performed in accordance with the Declaration of Helsinki as well as relevant guidelines and regulations. The patients/participants provided their written informed consent to participate in this study. All animal experiments were approved by the Malmö-Lund Animal Care Ethics Committee (M17009-18).

AUTHOR CONTRIBUTIONS

Conceptualization: AE, LT, ABS, and JB; Methodology: LT, JB, ABS, RKVB, and JSE; Investigation: LT, JB, and RKVB, JSE; Funding acquisition: AE, ABS, and LT; Project administration: AE, LT Supervision: AE, LT; Writing—original draft: LT, JB; Writing—review and editing: LT, JB, ABS, AE, RKVB, and JSE.

Foundation 2019-0160 (AE); The Swedish Government Funds for Clinical Research 46402 (ALF; AE); The Alfred Österlund Foundation (AE); LU Innovation (ABS and LT); Royal Physiographic Society of Lund (LT); Tore Nilsons Stiftelse 2021-00936 (LT); and Lars Hiertas Minne Fund FO 2021-0284 (LT).

ACKNOWLEDGMENTS

We would like to acknowledge the kind donation of MEF cells from Maria Allhorn (Lund University). We would also like to acknowledge the assistance received from the Lund University Bioimaging Centre (LBIC). In addition, we would like to acknowledge the flow cytometry support received from Assoc. Prof. Oonagh Shannon (Lund University). Figures feature elements created in BioRender.com.

REFERENCES

1. Alexeeff, S. E., Litonjua, A. A., Sparrow, D., Vokonas, P. S., and Schwartz, J. (2007). Statin Use Reduces Decline in Lung Function: VA Normative Aging Study. *Am. J. Respir. Crit. Care Med.* 176, 742–747. doi:10.1164/rccm.200705-656OC
2. Baratella, E., Ruaro, B., Giudici, F., Wade, B., Santagiuliana, M., Salton, F., et al. (2021). Evaluation of Correlations between Genetic Variants and High- Resolution Computed Tomography Patterns in Idiopathic Pulmonary Fibrosis. *Diagn. (Basel)* 11, 762. doi:10.3390/diagnostics11050762
3. Berg, R. A., and Prockop, D. J. (1973). The Thermal Transition of a Non-hydroxylated Form of Collagen. Evidence for a Role for Hydroxyproline in Stabilizing the Triple-Helix of Collagen. *Biochem. Biophys. Res. Commun.* 52, 115–120. doi:10.1016/0006-291x(73)90961-3
4. Burnett, J. R., and Vasikaran, S. D. (2002). Cardiovascular Disease and Osteoporosis: Is There a Link between Lipids and Bone? *Ann. Clin. Biochem.* 39, 203–210. doi:10.1258/0004563021902134
5. Chakarov, S., Lim, H. Y., Tan, L., Lim, S. Y., See, P., Lum, J., et al. (2019). Two Distinct Interstitial Macrophage Populations Coexist across Tissues in Specific Subtissular Niches. *Science* 363, 363eaau0964. doi:10.1126/science.aau0964
6. Chang, X., Xing, L., Wang, Y., Yang, C. X., He, Y. J., Zhou, T. J., et al. (2020). Monocyte-derived Multipotent Cell Delivered Programmed Therapeutics to Reverse Idiopathic Pulmonary Fibrosis. *Sci. Adv.* 6, eaba3167. doi:10.1126/sciadv.aba3167
7. Chen, X., Abair, T. D., Ibanez, M. R., Su, Y., Frey, M. R., Dise, R. S., et al. (2007). Integrin Alpha1beta1 Controls Reactive Oxygen Species Synthesis by Negatively Regulating Epidermal Growth Factor Receptor-Mediated Rac Activation. *Mol. Cell Biol.* 27, 3313–3326. doi:10.1128/MCB.01476-06
8. Clendening, J. W., Pandyra, A., Boutros, P. C., El Ghamrasni, S., Khosravi, F., Trentin, G. A., et al. (2010). Dysregulation of the Mevalonate Pathway Promotes Transformation. *Proc. Natl. Acad. Sci. U. S. A.* 107, 15051–15056. doi:10.1073/pnas.0910258107
9. Cutolo, M., Ruaro, B., Montagna, P., Brizzolara, R., Stratta, E., Trombetta, A. C., et al. (2018). Effects of Selexipag and its Active Metabolite in Contrasting the Profibrotic Myofibroblast Activity in Cultured Scleroderma Skin Fibroblasts. *Arthritis Res. Ther.* 20, 77. doi:10.1186/s13075-018-1577-0
10. de Jong, S., van Veen, T. A. B., de Bakker, J. M. T., and van Rijen, H. V. M. (2012). Monitoring Cardiac Fibrosis: a Technical Challenge. *Neth. Heart J.* 20, 44–48. doi:10.1007/s12471-011-0226-x
11. Dunford, J. E., Thompson, K., Coxon, F. P., Luckman, S. P., Hahn, F. M., Poulter, C. D., et al. (2001). Structure-Activity Relationships for Inhibition of Farnesyl Diphosphate Synthase *In Vitro* and Inhibition of Bone Resorption *In Vivo* by Nitrogen-Containing Bisphosphonates. *J. Pharmacol. Exp. Ther.* 296, 235. Available at: http://jpet.aspetjournals.org/content/296/2/235.abstract.
12. Dunstan, C. R., Felsenberg, D., and Seibel, M. J. (2007). Therapy Insight: the Risks and Benefits of Bisphosphonates for the Treatment of Tumor-Induced Bone Disease. *Nat. Clin. Pract. Oncol.* 4, 42–55. doi:10.1038/ncponc0688
13. Fernández, A. B., Karas, R. H., Alsheikh-Ali, A. A., and Thompson, P. D. (2008). Statins and Interstitial Lung Disease: a Systematic Review of the Literature and of Food and Drug Administration Adverse Event Reports. *Chest* 134, 824–830. doi:10.1378/chest.08-0943
14. Fetro, C., and Scherman, D. (2020). Drug Repurposing in Rare Diseases: Myths and Reality. *Therapies* 75, 157–160. doi:10.1016/j.therap.2020.02.006
15. Gruenbacher, G., and Thurnher, M. (2017). Mevalonate Metabolism Governs Cancer Immune Surveillance. *Oncoimmunology* 6, e1342917. doi:10.1080/2162402X.2017.1342917
16. Guilliams, M., Thierry, G. R., Bonnardel, J., and Bajenoff, M. (2020). Establishment and Maintenance of the Macrophage Niche. *Immunity* 52, 434–451. doi:10. 1016/j.immuni.2020.02.015
17. Hampton, R., Dimster-Denk, D., and Rine, J. (1996). The Biology of HMG-CoA Reductase: the Pros of Contra-regulation. *Trends Biochem. Sci.* 21, 140–145. doi:10.1016/S0968-0004(96)80168-X
18. Henderson, N. C., Rieder, F., and Wynn, T. A. (2020). Fibrosis: from Mechanisms to Medicines. *Nature* 587, 555–566. doi:10.1038/s41586-020-2938-9
19. Hu, B., and Phan, S. H. (2013). Myofibroblasts. *Curr. Opin. Rheumatol.* 25, 71–77. doi:10.1097/BOR.0b013e32835b1352
20. Huang, R., Wang, X., Zhou, Y., and Xiao, Y. (2017). RANKL-induced M1 Macrophages Are Involved in Bone Formation. *Bone Res.* 5, 17019. doi:10.1038/boneres.2017.19
21. Ichikawa, T., Hirahara, K., Kokubo, K., Kiuchi, M., Aoki, A., Morimoto, Y., et al. (2019). $CD103^{hi}$ T_{reg} Cells Constrain Lung Fibrosis Induced by $CD103^{lo}$ Tissue- Resident Pathogenic CD4 T Cells. *Nat. Immunol.* 20, 1469–1480. doi:10.1038/s41590-019-0494-y
22. Kaneko, J., Okinaga, T., Hikiji, H., Ariyoshi, W., Yoshiga, D., Habu, M., et al. (2018). Zoledronic Acid Exacerbates Inflammation through M1 Macrophage Polarization. *Inflamm. Regen.* 38, 16. doi:10.1186/s41232-018-0074-9
23. Kim, H. Y., Kim, D. K., Bae, S.-H., Gwak, H., Jeon, J. H., Kim, J. K., et al. (2018). Farnesyl Diphosphate Synthase Is Important for the Maintenance of Glioblastoma Stemness. *Exp. Mol. Med.* 50, 1–12. doi:10.1038/s12276-018-0166-2
24. Kreuter, M., Bonella, F., Maher, T. M., Costabel, U., Spagnolo, P., Weycker, D., et al. (2017). Effect of Statins on Disease-Related Outcomes in Patients with Idiopathic Pulmonary Fibrosis. *Thorax* 72, 148–153. doi:10.1136/thoraxjnl- 2016-208819
25. Kreuter, M., Costabel, U., Richeldi, L., Cottin, V., Wijsenbeek, M., Bonella, F., et al. (2018). Statin Therapy and Outcomes in Trials of Nintedanib in Idiopathic Pulmonary Fibrosis. *Respiration* 95, 317–326. doi:10.1159/000486286
26. Larson-Casey, J. L., Deshane, J. S., Ryan, A. J., Thannickal, V. J., and Carter, A. B. (2016). Macrophage Akt1 Kinase-Mediated Mitophagy Modulates Apoptosis Resistance and Pulmonary Fibrosis. *Immunity* 44, 582–596. doi:10.1016/j. immuni.2016.01.001
27. Larson-Casey, J. L., Murthy, S., Ryan, A. J., and Carter, A. B. (2014). Modulation of the Mevalonate Pathway by Akt Regulates Macrophage Survival and Development of Pulmonary Fibrosis. *J. Biol. Chem.* 289, 36204–36219. doi:10.1074/jbc.M114.593285
28. Larson-Casey, J. L., Vaid, M., Gu, L., He, C., Cai, G. Q., Ding, Q., et al. (2019). Increased Flux through the Mevalonate Pathway Mediates Fibrotic Repair without Injury. *J. Clin. Investigation* 129, 4962–4978. doi:10.1172/JCI127959
29. Lederer, D. J., and Martinez, F. J. (2018). Idiopathic Pulmonary Fibrosis. *N. Engl.J. Med.* 378, 1811–1823. doi:10.1056/nejmra1705751
30. Liu, H., Wang, S.-H., Chen, S.-C., Chen, C.-Y., and Lin, T.-M. (2019). Zoledronic Acid Blocks the Interaction between Breast Cancer Cells and Regulatory T-Cells. *BMC Cancer* 19, 176. doi:10.1186/s12885-019-5379-9
31. Martinez, F. J., Collard, H. R., Pardo, A., Raghu, G., Richeldi, L., Selman, M., et al. (2017). Idiopathic Pulmonary Fibrosis. *Nat. Rev. Dis. Prim.* 3, 17074. doi:10. 1038/nrdp.2017.74
32. Osborn-Heaford, H. L., Ryan, A. J., Murthy, S., Racila, A.-M., He, C., Sieren, J. C., et al. (2012). Mitochondrial Rac1 GTPase Import and Electron Transfer from Cytochrome C Are Required for Pulmonary Fibrosis. *J. Biol. Chem.* 287, 3301–3312. doi:10.1074/jbc.M111.308387
33. Papadimitriou, T.-I., van Caam, A., van der Kraan, P. M., and Thurlings, R. M. (2022). Therapeutic Options for Systemic Sclerosis: Current and Future Perspectives in Tackling Immune-Mediated Fibrosis. *Biomedicines* 10, 316. doi:10.3390/biomedicines10020316
34. Piera-Velazquez, S., and Jimenez, S. A. (2018). Simultaneous Inhibition of C-Abl and Src Kinases Abrogates the Exaggerated Expression of Profibrotic Genes in Cultured Systemic Sclerosis Dermal Fibroblasts. *Clin. Exp. Rheumatol.* 113, 36 Politiek, F. A., and Waterham, H. R. (2021). Compromised Protein Prenylation as Pathogenic Mechanism in Mevalonate Kinase Deficiency. *Front. Immunol.* 12,724991. doi:10.3389/fimmu.2021.724991

35. Raghu, G., Collard, H. R., Egan, J. J., Martinez, F. J., Behr, J., Brown, K. K., et al. (2011). An Official ATS/ERS/JRS/ALAT Statement: Idiopathic Pulmonary Fibrosis: Evidence-Based Guidelines for Diagnosis and Management. *Am. J. Respir. Crit. Care Med.* 183, 788–824. doi:10.1164/rccm.2009-040GL
36. Raghu, G., Flaherty, K. R., Lederer, D. J., Lynch, D. A., Colby, T. V., Myers, J. L., et al. (2019). Use of a Molecular Classifier to Identify Usual Interstitial Pneumonia in Conventional Transbronchial Lung Biopsy Samples: a Prospective Validation Study. *Lancet Respir. Med.* 7, 487–496. doi:10.1016/S2213-2600(19)30059-1
37. Rosen, L. S., Gordon, D., Kaminski, M., Howell, A., Belch, A., Mackey, J., et al. (2003). Long-term Efficacy and Safety of Zoledronic Acid Compared with Pamidronate Disodium in the Treatment of Skeletal Complications in Patients with Advanced Multiple Myeloma or Breast Carcinoma. *Cancer* 98, 1735–1744. doi:10.1002/cncr.11701
38. Ruaro, B., Soldano, S., Smith, V., Paolino, S., Contini, P., Montagna, P., et al. (2019). Correlation between Circulating Fibrocytes and Dermal Thickness in Limited Cutaneous Systemic Sclerosis Patients: a Pilot Study. *Rheumatol. Int.* 39, 1369–1376. doi:10.1007/s00296-019-04315-7
39. Schafer, M. J., White, T. A., Iijima, K., Haak, A. J., Ligresti, G., Atkinson, E. J., et al. (2017). Cellular Senescence Mediates Fibrotic Pulmonary Disease. *Nat. Commun.* 8, 1–11. doi:10.1038/ncomms14532
40. Skibba, M., Drelich, A., Poellmann, M., Hong, S., and Brasier, A. R. (2020). Nanoapproaches to Modifying Epigenetics of Epithelial Mesenchymal Transition for Treatment of Pulmonary Fibrosis. *Front. Pharmacol.* 11, 607689. doi:10.3389/fphar.2020.607689
41. Spagnolo, P., Tzouvelekis, A., and Bonella, F. (2018). The Management of Patients with Idiopathic Pulmonary Fibrosis. *Front. Med.* 5, 148. doi:10.3389/fmed.2018. 00148
42. Tanner, L., and Single, A. B. (2019). Animal Models Reflecting Chronic Obstructive Pulmonary Disease and Related Respiratory Disorders: Translating Pre-clinical Data into Clinical Relevance. *J. Innate Immun.* 12, 203–225. doi:10.1159/ 000502489
43. Tashiro, J., Rubio, G. A., Limper, A. H., Williams, K., Elliot, S. J., Ninou, I., et al. (2017). Exploring Animal Models that Resemble Idiopathic Pulmonary Fibrosis. *Front. Med. (Lausanne)* 4, 118. doi:10.3389/fmed.2017.00118
44. Tsou, P.-S., Haak, A. J., Khanna, D., and Neubig, R. R. (2014). Cellular Mechanisms of Tissue Fibrosis. 8. Current and Future Drug Targets in Fibrosis: Focus on Rho GTPase-Regulated Gene Transcription. *Am. J. Physiol. Cell Physiol.* 307, C2–C13. doi:10.1152/ajpcell.00060.2014
45. Upagupta, C., Shimbori, C., Alsilmi, R., and Kolb, M. (2018). Matrix Abnormalities in Pulmonary Fibrosis. *Eur. Respir. Rev.* 27, 180033. doi:10.1183/16000617. 0033-2018
46. Vannella, K. M., and Wynn, T. A. (2017). Mechanisms of Organ Injury and Repair by Macrophages. *Annu. Rev. Physiol.* 79, 593–617. doi:10.1146/annurev- physiol-022516-034356
47. Waghray, M., Cui, Z., Horowitz, J. C., Subramanian, I. M., Martinez, F. J., Toews, G. B., et al. (2005). Hydrogen Peroxide Is a Diffusible Paracrine Signal for the Induction of Epithelial Cell Death by Activated Myofibroblasts. *FASEB J.* 19, 1–16. doi:10.1096/fj.04-2882fje
48. Watts, N. B., and Diab, D. L. (2010). Long-term Use of Bisphosphonates in Osteoporosis. *J. Clin. Endocrinol. Metabolism* 95, 1555–1565. doi:10.1210/jc. 2009-1947
49. Wynn, T. A., and Ramalingam, T. R. (2012). Mechanisms of Fibrosis: Therapeutic Translation for Fibrotic Disease. *Nat. Med.* 18, 1028–1040. doi:10.1038/nm. 2807
50. Wynn, T. A., and Vannella, K. M. (2016). Macrophages in Tissue Repair, Regeneration, and Fibrosis. *Immunity* 44, 450–462. doi:10.1016/j.immuni. 2016.02.015
51. Xu, J.-F., Washko, G. R., Nakahira, K., Hatabu, H., Patel, A. S., Fernandez, I. E., et al. (2012). Statins and Pulmonary Fibrosis: the Potential Role of NLRP3 Inflammasome Activation. *Am. J. Respir. Crit. Care Med.* 185, 547–556. doi:10. 1164/rccm.201108-1574OC
52. Xue, H., Li, J., Xie, H., and Wang, Y. (2018). Review of Drug Repositioning Approaches and Resources. *Int. J. Biol. Sci.* 14, 1232–1244. doi:10.7150/ijbs. 24612
53. Zeng, P.-Y., Rane, N., Du, W., Chintapalli, J., and Prendergast, G. C. (2003). Role for RhoB and PRK in the Suppression of Epithelial Cell Transformation by Farnesyltransferase Inhibitors. *Oncogene* 22, 1124–1134. doi:10.1038/sj.onc. 1206181
54. Zhang, J., Lu, J., Xie, H., Wang, D., Ni, H., Zhu, Y., et al. (2019). circHIPK3 Regulates Lung Fibroblast-To-Myofibroblast Transition by Functioning as a Competing Endogenous RNA. *Cell Death Dis.* 10, 182. doi:10.1038/s41419-019-1430-7
55. Zhang, L., Wang, Y., Wu, G., Xiong, W., Gu, W., and Wang, C.-Y. (2018). Macrophages: Friend or Foe in Idiopathic Pulmonary Fibrosis? *Respir. Res.* 19, 1–10. doi:10.1186/s12931-018-0864-2
56. Zhao, C.-Z., Zhao, X.-M., Yang, J., Mou, Y., Chen, B., Wu, H.-D., et al. (2016). Inhibition of Farnesyl Pyrophosphate Synthase Improves Pressure Overload Induced Chronic Cardiac Remodeling. *Sci. Rep.* 6, 39186. doi:10.1038/srep39186
57. Zhou, Y., Peng, H., Sun, H., Peng, X., Tang, C., Gan, Y., et al. (2014). Chitinase 3-like 1 Suppresses Injury and Promotes Fibroproliferative Responses in Mammalian Lung Fibrosis. *Sci. Transl. Med.* 6, 240ra76. doi:10.1126/scitranslmed.3007096

14

Club Cell Loss as a Feature of Bronchiolization in ILD

*Paul Reynaud[1], Engi Ahmed[1,2], Isabelle Serre[3], Lucie Knabe[1], Sébastien Bommart[4], Carey Suehs[1], Isabelle Vachier[1], Jean Philippe Berthet[5], Micaela Romagnoli[6], Charlotte Vernisse[1,2], Jean Pierre Mallet[1], Anne Sophie Gamez[1] and Arnaud Bourdin[1,2]**

[1] Department of Respiratory Diseases, Univ Montpellier, CHU Montpellier, Montpellier, France, [2] PhyMedExp, Univ Montpellier, CNRS, INSERM, CHU Montpellier, Montpellier, France, [3] Department of Pathology, Univ Montpellier, CHU Montpellier, Montpellier, France, [4] Department of Radiology, Univ Montpellier, CHU Montpellier, Montpellier, France, [5] Pulmonology Unit, Ospedale Ca'Foncello, AULSS2 Marca Trevigiana, Trevise, Italy, [6] Department of Cardiac, Thoracic and Vascular Surgery, Univ Nice, CHU Nice, Nice, France

***Correspondence:**
Arnaud Bourdin
a-bourdin@chu-montpellier.fr

Background: Distal airway metaplasia may precede honeycombing in progressive fibrosing interstitial lung disease (ILD). The SCGB1A1$^+$ bronchiolar-specific club cell may play a role in this aberrant regenerative process.

Objective: To assess the presence of club cells in the small airways of patients suffering from ILD.

Methods: Small airways (internal diameter <2 mm) in lung samples [surgical lung biopsy (SLB) and/or transbronchial lung cryobiopsy (TBLC)] from 14 patients suffering from ILD and 10 controls were morphologically assessed and stained for SCGB1A1. SCGB1A1 was weighted by epithelial height as a marker of airway generation (SCGB1A1/EH). Correlations between clinical, functional, and high-resolution CT (HRCT) prognostic factors and histomorphometry were assessed.

Results: Small airways from samples with ILD patterns were significantly less dense in terms of SCGB1A1$^+$ cells [0.064 (0.020–0.172)] as compared to controls' sample's small airways [0.393 (0.082–0.698), $p < 0.0001$]. Usual interstitial pneumonia (UIP) patterns most frequently contained small airways with limited or absent SCGB1A1 expression (SCGB1A1/EH <0.025): UIP (18/33; 55%) as compared with non-UIP patterns (4/31; 13%) or controls (0/29; 0%): $p < 0.0001$. In addition, correlations with HRCT indicated a significant negative relationship between SCGB1A1 and bronchiectasis as a feature of bronchiolization (Rho −0.63, $p < 0.001$) and a positive relationship with both forced vital capacity (FVC) and Hounsfield unit (HU)-distribution pattern in kurtosis (Rho 0.38 and 0.50, respectively, both $p < 0.001$) as markers of fibrotic changes.

Conclusion: Compared with controls, the small airways of patients with ILD more often lack SCGB1A1, especially so in UIP. Low densities of SCGB1A1-marked cells correlate with bronchiectasis and fibrotic changes. Further research investigating SCGB1A1 staining as a pathological feature of the bronchiolization process is merited.

Keywords: club (clara) cell, idiopathic pulmonary fibrosis, metaplasia, SCGB1A1, bronchiolization, interstitial lung disease

INTRODUCTION

Interstitial lung disease (ILD) are devastating affections nearly constantly leading to respiratory failure and death. The early phases of the disease are hallmarked by progressive fibrosis in the peripheral zones of the lung, which is associated with lung function decline (1). High-resolution CT (HRCT) has become the gold standard for diagnosing such fibrotic changes and characterizing their progression (2). Notably, the presence of traction bronchiectasis (the enlargement of small airways by traction) is now considered a red flag for subpleural fibrotic changes. Interestingly, histomorphological assessments of these fibrotic areas consistently report bronchiolar metaplasia of unclear origin (3). The latter "bronchiolization" may represent aberrant regeneration of the lung in a profibrotic environment, where distal airway precursors never reach their potential as functional alveoli (4). The result is the presence of proximal features in the distal compartment currently detectable only *via* histopathology (5).

Club cells are thought to be highly expressed at the small airway level (6), where they are supposed to play a protective role against noxious inhaled particles. Among the latter, cigarette smoke and occupational dust have also been implicated in the pathogenesis of idiopathic pulmonary fibrosis (IPF) (7, 8). Interestingly, club cells were also attributed an accessory stem cell role at the small airway level, but this role has mostly been evidenced in animal models at the bronchoalveolar duct junction, where they are preferentially located (9). Due to recent advances in single-cell biology, it is now clear that these cells are heterogeneous and not all are playing the same role. Currently, they are considered as differentiation of basal cells, and the transition from basal to club cells has been ontogenically evidenced. Additionally, club cells are situated at the crossroads of the epithelial phenotype. Their natural trend is to progressively acquire features of goblet cells, but some can also move toward ciliogenesis. Whether or not appropriate transition pathways are failing during the bronchiolisation process remain unclear.

New opportunities for lung tissue sampling are provided by the arrival of transbronchial lung cryobiopsies (TBLC). Beyond clinical and technical considerations, it seems that TBLC, as compared to traditional surgical lung biopsies (SLB), samples airway-centered, more proximal tissue, and this is likely to change not only the pathological patterns and eventually the final pathological diagnosis but also the representation of the different compartments. In particular, airways contained in TBLC samples are more likely to represent earlier generations than those taken in the more peripheral SLB samples (10). Intuitively, the small airways present in TBLC samples might then be less frequently affected by bronchiolization. Given the relationship between this process and the fibrotic changes affecting the lung in progressing ILD, these pathological changes may have some diagnostic and/or prognostic value identifiable by clinical correlations in a cross-sectional study.

The objective of this study was to assess the presence of club cells in the small airways of patients suffering from ILD by combining pathology, physiology, and HRCT data.

We hypothesized that "protective" club cells characterized by their specific protein SCGB1A1 might be deficient in fibrotic diseases and particularly at the site where bronchiolar metaplasia occurs.

MATERIALS AND METHODS

CryoPID [NCT02763540] was a prospective trial evaluating the diagnostic concordance between TBLC and SLB, which were performed sequentially in the same patients between January 2016 and March 2018 at the Montpellier University Hospital (11). The study included patients with ILD requiring an SLB as per a multidisciplinary approach decision, given an undefined HRCT pattern. For the current histology assessment, 14 CryoPID patients were compared with 10 control subjects randomly selected from the bio-bank of the Montpellier University Hospital. Pathological patterns reported from SLB and TBLC together by a pathologist involved in the present study were used. Controls had normal lung function, were free of chronic respiratory disease, and matched, as well as a possibility for smoking, in gender and age with the ILD population. They had undergone a lobar resection for a colic metastasis in the last 3 years. Lung parenchyma at a large distance from the metastasis was analyzed.

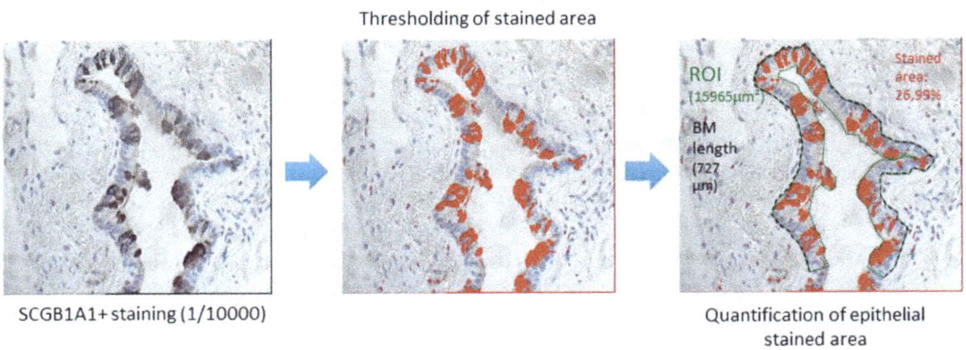

FIGURE 1 | After SCGB1A1 staining, small airway epithelia were isolated *via* thresholding, perimeters, thickness/height, and by the area quantified.

Briefly, lung samples were fixed in 4% formalin at pH 7.4 and embedded in paraffin. Three-millimeter-thick sections were stained by H&E. Lung samples were anonymized and blindly assessed by an expert pathologist (TVC). Serial sections were used for SCGB1A1 immunostaining (dilution 1/10,000; Biovendor, Czech Republic). For some slides, a Bleu Alcian staining could also be performed.

Small airways (identified by an internal diameter of 2 mm or less) were assessed in all samples. Morphometry was assessed using the Cell P software (Olympus, Tokyo, Japan). Bronchiolization was referred to small airways with evidence of proximal features, including the presence of ciliated and/or goblet cells, as per the previously published standards (12, 13). Epithelial area, epithelial height (EH), and the percentage of SCGB1A1$^+$ immune-stained area were determined for each small airway. The SCGB1A1$^+$/EH ratio was computed to adjust for variations known to affect club cell density through airway generation (**Figure 1**). The small airway density for each sample was based on a semi-quantitative scale ranging from 0 (absence of small airways) to 5 (highest small airway density). The absence or near-absence of club cells was defined by a SCGB1A1/EH ratio <0.025 by taking into account the background noise.

Prognostic factors were recorded and included clinical (age, gender, smoking history), biological/laboratory [arterial oxygen pressure (PaO_2), bronchoalveolar lavage cellularity (BAL)], and functional [forced vital capacity (FVC), diffusing capacity of the lungs for carbon monoxide (DLCO)] criteria.

A visual tomodensitometric analysis scored fibrotic changes (honeycombing and reticulations), intensity, and the spread of ground-glass opacity (GGO) (14), as well as the extent of bronchiectasis [ranking the severity of bronchiectasis by a lobe on a scale ranging from 0 to 3 (15) by acquiring consensus among two experienced thoracic senior radiologists (SB and GD)].

Automatic quantification *via* the Thoracic VCAR software (GE HealthCare, USA) was also performed, classifying pixels from the whole lung (WL) volume into four groups as proposed by Shin et al. (16) (< −950 HU: "emphysema," −950 to −700 HU "functional parenchyma," −700 to −500 HU "interstitial disease," > −500 HU "extra parenchymal"). Three prognostic variables were then derived: total lung capacity (TLC), percentage of normal lung (%NL), and mean lung attenuation (MLA) (17). Pulmonary attenuation distribution histograms were obtained for assessing skewness and kurtosis, previously reported as having the prognostic value (18).

TABLE 1 | Population characteristics.

	ILD [Median (IQR25–75)]	Controls [Median (IQR25–75)]	*p*-value
N	14	10	
Age (years)	63 [43.5–65]	64 [57.5–67.5]	0.21
Gender (W/M)	10 vs. 04	3 vs. 7	0.0987
Weight (kg)	65.5 [60.65–81.75]	65 [62.25–83.75]	0.49
Height (cm)	160 [158.5–170]	166.5 [160–170]	0.44
Smoking history (p.y)	2.5 [0–28.75]	19 [1.25–30]	0.77
Smoking status (current-former-never)	1/5/8	1/5/4	
Positive autoantibodies	0	0	
PaO_2 (mmHg)	84.2 [75.75–88.28]	88.65 [81.29–93.5]	0.15
FVC (l)	2.3 [1.74–3.31]	3.43 [2.75–4.07]	0.027*
FVC (% pred values)	84.5 [68.5–2.77]	100 [92.25–107.5]	0.004*
FEV1 (l)	2.1 [1.59–2.77]	2.39 [2.02–3.39]	0.077
FEV1 (% pred values)	84 [72.75–90]	95.5 [86–110.8]	0.010*
TLC (l)	3.69 [3.55–4.49]	6.23 [6.16–6.59]	0.001*
TLC (% pred values)	77.5 [66.25–84.75]	103 [101–106]	0.00005*
RV (l)	1.57 [1.31–1.79]	2.64 [2.58–3.12]	0.0002*
RV (% pred values)	89 [65–102]	116 [100–121]	0.0049*
TLCO (% pred values)	56 [40–60]	76 [70–80]	0.0097*
KCO	79 [73–96]	85 [78–103]	0.58
Kurtosis	6.33 [4.32–7.48]	14.77 [13.78–17.16]	0.0017*
Skewness	2.29 [2.02–2.53]	3.59 [3.39–3.85]	0.00014*
Whole lung (WL)	3.44 [2.79–4.12]	5.61 [3.54–6.17]	0.1095
% Normal lung (NL)	79.98 [71.14–82.04]	88.72 [88.2–90.25]	0.00045
Mean lung attenuation (Hounsfield)	−764 [−796 to −720]	−838 [−859 to −819]	0.0012*
Fibrotic score	15 [10–22.5]	0 [0–0]	0.00006*
Ground glass opacity	5 [5–5]	0 [0–0]	0.059
Bronchiectasis score	6 [5.25–8]	0 [0–0]	0.00003*

%NL, percentage of normal lung; BMI, body mass index; CT, computed tomography; DLCO, diffusing capacity of the lungs for carbon monoxide; FEV1, forced expiratory volume in 1 s; FVC, forced vital capacity; ILD, interstial lung disease; IQR, interquartile range; KCO, transfer coefficient of the lung for carbon monoxide; MLA, mean lung attenuation; N, number; PaO_2, arterial oxygen pressure; RV, residual volume; SD, standard deviation; TLC, total lung capacity.

$^*p < 0.05$.

Statistical Analysis

Parametric and non-parametric tests were used to describe and compare normally and non-normally distributed data as appropriate. Spearman's correlation coefficients were computed for testing variable relationships.

RESULTS

Population Description

Fourteen patients with ILD and 10 controls were studied (**Table 1**). As expected, patients with ILD had worse pulmonary function tests and higher HRCT semi-quantitative scores. Of note, as these patients were deemed eligible for SLB, most had a mild functional impairment, suggesting that many were at an early stage of the disease. As previously reported (11), discrepancies in the pathological diagnosis between SLB and TBLC existed, potentially leading to different final diagnoses during a second multidisciplinary assessment (**Table 2**). For subsequent classification as usual interstitial pneumonia (UIP) and non-UIP, only samples with a clear and confirmed (high level of confidence) UIP pattern were retained.

Among patients with ILD, the mean SLB sample size was 49.5 mm [41.5–60] compared to 7 mm (6–8) ($p < 0.00001$) for TBLC. A significant difference in the semi-quantitative scoring of small airway density between SLB and TBLC sample was found (**Table 3**). No difference was found between TBLC and SLB

TABLE 2 | Blinded histology and multidisciplinary diagnostic results for each patient.

Patient	Histology diagnosis based on TBLC	Histology diagnosis based on SLB	Diagnosis based on MDA 1 (before histology)	Diagnosis based on MDA 2 (after histology)
1	UIP	UIP	Possible UIP	CHP
2	Non-diagnostic	PLCH	DIP	PLCH
3	UIP	CHP	NSIP	IPF
4	UIP	NSIP	No classification	NSIP
5	RB-ILD	RB-ILD	RB-ILD	RB-ILD
6	Non-diagnostic	UIP	NSIP	IPF
7	PLCH	UIP	Possible UIP	IPF
8	NSIP	NSIP	Fibrotic NSIP	NOS
9	UIP	UIP	NSIP	IPF
10	Non-diagnostic	ALI	NSIP	NOS
11	NSIP	LP	Sarcoidosis	CVID
12	UIP	NSIP	NSIP	NSIP
13	Non-diagnostic	UIP	CHP	IPF
14	UIP	UIP	Possible UIP	IPF

CHP, chronic hypersensitivity pneumonitis; CVID, common variable immune deficiency; DIP, desquamative interstitial pneumonia; HP, hypersensitivity pneumonitis; IPF, idiopathic pulmonary fibrosis; LP, lymphoid process; MDA1, a first multidisciplinary assessment; MDA2, the final multidisciplinary assessment; NOS, not otherwise specified; NSIP, non-specific interstitial pneumonia; OP, organizing pneumonia; PLCH, pulmonary Langerhans cell histiocytosis; RB-ILD, respiratory bronchiolitis-associated interstitial lung disease; SLB, surgical lung biopsy; TBLC, transbronchial lung cryobiopsy; UIP, usual interstitial pneumonia.

TABLE 3 | Samples characteristics.

	SLB (controls)	SLB (ILD)	TBLC (ILD)	*p*-value
N	10	14	14	
Number of small airways assessed	32	35	31	
Small airway density [semi quantitative score (0 = minimal; 5 = maximal)]	2.1 ± 0.1	2.4 ± 0.6	0.4 ± 0.3	0.04
Epithelial area (mean ± SD per bronchiole. μm²)	20,818 ± 9,040	26,738 ± 11,733	19,638 ± 11,216	ns
Epithelial height (mean ± SD per bronchiole. μm)	37.8 ± 7.8	39.5 ± 11.9	35.8 ± 11.4	ns
SCGB1A1⁺ stained area	19.7 (4.2–27.7)	3.6 (1.6–7.4)	0.9 (0.3–2.9)	<0.0001
SCGB1A1⁺/EH	0.5 (0.1–0.7)	0.1 (0.0–0.2)	0.0 (0.0–0.1)	0.02
% airway without club cells§	0 (0/32)	14 (5/35)	55 (17/31)	0.01

§ *Defined by SCGB1A1+/EH ratio < 0.025.*

regarding club cell representation in the small airways. Fewer airways positively stained for SCGB1A1 in ILD, in particular, for those with a pathological UIP pattern, and in general, this staining was less intense (**Figure 2A**). This decrease persisted after adjusting on epithelial height as a surrogate marker of the generation of the airway assessed. Hence, SCGB1A1/EH was statistically lower in the small airways of samples from patients with ILD vs. controls (**Figure 2B**; the Kruskal-Wallis test, $p = 7.598e\text{-}07$).

Moreover, sparsely stained airways (defined as SCGB1A1/EH <0.025) were significantly more represented in the UIP pathological patterns [UIP 18/33 vs. non-UIP 4/31 ($p = 0.0027$)] (**Table 2** and **Figure 3**).

The tested prognostic correlations are provided in **Figure 4**. Interestingly, statistically significant non-parametric correlations were found between SCGB1A1/EH and two surrogate markers of lung fibrosis. First, a correlation was found with the kurtosis value of the histogram distribution of lung attenuation assessed at HRCT (Rho = 0.50, $p < 0.001$). The less the lung is involved by fibrosis, the greater the club cell density found in the small airways, as the kurtosis value decreases with the extent of fibrosis in ILD (18). Second, SCGB1A1/EH also positively correlated with FVC (Rho = 0.38, $p < 0.001$), as expected.

The negative correlation found between SCGB1A1/EH and the bronchiectasis scores (Rho = −0.63, $p < 0.001$) is also represented in **Figure 4**. The latter indicates that fewer club cells were present in the small airways of patients with more intense bronchiectasis.

DISCUSSION

With the aim of understanding the mechanisms of bronchiolization, we found that club cells are absent or nearly absent from these aberrant small airways in the most subpleural areas of fibrotic lungs. This was particularly true in ILD where a UIP pattern could be identified. Bronchiolized areas seem to fit with small airways saliently featuring proximal differentiation patterns very close to terminal airspaces. As expected, both TBLC and SLB could identify these patterns, even though the density of small airways in TBLC is largely lower. Interestingly, the correlation between these bronchiolization patterns (highlighted by the absence of club cells) and clinical prognostic markers (such as HRCT kurtosis and bronchiectasis), as well as physiology (FVC), was demonstrated.

Most of our results were driven by a particularly high number of unstained or sparsely stained airways in lung samples from patients with a UIP pattern. Most of these pauci-SCGB1A1 small airways displayed features of bronchiolar metaplasia. Interestingly, they were referred to as "bronchiolizing areas" in the routine pathology report.

Fukumoto et al. hypothesized that this phenomenon may indicate an impaired differentiation with aberrant proliferation (19). The latter hypothesis is supported by the morphologic appearance of these areas where proximal features are found where they should not be.

The underexpression of the club cell-specific protein SCGB1A1 may be directly linked to the bronchiolization process, as already supposed by Jensen-Taubman (20). A blockade in the

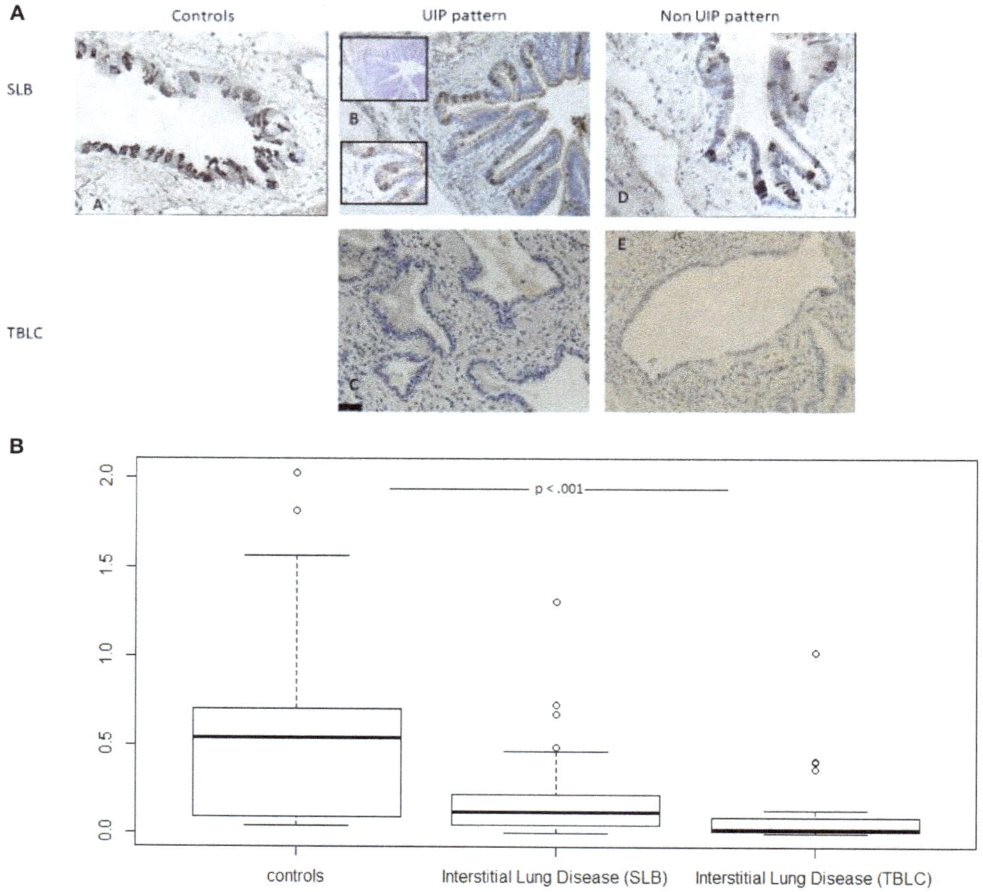

FIGURE 2 | (A) Small airways are immune-stained for SCGB1A1 in controls, UIP, and non-UIP patterns. Upper left: (A) SLB from a control (no TBLC were available in this group). Middle row: (B) Very limited staining in some (left lower part) but not all small airways sampled by SLB; Inserts are: Serial cut with a Blue Alcian staining suggestive of the presence of mucin-costaining and a higher magnification suggestive of goblet cell morphology for SCGB1A1 positively stained epithelial cells. Ectasic small airway from a TBLC UIP pattern with bronchiolar metaplasia nearly free of staining despite abundant mucostasis. Right: SCGB1A1 stained small airways obtained by SLB (D) and by TBLC (E) in non-UIP patterns. **(B)** Box plots demonstrating group differences (Control vs. ILD for SLB and TBLC) for SCGB1A1 staining variables. TBLC, transbronchial lung cryobiopsies; SLB, surgical lung biopsy; UIP, usual interstitial pneumonia; ILD, interstitial lung disease.

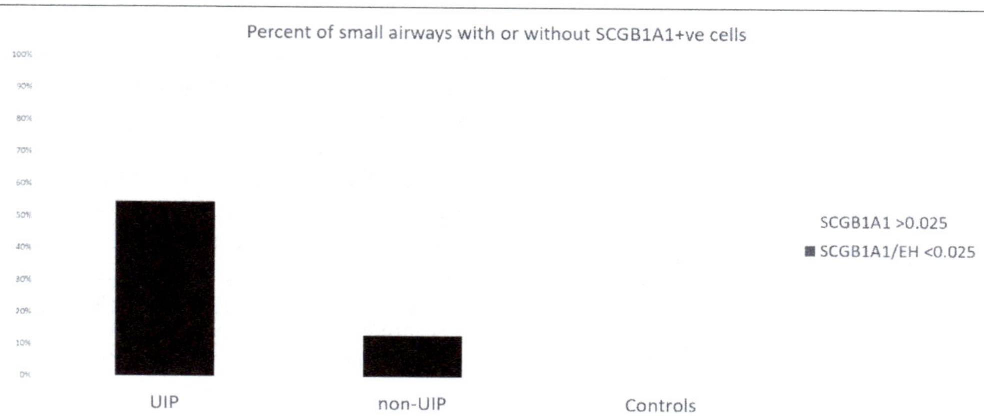

FIGURE 3 | The proportion of samples with SCGB1A1/EH <0.025 was used to define the absence of positive staining [UIP 18/33 vs. non-UIP 4/31 ($p = 0.0027$)].

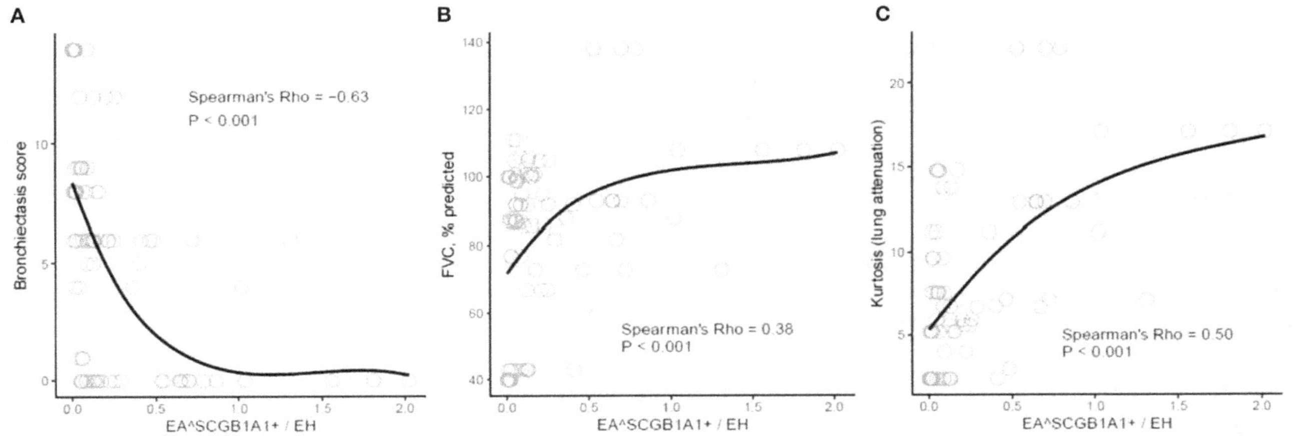

FIGURE 4 | Scatterplots demonstrating the relationships between selected pulmonary function variables [bronchiectasis score **(A)**, % predicted forced vital capacity (FVC, % predicted) **(B)**, and kurtosis of lung attenuation scores **(C)**] and % epithelial area of small airways that stains SCGB1B1$^+$ weighted by epithelial height (EA$^{SCGB1B1+}$/EH). Smoothing is performed *via* a local loess estimator (in black). Spearman's correlation statistics (Rho and FDR-corrected *p*-value) are provided.

notch pathway might be involved in this ontogenically impaired process, as the notch is critically involved in basal to club cell transitioning (21). Wnt/β-catenin pathways were also shown to be involved.

This mechanism may help accelerate the paradigm shift that is already in motion, where instead of envisioning bronchiolization and bronchiectasis as a consequence of fibrosis, they are now understood to be an active part of the fibrotic process [as again recently suggested (4)].

Senescence may play a key role in the fibrotic process characteristic of UIP (22) possibly *via* this bronchiolization. Aberrantly proliferating cells can lead to both replicative and premature senescence (23), possibly leading to these poorly differentiated airways. The secretion of senescence-associated secretory protein (SASP), mainly interleukin-8, has already been shown to be involved (24).

Our study has several limits. Few patients were included due to the particular procedures used in the CryoPID study. Our patient group was so heterogeneous that artificially gathering patients from a "non-UIP" group was required. Moreover, staining for MUC5B, a validated bronchiolization marker, would have been of great interest to increase confidence in the mechanism and further characterize the phenotype of the remaining club cells. As shown by Best et al. (25), a higher proportion of SCGB1A1$^+$/MUC5B$^+$ cells is observed in IPF, highly expressing genes related to mucins and chemoattractant cytokines for immune cells. Though we missed this opportunity, we nonetheless had attempted the Bleu Alcian staining in a few slides when some unused material was available; the latter suggested convergent findings and merits further investigation.

Of note, we decided to focus our analysis at the sample level (as opposed to the patient level) to take into account the regional heterogeneity of the fibrotic process where zones of normal appearance are classically neighboring the involved tissue (6). This was also justified by the aim of comparing TBLC and SLB in this regard. Correlations were tested at the individual level by expressing SCGB1A1 as a mean and our findings remained consistent.

There are a few steps left to definitively demonstrate that bronchiolization precedes the fibrotic process. Recently, by matching micro-CT imaging with histology, Verleden et al. showed that small airway involvement is the most striking finding in the early IPF stages, suggesting that the disease starts at this level (4).

Our study also supports that the bronchiolization process is key in the course of the disease as we could find correlations with two different HRCT-derived parameters. Kurtosis refers to the tailedness of the distribution histogram of lung attenuation, and this value was suggested to be a surrogate of interstitial changes (25). A significant negative relationship between the expression of the club cell marker SCGB1A1 and the bronchiectasis score was also found; an intuitively-expected finding enhancing the concept that bronchiectasis found at HRCT is related to the bronchiolization process hallmarked by the absence of club cells. Convincingly, a significant correlation was also found with FVC, a physiological marker more than relevant in interstitial lung diseases.

In summary, we demonstrated that bronchiolization, a typical characteristic of ILD and of UIP in particular, is also hallmarked by the absence of club cells. This suggests that an impaired transition process affected epithelial cell fate.

Pauci-SCGB1A1 staining status merits further study as a potential marker of bronchiolization in ILD.

ETHICS STATEMENT

The studies involving human participants were reviewed and approved by CPP Ile de France. The patients/participants provided their written informed consent to participate in this study.

AUTHOR CONTRIBUTIONS

AB elaborated the study, enrolled patients, performed biopsies, participated to the interpretation of the data, and the writing of the manuscript. PR participated to the study, enrolled patients, performed biopsies, acquisition of data, immunostaining, morphometry, HRCT analysis, and the writing of the manuscript. EA participated to the study, enrolled patients, performed biopsies, acquisition of data, and the writing of the manuscript. IS participated to the study, assessed biopsies, and contributed to the immunostaining. LK, CV, CS, and IV participated to the study, interpretation of the data, and the writing of the manuscript. SB participated to HRCT analysis. MR, JB, JM, and AG participated to the study, enrolled patients, and performed biopsies. All authors contributed to the article and approved the submitted version.

REFERENCES

1. Olson AL, Gifford AH, Inase N, Fernández Pérez ER, Suda T. The epidemiology of idiopathic pulmonary fibrosis and interstitial lung diseases at risk of a progressive-fibrosing phenotype. *Eur Respir Rev.* (2018) 27:180077. doi: 10.1183/16000617.0077-2018
2. Sverzellati N, Brillet P-Y. When Deep Blue first defeated Kasparov: is a machine stronger than a radiologist at predicting prognosis in idiopathic pulmonary fibrosis? *Euro Respir J.* (2017) 49:1602144. doi: 10.1183/13993003.02144-2016
3. Visscher DW, Myers JL. Histologic spectrum of idiopathic interstitial pneumonias. *Proc Am Thorac Soc.* (2006) 3:322–9. doi: 10.1513/pats.200602-019TK
4. Verleden SE, Tanabe N, McDonough JE, Vasilescu DM, Xu F, Wuyts WA, et al. Small airways pathology in idiopathic pulmonary fibrosis: a retrospective cohort study. *Lancet Respir Med.* (2020) 8:573–84. doi: 10.1016/S2213-2600(19)30356-X
5. Plantier L, Crestani B, Wert SE, Dehoux M, Zweytick B, Guenther A, et al. Ectopic respiratory epithelial cell differentiation in bronchiolised distal airspaces in idiopathic pulmonary fibrosis. *Thorax.* (2011) 66:651–7. doi: 10.1136/thx.2010.151555
6. Boers JE, Ambergen AW, Thunnissen FB. Number and proliferation of clara cells in normal human airway epithelium. *Am J Respir Crit Care Med.* (1999) 159:1585–91. doi: 10.1164/ajrccm.159.5.9806044
7. Akram KM, Lomas NJ, Spiteri MA, Forsyth NR. Club cells inhibit alveolar epithelial wound repair via TRAIL-dependent apoptosis. *Euro Respir J.* (2013) 41:683–94. doi: 10.1183/09031936.00213411
8. Singh G, Katyal SL. Clara cells and clara cell 10 kD protein (CC10). *Am J Respir Cell Mol Biol.* (1997) 17:141–3. doi: 10.1165/ajrcmb.17.2.f138
9. Rawlins EL, Okubo T, Xue Y, Brass DM, Auten RL, Hasegawa H, et al. The role of Scgb1a1+ Clara cells in the long-term maintenance and repair of lung airway, but not alveolar, epithelium. *Cell Stem Cell.* (2009) 4:525–34. doi: 10.1016/j.stem.2009.04.002
10. Colby TV, Tomassetti S, Cavazza A, Dubini A, Poletti V. Transbronchial cryobiopsy in diffuse lung disease: update for the pathologist. *Arch Pathol Lab Med.* (2017) 141:891–900. doi: 10.5858/arpa.2016-0233-RA
11. Romagnoli M, Colby TV, Berthet J.-P, Gamez AS, Mallet J.-P, Serre I, et al. Poor concordance between sequential transbronchial lung cryobiopsy and surgical lung biopsy in the diagnosis of diffuse interstitial lung diseases. *Am J Respir Crit Care Med.* (2019) 199:1249–56. doi: 10.1164/rccm.201810-1947OC
12. Nettesheim P, Szakal AK. Morphogenesis of alveolar bronchiolization. *Lab Invest.* (1972) 26:210–9.
13. Allen TC. Pathology of small airways disease. *Arch Pathol Lab Med.* (2010) 134:702–18. doi: 10.5858/134.5.702
14. Shin KM, Lee KS, Chung MP, Han J, Bae YA, Kim TS, et al. Prognostic determinants among clinical, thin-section CT, and histopathologic findings for fibrotic idiopathic interstitial pneumonias: tertiary hospital study. *Radiology.* (2008) 249:328–37. doi: 10.1148/radiol.2483071378
15. Edey AJ, Devaraj AA, Barker RP, Nicholson AG, Wells AU, Hansell DM. Fibrotic idiopathic interstitial pneumonias: HRCT findings that predict mortality. *Eur Radiol.* (2011) 21:1586–93. doi: 10.1007/s00330-011-2098-2
16. Shin KE, Chung MJ, Jung MP, Choe BK, Lee KS. Quantitative computed tomographic indexes in diffuse interstitial lung disease: correlation with physiologic tests and computed tomography visual scores. *J Comput Assist Tomogr.* (2011) 35:266–71. doi: 10.1097/RCT.0b013e31820ccf18
17. Ohkubo H, Kanemitsu Y, Uemura T, Takakuwa O, Takemura M, Maeno K, et al. Normal lung quantification in usual interstitial pneumonia pattern: the impact of threshold-based volumetric CT analysis for the staging of idiopathic pulmonary fibrosis. *PLoS ONE.* (2016) 11:e0152505. doi: 10.1371/journal.pone.0152505
18. Lynch DA. Quantitative CT of fibrotic interstitial lung disease. *Chest.* (2007) 131:643–4. doi: 10.1378/chest.06-2955
19. Fukumoto J, Soundararajan R, Leung J, Cox R, Mahendrasah S, Muthavarapu N, et al. The role of club cell phenoconversion and migration in idiopathic pulmonary fibrosis. *Aging.* (2016) 8:3091–105. doi: 10.18632/aging.101115
20. Jensen-Taubman SM, Steinberg SM, Linnoila RI. Bronchiolization of the alveoli in lung cancer: pathology, patterns of differentiation and oncogene expression. *Int J Cancer.* (1998) 75:489–96. doi: 10.1002/(SICI)1097-0215(19980209)75:4<489::AID-IJC1>3.0.CO;2-P
21. Gras D, Chanez P, Vachier I, Petit A, Bourdin A. Bronchial epithelium as a target for innovative treatments in asthma. *Pharmacol Ther.* (2013) 140:290–305. doi: 10.1016/j.pharmthera.2013.07.008
22. Alder JK, Chen JJ.-L, Lancaster L, Danoff S, Su S.-c, Cogan JD, et al. Short telomeres are a risk factor for idiopathic pulmonary fibrosis. *Proc Natl Acad Sci USA.* (2008) 105:13051–6. doi: 10.1073/pnas.0804280105
23. Adnot S, Amsellem V, Boyer L, Marcos E, Saker M, Houssaini A, et al. Telomere dysfunction and cell senescence in chronic lung diseases: therapeutic potential. *Pharmacol Ther.* (2015) 153:125–34. doi: 10.1016/j.pharmthera.2015.06.007
24. Chilosi M, Carloni A, Rossi A, Poletti V. Premature lung aging and cellular senescence in the pathogenesis of idiopathic pulmonary fibrosis and COPD/emphysema. *Transl Res.* (2013) 162:156–73. doi: 10.1016/j.trsl.2013.06.004
25. Best AC, Meng J, Lynch AM, Bozic CM, Miller D, Grunwald GK, et al. Idiopathic pulmonary fibrosis: physiologic tests, quantitative CT indexes, and CT visual scores as predictors of mortality. *Radiology.* (2008) 246:935–40. doi: 10.1148/radiol.2463062200

15

Research Progress in the Molecular Mechanisms, Therapeutic Targets and Drug Development of Idiopathic Pulmonary Fibrosis

Hongbo Ma[1,2†], *Xuyi Wu*[1,3†], *Yi Li*[1,3] *and Yong Xia*[1,3*]

[1]*Department of Rehabilitation Medicine, State Key Laboratory of Biotherapy and Cancer Center, National Clinical Research Center for Geriatrics, West China Hospital, Sichuan University, Chengdu, China,* [2]*West China School of Pharmacy, Sichuan University, Chengdu, China,* [3]*Key Laboratory of Rehabilitation Medicine in Sichuan Province/Rehabilitation Medicine Research Institute, Chengdu, China*

***Correspondence:**
Yong Xia
yxia4@scu.edu.cn

†*These authors have contributed equally to this work and share first authorship*

Idiopathic pulmonary fibrosis (IPF) is a fatal interstitial lung disease. Recent studies have identified the key role of crosstalk between dysregulated epithelial cells, mesenchymal, immune, and endothelial cells in IPF. In addition, genetic mutations and environmental factors (e.g., smoking) have also been associated with the development of IPF. With the recent development of sequencing technology, epigenetics, as an intermediate link between gene expression and environmental impacts, has also been reported to be implicated in pulmonary fibrosis. Although the etiology of IPF is unknown, many novel therapeutic targets and agents have emerged from clinical trials for IPF treatment in the past years, and the successful launch of pirfenidone and nintedanib has demonstrated the promising future of anti-IPF therapy. Therefore, we aimed to gain an in-depth understanding of the underlying molecular mechanisms and pathogenic factors of IPF, which would be helpful for the diagnosis of IPF, the development of anti-fibrotic drugs, and improving the prognosis of patients with IPF. In this study, we summarized the pathogenic mechanism, therapeutic targets and clinical trials from the perspective of multiple cell types, gene mutations, epigenetic and environmental factors.

Keywords: idiopathic pulmonary fibrosis, cells crosstalk, gene mutations, epigenetics, emerging drugs

1 INTRODUCTION

Idiopathic pulmonary fibrosis (IPF) is a progressive, life-threatening, interstitial lung disease of unknown pathogenesis. IPF has a familial and sporadic onset with a poor prognosis, and death usually occurs within 2–5 years of diagnosis due to secondary respiratory failure (Noble et al., 2012). CT imaging of IPF usually shows a typical usual interstitial pneumonia (UIP) pattern, characterized by irregular reticular opacities with obligatory honeycombing, associated with traction bronchiectasis. IPF also exhibits histological features of UIP/IPF pattern characterized by architecture remodeling due to dense fibrosis with frequent honeycombing, patchy lung involvement by fibrosis, subpleural and/or paraseptal distribution, fibroblast foci at the edge of dense scars (Spagnolo et al., 2018; Baratella et al., 2021). Although the etiology of IPF is unknown, various imbalances centered on alveolar epithelial cell/fibroblast apoptosis imbalance has been shown to play an important role in the pathogenesis of IPF (Wang et al., 2021). Therefore, it is necessary to understand the respective roles and interactions of alveolar epithelial cells, fibroblasts,

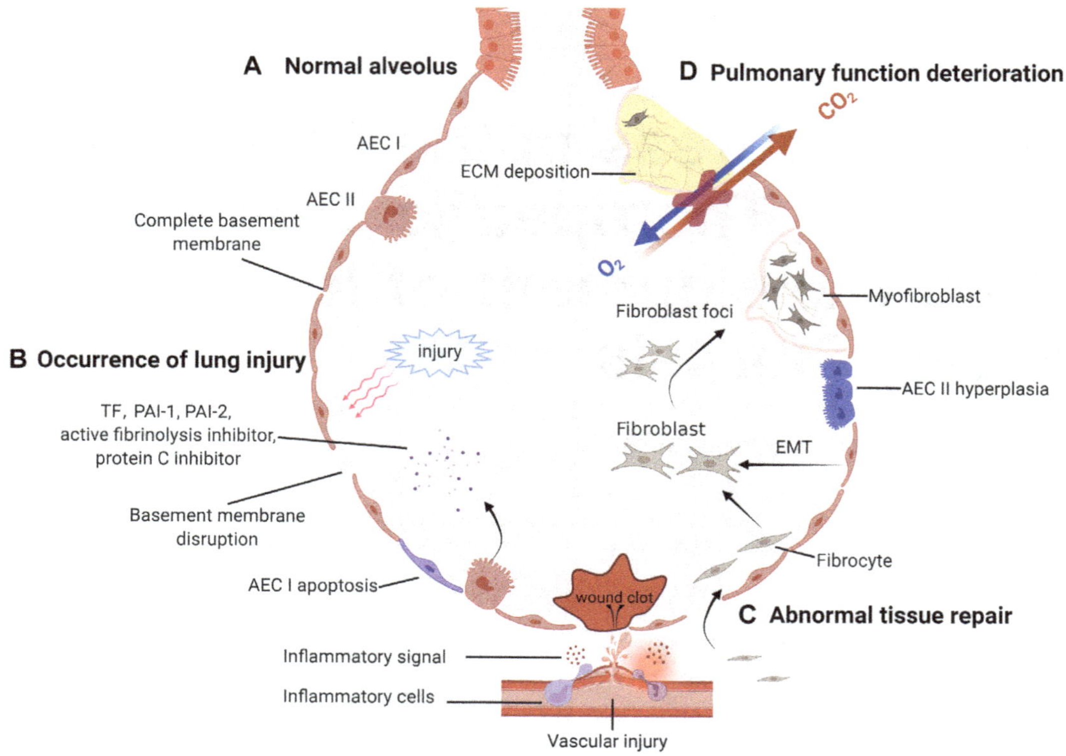

FIGURE 1 | The pathological process of idiopathic pulmonary fibrosis. **(A)** After normal alveoli are damaged and abnormally repaired, irreversible lung function deterioration occurs. Normal alveolus has a complete basement membrane and gas exchange function. **(B)** When the basement membrane continuity is disrupted by external injury, the damaged capillaries and activated AECs release inflammatory signals and coagulation factors, forming a local inflammatory microenvironment. **(C)** If the damage persists, abnormal repair will be initiated. Lung mesenchymal progenitors, fibrocytes recruited to the lung, and endothelial cells undergoing EMT can aggregate to form fibroblasts foci and differentiate into matrix-secreting myofibroblasts. To compensate for the local blood supply to the alveoli, new blood vessels are gradually formed. **(D)** As fibroblast foci increased, more ECM was deposited and cross-linked together, triggering a deterioration in lung compliance and gas exchange function.

immune cells, and extracellular matrix (ECM) in the complex crosstalk. In addition, we discuss potential factors affecting these pro-fibrotic cells, including genetic mutations, epigenetic alterations, environmental factors and aging, with the aim of finding the underlying cause of the disease. The currently approved IPF treatment drugs are pirfenidone and nintedanib, both of which can slow the progression of IPF, but there is no evidence that they can reverse IPF-related pulmonary fibrosis (Chu et al., 2020). Lung transplantation is the only option for patients with end-stage IPF (Lederer and Martinez, 2018; Villavicencio et al., 2018). Therefore, there is a necessity to develop novel agents for the treatment of IPF. This article reviews the roles of various cells and extracellular matrix associated with pathogenic mechanisms, potential pathogenic factors, and the latest information on clinical trials of IPF.

2 THE PATHOLOGICAL PROCESS OF IDIOPATHIC PULMONARY FIBROSIS

The current paradigm suggests that IPF occurs as a result of epithelial injury and dysregulation of the epithelial/mesenchymal crosstalk, which continuously activates multiple interconnected downstream profibrotic pathways, ultimately leading to an abnormal repair response and decreased lung function (Spagnolo et al., 2021).

In the next sections, we provide a brief overview of the pathogenic mechanisms of IPF (**Figure 1**). Damage to alveolar epithelial cells in response to external stimuli leads to disruption of the basement membrane and release of large amounts of cytokines. Many cytokines (interleukins, chemokines, and growth factors) are released by alveolar epithelial cells (AEC) to recruit and activate inflammatory cells and fibroblasts (Phan et al., 2021; She et al., 2021). Coagulation factors (tissue factor (TF), plasminogen activation inhibitors (PAI 1 and PAI 2), fibrinolysis inhibitors and protein C inhibitors) induce a microenvironment that promotes coagulation and inhibits fiber degradation (King et al., 2011; Selman and Pardo, 2014; Betensley et al., 2016). In addition to microenvironmental changes in the lung, cellular processes (apoptosis, senescence, epithelial-mesenchymal transition, endothelial-mesenchymal transition, and epithelial cell migration) have been shown to play a key role in IPF-associated tissue remodeling (Phan et al., 2021). In addition, fibroblasts differentiate into myofibroblasts and secrete large amounts of extracellular matrix, which eventually leads to the formation of fibroblast foci and the development of pulmonary fibrosis (Yagihashi et al., 2016). In conclusion, following injury to the AEC, the lung microenvironment and cellular processes are altered, which initiates abnormal repair and ultimately leads to the development of IPF and pulmonary function deterioration.

3 IMPORTANT CELLS AND EXTRACELLULAR MATRIX INVOLVED IN THE PATHOGENESIS OF IPF

There are AECs, alveolar capillary endothelial cells, immune cells, fibroblasts, and mesenchymal progenitor cells near the alveoli. These cells maintain the homeostasis of the alveolar environment under normal physiological conditions. However, in the pathophysiological process of IPF, the intercellular crosstalk

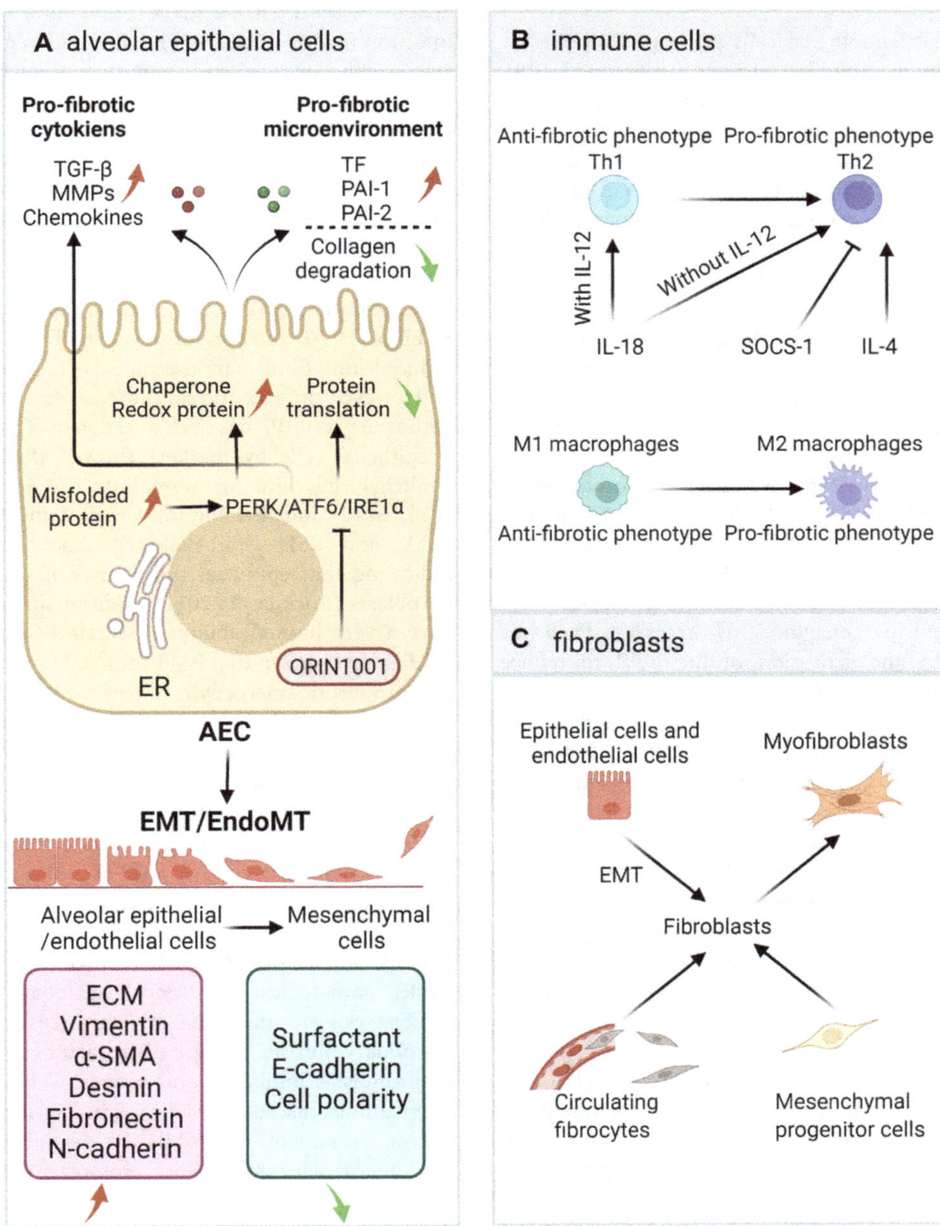

FIGURE 2 | A schematic view of the roles of AECs, immune cells and fibroblasts. **(A)** Alveolar epithelial cells/endothelial cells participate in IPF via ER stress/UPR, EMT, coagulation cascade, and the secretion of a variety of signaling factors. **(B)** The balance of Th1/Th2 and M1/M2. **(C)** The sources of fibroblasts and the fibroblast-to-myofibroblasts differentiation.

leads to reprogramming of cell phenotype. AECs, endothelial cells, and immune cells work together through multiple signaling pathways to regulate fibroblast phenotype. Then, fibroblasts recruitment, proliferation, differentiation, and secretion of extracellular matrix directly lead to fibrosis and exhaustion of pulmonary function. therefore, it is necessary to clarify the roles of various cells and extracellular matrix in the development of IPF.

3.1 Alveolar Epithelial Cells and Endothelial Cells

Alveolar epithelial cells/endothelial cells participate in IPF via various ways, including unfolded protein response (UPR), Epithelial-mesenchymal transition (EMT), coagulation cascade, angiogenesis, and the secretion of a variety of signaling factors (such as TGF-β) (Margaritopoulos et al., 2017; Upagupta et al., 2018; Chanda et al., 2019; Hill et al., 2019; Salton et al., 2019; Selman and Pardo, 2020). In this section, we show how AECs are involved in pulmonary fibrosis (**Figure 2A**).

3.1.1 Unfolded Protein Response

The UPR of AEC is one of the underlying mechanisms for the development of IPF. As an important site for cellular protein synthesis, the ER (endoplasmic reticulum) must maintain relative homeostasis. Under pathological conditions [e.g., viral infection, smoking, asbestos exposure, ROS, hypoxia, senescence, mechanical stretching, proteasome dysfunction, and autophagy disorders (Burman et al., 2018)], misfolded proteins accumulate in the ER of AECs, resulting in ER stress. To restore protein metabolism homeostasis, PERK/ATF6/IRE1α (Protein kinase R-like endoplasmic reticulum kinase/activating transcription factor 6/inositol-requiring enzyme 1α) receptors will be activated, followed by the activation of the UPR to reduce overall protein translation and increase the expression of chaperone and redox proteins. The UPR/ER stress regulates AEC apoptosis and EMT (Burman et al., 2018). However, UPR can also participate in pulmonary fibrosis by increasing the expression of profibrotic mediators, such as TGF-β1, platelet-derived growth factor (PDGF), CXCL12, and CCL2 (Zolak and de Andrade, 2012; Wolters et al., 2014). Because the upstream targets of the UPR/ER stress are of great significance for the maintenance of cell survival and organ development, pathways targeting upstream molecules may cause severe cytotoxicity. Therefore, targeting downstream molecular pathways or chaperones seems to be a better choice. (Burman et al., 2018). Currently, ORIN1001, which targets inositol-requiring transmembrane kinase endoribonuclease-1α (IRE1α), is undergoing a phase I clinical trial for the treatment of IPF(NCT04643769). The crosstalk between autophagy and endoplasmic reticulum stress is important in pulmonary fibrosis (Ghavami et al., 2018; Maciel et al., 2018). Therapeutic approaches targeting autophagy have been shown to have great potential in cancer and aging (Xia et al., 2021; Cassidy and Narita, 2022). Interestingly, studies have found that autophagy also plays an important role in IPF. TGF-β can inhibit autophagy in fibroblasts, while rapamycin and Tubastatin can promote autophagy and inhibit bleomycin-mediated pulmonary fibrosis (Patel et al., 2012; Saito et al., 2017).

3.1.2 Epithelial-Mesenchymal Transition

EMT refers to a process in which AECs gradually lose their epithelial characteristics under specific stimuli and conditions, with the subsequent appearance of interstitial cells characteristics. During this process, AECs are reprogrammed with changes in secretory phenotype, cytoskeletal proteins, intercellular junctions, and cell polarity (Salton et al., 2019). The conditions that induce EMT in AECs include alveolar epithelial cell injury and abnormal apoptosis, the UPR/ER stress, mechanical stress, smoking, and infection (Salton et al., 2019). Under the repeated stimuli, AECs are severely damaged and cannot complete repair processes and re-epithelialization normally, resulting in reprogramming and manifesting as abnormal repair processes (Salton et al., 2020). TGF-β, epidermal growth factor (EGF), fibroblast growth factor (FGF), IL-1, connective tissue growth factor factors (CTGF), insulin-like growth factor-2 (IGF-2), nuclear factor-kb (NF-kB) and Wnt can activate the transcription factors SNAIL, TWIST1 and ZEB through a variety of cytokine pathways to directly initiate EMT (Salton et al., 2019). FGFR1-3 inhibitor SKLB-YTH-60 ameliorates EMT and fibrosis in bleomycin-induced lung fibrosis mouse models (Liu et al., 2021).

However, in recent years, the central role of EMT in the pathogenesis of IPF has been questioned. The localization of type 2 epithelial cells by markers showed that the conversion of epithelial cells into myofibroblasts was incomplete (Gjorevski et al., 2012) and that the marker protein of myofibroblasts, α-SMA, and EMT epithelial cells could not be colocalized, indicating that epithelial cells may not completely convert to fibroblasts (Rock et al., 2011); additionally, mesenchymal AECs have a very limited ability to secrete ECM (Yao et al., 2019). Studies have shown that EMT indirectly promotes the formation of a profibrotic microenvironment through the dysregulation of paracrine signals between epithelial cells and mesenchymal cells (Hill et al., 2019; Yao et al., 2019). Therefore, although there is a large amount of evidence that EMT does exist in IPF, due to the latest lineage tracing results, EMT is more regarded as an indirect process. Nevertheless, the profibrotic microenvironment that regulates the occurrence of EMT is still quite promising in the inhibition of IPF (Hill et al., 2019).

3.1.3 Coagulation Cascade and Angiogenesis

Under pathological conditions, the coagulation cascade and angiogenesis are important driving forces for the promotion of pulmonary fibrosis. Because tissue factor can activate PAI 1, PAI 2, fibrinolysis inhibitors and protein C inhibitors through the coagulation cascade, resulting in a local pro-coagulation microenvironment, it inhibits the degradation of the ECM in this microenvironment and promotes the differentiation of fibrocytes (King et al., 2011; Selman and Pardo, 2014; Betensley et al., 2016). IPF patients have a relatively lower number of endothelial progenitor cells, which may potentially contribute to suppressed repair of the damaged pulmonary endothelium and thereby may drive the sequence of events in profibrogenic direction (Malli et al., 2013). Besides, it is reported that compensatory pro-angiogenic VEGF increases, which is a pro-fibrotic mediator (Malli et al., 2013).

3.1.4 Pro-Fibrotic Secretory Phenotype of AEC

In addition to the above pathways, AECs also participate in pulmonary fibrosis through the secretion of a variety of mediators, including growth factor (TGF-β, PDGF/CTGF/IGF-I/insulin-like growth factor binding proteins 3 and 5), matrix metalloproteinases (MMP1/MMP2/MMP7), chemokines (CCL17/CCL2/CXCL12), pigment epithelium-derived factor, autotaxin, sphingosine-1-phosphate, neuregulin (NRG) 1α, growth and differentiation factor 15 (GDF15), transmembrane protease serine 4 (TMPRSS4), tumor necrosis factor-alpha (TNF-α), osteopontin, and angiotensinogen. Mareike Lehmann et al. summarized the possible roles of these cytokines in detail in the occurrence and development of IPF (Selman and Pardo, 2020).

3.2 Immune Cells

A large number of studies have demonstrated that immune cells play a role in IPF. However, anti-inflammatory therapies, i.e., TNF-α monoclonal antibodies (Utz et al., 2003; Raghu et al., 2008) and glucocorticoids (Raghu et al., 2012), fail to achieve primary outcomes in clinical trials. Neither of these promising conventional treatments prevent a decline in forced vital capacity (FVC) or the progression of pulmonary fibrosis or benefit survival. In addition, a phase 3, randomized, double-blind, placebo-controlled study including 826 participants (NCT00075998) showed that the subcutaneous injection of IFNγ-1b neither improved the FVC of patients nor prolonged the survival time of patients. These clinical trials are important milestones for clinical treatment strategies for IPF, causing a shift from traditional anti-inflammatory treatment to simultaneous interventions for multiple pathogenic links. Past treatments generally treated inflammation as a whole while ignoring the dual profibrotic/antifibrotic roles of different inflammatory factors and different inflammatory cells. Perhaps by further distinguishing the roles of different inflammatory factors and pathways involved in different inflammatory cells, more precise therapeutic targets can be found. Therefore, inflammation, as one of the potential pathogeneses of IPF, remains an important focus of research.

With the deepening of research in the field of immunization, the role of immune factors in IPF has received increasing attention. Although the diagnostic criteria for IPF require the exclusion of autoimmune diseases as the underlying pathogenesis, many IPF patients still have unexplained elevated autoantibodies, and some autoantibodies are associated with acute exacerbations of IPF (AE-IPF) (Ogushi et al., 2001; Kurosu et al., 2008; Taillé et al., 2011; Kahloon et al., 2013). To inhibit the function of B cells, Ianalumab (B-cell activating factor receptor mAb) and Rituximab (CD20 mAb) have entered phase II clinical trials.

Heukels conducted a detailed review on the role of each immune cell in IPF and the correlation of each cell type with the development of fibrosis (Heukels et al., 2019). Nevertheless, the mechanism of action of some immune cells in the pathogenesis of IPF is still not very clear. The following subsections introduce the roles of the Th1/Th2 balance and the M1/M2 balance in IPF, although these paradigms simplify the role of immune cells (**Figure 2B**).

3.2.1 Th1/Th2 Balance

Th1 (helper T cell type 1) cells are helper T cells produced by $CD4^+$ cells under IFN-γ/IL-12 induction. CXC chemokine receptor 3 expressed by Th1 cells can recognize interferon-inducible T cell a chemoattractant (I-TAC), interferon g-inducible protein of 10 kD (IP-10), and monokine induced by interferon gamma (Mig) (Sumida et al., 2008). The main function of Th1 is to secrete IFN-γ. IFN-γ is considered to be antifibrotic and can reduce the production of ECM (Bouros et al., 2006; Smaldone, 2018).

Th2 (helper T cell type 2) are helper T cells produced by $CD4^+$ cells under IL-4 induction. Th2 cells that express CC chemokine receptor 4 can recognize thymus- and activation-regulated chemokines (TARCs) and macrophage-derived chemokines (MDCs) (Sumida et al., 2008). The main function of Th2 cells is to secrete IL-4/IL-5/IL-13; these interleukins are considered to promote fibrosis (Romagnani, 2000).

Th2 polarization has been observed in IPF. In the BALF of IPF patients and in systemic circulation, the levels of Th1 cells and their secretion of IFN-γ are relatively low, and the levels of Th2 cells and their secretion of IL-4/IL-5/IL-13 are relatively high (Hams et al., 2014). In addition, in a bleomycin-induced mouse model, an increase in IFN-γ levels and a reduction in pulmonary fibrosis were observed after the administration of IL-12, an inducer of Th1 cells; in contrast, an increase in fibroblast proliferation and fibrosis was found with the use of IL-4, an inducer of Th2 cells (Hams et al., 2014; Passalacqua et al., 2017).

The inhibition of Th2 polarization is a possible direction for the treatment of IPF. Many factors can cause Th2 polarization. Galectin-1 and prostaglandin E2 promote Th2 polarization by inducing Th1 apoptosis and reducing the synthesis of Th1 inducers (Kaliński et al., 1997; Cedeno-Laurent and Dimitroff, 2012; Corapi et al., 2018), and suppressor of cytokine signaling-1 (SOCS-1) inhibits the expression of Th2 inducers to prevent excessive Th2 cell accumulation (Bao et al., 2014). Among the interleukins that regulate Th1 and Th2 differentiation, IL-18 is notable; the polarization direction mediated by IL-18 is regulated by IL-12. Under the synergistic effect of IL-12, IL-18 induces Th1 cells to produce IFN-γ, IL-12, and GM-CSF and upregulate the expression of IL-2Rα to promote an inflammatory response. In contrast, in the absence of IL-12, IL-18 induces the production of Th2-related cytokines, such as IL-13/IL-4, by T cells, NK cells, basophil cells, and mast cells and promotes the differentiation of Th2 cells (Wawrocki et al., 2016). IL-4 is another important interleukin that promotes Th2 differentiation and is an important marker of type 2 immunity. Studies have shown that significant polymorphisms are found in the IL-4 promoter of IPF patients and that these polymorphisms are strongly associated with IPF (Vasakova et al., 2006). In addition to cytokine therapy, a study used the serum IFN-γ/IL-4 ratio to represent the Th1/Th2 balance to predict the development of IPF and found that the IFN-γ/IL-4 ratio was associated with symptoms, imaging changes, FEV1 (forced expiratory volume in one second), FVC (Forced vital capacity), TLC (total lung capacity), and 6-min walking distance in IPF patients and can predict IPF progression (Peng et al., 2013).

3.2.2 M1/M2 Balance

In addition to the Th1/Th2 balance, the balance of macrophage subpopulations also plays an important role in the pathogenesis of IPF. Because cytokines secreted by Th1/Th2 cells greatly affect the differentiation of M1/M2 macrophages, Th1/Th2 cells and M1/M2 macrophages interact with each other to jointly shape the type 1 and type 2 immune microenvironments (Wang et al., 2021).

The main function of M1 (type I macrophages) is to respond to lipopolysaccharide (LPS), IL-1, and IL-6. They can secrete type 1 immune factors such as IL-12, induced nitric oxide synthase (iNOS), TNF-α, IL-1β, IL-23, IL-6, and CXCL10 (Liu G. et al., 2019), thereby playing a role in the early stage of inflammation. The main function of M2 (type II macrophages) is to respond to type 2 immune factors (IL-4, IL-10, and IL-13), glucocorticoids, and immune complexes. They can secrete cytokines that promote tissue repair, limit inflammation (Martinez et al., 2008; Zhang et al., 2018; Liu G. et al., 2019), participate in immune regulation, suppress immune responses, and remodel tissue. M2 macrophages can also be divided into M2a, M2b, and M2c macrophages based on induction conditions and functions (Martinez et al., 2008).

M2 polarization is one of the important links in the occurrence and development of pulmonary fibrosis. The M2-mediated type 2 immune response is an important component of pulmonary fibrosis. M2 macrophages provide an important microenvironment for pulmonary fibrosis by secreting profibrotic substances such as CCL18, IL-10, TIMP1 (tissue inhibitors of metalloproteinases 1), TGF-β, FGF, PDGFα, IGF1, and VEGF (Prasse et al., 2006; Heukels et al., 2019; Wang et al., 2021). Macrophages can not only secrete chemokines to recruit other cells (like CCL18), but also are attracted by chemokines themselves. CCL2 and CCL3 are important signaling molecules involved in monocyte/macrophage recruitment and help macrophages migrate to the lungs. Therefore, the antagonism of CCL2 and CCL3 may have an antifibrotic effect (Iyonaga et al., 1994; Suga et al., 1999; Deshmane et al., 2009).

3.3 Fibroblasts and Myofibroblasts

Fibrocytes are monocyte progenitor cells with differentiation potential derived from bone marrow; these cells can differentiate into adipocyte cells, chondrocytes, osteoblasts, and fibroblasts under the action of different tissue environments and humoral factors. In the *in vitro* environment, CD45+/CD34+ primary bone marrow fibrocytes were stimulated by the ECM of IPF patients; then the hematopoietic surface antigens CD45 and CD34 rapidly disappeared, and mesenchymal markers, i.e., α-SMA, rapidly increased. The fibrocytes transformed into fibroblasts with a contractility like that of smooth muscle cells and a strong ability to synthesize ECM (Mori et al., 2005; Lama and Phan, 2006; Kage and Borok, 2012; Chong et al., 2019). In addition to the ECM of IPF patients, TGF-β, endothelin, CTGF, interleukins (IL-3 and IL-4), serum response factors (Shi-Wen et al., 2004) and microRNA (miRNA-21, miRNA-22, miRNA-29, miRNA-125b, miRNA-126, miRNA-130a and miRNA-132, miRNA-142a) (Pandit et al., 2011; Wang et al., 2012; Cushing et al., 2015; Kuse et al., 2020) have been shown to be associated with the differentiation of fibrocytes into fibroblasts. After getting activated, fibroblasts proliferate, differentiate, resist apoptosis and can directly lead to IPF through the secretion of profibrotic factors and the remodeling of the ECM (Selman et al., 2000). Under normal circumstances, the secretion and degradation of the ECM by fibroblasts are in a dynamic balance. However, when exposed to inflammation and environmental stress, fibroblasts are reprogrammed and continue to be active and resist apoptosis (Filer and Buckley, 2013), ultimately leading to an increase in the relative rate of ECM synthesis. In patients, the number of fibrocytes and fibroblasts in the lung is positively correlated with collagen deposition and the progression of pulmonary fibrosis. When fibroblast foci start to cross-link with each other, patient lung function may decrease substantially (Snijder et al., 2019).

Although fibroblast is the chief culprit in pulmonary fibrosis, its source is still unclear. Possible sources include peripheral recruitment, mesenchymal progenitor cells in lung tissues, and EMT (**Figure 2C**). When local lung injury occurs, epithelial cells and endothelial cells are activated and release chemokines. Through chemokine ligand–receptor pathways (including CXCL12/SDF1-CXCR4, CCL21-CCR7 and CCL2-CCR2) (Chong et al., 2019), many circulating fibrocytes and mesenchymal progenitor cells are recruited into local tissues and undergo phenotypic transformation to become fibroblasts. In the lungs of IPF patients, there is a high level of CXCL12/CXCR4 (Mehrad et al., 2007), which is conducive to the recruitment of circulating fibrocytes to the lungs along the concentration gradient of chemokines. In addition, AECs that cannot re-epithelialize can convert into interstitial AECs through EMT, leading to a decrease in intercellular junctions and epithelial features. However, the contribution of epithelial EMT in pulmonary fibrosis is still controversial (Salton et al., 2020). In addition, local fibrocytes and fibroblasts can self-proliferate rapidly. Under the influence of cytokines, growth factors and TIMPs, local fibroblasts in IPF can resist apoptosis and continue to proliferate (Andersson-Sjöland et al., 2011).

3.4 Extracellular Matrix

In IPF, ECM remodeling and collagen deposition are the classical pathological features of the disease. ECM is mainly produced by fibroblasts/myofibroblasts, epithelial cells, inflammatory cells, and mesenchymal progenitor cells.

ECM has complex functions in IPF (**Figure 3**). ECM has a certain degree of mechanical stiffness, which plays an important role in the sclerosis of lung tissues (Elowsson Rendin et al., 2019). Besides, ECM also serves as a pool for variety of growth factors (bFGF, VEGF), stimulating factors (GM-CSF, M-CSF), and interleukins (IL-1, IL-8), allowing signal exchange with different cells (Andersson-Sjöland et al., 2011). The mechanical force of the ECM itself can also directly participate

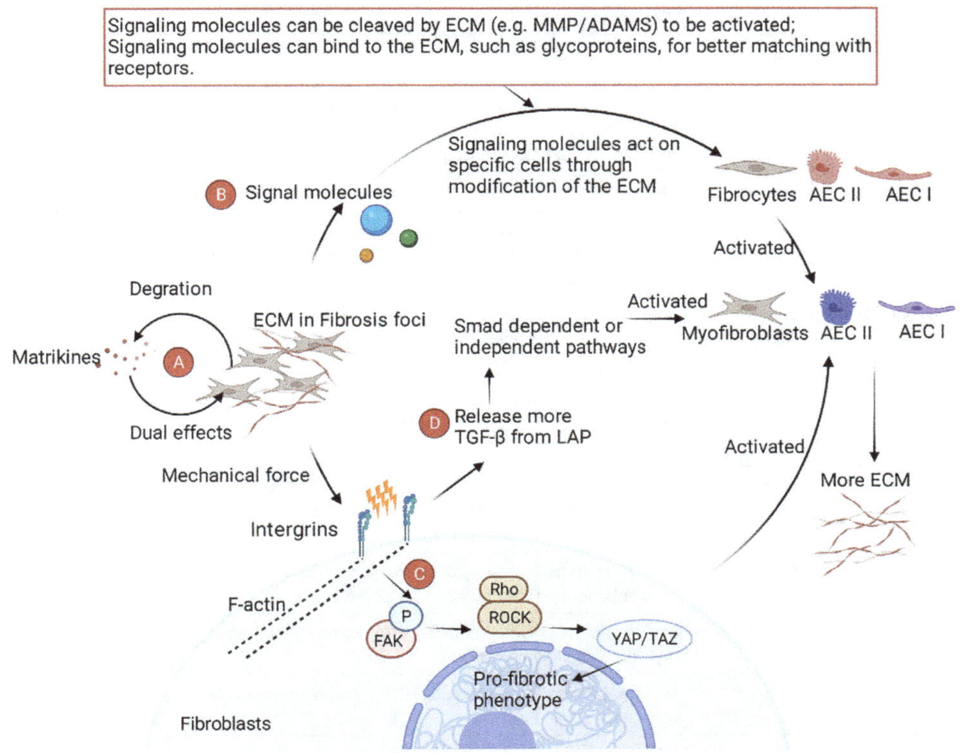

FIGURE 3 | A schematic view of the role of ECM in IPF. **(A)** Matrkines, which contain multiple degradation products of the ECM, exert dual pro- and anti-fibrotic roles in IPF. **(B)** The ECM is involved in the phenotypic reprogramming of fibroblasts and AECs by modifying key signaling molecules. **(C)** After binding specific ECM ligands to the ectodomain of integrins, integrins bind to the cytoskeleton and various signaling proteins through their cytoplasmic tails, translating the mechanical force of cytoskeleton contraction and ECM stiffness into biochemical signals. **(D)** Integrins activate TGF-β-dependent fibrosis by releasing TGF-β through stretch force generated by actin-cytoskeleton interactions.

in pulmonary fibrosis through mechanoreceptors and some cellular pathways. Under the action of mechanical force, α6 integrin (Rahaman et al., 2014) and the transient receptor potential vanilloid 4 (TRPV4) channel (Chen et al., 2016) act as sensors to detect mechanical stimulation signals and transfer the signals into myofibroblasts. Subsequently, F-actin contracts, resulting in the phosphorylation of focal adhesion kinase (FAK). Phosphorylated FAK activates Rho kinase (ROCK) by binding Rho to ROCK. This step activates yes-associated protein (YAP)/transcriptional coactivator with PDZ-binding motif (TAZ), which ultimately activates the transcription, translation, and expression of profibrotic genes in the nucleus. In addition to the FAK-ROCK-YAP/TAZ axis, mechanical force can also release TGF-β bound by latency-associated peptide (LAP), thus activating the TGF-β-Smad dependent/independent pathway in fibroblasts and AECs and directly participating in myofibroblast differentiation (Upagupta et al., 2018).

Matrikines, the degradation product of the ECM, also have special biological activities in lung diseases (Burgess and Weckmann, 2012). Matrikines are biologically active fragments derived from the degradation of ECM. These biologically active fragments exert dual biological properties by binding to integrins, heparan sulfate proteoglycans, and growth factor receptors. For example, endotrophin (the degradation product of collagen VI) promotes fibrosis, while endostatin (the degradation product of collagen XVIII) has antifibrosis effects (Ricard-Blum and Salza, 2014).

ECM includes the core matrisome and associated matrisomes. Core matrisomes include collages, ECM glycoproteins, and ECM proteoglycans. Associated matrisomes include ECM regulators, ECM-affiliated proteins, and secreted factors (Kreus et al., 2021). In the ECM of IPF patients, laminins and collagen IV associated with the basement membrane decreased, while the vast majority of core matrisomes showed an increasing trend (Elowsson Rendin et al., 2019). Although there have been numerous studies, very little is known about the role of some mediators in IPF. The various substances in the ECM are described in detail below.

3.4.1 Collagen

Collagen is the main component of ECM. Collagen is derived from activated (myo)fibroblasts, fibrocytes, epithelial cells (which can transform into mesenchymal cells through EMT), mesenchymal stromal cells, and pericytes. The vast majority of interstitial and fibrillar collagens (mainly collagen I and collagen III) are secreted by (myo)fibroblasts. These collagens constitute the main frame of the ECM and

TABLE 1 | The potential role of MMPs/TIMPs in IPF.

MMPs	Cellular Sources	Pro/ Antifibrotic	Mechanism	Ref
MMP1	AEC, macrophage	Profibrotic	MMP1 Induces lung alveolar epithelial cell migration and proliferation, protects from apoptosis, and represses mitochondrial oxygen consumption by activation of HIF-1α	Herrera et al. (2013)
MMP2	BECs, AECs, fibroblasts, fibrocytes	Profibrotic	MMP2 damages the integrity of alveolar walls, regulates EMT, and involves in activation of TGF-β	Nguyen et al. (2001); Wu et al. (2007); Lam et al. (2014)
MMP3	BECs, AECs, macrophage, fibroblasts	Profibrotic	MMP3 activates the β-catenin and TGF-β pathway, induces EMT, releases endothelin	Wu et al. (2007); Richter et al. (2009); Yamashita et al. (2011)
MMP7	Lung epithelial cell, fibroblast	Pro/ Antifibrotic	MMP7 regulates osteopontin, mediates E-cadherin ectodomain shedding, and regulates anti-inflammatory and antifibrotic pulmonary dendritic cells	McGuire et al. (2003); Pardo et al. (2005); Manicone et al. (2009)
MMP8	blood monocytes, AM, BECs, AECs, fibrocytes	Profibrotic	MMP8 reduces the levels of IL-10, IP-10 and MIP-1a, affects the migration of fibrocytes mediated by PDGF-B or stromal cell-derived factor-1α	García-Prieto et al. (2010); Craig et al. (2013)
MMP9	AECs, neutrophils, AM, fibrocytes, fibroblasts	Profibrotic	MMP9 production is related to TGF-β1. MMP9 cleaves SP-D; MMP9 involves in macrophage-induced fibroblast migration and TGF-β1/Smad2-dependent EMT.	Murthy et al. (2010); Bratcher et al. (2012); Li et al. (2019); Zhang et al. (2019)
MMP10	AM, BECs, AECs	Antifibrotic	MMP10 involves in the migration of macrophages and macrophage-mediated collagenase degradation	Murray et al. (2013); Rohani et al. (2015)
MMP11	furin-like proconvertase enzyme	Profibrotic	MMP11 activates Notch pathway and promotes fibroblasts to myofibroblasts differentiation	Aoyagi-Ikeda et al. (2011)
MMP14	AECs, AM, and endothelial cells	Antifibrotic	MMP14 involves in activation of TGF-β, fibroblast-dependent collagenolysis and invasion	Sabeh et al. (2009); Xiong et al. (2017)
MMP19	monocytes, AM, fibrocyte, AEC	Antifibrotic	MMP19 promotes wound healing and cell migration by inducing PTSG2 (prostaglandin endoperoxide synthase 2); MMP19 regulates ECM formation, migration, proliferation, and autophagy of fibroblasts	Yu et al. (2012); Jara et al. (2015)
MMP28	Macrophages	Profibrotic	MMP28 promotes M2 polarization and TGF-β-dependent EMT.	Jara et al. (2015)

increase the mechanical stiffness of fibrotic tissue (Snijder et al., 2019). Currently, it is believed that type III collagen plays a role in the early disease stage and that type I collagen is associated with the deterioration of lung function in the late disease stage due to its involvement in collagen crosslinking mediated by lysyl oxidase (LOX) family enzymes (Rock et al., 2011). In view of the important contribution of collagen to the mechanical stiffness of pulmonary fibrosis, collagen turnover has naturally become an important means for monitoring disease progression and predicting patient prognosis. Increased concentrations of the collagen degradation markers type 1/3/6 collagen, and C-reactive protein are associated with an increased risk of overall mortality, and elevated levels of the collagen synthesis markers Pro-C3 and Pro-C6 are associated with IPF progression (Organ et al., 2019; Jessen et al., 2021).

3.4.2 Glycoproteins and Proteoglycans

There are relatively few studies on ECM glycoproteins and proteoglycans. In a radiation-induced pulmonary fibrosis model, the glycoprotein glectin-3 produced by type I AECs increased dramatically (Kasper and Hughes, 1996). In recent years, studies on proteoglycans have shown that the proteoglycan decorin reduces pulmonary fibrosis by antagonizing TGF-β and antagonizing CTGF-mediated collagen deposition (Nikaido et al., 2018). In addition, the proteoglycan lumican directly acts in the differentiate of monocytes into fibroblasts through an integrin-dependent pathway (Pilling et al., 2015). Chondroitin sulfate type E (CS-E), another proteoglycan, inhibits the expression of α-SMA, CTGF, LOXL2, and CCL2/MCP-1 by silencing the genes of CS-E and the related enzyme carbohydrate sulfotransferase 15 (CHST15) through miRNA (Kai et al., 2017). Syndecan-4 is a heparan sulfate proteoglycan. Silencing of syndecan-4 can reduce SMA-α and collagen deposition (Tanino et al., 2019). In addition, proteoglycans assist other factors in producing biological effects. For example, FXIIa must bind to the proteoglycan heparan sulfate to stimulate the migration of human lung fibroblasts (Wujak et al., 2015).

3.4.3 ECM Regulators

ECM regulators include serine protease inhibitors, cystatins, TIMPs, MMPs (Kreus et al., 2021), a disintegrin and metalloproteinases (ADAMs), and crosslinking enzymes (Ricard-Blum and Salza, 2014; Liu et al., 2016); these molecules are mainly involved in the regulation of ECM decomposition. MMPs/TIMPs play an important role in

TABLE 2 | Genetic mutations associated with IPF.

Targets	Physiological function of the target site	Potential pathogenic mechanisms of gene mutations	Clinical significance	Ref
TERT and TERC	TERT and TERC are important components of the telomerase complex	Telomere shortening may affect the turnover and healing of AEC.	TERT (rs2736100) and TERC (6793295) mutations are associated with IPF susceptibility	Armanios et al. (2007); Borie et al. (2016)
DKC1	DKC1, a pseudouridine synthase, is involved in the synthesis of non-coding ribonucleic acids	Mutations in DKC1 can shorten telomeres in alveolar epithelial cells and affect the stability of telomerase RNA.	DKC1 mutations cause dyskeratosis congenita and pulmonary fibrosis	Kropski et al. (2017); Gaysinskaya et al. (2020)
TIN2	TIN2 is an important component of the shelterin complex	Mutations in TIN2 can shorten telomeres	Heterozygous mutations in TINF2 causes IPF	Fukuhara et al. (2013)
PARN	PARN, a 3′exoribonuclease, is responsible for telomere maturation	PARN mutations lead to shortened telomeres	PARN mutations and telomere shortening are associated with leukopenia	Stuart et al. (2015)
RTEL	RTEL is a DNA helicase crucial for unwinding the T-loop structure	Loss of functional RTEL1 leads to cleavage of the telomeric end proximal to the T-loop by endonuclease SLX4, leading to release of T-loops and shortened telomere	RTEL and telomere shortening are associated with leukopenia	Cogan et al. (2015); Stuart et al. (2015)
NAF1	NAF1, a box H/ACA RNA biogenesis factor, is required for stability and assembly into a mature telomerase holoenzyme complex	NAF1 mutations can reduce telomerase RNA levels, resulting in shorter telomeres	Pulmonary fibrosis-emphysema in NAF1 mutation patients is telomere-mediated	Stanley et al. (2016a)
OBFC1	OBFC1 associates with TPP1 and is implicated in telomere length regulation	N.A.	rs11191865 was associated with a lower risk of IPF.	Fingerlin et al. (2013)
MUC5B	Mucin 5B is involved in mucosal clearance along with surfactant protein C and ciliates	Excess Mucin may increase the retention of harmful particles in the lung and interfere with the normal developmental pathway and alveolar epithelial repair	rs35705950 was the strongest genetic risk factor for IPF, but was associated with lower mortality. MUC5B and MUC5AC expression was increased in patients with IPF.	Peljto et al. (2013); Conti et al. (2016); Evans et al. (2016)
SFTPC	SFTPC regulates alveolar surface tension	SFTPC mutations may promote lung fibrosis by inducing endoplasmic reticulum stress and apoptotic cell death in AEC II.	SFPTC mutations are associated with familial and sporadic IPF onsets	Ono et al. (2011); Venosa et al. (2017)
SFTPA2	SFTPA is involved in the intrinsic immunity of the lung	SFTPA mutant mouse models exhibit intracellular retention of SFTPA and enhanced ER stress	Mutations in SFTPA2 leads to the trafficking of several proteins and causes the development of IPF.	Yongyu Wang et al. (2009); Maitra et al. (2010); Guenther et al. (2019)
ABCA3	A type of phospholipid carrier, involved in the secretion and transport of surface-active substances in AEC II.	ABCA3 mutations may induce ER stress and proteostasis failure through misfolded alveolar surface-active substances	Heterozygous variants of the ABCA3 gene are associated with IPF susceptibility. pG1205R, an ABCA3 gene allele, is more frequently expressed in patients with IPF and ILDs	Zhou et al. (2017); Manali et al. (2019)
ATP11A	ATP11A encodes ABCA1, a transmembrane protein with general transport function	N.A.	rs1278769 was associated with a lower risk of IPF.	Fingerlin et al. (2013)
IL1RN	IL-1RN is a competitive antagonist of IL-1R receptor	MSC exerts anti-inflammatory and anti-fibrotic effects via IL-1RN.	The proportion of IL-1RN gene polymorphisms in patients with fibrosing alveolitis was more	Whyte et al. (2000); Ortiz et al. (2007)
IL-4	IL-4 is associated with type 2 immunity	IL-4 gene polymorphisms may promote a Th2 cytokine environment with exaggerated fibroproliferative healing	Higher percentage of IL-4 gene polymorphisms in IPF patients	Vasakova et al. (2013)
IL-8	IL-8 is a chemokine secreted by macrophages and is involved in the recruitment of neutrophils	IL-8 increases the fibrogenicity of mesenchymal progenitor cells and is involved in the proliferation, activation, and recruitment of mesenchymal cells	IL-8 gene diversity is associated with lung alveolitis and lung function decline	Ziegenhagen et al. (1998); Yang et al. (2018)
TLR3	TLR3 is known as one of the innate immunity receptors, which mediate	Defective TLR3 L412F gene activates abnormal inflammation and promotes fibroplasia in IPF, which may be	rs3775291 increase the risk for IPF patients and also reduces forced volume capacity (FVC)	O'Dwyer et al. (2013); O'Dwyer et al. (2015); Evans et al. (2016)

(Continued on following page)

TABLE 2 | (*Continued*) Genetic mutations associated with IPF.

Targets	Physiological function of the target site	Potential pathogenic mechanisms of gene mutations	Clinical significance	Ref
	inflammation, tissue injury and viral infection	associated with dysregulation of fibroblast proliferation mediated by a sluggish IFN-β response		
TOOLIP	TOLLIP is involved in the signaling pathway of TGF-β, TLR and ILs	rs3750920 may lead to unregulated TLR signaling pathway	rs5743890 was associated with a lower susceptibility to IPF, whereas rs5743894 was associated with a higher susceptibility to IPF. The rs3750920 polymorphism was associated with the efficacy of NAC. rs5743890 was associated with increased IPF morbidity and mortality	Noth et al. (2013); Oldham et al. (2015)
HLA-DRB1	HLA gene encodes major histocompatibility complex (MHC)	N.A.	HLA-DRB1*1501 is related to greater differences in gas exchanges and immunogenic process	Xue et al. (2011); Zhang et al. (2015)
MDGA2	MDGA2 encodes a paralogue for ICAM, which has been shown to be a potential biomarker of IPF disease activity	N.A.	rs7144383 was associated with a higher risk of IPF.	Noth et al. (2013)
DSP	DSP, a desmosomal protein, is mainly expressed in the airway epithelium and is involved in cell adhesion	rs2076304 might influence the binding of RHOXF1	rs2076304 and rs2076295 increased the IPF risk and rs2744371 decreased the IPF sub-risk	Mathai et al. (2016); Wang et al. (2018)
DPP9	DPP9 is a serine protease that belongs to a member of the S9B family. DPP9 is expressed in epithelial cells and is involved in cell adhesion, cell migration and apoptosis	N.A.	rs12610495 is associated with IPF susceptibility	Fingerlin et al. (2013); Zhou and Wang, (2016)
SPPL2C	SPPL2C is a transmembrane GxGD type of cleavage proteases	N.A.	rs17690703 was also known to reduce FVC in IPF. A low survival rate and mortality were reported in people with greater gene SPPL2C expression	Wu et al. (2016); Lorenzo-Salazar et al. (2019)
AKAP13	AKAP13 is a Rho guanine nucleotide exchange factor regulating activation of RhoA	AKAP13 mutations may affect the RhoA/ROCK signaling pathway	rs62025270 was associated with increased production of AKAP13, but no correlation with survival was observed	Allen et al. (2017)
FAM13A	FAM13A contains a protein domain called Rho GTPase activating protein (Rho GAP)	FAM13A mutation may affect the RhoA/ROCK signaling pathway	The rs2609255 was associated with higher mortality rate. The FAM13A allele was associated with worse disease and lower DLCO.	Hirano et al. (2017); van Moorsel, (2018); Ruffin et al. (2020)
MAPT	MAPT encodes Tau protein, a microtubule-associated protein	N.A.	rs1981997 is associated with a lower risk of IPF.	Fingerlin et al. (2013); van Moorsel, (2018)

IPF and are directly involved in ECM remodeling. MMPs belong to zinc-dependent endopeptidases of the M10A subfamily, and 24 gene subtypes are expressed in the human body. As a crucial component of ECM, MMPs participate in the formation and progression of IPF via many pathways, especially TGF-β signaling pathway. Many studies have focused on MMPs and explored their potential value in resisting IPF (**Table 1**). Although the pathological processes of MMPs and IPF have been verified, there are no MMP inhibitors for the treatment of IPF in the clinic (Yue et al., 2021).

ECM contains a variety of signal molecules secreted by cells; therefore, the ECM is a transfer station for signal exchange. In IPF, the signaling molecules from different cells constitute a complex signaling network through the bridge function of the ECM. Upstream signals are modified and regulated by positive feedback in the ECM; this feedback, e.g., the TGF-β pathway and Rho/ROCK signaling, can affect the transcription and translation of ECM-related genes and eventually lead to pulmonary fibrosis (Snijder et al., 2019).

Although there have been many studies on active fragments, the roles of these active products in IPF are still not clear. In recent years, the ECM has shown extraordinary clinical and scientific value in the fields of anti-infection, anti-angiogenesis, and wound healing (Ricard-Blum and Salza, 2014; Ricard-Blum and Vallet, 2019). Therefore, research on active fragments and their derivatives as targets for antifibrosis therapies is innovative and has great potential.

4 UNDERLYING FACTORS ASSOCIATED WITH THE PATHOGENESIS OF IPF

4.1 Genetic Susceptibility and Epigenetic Alterations in the Development of IPF

A growing number of studies have shown that genetic mutations are associated with susceptibility, diagnosis, progression, prognosis, and adverse effects of treatment in IPF. The proportion of patients carrying genetic mutations in IPF may be underestimated. A cohort study showed that up to 36% of patients with IPF have familial genetic mutations (Barros et al., 2019). In addition, IPF mutations are present in nearly 40% of sporadic pulmonary fibrosis cases (Wolters et al., 2014). These common and rare genetic mutations mainly include mutations in telomeres, alveolar surfactant and muco-ciliary transportation system, immune and cytokine-related genes, cell adhesion and cell integrity-related genes (**Table 2**). MUC5B and telomere related gene mutations are more common in IPF patients, which has inspired a very large number of studies to explore the pathogenic mechanisms of gene mutations (Evans et al., 2016; Zhang et al., 2021). Besides, genetic variants have been associated with the imaging presentation of IPF. Patients with TERT mutations were more likely to exhibit the classical UIP pattern compared to patients without mutations with two-year-follow up (Baratella et al., 2021).

Notably, the majority of existing studies still remain to verify the correlation between mutations and IPF susceptibility, and there are only a few studies related to the causality and pathogenesis of IPF. Moreover, further research needs to focus on how to cross the gap between genetic testing and clinical treatment. Drugs targeting histone modifications and DNA modifications have also shown potential in preclinical studies, so we will also cover the role of epigenetics in IPF in the next sections.

4.1.1 Genetic Mutations in Telomeres

Telomeres are a TTAGGG repeat sequence at the end of human chromosomes, whose function is to stabilize the chromosome, prevent fusion of chromosome ends, protect structure of chromosomes, and determine cell life span, but telomerase activity in adult human cells is extremely low (Lister-Shimauchi et al., 2022).

Telomeres are protected by the shelterin complex, which consists of the protein components TRF1, TRF2, RAP1, TIN2, TPP1, and POT1. The ends of telomeres are bonded with telomerase, which is comprised of the catalytic subunit of TERT, the telomerase RNA component of TERC, and accessory proteins. The telomerase exerts its effects by adding telomeric sequences to the telomeric ends (Zhang et al., 2021). Telomere shortening is one of the important phenotypes of IPF. Telomere length of half of IPF patients rank in the lowest 1% of their age group (Stanley et al., 2016b). And telomeres are shorter in IPF patients than in other interstitial pneumonia (Snetselaar et al., 2015). However, it is questionable whether the cause of telomere shortening in IPF patients necessarily stems from telomere gene mutations. In patients with sporadic and familial pulmonary fibrosis, telomere shortening is present regardless of the presence of known telomere related gene mutations (Snetselaar et al., 2015). A possible reason for this is the presence of other unknown genetic mutations that can shorten telomere length.

The causal relationship between mutation-mediated telomere shortening and the development of IPF is inconclusive because not all individuals carrying a known telomere defective gene develop telomere shortening and IPF (Hoffman et al., 2018). Firstly, telomere gene defects in different cells may lead to different outcomes. systematically TERT knock-out does not induce spontaneous pulmonary fibrosis in mice, but can increase susceptibility to bleomycin (Degryse et al., 2012), while mesenchymal-specific TERT knock-out can alleviate bleomycin-induced pulmonary fibrosis (Liu et al., 2015); and AEC II-specific TERT defect reduces AEC II proliferation and induces AEC II cell senescence (Liu T. et al., 2019). Secondly, telomere gene defect-mediated DNA damage may be slow, which requires multiple generations of mice to become apparent (Blasco et al., 1997). Thirdly, due to the heterogeneity of the clinical manifestations, even the same genetic mutations may have different phenotypes, leading to the appearance of extra-pulmonary pathological features (rather than interstitial lung disease) (Borie et al., 2016). Fourthly, telomere length may differ in peripheral blood leukocytes and lung tissue (Snetselaar et al., 2017). Therefore, before telomere length measurements can be applied to clinical decisions, there is a need to clarify the effect of telomere length on different cells, the optimal sample type, and the corresponding intrapulmonary/extrapulmonary clinical manifestations.

The mechanism by which telomerase gene mutations lead to IPF is unclear. Available data suggest that cellular senescence or death of alveolar stem cells induced by telomere dysfunction is implicated in pulmonary fibrosis (Zhang et al., 2021). Knockdown of telomerase related genes leads to lung stem cell regenerative capacity and the senescence/death of AEC II (Jackson et al., 2011; Alder et al., 2015; Snetselaar et al., 2017; Wang et al., 2020). In addition, knockdown of telomerase related genes leads to elevated SASP (including TGF-β) levels and lung inflammation mediated by intrinsic immune cell infiltration (Chen et al., 2015; Povedano et al., 2015; Naikawadi et al., 2016; Liu et al., 2018).

Telomere length and specific telomere gene defects are instructive for susceptibility, diagnosis, progression, prognosis, and early warning of adverse effects in IPF. Shorter telomere length as an independent predictor is associated with worse survival and more pronounced imaging changes in IPF patients (Stuart et al., 2014; Newton et al., 2016; Ley et al., 2017). Pirfenidone treatment did not improve FVC and DLCO in IPF patients carrying TERT/TERC mutations (Justet et al., 2018). The relationship between TERT/TERC mutations and resistance to drug therapy needs to be further validated. Patients carrying telomere-related mutations may be at higher risk for complications after lung transplantation, such as death,

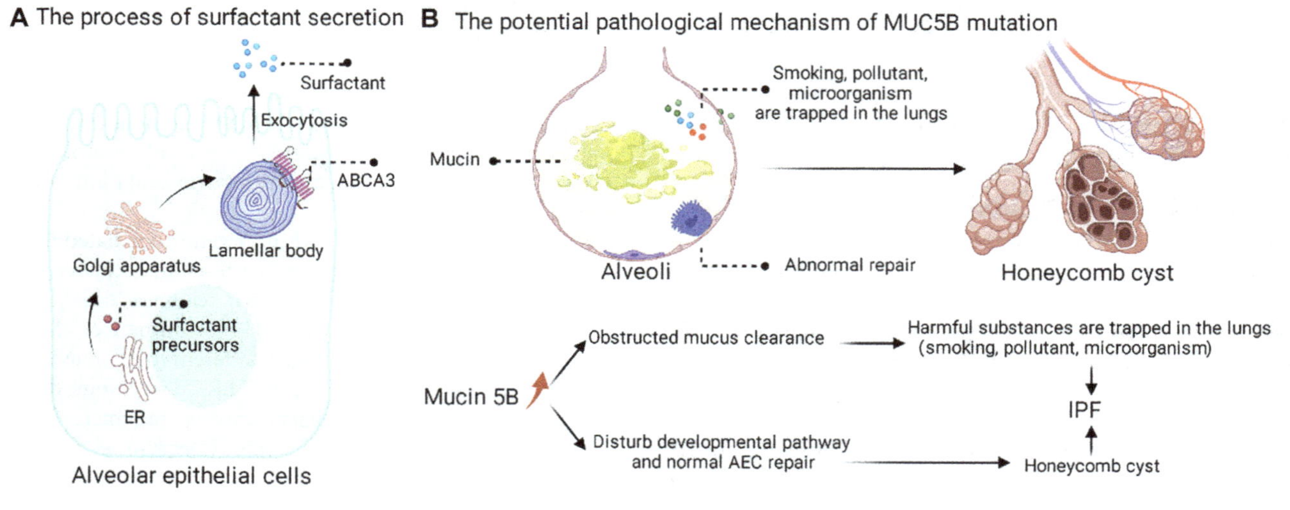

FIGURE 4 | The process of surfactant secretion and the potential pathological mechanism of MUC5B mutation. **(A)** The surfactant precursors are synthesized on the endoplasmic reticulum, followed by Golgi modifications, and finally secreted into the periphery by cytosolic exocytosis of the lamellar body. **(B)** MUC5B mutation may promote the retention of harmful substances in the lung and interfere with the normal repair of AEC.

chronic lung allograft dysfunction, renal disease, CMV complications (Popescu et al., 2019; Swaminathan et al., 2019), hematological complications (Silhan et al., 2014; Borie et al., 2015), anemia, leukopenia, recurrent lower respiratory tract infections (Tokman et al., 2015).

Drugs that target telomeres have also shown therapeutic potential. GRN510, a telomerase agonist, reduces inflammatory infiltration and collagen deposition in a mouse model of bleomycin-induced pulmonary fibrosis (Le Saux et al., 2013). PAP-associated domain-containing protein 5 (PAPD5) is involved in the degradation of TERC RNA. BCH001 (a PAPD5 inhibitor) and RG7834 (a PAPD5/7 inhibitor) rescue the TERC levels and telomerase activity in the cellular model of dyskeratosis congenital (Nagpal et al., 2020; Shukla et al., 2020). One study reported that hormones may regulate telomerase activity through an imperfect oestrogen response element within the TERT promoter (Bayne and Liu, 2005), which has inspired a series of subsequent clinical trials of hormones for IPF. Danazol, a synthetic androgen, was shown to increase telomere length and stabilize DLCO and FVC in a small-scale clinical trial (Townsley et al., 2016a; Townsley et al., 2016b). Danazol is currently in phase II clinical trials for plumonary fibrosis (NCT04638517). However, hepatotoxicity and worsening pulmonary fibrosis associated with long-term use of Danazol has been reported after danazol initiation and withdrawal (Chambers et al., 2020). Therefore, lower doses of danazol (200 mg) are being used in clinical trials to reduce hepatotoxicity. Nandrolone Decanoate, an anabolic androgenic steroid, is undergoing phase I/II clinical trials (NCT02055456). Telomerase reactivation therapy still has a long way to go before it becomes a therapeutic option, especially in terms of the serious adverse effects associated with hepatotoxicity. Whether peripheral blood telomere length can be used as a substitute outcome for pulmonary telomere length and how effective is telomerase reactivation therapy for IPF are still awaiting the results of current clinical trials.

In summary, details remain unclear in the complex field of the role telomeres play in the pathogenesis of ILDs and no clinical trials employing gene therapy have been initiated in patients with telomeropathies. Hopefully, adeno-associated virus-9 (AAV9)-mediated gene therapy has been reported to be successful in mouse models (Bär et al., 2016), and perhaps a telomerase-directed therapeutic strategy may be used for the treatment of IPF in the future.

4.1.2 Genetic Mutations in Alveolar Surfactant/Mucin

Phospholipids and four surfactant proteins (SFTPA, B, C, D) can be secreted by AEC II. The process of surfactant secretion is shown (**Figure 4A**). ATP-binding cassette subfamily A member 3 (ABCA3) is essential for the intracellular synthesis of alveolar surface-active substances (Mulugeta et al., 2015). Among four surfactant, genetic mutations of SFTPA (Wang Y. et al., 2009; Guenther et al., 2019), SFTPC (Venosa et al., 2017) and ABCA3(Zhou et al., 2017; Manali et al., 2019) have been identified in IPF patients. Although SFTPA is not directly involved in the formation of alveolar surface-active tension, it plays an important role in intrinsic lung immunity. Mouse models with SFTPA mutations exhibit intracellular retention of SFTPA and enhanced ER stress (Wang Y. et al., 2009; Maitra et al., 2010). Molecular signatures of UPR signaling and apoptotic activation associated with SFTPC have been reported in patients with IPF (Korfei et al., 2008; Lawson et al., 2008). Patients with pure mutations in ABCA3 and ABCA3-deficient mice exhibit a complete lack of alveolar surface-active substance, deformation of lamellar bodies, and death from respiratory distress shortly after birth (Shulenin et al., 2004; Cheong et al., 2007; Fitzgerald et al., 2007; Wambach et al., 2014). In lung disease, there are also reports of ABCA3 heterozygous mutations that appear to interact with SFTPC mutations (Bullard and Nogee, 2007; Crossno et al., 2010). ABCA3 mutations may induce ER stress and proteostasis failure through misfolded alveolar surface-active substances (Cheong et al., 2006; Matsumura et al., 2006; Weichert et al., 2011).

The MUC5B promoter variant, rs35705950, as the strongest genetic risk factor and common variation, was found in up to 30% of IPF (Evans et al., 2016). The rs35705950 mutation leads to increased Muc5B expression, but a causal relationship between mucus and progression of pulmonary fibrosis disease has not been established. Christopher M. Evans proposed two hypotheses for the pathogenic mechanism of MUC5B mutations (**Figure 4B**) (Evans et al., 2016). The first possible mechanism is that overexpression of Muc5B at the bronchoalveolar junction impairs mucociliary clearance, which in turn promotes prolonged retention of harmful particles (e.g., air pollutants, cigarette smoke, microorganisms, etc.) in the lung and induces fibrosis in the lung tissue. The second possible mechanism is that overexpression of Muc5B may lead to fibrosis and cellulitic cyst formation by interfering with the normal developmental pathway and alveolar epithelial repair. In summary, the overexpression of MUC5B at the bronchoalveolar junction in IPF patients led us to recognize that the peripheral airway also seems to influence interstitial fibrosis.

4.1.3 Genetic Mutations in Inflammatory Regulators

Genetic mutations in cytokines have also been reported in patients with IPF. IL1RN gene polymorphisms may be associated with susceptibility to fibrosing alveolitis, a disease characterized by interstitial lung fibrosis (Whyte et al., 2000). Mesenchymal stem cells (MSC) can exert anti-inflammatory and anti-fibrotic effects via IL-1RN (Ortiz et al., 2007). Association between genetic polymorphisms of IL-4 and IPF has been reported (Riha et al., 2004). IL-4 may be pro-fibrotic by promoting type 2 immunity. IL-8 gene diversity is associated with lung alveolitis and lung function decline (Ziegenhagen et al., 1998). IL-8 increases the fibrogenicity of mesenchymal progenitor cells and is involved in the proliferation, activation, and recruitment of mesenchymal cells (Yang et al., 2018). TLR3 (Toll-like receptor 3) mutation rs3775291 increase the risk for IPF patients and also reduces forced volume capacity (FVC) (Evans et al., 2016). Defectiveness of the gene TLR3 L412F causes aberrant inflammation and fibroblasts proliferation in IPF, which may be related to dysregulation of fibroblast proliferation mediated by a sluggish IFN-β response (O'Dwyer et al., 2013). The different mutations of TOOLIP (TOLL interacting protein) may be associated with different IPF susceptibility. The rs5743890 was associated with lower IPF susceptibility, while the rs5743894 was associated with higher IPF susceptibility (Oldham et al., 2015). In addition, rs5743890 was associated with increased morbidity and mortality in IPF (Noth et al., 2013). rs3750920 polymorphism is associated with the efficacy of N-Acetyl-L-cysteine (NAC) (Oldham et al., 2015). It is important to note that different studies with different populations and specimens may reach different conclusions. In a study conducted in China, except for the polymorphisms of HLA haplotype, none of the other cytokines showed an association for IPF susceptibility (Zhang et al., 2015). Therefore, the study of genetic polymorphisms of cytokines should pay more attention to the reproducibility of experimental results.

In recent years, the launch of pirfenidone and nintedanib has witnessed breakthroughs in the signaling pathways of cytokines and growth factors in the treatment of IPF, however, studies focusing on cytokine and immune-related gene polymorphisms need to be further developed.

4.1.4 Other Potential Genetic Mutations Associated With IPF

In recent years, with the availability of next-generation sequencing technologies, more and more novel mutations have been identified in IPF patients. The mutations of the gene DSP (Mathai et al., 2016; Wang et al., 2018) and DPP9 (associated with cell adhesion) (Fingerlin et al., 2013; Zhou and Wang, 2016), AKAP13 166] and FAM13A (associated with RhoA/ROCK signaling pathway) (Hirano et al., 2017; van Moorsel, 2018), and SPPL2C (associated with intramembrane proteases) (Wu et al., 2016; Lorenzo-Salazar et al., 2019) were reported to be a risk of IPF susceptivity, progression and prognosis. However, the pathogenesis of these mutations remains unclear, and current studies are limited to correlation analysis (**Table 2**).

4.1.5 DNA Methylation

DNA methylation is a chemical modification process in which a specific base on the DNA sequence acquires a methyl group by covalent bonding with S-adenosyl methionine (SAM) as the methyl donor. DNA methylation is catalyzed by DNA methyltransferase (DNMT). In humans, DNA methylation occurs mainly at the fifth carbon atom of cytosine in CpG dinucleotides. It is generally believed that DNA methylation can inhibit the transcription and expression of the gene.

Global methylation and methylation of specific gene have been shown to be involved in the pathogenesis of IPF. Global DNA methylation analysis based on whole lung tissue showed that DNMT expression was increased in IPF, and DNA methylation of 16 genes (including CLDN5, ZNF467, TP53INP1 and DDAH1) was associated with decreased mRNA expression (Sanders et al., 2012). In order to clarify the contribution of specific cell types to IPF, single-cell-based or cell-type-specific sequencing is necessary. The global DNA methylation analysis based on fibroblasts showed that cells derived from IPF patients differ in the methylation of multiple CpG sites (including CDKN2B, CARD10, and MGMT) (Huang et al., 2014). Hypermethylation of specific genes not only can suppress the expression of some genes [Thy-1, COX-2, PTGER2, $p14^{ARF}$, IP-10 (Zhou et al., 2020), SFRP1/4, CDKN2B (Xue et al., 2021)], but also can promote the expression of some genes [α-SMA, MeCP2, KCNMB1 (Xue et al., 2021)], which eventually leads to the development of IPF (**Figure 5A**). Decitabine, a DNMT inhibitor, reduced fibrotic gene and DNMT-1 expression, enhanced miR-17–92 cluster expression (Dakhlallah et al., 2013). PGE2 has the capacity to limit fibrosis through its inhibition of numerous functions of these fibroblasts, and

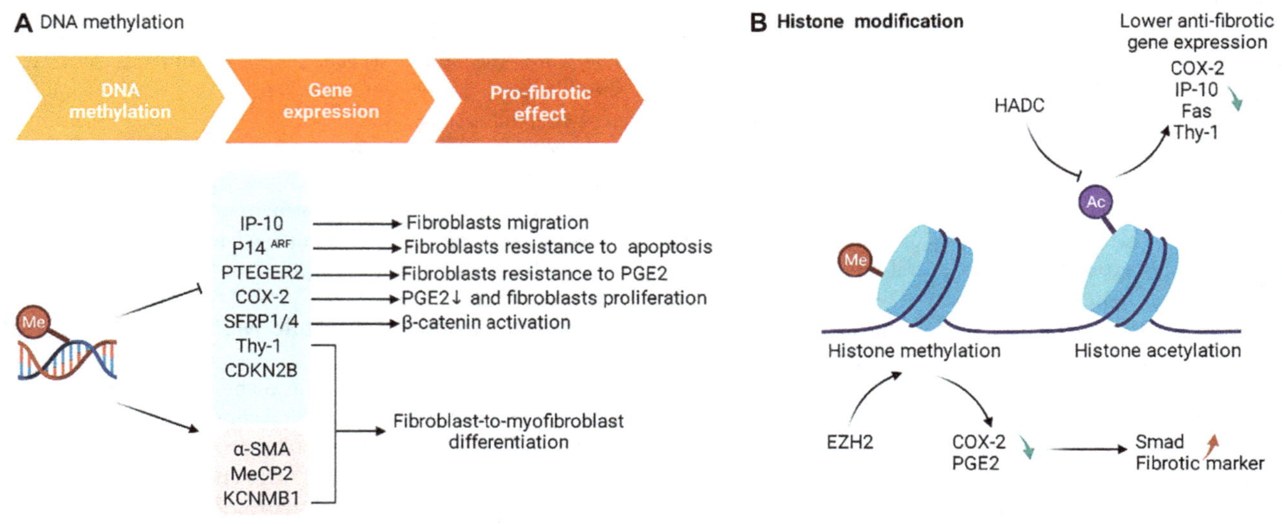

FIGURE 5 | The roles of DNA methylation and histone modification in IPF. **(A)** DNA methylation affects the expression of gene associated with fibrosis and produces a pro-fibrotic effect. **(B)** EZH2 and HADC induce changes in gene expression associated with fibrosis by affecting histone modifications.

TABLE 3 | Drugs targeting histone modification in IPF.

Drugs	Targets	Cell or animal model	Mechanism of action	Ref
3-DZNeP	EZH2/G9a inhibitor	BLM mice and LL29 cell	Reduce p-Smad2/3 nuclear translocations *in vitro* and downregulate α-SMA, COL1A1 and COL3A1 expression *in vivo*. Restore COX-2 expression and PGE2 production	Coward et al. (2014); Xiao et al. (2016)
A6	p300i	BLM mice; lung fibroblast cells	Decrease histone acetylation and pro-fibrotic gene expression *in vitro*, and reduce collagen deposition *in vivo*	Hwang et al. (2020)
Ac-SDKP	α-TAT1	MRC5/A549 cell	Promote apoptosis	Shifeng et al. (2019)
Romidepsin	HDACi	BLM mice	Inhibit LOX expression	Conforti et al. (2017)
LBH589	pan-HDACi	Primary IPF	Reduce expression of genes associated with ECM synthesis, proliferation and cell survival and suppress HDAC7 level	Korfei et al. (2015)
CG-745	HDACi	BLM/PHMG mice	Inhibit collagen production, inflammatory cell accumulation, and cytokines release	Kim et al. (2019)
Entinostat and vorinostat	HDACi	HFL-1 cell	Upregulate XPLN mRNA expression and reverse TGF-β-induced SPARC expression	Kamio et al. (2017)
TSA	pan-HDACi	NHLF cell	Reduce p-Akt level to inhibit TGF-β-mediated α-SMA expression	Guo et al. (2009)
SAHA	pan-HDACi	HLF cell	Promote the differentiation of fibroblasts into myofibroblasts and collagen deposition	Z Wang et al. (2009)
SpA	HDACi	Primary IPF	Inhibit the proliferation of IPF fibroblasts by increasing p21 expression	Davies et al. (2012)
JQ1	Bromodomain protein inhibitor	IPF fibroblasts	Bromodomain protein is the "Reader" of acetylated lysine in histone, and it is the only protein domain that can recognize and bind acetylated lysine in histone	Filippakopoulos et al. (2010)

Decitabine restored PGE2 responsiveness in fibrotic fibroblasts (Huang et al., 2010).

4.1.6 Histone Modification

Nucleosome, the basic unit of chromatin, is comprised of 146–147 base pairs of DNA and a histone octamer with one H2A-H2B tetramer and two H3-H4 dimers (Jenuwein and Allis, 2001).

The N- and C-terminal tails of H3 and H4 are the most frequently modified regions. The types of modifications include methylation, acetylation, phosphorylation, SUMOylation, and ubiquitination. The histone mark is named according to the histone, the modification site of these tails, and the type of modification. Histone modifications can change the electronic charge and structure of DNA-bound histone tails, thus altering chromatin state and gene expression (Kouzarides, 2007). The effect of histone acetylation and methylation in IPF has been extensively studied, and a large number of agents have been designed and validated in preclinical studies (**Figure 5B**).

Histone methylation is catalyzed by the histone methyltransferase (HMT), which uses S-adenosyl methionine (SAM) as the substrate to transfer methyl groups onto the lysine residues of histones. Methylation of H3K4, H3K36, and H3K79 is thought to be associated with gene activation, while H3K9, H3K27, and H4K20 are thought to be associated with gene inactivation (Black et al., 2012). Inhibition of EZH2, an H3K27me-specific methyltransferase, by 3-DZNeP and BIX01294 increased the expression of COX-2 and PGE2, and suppressed the expression of Smad signaling and fibrosis markers (Coward et al., 2014; Xiao et al., 2016).

Histone acetyltransferases (HATs) promote histone acetylation, while histone deacetylases (HDACs) reduce histone acetylation. Histone acetylation is thought to be associated with gene activation (Clayton et al., 1993). In addition, sirtuins (SIRTs) are a family of deacetylases. SIRT1 inhibits the expression of aging-related secretions by deacetylating the SASP gene (Hayakawa et al., 2015). Inhibition of SIRT3 expression promotes fibrosis in human lung fibroblasts (Sosulski et al., 2017). Histone deacetylation is associated with the repression of anti-fibrotic genes, which includes COX-2 (Coward et al., 2009), IP-10 (Coward et al., 2010), Fas (Huang et al., 2013), Thy-1 (Sanders et al., 2011).

Inhibition of histone deacetylation may have anti-pulmonary fibrosis effects. HDACi consists of a zinc-binding-group, a hydrophobic group for protein recognition and interaction, and a linker connecting both of them (Wang and Dymock, 2009). A large number of agents targeting histone modification have already demonstrated antifibrotic effects in preclinical trials or in cell levels (**Table 3**).

4.2 Environment Factors

Environmental factors such as asbestos, metal dust, stone dust, wood dust, chemotherapy and allergen exposure are important causes of IPF (Taskar and Coultas, 2006). Epidemiological surveys have shown that 38% of IPF patients were exposed to high-risk environments; however, it is uncertain whether these factors directly lead to the occurrence of IPF (Behr et al., 2015; Wuyts et al., 2018).

Smoking is a relatively special environmental factor. Both direct smoking and indirect smoking are independent exposure factors, and the correlation between the direct/indirect smoking and IPF increase with the increase of smoking in dose (Bellou et al., 2021). Interestingly, according to the German S2K guidelines, although 60%–70% of patients had a history of smoking, less than 7% of patients were active smokers when they developed IPF symptoms. In other words, most patients developed the disease several years after quitting smoking; the average time interval was 21 years (Behr et al., 2021). This indicates that across such a long period of time, the injury caused by smoking may continue to progress or transform into IPF.

4.3 Body Aging and Cell Senescence

According to epidemiological surveys, advanced age is one of the most relevant demographic factors for IPF (Sgalla et al., 2018). The incidence of IPF in elderly men over 50 years of age is significantly higher than that in younger men (Raghu et al., 2018). However, the mechanism of how senescence leads to IPF is still unclear. In a mouse model of fibrosis, researchers observed a series of signs of cellular senescence, including elevated senescence-associated β-galactosidase (SA-β-Gal) in lysosomes and elevated reactive oxygen species (ROS) in mitochondria, an increase in cell cycle arrest proteins such as P53/P21/P16, an increase in the apoptosis-related protein BCL-2/Bax ratio, and an increase in DNA damage in the nucleus (Blokland et al., 2020). In addition, a variety of senescence-associated secretory phenotypes (SASPs) have been observed in animal models of pulmonary fibrosis, and these SASP components are known to include powerful profibrotic molecules such as TGF-β (Cho and Stout-Delgado, 2020; Rana et al., 2020). Similarly, studies have found that the lung fibroblasts of elderly IPF patients exhibit the above characteristics (Álvarez et al., 2017). Therefore, although there is a lack of human research evidence that senescence directly causes IPF, epidemiological data from both animal experiments and cell experiments suggest that IPF is a senescence-related disease.

The main manifestations of lung senescence are decreased lung tissue elasticity, decreased effective lung volume, the thickening of intercellular substances, and decreased lung function. Cell senescence mainly manifests as cell morphology and structure disorder, cell dysfunction, and cell growth/proliferation arrest (Rana et al., 2020).

The mechanism of pulmonary fibrosis caused by aging is not very clear, but there are quite a few theories to explain the mechanism of senescence in IPF. Cell senescence can disrupt of a variety of processes and generate imbalances (for example, shortened telomeres and DNA damage, oncogene activation, redox imbalances, mitochondrial dysfunction, lysosomal and proteasome dysfunction, ER stress), resulting in increased SASP, myofibroblast resistance to apoptosis, and stem cell depletion, ultimately manifesting as abnormal repair at the lung injury site (e.g., failure of the alveolar epithelium to regenerate properly and ECM deposition) (Sgalla et al., 2018; Glass et al., 2020; Liu and Liu, 2020; Merkt et al., 2020). Aging has been reported to reprogram the hematopoietic-vascular niche to impede regeneration and promote fibrosis (Chen et al., 2021).

Because senescent cells that resist apoptosis can continuously produce profibrotic cytokines, which in turn aggravate pulmonary fibrosis, the induction of apoptosis in senescent cells (e.g., dasatinib/quercetin, ABT-263, and NOX4 inhibitors) or selective antagonism of profibrotic senescence-related factors (e.g., IL-6, TGF-β or leukotrienes) may help to alleviate IPF (Merkt et al., 2020). Many antiaging drugs have passed preclinical animal studies and entered clinical trials. For example, dasatinib (D) and quercetin (Q) can promote the apoptosis of senescent cells. The DQ combination regimen has been investigated in a phase I clinical trial (NCT02874989). A total of 14 patients were enrolled in the trial; except for one patient who had severe adverse reactions (bacterial pneumonia), the remaining patients tolerated the treatment well, and improvements in parameters such as 6-min walking distance, 4-m gait speed, and chair stand time were reported (Schafer et al., 2017; Justice et al., 2019). Interestingly, Nifurtimox (NIF), originally used to treat diarrhea, has been reported to improve pulmonary fibrosis by blocking the production of myofibroblasts (Gan et al., 2022).

TABLE 4 | Summary of emerging therapeutic targets for IPF in drug discovery.

Therapeutic targets	Mechanism	Ref
TGF-β	TGF-β is a powerful pro-fibrotic mediator	Ong et al. (2021)
αvβ6 Integrin	Integrin αvβ6 binds to an arginine-glycine-aspartic (RGD) sequence on LAP to activate latent form TGF-β1	Munger et al. (1999)
CTGF/CNN2	As a co-regulator of TGF-β in the pulmonary fibrosis microenvironment, CTGF can cooperate with TGF-β to participate in abnormal tissue repair processes including ECM production, fibroblast activation and differentiation	Lipson et al. (2012)
Galectin-3	Modulate macrophage phenotype/Gal-3 expression and fibroblast activation, reduce the effects of key profibrotic growth factors that act on myofibroblasts, and inhibiting EMT.	Humphries et al. (2021)
Leukotrienes	Leukotrienes have profibrotic effects by inducing fibroblast migration, proliferation, and matrix protein synthesis	Antoniou et al. (2007)
ATX-LPA-LPAR	The binding of LPA-to-LPAR can promote apoptosis of epithelial cells, regulation of endothelial permeability, activation of αvβ6 integrin-mediated TGF-β signaling, secretion of IL-8, recruitment and survival of fibroblasts. ATX is the key enzyme for LPA synthesis	Tager et al. (2008); Ninou et al. (2018); Suryadevara et al. (2020)
SPHK1-S1P-S1PR	The binding of S1P-to-S1PR can lead to mitochondrial reactive oxygen species (mtROS) and promote YAP1 to enter cell nuclei, affecting the differentiation of myofibroblasts and matrix remodeling. SPHK1 is the key enzyme for S1P synthesis	Huang et al. (2020)
PTX-2/SAP	As a ligand for the Fcγ receptor, PTX-2 downregulates monocyte and macrophage activity (especially M2)	Castaño et al. (2009)
JAK	JAK/STAT is a downstream pathway of IL-6, IL-11, IL-13, PDGF, TGF-β1 and FGF. The effect of JAK/STAT phosphorylation on cellular fibrotic processes includes proliferation, senescence, autophagy, endoplasmic reticulum stress, or epithelial/fibroblast to mesenchymal transition	Montero et al. (2021)
Src	Src is a group of nonreceptor tyrosine kinases, which participate in the TGF-β pathway by activating FAK.	Hu et al. (2014)
PI3K/Akt/mTOR	PI3K/Akt/mTOR plays a critical role in cell survival, growth, proliferation, protein synthesis, and EMT. *In vitro*, mTOR inhibitors can reduce TGF-β-induced fibroblast proliferation and type I collagen synthesis	Hennessy et al. (2005); Mercer et al. (2016); Lawrence and Nho, (2018)
Smo receptor	Smo is an important mediator of hedgehog signaling which is reactivated in adulthood within IPF	Effendi and Nagano, (2021)
Nitric oxide synthase	Activated macrophages, contributing to the cellular injury mediated by ROS, produce both nitric oxide (NO) and peroxynitrite	Giri, (2003)
GPR40/GPR84	GPR40 and GPR84 are G protein coupled receptors with free fatty acid ligands and are associated with metabolic and inflammatory disorders. PR40 agonist and GPR84 antagonists act on cells that involved in fibrotic pathways: macrophages, fibroblasts, and epithelial cells, and finally reduce inflammation	Gagnon et al. (2018)
LOX and LOXL	Lysyl oxidase (LOX) and LOX-like (LOXL) are enzymes involved in collagen cross-linking	Chen et al. (2019)

5 RECENT PROGRESS IN THERAPEUTIC TARGETS AND NEW DRUG DEVELOPMENT FOR IPF

Pirfenidone and nintedanib are two drugs approved by the FDA for the treatment of IPF. They can delay lung function deterioration and prolong patient survival in IPF patients. Although the launch of Pirfenidone and nintedanib has demonstrated the feasibility of drug treatment for IPF, they do not reverse pulmonary fibrosis and their efficacy in patients with end-stage IPF is not fully clear. Therefore, there is a need to develop additional anti-pulmonary fibrosis drugs. The development of drugs for some specific targets is currently underway, which will be described in the following sections. In addition, drug combinations for antifibrotic therapy are worth investigating. Immune checkpoint inhibitors (ICIs), either as single agents or in combination regimens, have shown great success in clinical treatment (Wu et al., 2022). A case reports indicates that the addition of nintedanib to ICIs therapy might prevent drug-induced pneumonitis or acute exacerbation of IPF (Yamakawa et al., 2019).

5.1 Summary of Emerging Therapeutic Targets for IPF in Drug Discovery

In this section we briefly describe the current therapeutic targets in clinical trials and the latest clinical trial developments. We summarize the emerging therapeutic targets and representative mechanisms in the development of IPF (**Table 4**).

TGF-β plays an important role in the pathogenesis of IPF by stimulating the activation and proliferation of fibroblasts (Ong et al., 2021). Both anti-TGF-β mAb and anti-TGF-β mRNA nucleic acid have entered clinical trials (NCT00125385 and NCT03727802, respectively). Monoclonal antibodies against integrins that activate latent TGF-β have also entered phase II clinical trials (NCT04072315 and NCT04396756). Tyrosine kinase inhibitors targeting the TGF-β receptor have also entered phase II clinical trials (NCT03832946). Other growth factors (PDGF, VEGF, FGF, EGF, CTGF) are also involved in the process of pulmonary fibrosis. The mAb targeting CTGF, Pamrevlumab, demonstrated clinical benefit in phase II clinical trials and is now in phase III clinical trials (NCT03955146 and NCT04419558).

Chemokines and interleukins are also involved in recruitment of pro-fibrotic cells and formation of pro-fibrotic microenvironment, as we discussed in our previous paper (Ma et al., 2022). However, CCL2, a key chemokine for monocyte/macrophage migration and infiltration, failed to demonstrate clinical benefit in a phase II clinical trial (NCT00786201). Anti-IL-13 therapy didn't contribute to lung function in patients with IPF (NCT02345070 and NCT01872689) or was terminated due to Lack of evidence of efficacy (NCT01266135 and NCT01266135).

Leukotrienes have profibrotic effects by inducing fibroblast migration, proliferation, and matrix protein synthesis (Antoniou et al., 2007). MN-001/Tipelukast, leukotriene receptor antagonist, is undergoing phase II clinical trial (NCT02503657).

As lipid proinflammatory mediators, The ATX-LPA-LPAR axis and SPHK1-S1P-S1PR axis have also been reported as targets of IPF. LPA and S1P have been demonstrated to promote the development of fibrosis (Tager et al., 2008; Ninou et al., 2018; Huang et al., 2020; Suryadevara et al., 2020). BMS-986278 (LPA1R antagonist) has entered phase II clinical trials (NCT04308681).

PTX-2, a ligand for the Fcγ receptor, can downregulate monocyte and macrophage activity (especially M2) (Castaño et al., 2009). PRM-151, a recombinant human pentraxin-2, has entered phase II clinical trials (NCT04594707 and NCT04552899).

Multiple cellular signaling pathways play a crucial role in the development of IPF. JAK/STAT signaling (Montero et al., 2021), receptor-type tyrosine kinase/non-receptor-type tyrosine kinase signaling (e.g., Src) (Hu et al., 2014), PI3K/Akt/mTOR signaling (Hennessy et al., 2005; Mercer et al., 2016; Lawrence and Nho, 2018), and Hedgehog signaling (Effendi and Nagano, 2021) comprise complex fibrosis regulatory signaling pathway. In our previous reviews, we have discussed the aforementioned signaling pathways (Ma et al., 2022).

There are also drugs in clinical trials targeting oxidative stress (Giri, 2003), GPR40/GPR84 (Gagnon et al., 2018), and collagen cross-linking enzymes (Chen et al., 2019).

5.2 Summary of Ongoing Clinical Trials for IPF

We searched clinical trials in recent years and summarized the anti-IPF drugs undergoing clinical trials and their mechanisms of action (**Table 5**). We also update the latest clinical trial progress for these drugs.

TABLE 5 | Ongoing clinical trials about some investigational compounds for IPF.

Targets	Drugs	Clinical trial information
LPC-ATX-LPA	BMS-986278 (LPA1R antagonist)	Phase 2 (recruiting, NCT04308681)
PTX-2/SAP	PRM-151(Intravenous recombinant human pentraxin-2)	Phase 3 (recruiting, NCT04594707, NCT04552899)
CTGF/CNN2	FG-3019/Pamrevlumab (CTGF mAb)	Phase 3 (recruiting, NCT04419558, NCT03955146)
Galectin 3	TD139 (small-molecule antagonist of Galectin-3)	Phase 2 (recruiting, NCT03832946)
Oxidative stress	Niacin (nicotinic acid)	Phase 2 (recruiting, NCT0386592)
	Setanaxib/GKT137831(NOS1/4 inhibitor)	Phase 2 (recruiting, NCT03865927)
JNK	Jaktinib Dihydrochloride Monohydrate (JNK1/2 inhibitor)	Phase 2 (recruiting, NCT04312594)
	CC-90001 (JNK1/2 inhibitor)	Phase 2 (active, not recruiting, NCT03142191)
Src	Saracatinib (Src kinase inhibitor)	Phase 1/2 (recruiting, NCT04598919)
Hedgehog pathways	taladegib/ENV-101(Smo receptor inhibitor)	Phase 2 (not yet recruiting, NCT04968574)
Leukotrienes	MN-001/Tipelukast (leukotriene receptor antagonist)	Phase 2(Active, not recruiting, NCT02503657)
LOXL2	EGCG (irreversible inhibitor of both LOXL2 and TGF-β receptors 1 and 2 kinase)	Early Phase 1 (recruiting, NCT03928847)
IRE1	ORIN1001(IRE1 inhibitor)	Phase 1 (recruiting, NCT04643769)
PDE4b	BI 1015550(PDE4b inhibitor)	Phase 2 (active, not recruiting, NCT04419506)
NDMA	NP-120/Ifenprodil (N-methyl-d-aspartate (NDMA) receptor glutamate receptor antagonist)	Phase 2 (recruiting, NCT04318704)
B cell	Ianalumab/VAY736(B-cell activating factor receptor mAb)	Phase 2 (active, not recruiting, NCT03287414)
	Rituximab (CD20 chimeric mAb)	Phase 2 (active, not recruiting, NCT01969409); Phase 2 (recruiting, NCT03584802); Phase 2 (recruiting, NCT03286556); Phase2 (recruiting, NCT03500731)
Traditional medicine	Jin-shui Huan-xian granule	Not Applicable (recruiting, NCT04187690)
	Fuzheng Huayu tablet	Phase 2 (recruiting, NCT04279197)

6 CONCLUSION AND OUTLOOK

The research on the pathogenesis of IPF has made considerable progress. After years of basic and clinical studies, the pathogenesis of IPF has changed from simple inflammation to abnormal epithelial-mesenchymal crosstalk and other common pathogenic mechanisms. Based on this pathological mechanism, many studies have systematically studied the key roles of fibrocytes/(myo)fibroblasts, epithelial/endothelial cells, and ECM in the pathogenesis of IPF. With the progresses in understanding the key role of genetics and epigenetics in IPF, researchers have found that an increasing number of genetic loci and their apparent modifications are related to the maintenance of lung homeostasis although the effects of gene mutations and epigenetics on IPF still need further study.

The advent of pirfenidone and nintedanib is undoubtedly a sensational event in the field of IPF treatment, but they also have some major limitations, such as insufficient curative effect and poor pharmacokinetic properties. In addition, combination therapy based on them needs to be further studied. The number of clinical trials for therapies targeting cytokines, growth factors, and their signaling pathways is increasing rapidly. Furthermore, drugs targeting MMPs, telomerase activity, and epigenetic modifications need to be further developed.

Although IPF is idiopathic by definition, this deadly disease may become less mysterious with the progress in the understanding of the pathogenesis of IPF. The number of observed therapeutic targets is increasing, as well as the number of new drugs entering clinical trials. For patients with IPF, these advances described in this review show that slowing the IPF progression, prolonging their lives, and improving their quality of life might be possible in the future.

AUTHOR CONTRIBUTIONS

HM contributed to the conception of this review and preparation of the manuscript, tables, and figures; XW collected information about the clinical trials; YL revised the tables and figures; YX contributed to the conception, supervision, and revision of the manuscript. All authors have approved the final article and are included in the disclosure.

REFERENCES

1. Álvarez, D., Cárdenes, N., Sellarés, J., Bueno, M., Corey, C., Hanumanthu, V. S., et al. (2017). IPF Lung Fibroblasts Have a Senescent Phenotype. *Am. J. Physiol. Cell. Mol. Physiol.* 313 (6), L1164–l1173. doi:10.1152/ajplung.00220.2017
2. Alder, J. K., Barkauskas, C. E., Limjunyawong, N., Stanley, S. E., Kembou, F., Tuder, R. M., et al. (2015). Telomere Dysfunction Causes Alveolar Stem Cell Failure. *Proc. Natl. Acad. Sci. U. S. A.* 112 (16), 5099–5104. doi:10.1073/pnas.1504780112
3. Allen, R. J., Porte, J., Braybrooke, R., Flores, C., Fingerlin, T. E., Oldham, J. M., et al. (2017). Genetic Variants Associated with Susceptibility to Idiopathic Pulmonary Fibrosis in People of European Ancestry: A Genome-wide Association Study. *Lancet Respir. Med.* 5 (11), 869–880. doi:10.1016/s2213-2600(17)30387-9
4. Andersson-Sjöland, A., Nihlberg, K., Eriksson, L., Bjermer, L., and Westergren- Thorsson, G. (2011). Fibrocytes and the Tissue Niche in Lung Repair. *Respir. Res.* 12 (1), 76. doi:10.1186/1465-9921-12-76
5. Antoniou, K. M., Pataka, A., Bouros, D., and Siafakas, N. M. (2007). Pathogenetic Pathways and Novel Pharmacotherapeutic Targets in Idiopathic Pulmonary Fibrosis. *Pulm. Pharmacol. Ther.* 20 (5), 453–461. doi:10.1016/j.pupt.2006. 01.002
6. Aoyagi-Ikeda, K., Maeno, T., Matsui, H., Ueno, M., Hara, K., Aoki, Y., et al. (2011). Notch Induces Myofibroblast Differentiation of Alveolar Epithelial Cells via Transforming Growth Factor-{beta}-Smad3 Pathway. *Am. J. Respir. Cell. Mol. Biol.* 45 (1), 136–144. doi:10.1165/rcmb.2010-0140oc
7. Armanios, M. Y., Chen, J. J., Cogan, J. D., Alder, J. K., Ingersoll, R. G., Markin, C., et al. (2007). Telomerase mutations in families with idiopathic pulmonary fibrosis. *N. Engl. J. Med.* 356 (13), 1317–1326. doi:10.1056/NEJMoa066157
8. Bär, C., Povedano, J. M., Serrano, R., Benitez-Buelga, C., Popkes, M., Formentini, I., et al. (2016). Telomerase Gene Therapy Rescues Telomere Length, Bone Marrow Aplasia, and Survival in Mice with Aplastic Anemia. *Blood* 127 (14), 1770–1779. doi:10.1182/blood-2015-08-667485
9. Bao, Z., Zhang, Q., Wan, H., He, P., Zhou, X., and Zhou, M. (2014). Expression of Suppressor of Cytokine Signaling 1 in the Peripheral Blood of Patients with Idiopathic Pulmonary Fibrosis. *Chin. Med. J. Engl.* 127 (11), 2117–2120.
10. Baratella, E., Ruaro, B., Giudici, F., Wade, B., Santagiuliana, M., Salton, F., et al. (2021). Evaluation of correlations between genetic variants and high-resolution computed tomography patterns in idiopathic pulmonary fibrosis. *Diagnostics* 11 (5), 762. doi:10.3390/diagnostics11050762
11. Barros, A., Oldham, J., and Noth, I. (2019). Genetics of idiopathic pulmonary fibrosis. *Am. J. Med. Sci.* 357 (5), 379–383. doi:10.1016/j.amjms.2019.02.009
12. Bayne, S., and Liu, J. P. (2005). Hormones and Growth Factors Regulate Telomerase Activity in Ageing and Cancer. *Mol Cell Endocrinol.* 240 (1–2), 11–22. doi:10.1016/j.mce.2005.05.009
13. Behr, J., Günther, A., Bonella, F., Dinkel, J., Fink, L., Geiser, T., et al. (2021). S2K guideline for diagnosis of idiopathic pulmonary fibrosis. *Respiration* 100 (3), 238–271. doi:10.1159/000512315
14. Behr, J., Kreuter, M., Hoeper, M. M., Wirtz, H., Klotsche, J., Koschel, D., et al. (2015). Management of Patients with Idiopathic Pulmonary Fibrosis in Clinical Practice: The INSIGHTS-IPF Registry. *Eur. Respir. J.* 46 (1), 186–196. doi:10. 1183/09031936.00217614
15. Bellou, V., Belbasis, L., and Evangelou, E. (2021). Tobacco smoking and risk for pulmonary fibrosis: A prospective cohort study from the UK biobank. *Chest* 160 (3), 983–993. doi:10.1016/j.chest.2021.04.035
16. Betensley, A., Sharif, R., and Karamichos, D. (2016). A systematic review of the role of dysfunctional wound healing in the pathogenesis and treatment of idiopathic pulmonary fibrosis. *J. Clin. Med.* 6 (1), 2. doi:10.3390/jcm6010002
17. Black, J. C., Van Rechem, C., and Whetstine, J. R. (2012). Histone Lysine Methylation Dynamics: Establishment, Regulation, and Biological Impact. *Mol. Cell.* 48 (4), 491–507. doi:10.1016/j.molcel.2012.11.006
18. Blasco, M. A., Lee, H. W., Hande, M. P., Samper, E., Lansdorp, P. M., DePinho, R. A., et al. (1997). Telomere Shortening and Tumor Formation by Mouse Cells Lacking Telomerase RNA. *Cell.* 91 (1), 25–34. doi:10.1016/s0092-8674(01) 80006-4
19. Blokland, K. E. C., Pouwels, S. D., Schuliga, M., Knight, D. A., and Burgess, J. K. (2020). Regulation of Cellular Senescence by Extracellular Matrix during Chronic Fibrotic Diseases. *Clin. Sci. (Lond)* 134 (20), 2681–2706. doi:10.1042/ cs20190893

20. Borie, R., Kannengiesser, C., Hirschi, S., Le Pavec, J., Mal, H., Bergot, E., et al. (2015). Severe Hematologic Complications after Lung Transplantation in Patients with Telomerase Complex Mutations. *J. Heart Transpl.* 34 (4), 538-546. doi:10.1016/j.healun.2014.11.010
21. Borie, R., Tabèze, L., Thabut, G., Nunes, H., Cottin, V., Marchand-Adam, S., et al. (2016). Prevalence and Characteristics of TERT and TERC Mutations in Suspected Genetic Pulmonary Fibrosis. *Eur. Respir. J.* 48 (6), 1721–1731. doi:10.1183/13993003.02115-2015
22. Bouros, D., Antoniou, K. M., Tzouvelekis, A., and Siafakas, N. M. (2006). Interferon-gamma 1b for the Treatment of Idiopathic Pulmonary Fibrosis. *Expert Opin. Biol. Ther.* 6 (10), 1051–1060. doi:10.1517/14712598.6.10.1051
23. Bratcher, P. E., Weathington, N. M., Nick, H. J., Jackson, P. L., Snelgrove, R. J., and Gaggar, A. (2012). MMP-9 Cleaves SP-D and Abrogates its Innate Immune Functions *In Vitro*. *PLoS One* 7 (7), e41881. doi:10.1371/journal.pone.0041881
24. Bullard, J. E., and Nogee, L. M. (2007). Heterozygosity for ABCA3 Mutations Modifies the Severity of Lung Disease Associated with a Surfactant Protein C Gene (SFTPC) Mutation. *Pediatr. Res.* 62 (2), 176–179. doi:10.1203/PDR.0b013e3180a72588
25. Burgess, J. K., and Weckmann, M. (2012). Matrikines and the Lungs. *Pharmacol. Ther.* 134 (3), 317–337. doi:10.1016/j.pharmthera.2012.02.002
26. Burman, A., Tanjore, H., and Blackwell, T. S. (2018). Endoplasmic Reticulum Stress in Pulmonary Fibrosis. *Matrix Biol.* 68-69, 355–365. doi:10.1016/j.matbio.2018. 03.015
27. Cassidy, L. D., and Narita, M. (2022). Autophagy at the Intersection of Aging, Senescence, and Cancer. *Mol. Oncol.* doi:10.1002/1878-0261.13269
28. Castaño, A. P., Lin, S. L., Surowy, T., Nowlin, B. T., Turlapati, S. A., Patel, T., et al. (2009). Serum Amyloid P Inhibits Fibrosis through Fc Gamma R-dependent Monocyte-Macrophage Regulation *In Vivo*. *Sci. Transl. Med.* 1 (5), 5ra13. doi:10.1126/scitranslmed.3000111
29. Cedeno-Laurent, F., and Dimitroff, C. J. (2012). Galectin-1 Research in T Cell Immunity: Past, Present and Future. *Clin. Immunol.* 142 (2), 107–116. doi:10.1016/j.clim.2011.09.011
30. Chambers, D. C., Lutzky, V. P., Apte, S. H., Godbolt, D., Feenstra, J., and Mackintosh, J. (2020). Successful Treatment of Telomeropathy-Related Interstitial Lung Disease with Immunosuppression and Danazol. *Respirol. Case Rep.* 8 (6), e00607. doi:10.1002/rcr2.607
31. Chanda, D., Otoupalova, E., Smith, S. R., Volckaert, T., De Langhe, S. P., and Thannickal, V. J. (2019). Developmental Pathways in the Pathogenesis of Lung Fibrosis. *Mol. Asp. Med.* 65, 56–69. doi:10.1016/j.mam.2018.08.004
32. Chen, H., Qu, J., Huang, X., Kurundkar, A., Zhu, L., Yang, N., et al. (2016). Mechanosensing by the α6-integrin Confers an Invasive Fibroblast Phenotype and Mediates Lung Fibrosis. *Nat. Commun.* 7, 12564. doi:10.1038/ncomms12564
33. Chen, L., Li, S., and Li, W. (2019). LOX/LOXL in Pulmonary Fibrosis: Potential Therapeutic Targets. *J. Drug Target* 27 (7), 790–796. doi:10.1080/1061186x.2018.1550649
34. Chen, R., Zhang, K., Chen, H., Zhao, X., Wang, J., Li, L., et al. (2015). Telomerase deficiency causes alveolar stem cell senescence-Associated low-Grade inflammation in lungs. *J. Biol. Chem.* 290 (52), 30813–30829. doi:10.1074/jbc.M115.681619
35. Chen, Y., Pu, Q., Ma, Y., Zhang, H., Ye, T., Zhao, C., et al. (2021). Aging reprograms the hematopoietic-vascular niche to impede regeneration and promote fibrosis. *Cell. Metab.* 33 (2), 395–e4. e394. doi:10.1016/j.cmet.2020.11.019
36. Cheong, N., Madesh, M., Gonzales, L. W., Zhao, M., Yu, K., Ballard, P. L., et al. (2006). Functional and Trafficking Defects in ATP Binding Cassette A3 Mutants Associated with Respiratory Distress Syndrome. *J. Biol. Chem.* 281 (14), 9791–9800. doi:10.1074/jbc.M507515200
37. Cheong, N., Zhang, H., Madesh, M., Zhao, M., Yu, K., Dodia, C., et al. (2007). ABCA3 Is Critical for Lamellar Body Biogenesis *In Vivo*. *J. Biol. Chem.* 282 (33), 23811–23817. doi:10.1074/jbc.M703927200
38. Cho, S. J., and Stout-Delgado, H. W. (2020). Aging and lung disease. *Annu. Rev. Physiol.* 82, 433–459. doi:10.1146/annurev-physiol-021119-034610
39. Chong, S. G., Sato, S., Kolb, M., and Gauldie, J. (2019). Fibrocytes and Fibroblasts- Where Are We Now. *Int. J. Biochem. Cell. Biol.* 116, 105595. doi:10.1016/j. biocel.2019.105595
40. Chu, K. A., Yeh, C. C., Kuo, F. H., Lin, W. R., Hsu, C. W., Chen, T. H., et al. (2020). Comparison of Reversal of Rat Pulmonary Fibrosis of Nintedanib, Pirfenidone, and Human Umbilical Mesenchymal Stem Cells from Wharton's Jelly. *Stem Cell. Res. Ther.* 11 (1), 513. doi:10.1186/s13287-020-02012-y
41. Clayton, A. L., Hebbes, T. R., Thorne, A. W., and Crane-Robinson, C. (1993). Histone Acetylation and Gene Induction in Human Cells. *FEBS Lett.* 336 (1), 23–26. doi:10.1016/0014-5793(93)81601-u
42. Cogan, J. D., Kropski, J. A., Zhao, M., Mitchell, D. B., Rives, L., Markin, C., et al. (2015). Rare Variants in RTEL1 Are Associated with Familial Interstitial Pneumonia. *Am. J. Respir. Crit. Care Med.* 191 (6), 646–655. doi:10.1164/rccm.201408-1510OC
43. Conforti, F., Davies, E. R., Calderwood, C. J., Thatcher, T. H., Jones, M. G., Smart, D. E., et al. (2017). The Histone Deacetylase Inhibitor, Romidepsin, as a Potential Treatment for Pulmonary Fibrosis. *Oncotarget* 8 (30), 48737-48754. doi:10.18632/oncotarget.17114
44. Conti, C., Montero-Fernandez, A., Borg, E., Osadolor, T., Viola, P., De Lauretis, A., et al. (2016). Mucins MUC5B and MUC5AC in distal airways and honeycomb spaces: Comparison Among idiopathic pulmonary fibrosis/usual interstitial pneumonia, fibrotic nonspecific interstitial pneumonitis, and control lungs. *Am. J. Respir. Crit. Care Med.* 193 (4), 462–464. doi:10.1164/rccm.201507-1322LE
45. Corapi, E., Carrizo, G., Compagno, D., and Laderach, D. (2018). Endogenous galectin-1 in T lymphocytes regulates anti-prostate cancer immunity. *Front. Immunol.* 9, 2190. doi:10.3389/fimmu.2018.02190
46. Coward, W. R., Feghali-Bostwick, C. A., Jenkins, G., Knox, A. J., and Pang, L. (2014). A Central Role for G9a and EZH2 in the Epigenetic Silencing of Cyclooxygenase-2 in Idiopathic Pulmonary Fibrosis. *Faseb J.* 28 (7), 3183-3196. doi:10.1096/fj.13-241760
47. Coward, W. R., Watts, K., Feghali-Bostwick, C. A., Jenkins, G., and Pang, L. (2010). Repression of IP-10 by Interactions between Histone Deacetylation and Hypermethylation in Idiopathic Pulmonary Fibrosis. *Mol. Cell. Biol.* 30 (12), 2874–2886. doi:10.1128/mcb.01527-09
48. Coward, W. R., Watts, K., Feghali-Bostwick, C. A., Knox, A., and Pang, L. (2009). Defective Histone Acetylation Is Responsible for the Diminished Expression of Cyclooxygenase 2 in Idiopathic Pulmonary Fibrosis. *Mol. Cell. Biol.* 29 (15), 4325–4339. doi:10.1128/mcb.01776-08
49. Craig, V. J., Quintero, P. A., Fyfe, S. E., Patel, A. S., Knolle, M. D., Kobzik, L., et al. (2013). Profibrotic Activities for Matrix Metalloproteinase-8 during Bleomycin-Mediated Lung Injury. *J. Immunol.* 190 (8), 4283–4296. doi:10.4049/jimmunol.1201043
50. Crossno, P. F., Polosukhin, V. V., Blackwell, T. S., Johnson, J. E., Markin, C., Moore, P. E., et al. (2010). Identification of Early Interstitial Lung Disease in an Individual with Genetic Variations in ABCA3 and SFTPC. *Chest* 137 (4), 969–973. doi:10.1378/chest.09-0790
51. Cushing, L., Kuang, P., and Lü, J. (2015). The Role of miR-29 in Pulmonary Fibrosis. *Biochem. Cell. Biol.* 93 (2), 109–118. doi:10.1139/bcb-2014-0095
52. Dakhlallah, D., Batte, K., Wang, Y., Cantemir-Stone, C. Z., Yan, P., Nuovo, G., et al. (2013). Epigenetic Regulation of miR-17~92 Contributes to the Pathogenesis of Pulmonary Fibrosis. *Am. J. Respir. Crit. Care Med.* 187 (4), 397–405. doi:10. 1164/rccm.201205-0888OC
53. Davies, E. R., Haitchi, H. M., Thatcher, T. H., Sime, P. J., Kottmann, R. M., Ganesan, A., et al. (2012). Spiruchostatin A Inhibits Proliferation and Differentiation of Fibroblasts from Patients with Pulmonary Fibrosis. *Am. J. Respir. Cell. Mol. Biol.* 46 (5), 687–694. doi:10.1165/rcmb.2011-0040OC
54. Degryse, A. L., Xu, X. C., Newman, J. L., Mitchell, D. B., Tanjore, H., Polosukhin, V. V., et al. (2012). Telomerase Deficiency Does Not Alter Bleomycin-Induced Fibrosis in Mice. *Exp. Lung Res.* 38 (3), 124–134. doi:10.3109/01902148.2012. 658148
55. Deshmane, S. L., Kremlev, S., Amini, S., and Sawaya, B. E. (2009). Monocyte Chemoattractant Protein-1 (MCP-1): An Overview. *J. Interferon Cytokine Res.* 29 (6), 313–326. doi:10.1089/jir.2008.0027
56. Effendi, W. I., and Nagano, T. (2021). The Hedgehog signaling pathway in idiopathic pulmonary fibrosis: Resurrection time. *Int. J. Mol. Sci.* 23 (1), 171. doi:10.3390/ijms23010171
57. Elowsson Rendin, L., Löfdahl, A., Åhrman, E., Müller, C., Notermans, T., Michaliková, B., et al. (2019). Matrisome properties of scaffolds direct fibroblasts in idiopathic pulmonary fibrosis. *Int. J. Mol. Sci.* 20 (16), 4013. doi:10.3390/ijms20164013
58. Evans, C. M., Fingerlin, T. E., Schwarz, M. I., Lynch, D., Kurche, J., Warg, L., et al. (2016). Idiopathic pulmonary fibrosis: A genetic disease that involves mucociliary dysfunction of the peripheral airways. *Physiol. Rev.* 96 (4), 1567-1591. doi:10.1152/physrev.00004.2016
59. Filer, A., and Buckley, C. D. (2013). *Fibroblasts and fibroblast-like synoviocytes*, 215–231. doi:10.1016/b978-1-4377-1738-9.00015-3
60. Filippakopoulos, P., Qi, J., Picaud, S., Shen, Y., Smith, W. B., Fedorov, O., et al. (2010). Selective Inhibition of BET Bromodomains. *Nature* 468 (7327), 1067–1073. doi:10.1038/nature09504
61. Fingerlin, T. E., Murphy, E., Zhang, W., Peljto, A. L., Brown, K. K., Steele, M. P., et al. (2013). Genome-wide Association Study Identifies Multiple Susceptibility Loci for Pulmonary Fibrosis. *Nat. Genet.* 45 (6), 613–620. doi:10.1038/ng.2609

62. Fitzgerald, M. L., Xavier, R., Haley, K. J., Welti, R., Goss, J. L., Brown, C. E., et al. (2007). ABCA3 Inactivation in Mice Causes Respiratory Failure, Loss of Pulmonary Surfactant, and Depletion of Lung Phosphatidylglycerol. *J. Lipid Res.* 48 (3), 621–632. doi:10.1194/jlr.M600449-JLR200
63. Fukuhara, A., Tanino, Y., Ishii, T., Inokoshi, Y., Saito, K., Fukuhara, N., et al. (2013). Pulmonary Fibrosis in Dyskeratosis Congenita with TINF2 Gene Mutation. *Eur. Respir. J.* 42 (6), 1757–1759. doi:10.1183/09031936.00149113
64. Gagnon, L., Leduc, M., Thibodeau, J. F., Zhang, M. Z., Grouix, B., Sarra-Bournet, F., et al. (2018). A newly discovered antifibrotic pathway regulated by two fatty acid receptors: GPR40 and GPR84. *Am. J. Pathol.* 188 (5), 1132–1148. doi:10.1016/j. ajpath.2018.01.009
65. Gan, C., Zhang, Q., Liu, H., Wang, G., Wang, L., Li, Y., et al. (2022). Nifuroxazide Ameliorates Pulmonary Fibrosis by Blocking Myofibroblast Genesis: A Drug Repurposing Study. *Respir. Res.* 23 (1), 32. doi:10.1186/s12931-022-01946-6
66. García-Prieto, E., González-López, A., Cabrera, S., Astudillo, A., Gutiérrez-Fernández, A., Fanjul-Fernandez, M., et al. (2010). Resistance to Bleomycin- Induced Lung Fibrosis in MMP-8 Deficient Mice Is Mediated by Interleukin-10. *PLoS One* 5 (10), e13242. doi:10.1371/journal.pone.0013242
67. Gaysinskaya, V., Stanley, S. E., Adam, S., and Armanios, M. (2020). Synonymous mutation in DKC1 causes telomerase RNA insufficiency manifesting as familial pulmonary fibrosis. *Chest* 158 (6), 2449–2457. doi:10.1016/j.chest.2020.07.025
68. Ghavami, S., Yeganeh, B., Zeki, A. A., Shojaei, S., Kenyon, N. J., Ott, S., et al. (2018). Autophagy and the Unfolded Protein Response Promote Profibrotic Effects of TGF-B1 in Human Lung Fibroblasts. *Am. J. Physiol. Cell. Mol. Physiol.* 314 (3), L493–l504. doi:10.1152/ajplung.00372.2017
69. Giri, S. N. (2003). Novel Pharmacological Approaches to Manage Interstitial Lung Fibrosis in the Twenty-First Century. *Annu. Rev. Pharmacol. Toxicol.* 43, 73–95. doi:10.1146/annurev.pharmtox.43.100901.135740
70. Gjorevski, N., Boghaert, E., and Nelson, C. M. (2012). Regulation of epithelial- mesenchymal transition by transmission of mechanical stress through epithelial tissues. *Cancer Microenviron.* 5 (1), 29–38. doi:10.1007/s12307-011-0076-5
71. Glass, D. S., Grossfeld, D., Renna, H. A., Agarwala, P., Spiegler, P., Kasselman, L. J., et al. (2020). Idiopathic Pulmonary Fibrosis: Molecular Mechanisms and Potential Treatment Approaches. *Respir. Investig.* 58 (5), 320–335. doi:10. 1016/j.resinv.2020.04.002
72. Guenther, K., Seeger, W., Guenther, A., and Korfei, M. (2019). Cellular Consequences of Uncharacterized Surfactant Protein-A2 (SFTPA2)-Gene Mutations Associated with Familial IPF and Lung Cancer. *J Eur. Respir. J.* 54 (Suppl. 63), OA1608. doi:10.1183/13993003.congress-2019.OA1608
73. Guo, W., Shan, B., Klingsberg, R. C., Qin, X., and Lasky, J. A. (2009). Abrogation of TGF-Beta1-Induced Fibroblast-Myofibroblast Differentiation by Histone Deacetylase Inhibition. *Am. J. Physiol. Cell. Mol. Physiol.* 297 (5), L864–L870. doi:10.1152/ajplung.00128.2009
74. Hams, E., Armstrong, M. E., Barlow, J. L., Saunders, S. P., Schwartz, C., Cooke, G., et al. (2014). IL-25 and Type 2 Innate Lymphoid Cells Induce Pulmonary Fibrosis. *Proc. Natl. Acad. Sci. U. S. A.* 111 (1), 367–372. doi:10.1073/pnas. 1315854111
75. Hayakawa, T., Iwai, M., Aoki, S., Takimoto, K., Maruyama, M., Maruyama, W., et al. (2015). SIRT1 Suppresses the Senescence-Associated Secretory Phenotype through Epigenetic Gene Regulation. *PLoS One* 10 (1), e0116480. doi:10.1371/ journal.pone.0116480
76. Hennessy, B. T., Smith, D. L., Ram, P. T., Lu, Y., and Mills, G. B. (2005). Exploiting the PI3K/AKT Pathway for Cancer Drug Discovery. *Nat. Rev. Drug Discov.* 4 (12), 988–1004. doi:10.1038/nrd1902
77. Herrera, I., Cisneros, J., Maldonado, M., Ramírez, R., Ortiz-Quintero, B., Anso, E., et al. (2013). Matrix Metalloproteinase (MMP)-1 Induces Lung Alveolar Epithelial Cell Migration and Proliferation, Protects from Apoptosis, and Represses Mitochondrial Oxygen Consumption. *J. Biol. Chem.* 288 (36), 25964–25975. doi:10.1074/jbc.M113.459784
78. Heukels, P., Moor, C. C., von der Thüsen, J. H., Wijsenbeek, M. S., and Kool, M. (2019). Inflammation and Immunity in IPF Pathogenesis and Treatment. *Respir. Med.* 147, 79–91. doi:10.1016/j.rmed.2018.12.015
79. Hill, C., Jones, M. G., Davies, D. E., and Wang, Y. (2019). Epithelial-mesenchymal Transition Contributes to Pulmonary Fibrosis via Aberrant Epithelial/ fibroblastic Cross-Talk. *J. Health Dis.* 3 (2), 31–35. doi:10.29245/2689-999x/2019/2.1149
80. Hirano, C., Ohshimo, S., Horimasu, Y., Iwamoto, H., Fujitaka, K., Hamada, H., et al. (2017). FAM13A Polymorphism as a Prognostic Factor in Patients with Idiopathic Pulmonary Fibrosis. *Respir. Med.* 123, 105–109. doi:10.1016/j. rmed. 2016.12.007
81. Hoffman, T. W., van Moorsel, C. H. M., Borie, R., and Crestani, B. (2018). Pulmonary Phenotypes Associated with Genetic Variation in Telomere-Related Genes. *Curr. Opin. Pulm. Med.* 24 (3), 269–280. doi:10.1097/mcp. 0000000000000475
82. Hu, M., Che, P., Han, X., Cai, G. Q., Liu, G., Antony, V., et al. (2014). Therapeutic Targeting of SRC Kinase in Myofibroblast Differentiation and Pulmonary Fibrosis. *J. Pharmacol. Exp. Ther.* 351 (1), 87–95. doi:10.1124/jpet.114.216044
83. Huang, L. S., Sudhadevi, T., Fu, P., Punathil-Kannan, P. K., Ebenezer, D. L., Ramchandran, R., et al. (2020). Sphingosine kinase 1/S1P signaling contributes to pulmonary fibrosis by activating hippo/YAP pathway and mitochondrial reactive oxygen species in lung fibroblasts. *Int. J. Mol. Sci.* 21 (6), 2064. doi:10. 3390/ijms21062064
84. Huang, S. K., Fisher, A. S., Scruggs, A. M., White, E. S., Hogaboam, C. M., Richardson, B. C., et al. (2010). Hypermethylation of PTGER2 Confers Prostaglandin E2 Resistance in Fibrotic Fibroblasts from Humans and Mice. *Am. J. Pathol.* 177 (5), 2245–2255. doi:10.2353/ajpath.2010.100446
85. Huang, S. K., Scruggs, A. M., Donaghy, J., Horowitz, J. C., Zaslona, Z., Przybranowski, S., et al. (2013). Histone Modifications Are Responsible for Decreased Fas Expression and Apoptosis Resistance in Fibrotic Lung Fibroblasts. *Cell. Death Dis.* 4 (5), e621. doi:10.1038/cddis.2013.146
86. Huang, S. K., Scruggs, A. M., McEachin, R. C., White, E. S., and Peters-Golden, M. (2014). Lung Fibroblasts from Patients with Idiopathic Pulmonary Fibrosis Exhibit Genome-wide Differences in DNA Methylation Compared to Fibroblasts from Nonfibrotic Lung. *PLoS One* 9 (9), e107055. doi:10.1371/ journal.pone.0107055
87. Humphries, D. C., Mills, R., Dobie, R., Henderson, N. C., Sethi, T., and Mackinnon, A. C. (2021). Selective myeloid depletion of galectin-3 offers protection against acute and chronic lung injury. *Front. Pharmacol.* 12, 715986. doi:10.3389/fphar. 2021.715986
88. Hwang, S. Y., Park, S. Y., Hong, J. Y., Lee, S. Y., Shin, J. H., Na, Y., et al. (2020). Field-based Rational Design of P300 Histone Acetyltransferase Inhibitor and Systematic Evaluation as an Anti-fibrotic Agent. *Chem. Commun. (Camb)* 56 (68), 9795–9798. doi:10.1039/d0cc03553j
89. Iyonaga, K., Takeya, M., Saita, N., Sakamoto, O., Yoshimura, T., Ando, M., et al. (1994). Monocyte Chemoattractant Protein-1 in Idiopathic Pulmonary Fibrosis and Other Interstitial Lung Diseases. *Hum. Pathol.* 25 (5), 455–463. doi:10. 1016/0046-8177(94)90117-1
90. Jackson, S. R., Lee, J., Reddy, R., Williams, G. N., Kikuchi, A., Freiberg, Y., et al. (2011). Partial Pneumonectomy of Telomerase Null Mice Carrying Shortened Telomeres Initiates Cell Growth Arrest Resulting in a Limited Compensatory Growth Response. *Am. J. Physiol. Lung Cell. Mol. Physiol.* 300 (6), L898–L909. doi:10.1152/ajplung.00409.2010
91. Jara, P., Calyeca, J., Romero, Y., Plácido, L., Yu, G., Kaminski, N., et al. (2015). Matrix Metalloproteinase (MMP)-19-deficient Fibroblasts Display a Profibrotic Phenotype. *Am. J. Physiol. Lung Cell. Mol. Physiol.* 308 (6), L511–L522. doi:10. 1152/ajplung.00043.2014
92. Jenuwein, T., and Allis, C. D. (2001). Translating the Histone Code. *Science* 293 (5532), 1074–1080. doi:10.1126/science.1063127
93. Jessen, H., Hoyer, N., Prior, T. S., Frederiksen, P., Karsdal, M. A., Leeming, D. J., et al. (2021). Turnover of Type I and III Collagen Predicts Progression of Idiopathic Pulmonary Fibrosis. *Respir. Res.* 22 (1), 205. doi:10.1186/s12931-021-01801-0
94. Justet, A., Thabut, G., Manali, E., Molina Molina, M., Kannengiesser, C., Cadranel, J., et al. (2018). Safety and Efficacy of Pirfenidone in Patients Carrying Telomerase Complex Mutation. *Eur. Respir. J.* 51 (3), 1701875. doi:10.1183/13993003.01875-2017
95. Justice, J. N., Nambiar, A. M., Tchkonia, T., LeBrasseur, N. K., Pascual, R., Hashmi, S. K., et al. (2019). Senolytics in Idiopathic Pulmonary Fibrosis: Results from a First-In-Human, Open-Label, Pilot Study. *EBioMedicine* 40, 554–563. doi:10. 1016/j.ebiom.2018.12.052
96. Kage, H., and Borok, Z. (2012). EMT and Interstitial Lung Disease: A Mysterious Relationship. *Curr. Opin. Pulm. Med.* 18 (5), 517–523. doi:10.1097/MCP. 0b013e3283566721
97. Kahloon, R. A., Xue, J., Bhargava, A., Csizmadia, E., Otterbein, L., Kass, D. J., et al. (2013). Patients with Idiopathic Pulmonary Fibrosis with Antibodies to Heat Shock Protein 70 Have Poor Prognoses. *Am. J. Respir. Crit. Care Med.* 187 (7), 768–775. doi:10.1164/rccm.201203-0506OC
98. Kai, Y., Tomoda, K., Yoneyama, H., Kitabatake, M., Nakamura, A., Ito, T., et al. (2017). Silencing of carbohydrate sulfotransferase 15 hinders murine pulmonary fibrosis development. *Mol. Ther. Nucleic Acids* 6, 163–172. doi:10.1016/j.omtn.2016.12.008

99. Kaliński, P., Hilkens, C. M., Snijders, A., Snijdewint, F. G., and Kapsenberg, M. L. (1997). IL-12-deficient Dendritic Cells, Generated in the Presence of Prostaglandin E2, Promote Type 2 Cytokine Production in Maturing Human Naive T Helper Cells. *J. Immunol.* 159 (1), 28–35.
100. Kamio, K., Azuma, A., Usuki, J., Matsuda, K., Inomata, M., Nishijima, N., et al. (2017). XPLN Is Modulated by HDAC Inhibitors and Negatively Regulates SPARC Expression by Targeting mTORC2 in Human Lung Fibroblasts. *Pulm. Pharmacol. Ther.* 44, 61–69. doi:10.1016/j.pupt.2017.03.003
101. Kasper, M., and Hughes, R. C. (1996). Immunocytochemical Evidence for a Modulation of Galectin 3 (Mac-2), a Carbohydrate Binding Protein, in Pulmonary Fibrosis. *J. Pathol.* 179 (3), 309–316. doi:10.1002/(SICI)1096-9896(199607)179:3<309:AID-PATH572>3.0.CO;2-D
102. Kim, Y. S., Cha, H., Kim, H. J., Cho, J. M., and Kim, H. R. (2019). The anti- fibrotic effects of CG-745, an HDAC inhibitor, in bleomycin and PHMG- induced mouse models. *Molecules* 24 (15), 2792. doi:10.3390/molecules24152792
103. King, T. E., Jr., Pardo, A., and Selman, M. (2011). Idiopathic Pulmonary Fibrosis. *Lancet* 378 (9807), 1949–1961. doi:10.1016/s0140-6736(11)60052-4
104. Korfei, M., Ruppert, C., Mahavadi, P., Henneke, I., Markart, P., Koch, M., et al. (2008). Epithelial Endoplasmic Reticulum Stress and Apoptosis in Sporadic Idiopathic Pulmonary Fibrosis. *Am. J. Respir. Crit. Care Med.* 178 (8), 838–846. doi:10.1164/rccm.200802-313OC
105. Korfei, M., Skwarna, S., Henneke, I., MacKenzie, B., Klymenko, O., Saito, S., et al. (2015). Aberrant Expression and Activity of Histone Deacetylases in Sporadic Idiopathic Pulmonary Fibrosis. *Thorax* 70 (11), 1022–1032. doi:10.1136/ thoraxjnl-2014-206411
106. Kouzarides, T. (2007). Chromatin Modifications and Their Function. *Cell.* 128 (4), 693–705. doi:10.1016/j.cell.2007.02.005
107. Kreus, M., Lehtonen, S., Skarp, S., and Kaarteenaho, R. (2021). Extracellular Matrix Proteins Produced by Stromal Cells in Idiopathic Pulmonary Fibrosis and Lung Adenocarcinoma. *PLoS One* 16 (4), e0250109. doi:10.1371/journal.pone. 0250109
108. Kropski, J. A., Young, L. R., Cogan, J. D., Mitchell, D. B., Lancaster, L. H., Worrell, A., et al. (2017). Genetic evaluation and testing of patients and families with idiopathic pulmonary fibrosis. *Am. J. Respir. Crit. Care Med.* 195 (11), 1423–1428. doi:10.1164/rccm.201609-1820PP
109. Kurosu, K., Takiguchi, Y., Okada, O., Yumoto, N., Sakao, S., Tada, Y., et al. (2008). Identification of Annexin 1 as a Novel Autoantigen in Acute Exacerbation of Idiopathic Pulmonary Fibrosis. *J. Immunol.* 181 (1), 756–767. doi:10.4049/ jimmunol.181.1.756
110. Kuse, N., Kamio, K., Azuma, A., Matsuda, K., Inomata, M., Usuki, J., et al. (2020). Exosome-derived microRNA-22 ameliorates pulmonary fibrosis by regulating fibroblast-To-myofibroblast differentiation *In vitro* and *In vivo*. *J. Nippon. Med. Sch.* 87 (3), 118–128. doi:10.1272/jnms.JNMS.2020_87-302
111. Lam, A. P., Herazo-Maya, J. D., Sennello, J. A., Flozak, A. S., Russell, S., Mutlu, G. M., et al. (2014). Wnt Coreceptor Lrp5 Is a Driver of Idiopathic Pulmonary Fibrosis. *Am. J. Respir. Crit. Care Med.* 190 (2), 185–195. doi:10.1164/rccm.201401-0079OC
112. Lama, V. N., and Phan, S. H. (2006). The Extrapulmonary Origin of Fibroblasts: Stem/progenitor Cells and beyond. *Proc. Am. Thorac. Soc.* 3 (4), 373–376. doi:10.1513/pats.200512-133TK
113. Lawrence, J., and Nho, R. (2018). The role of the mammalian target of rapamycin (mTOR) in pulmonary fibrosis. *Int. J. Mol. Sci.* 19 (3), 778. doi:10.3390/ ijms19030778
114. Lawson, W. E., Crossno, P. F., Polosukhin, V. V., Roldan, J., Cheng, D. S., Lane, K. B., et al. (2008). Endoplasmic Reticulum Stress in Alveolar Epithelial Cells Is Prominent in IPF: Association with Altered Surfactant Protein Processing and Herpesvirus Infection. *Am. J. Physiol. Lung Cell. Mol. Physiol.* 294 (6), L1119–L1126. doi:10.1152/ajplung.00382.2007
115. Le Saux, C. J., Davy, P., Brampton, C., Ahuja, S. S., Fauce, S., Shivshankar, P., et al. (2013). A Novel Telomerase Activator Suppresses Lung Damage in a Murine Model of Idiopathic Pulmonary Fibrosis. *PLoS One.* 8 (3), e58423. doi:10.1371/ journal.pone.0058423
116. Lederer, D. J., and Martinez, F. J. (2018). Idiopathic pulmonary fibrosis. *N. Engl. J. Med.* 378 (19), 1811–1823. doi:10.1056/NEJMra1705751
117. Ley, B., Newton, C. A., Arnould, I., Elicker, B. M., Henry, T. S., Vittinghoff, E., et al. (2017). The MUC5B Promoter Polymorphism and Telomere Length in Patients with Chronic Hypersensitivity Pneumonitis: An Observational Cohort-Control Study. *Lancet Respir. Med.* 5 (8), 639–647. doi:10.1016/s2213-2600(17)30216-3
118. Li, G., Jin, F., Du, J., He, Q., Yang, B., and Luo, P. (2019). Macrophage-secreted TSLP and MMP9 Promote Bleomycin-Induced Pulmonary Fibrosis. *Toxicol. Appl. Pharmacol.* 366, 10–16. doi:10.1016/j.taap.2019.01.011
119. Lipson, K. E., Wong, C., Teng, Y., and Spong, S. (2012). CTGF Is a Central Mediator of Tissue Remodeling and Fibrosis and its Inhibition Can Reverse the Process of Fibrosis. *Fibrogenes. Tissue Repair* 5 (Suppl. 1), S24. doi:10.1186/1755-1536-5-s1-s24
120. Lister-Shimauchi, E. H., McCarthy, B., Lippincott, M., and Ahmed, S. (2022). Genetic and epigenetic inheritance at telomeres. *Epigenomes* 6 (1), 9. doi:10.3390/epigenomes6010009
121. Liu, G., Zhai, H., Zhang, T., Li, S., Li, N., Chen, J., et al. (2019a). New Therapeutic Strategies for IPF: Based on the "Phagocytosis-Secretion-Immunization" Network Regulation Mechanism of Pulmonary Macrophages. *Biomed. Pharmacother.* 118, 109230. doi:10.1016/j.biopha.2019.109230
122. Liu, H., Wu, X., Gan, C., Wang, L., Wang, G., Yue, L., et al. (2021). A Novel Multikinase Inhibitor SKLB-YTH-60 Ameliorates Inflammation and Fibrosis in Bleomycin-Induced Lung Fibrosis Mouse Models. *Cell. Prolif.* 54 (7), e13081. doi:10.1111/cpr.13081
123. Liu, L., Yin, H., Huang, M., He, J., Yi, G., Wang, Z., et al. (2016). miR-21 Promotes Pulmonary Fibrosis in Rats via Down-Regulating the Expression of ADAMTS-*Xi Bao Yu Fen Zi Mian Yi Xue Za Zhi* 32 (12), 1636–1640.
124. Liu, R. M., and Liu, G. (2020). Cell Senescence and Fibrotic Lung Diseases. *Exp. Gerontol.* 132, 110836. doi:10.1016/j.exger.2020.110836
125. Liu, T., Gonzalez De Los Santos, F., Zhao, Y., Wu, Z., Rinke, A. E., Kim, K. K., et al. (2019b). Telomerase Reverse Transcriptase Ameliorates Lung Fibrosis by Protecting Alveolar Epithelial Cells against Senescence. *J. Biol. Chem.* 294 (22), 8861–8871. doi:10.1074/jbc.RA118.006615
126. Liu, T., Yu, H., Ding, L., Wu, Z., Gonzalez De Los Santos, F., Liu, J., et al. (2015). Conditional knockout of telomerase reverse transcriptase in mesenchymal cells impairs mouse pulmonary fibrosis. *PLoS One* 10 (11), e0142547. doi:10.1371/ journal.pone.0142547
127. Liu, Y. Y., Shi, Y., Liu, Y., Pan, X. H., and Zhang, K. X. (2018). Telomere Shortening Activates TGF-β/Smads Signaling in Lungs and Enhances Both Lipopolysaccharide and Bleomycin-Induced Pulmonary Fibrosis. *Acta Pharmacol. Sin.* 39 (11), 1735–1745. doi:10.1038/s41401-018-0007-9
128. Lorenzo-Salazar, J. M., Ma, S. F., Jou, J., Hou, P. C., Guillen-Guio, B., Allen, R. J., et al. (2019). Novel Idiopathic Pulmonary Fibrosis Susceptibility Variants Revealed by Deep Sequencing. *ERJ Open Res.* 5 (2), 00071–02019. doi:10.1183/23120541.00071-2019
129. Ma, H., Liu, S., Li, S., and Xia, Y. (2022). Targeting growth factor and cytokine pathways to treat idiopathic pulmonary fibrosis. *Front. Pharmacol.* 13. doi:10.3389/fphar.2022.918771
130. Maciel, M., Hernández-Barrientos, D., Herrera, I., Selman, M., Pardo, A., and Cabrera, S. (2018). Impaired Autophagic Activity and ATG4B Deficiency Are Associated with Increased Endoplasmic Reticulum Stress-Induced Lung Injury. *Aging (Albany NY)* 10 (8), 2098–2112. doi:10.18632/aging.101532
131. Maitra, M., Wang, Y., Gerard, R. D., Mendelson, C. R., and Garcia, C. K. (2010). Surfactant Protein A2 Mutations Associated with Pulmonary Fibrosis Lead to Protein Instability and Endoplasmic Reticulum Stress. *J. Biol. Chem.* 285 (29), 22103–22113. doi:10.1074/jbc.M110.121467
132. Malli, F., Koutsokera, A., Paraskeva, E., Zakynthinos, E., Papagianni, M., Makris, D., et al. (2013). Endothelial Progenitor Cells in the Pathogenesis of Idiopathic Pulmonary Fibrosis: An Evolving Concept. *PLoS One* 8 (1), e53658. doi:10. 1371/journal.pone.0053658
133. Manali, E. D., Legendre, M., Nathan, N., Kannengiesser, C., Coulomb-L'Hermine, A., Tsiligiannis, T., et al. (2019). Bi-allelic Missense ABCA3 Mutations in a Patient with Childhood ILD Who Reached Adulthood. *ERJ Open Res.* 5 (3), 00066–02019. doi:10.1183/23120541. 00066-2019
134. Manicone, A. M., Huizar, I., and McGuire, J. K. (2009). Matrilysin (Matrix Metalloproteinase-7) Regulates Anti-inflammatory and Antifibrotic Pulmonary Dendritic Cells that Express CD103 (alpha(E)beta(7)-integrin). *Am. J. Pathol.* 175 (6), 2319–2331. doi:10.2353/ajpath.2009.090101
135. Margaritopoulos, G. A., Lasithiotaki, I., and Antoniou, K. M. (2017). Toll-like Receptors and Autophagy in Interstitial Lung Diseases. *Eur. J. Pharmacol.* 808, 28–34. doi:10.1016/j.ejphar.2016.09.032
136. Martinez, F. O., Sica, A., Mantovani, A., and Locati, M. (2008). Macrophage Activation and Polarization. *Front. Biosci.* 13, 453–461. doi:10.2741/2692
137. Mathai, S. K., Pedersen, B. S., Smith, K., Russell, P., Schwarz, M. I., Brown, K. K., et al. (2016). Desmoplakin variants are associated with idiopathic pulmonary fibrosis. *Am. J. Respir. Crit. Care Med.* 193 (10), 1151–1160. doi:10.1164/rccm. 201509-1863OC
138. Matsumura, Y., Ban, N., Ueda, K., and Inagaki, N. (2006). Characterization and Classification of ATP-Binding Cassette Transporter ABCA3 Mutants in Fatal Surfactant Deficiency. *J. Biol. Chem.* 281 (45), 34503–34514. doi:10.1074/jbc. M600071200

139. McGuire, J. K., Li, Q., and Parks, W. C. (2003). Matrilysin (Matrix Metalloproteinase-7) Mediates E-Cadherin Ectodomain Shedding in Injured Lung Epithelium. *Am. J. Pathol.* 162 (6), 1831–1843. doi:10.1016/s0002-9440(10)64318-0
140. Mehrad, B., Burdick, M. D., Zisman, D. A., Keane, M. P., Belperio, J. A., and Strieter, R. M. (2007). Circulating Peripheral Blood Fibrocytes in Human Fibrotic Interstitial Lung Disease. *Biochem. Biophys. Res. Commun.* 353 (1), 104–108. doi:10.1016/j.bbrc.2006.11.149
141. Mercer, P. F., Woodcock, H. V., Eley, J. D., Platé, M., Sulikowski, M. G., Durrenberger, P. F., et al. (2016). Exploration of a Potent PI3 kinase/mTOR Inhibitor as a Novel Anti-fibrotic Agent in IPF. *Thorax* 71 (8), 701–711. doi:10. 1136/thoraxjnl-2015-207429
142. Merkt, W., Bueno, M., Mora, A. L., and Lagares, D. (2020). Senotherapeutics: Targeting Senescence in Idiopathic Pulmonary Fibrosis. *Semin. Cell. Dev. Biol.* 101, 104–110. doi:10.1016/j.semcdb.2019.12.008
143. Montero, P., Milara, J., Roger, I., and Cortijo, J. (2021). Role of JAK/STAT in interstitial lung diseases; molecular and cellular mechanisms. *Int. J. Mol. Sci.* 22 (12), 6211. doi:10.3390/ijms22126211
144. Mori, L., Bellini, A., Stacey, M. A., Schmidt, M., and Mattoli, S. (2005). Fibrocytes Contribute to the Myofibroblast Population in Wounded Skin and Originate from the Bone Marrow. *Exp. Cell. Res.* 304 (1), 81–90. doi:10.1016/j.yexcr.2004. 11.011
145. Mulugeta, S., Nureki, S., and Beers, M. F. (2015). Lost after Translation: Insights from Pulmonary Surfactant for Understanding the Role of Alveolar Epithelial Dysfunction and Cellular Quality Control in Fibrotic Lung Disease. *Am. J. Physiol. Lung Cell. Mol. Physiol.* 309 (6), L507–L525. doi:10.1152/ajplung. 00139.2015
146. Munger, J. S., Huang, X., Kawakatsu, H., Griffiths, M. J., Dalton, S. L., Wu, J., et al. (1999). The Integrin Alpha V Beta 6 Binds and Activates Latent TGF Beta 1: A Mechanism for Regulating Pulmonary Inflammation and Fibrosis. *Cell.* 96 (3), 319–328. doi:10.1016/s0092-8674(00)80545-0
147. Murray, M. Y., Birkland, T. P., Howe, J. D., Rowan, A. D., Fidock, M., Parks, W. C., et al. (2013). Macrophage Migration and Invasion Is Regulated by MMP10 Expression. *PLoS One* 8 (5), e63555. doi:10.1371/journal.pone.0063555
148. Murthy, S., Ryan, A., He, C., Mallampalli, R. K., and Carter, A. B. (2010). Rac1- mediated Mitochondrial H2O2 Generation Regulates MMP-9 Gene Expression in Macrophages via Inhibition of SP-1 and AP-1. *J. Biol. Chem.* 285 (32), 25062–25073. doi:10.1074/jbc.M109.099655
149. Nagpal, N., Wang, J., Zeng, J., Lo, E., Moon, D. H., Luk, K., et al. (2020). Small-Molecule PAPD5 Inhibitors Restore Telomerase Activity in Patient Stem Cells. *Cell Stem Cell* 26 (6), 896–909.e898. doi:10.1016/j.stem.2020.03.016
150. Naikawadi, R. P., Disayabutr, S., Mallavia, B., Donne, M. L., Green, G., La, J. L., et al. (2016). Telomere Dysfunction in Alveolar Epithelial Cells Causes Lung Remodeling and Fibrosis. *JCI Insight* 1 (14), e86704. doi:10.1172/jci.insight. 86704
151. Newton, C. A., Batra, K., Torrealba, J., Kozlitina, J., Glazer, C. S., Aravena, C., et al. (2016). Telomere-related Lung Fibrosis Is Diagnostically Heterogeneous but Uniformly Progressive. *Eur. Respir. J.* 48 (6), 1710–1720. doi:10.1183/13993003. 00308-2016
152. Nguyen, M., Arkell, J., and Jackson, C. J. (2001). Human Endothelial Gelatinases and Angiogenesis. *Int. J. Biochem. Cell. Biol.* 33 (10), 960–970. doi:10.1016/ s1357-2725(01)00007-3
153. Nikaido, T., Tanino, Y., Wang, X., Sato, Y., Togawa, R., Kikuchi, M., et al. (2018). Serum Decorin Is a Potential Prognostic Biomarker in Patients with Acute Exacerbation of Idiopathic Pulmonary Fibrosis. *J. Thorac. Dis.* 10 (9), 5346–5358. doi:10.21037/jtd.2018.08.60
154. Ninou, I., Magkrioti, C., and Aidinis, V. (2018). Autotaxin in pathophysiology and pulmonary fibrosis. *Front. Med. (Lausanne)* 5, 180. doi:10.3389/fmed.2018. 00180
155. Noble, P. W., Barkauskas, C. E., and Jiang, D. (2012). Pulmonary Fibrosis: Patterns and Perpetrators. *J. Clin. Investig.* 122 (8), 2756–2762. doi:10.1172/jci60323
156. Noth, I., Zhang, Y., Ma, S. F., Flores, C., Barber, M., Huang, Y., et al. (2013). Genetic Variants Associated with Idiopathic Pulmonary Fibrosis Susceptibility and Mortality: A Genome-wide Association Study. *Lancet Respir. Med.* 1 (4), 309–317. doi:10.1016/s2213-2600(13)70045-6
157. O'Dwyer, D. N., Armstrong, M. E., Kooblall, M., and Donnelly, S. C. (2015). Targeting Defective Toll-like Receptor-3 Function and Idiopathic Pulmonary Fibrosis. *Expert Opin. Ther. Targets* 19 (4), 507–514. doi:10.1517/14728222.2014.988706
158. O'Dwyer, D. N., Armstrong, M. E., Trujillo, G., Cooke, G., Keane, M. P., Fallon, P. G., et al. (2013). The Toll-like Receptor 3 L412F Polymorphism and Disease Progression in Idiopathic Pulmonary Fibrosis. *Am. J. Respir. Crit. Care Med.* 188 (12), 1442–1450. doi:10.1164/rccm.201304-0760OC
159. Ogushi, F., Tani, K., Endo, T., Tada, H., Kawano, T., Asano, T., et al. (2001). Autoantibodies to IL-1 Alpha in Sera from Rapidly Progressive Idiopathic Pulmonary Fibrosis. *J. Med. Investig.* 48 (3-4), 181–189.
160. Oldham, J. M., Ma, S. F., Martinez, F. J., Anstrom, K. J., Raghu, G., Schwartz, D. A., et al. (2015). TOLLIP, MUC5B, and the response to N-acetylcysteine Among individuals with idiopathic pulmonary fibrosis. *Am. J. Respir. Crit. Care Med.* 192 (12), 1475–1482. doi:10.1164/rccm.201505-1010OC
161. Ong, C. H., Tham, C. L., Harith, H. H., Firdaus, N., and Israf, D. A. (2021). TGF-β- induced Fibrosis: A Review on the Underlying Mechanism and Potential Therapeutic Strategies. *Eur. J. Pharmacol.* 911, 174510. doi:10.1016/j.ejphar. 2021.174510
162. Ono, S., Tanaka, T., Ishida, M., Kinoshita, A., Fukuoka, J., Takaki, M., et al. (2011). Surfactant Protein C G100S Mutation Causes Familial Pulmonary Fibrosis in Japanese Kindred. *Eur. Respir. J.* 38 (4), 861–869. doi:10.1183/09031936. 00143610
163. Organ, L. A., Duggan, A. R., Oballa, E., Taggart, S. C., Simpson, J. K., Kang'ombe, A. R., et al. (2019). Biomarkers of Collagen Synthesis Predict Progression in the PROFILE Idiopathic Pulmonary Fibrosis Cohort. *Respir. Res.* 20 (1), 148. doi:10.1186/s12931-019-1118-7
164. Ortiz, L. A., Dutreil, M., Fattman, C., Pandey, A. C., Torres, G., Go, K., et al. (2007). Interleukin 1 Receptor Antagonist Mediates the Antiinflammatory and Antifibrotic Effect of Mesenchymal Stem Cells during Lung Injury. *Proc. Natl. Acad. Sci. U. S. A.* 104 (26), 11002–11007. doi:10.1073/pnas. 0704421104
165. Pandit, K. V., Milosevic, J., and Kaminski, N. (2011). MicroRNAs in Idiopathic Pulmonary Fibrosis. *Transl. Res.* 157 (4), 191–199. doi:10.1016/j.trsl.2011. 01.012
166. Pardo, A., Gibson, K., Cisneros, J., Richards, T. J., Yang, Y., Becerril, C., et al. (2005). Up-regulation and Profibrotic Role of Osteopontin in Human Idiopathic Pulmonary Fibrosis. *PLoS Med.* 2 (9), e251. doi:10.1371/journal.pmed.0020251
167. Passalacqua, G., Mincarini, M., Colombo, D., Troisi, G., Ferrari, M., Bagnasco, D., et al. (2017). IL-13 and Idiopathic Pulmonary Fibrosis: Possible Links and New Therapeutic Strategies. *Pulm. Pharmacol. Ther.* 45, 95–100. doi:10.1016/j.pupt. 2017.05.007
168. Patel, A. S., Lin, L., Geyer, A., Haspel, J. A., An, C. H., Cao, J., et al. (2012). Autophagy in Idiopathic Pulmonary Fibrosis. *PLoS One* 7 (7), e41394. doi:10. 1371/journal.pone.0041394
169. Peljto, A. L., Zhang, Y., Fingerlin, T. E., Ma, S. F., Garcia, J. G., Richards, T. J., et al. (2013). Association between the MUC5B Promoter Polymorphism and Survival in Patients with Idiopathic Pulmonary Fibrosis. *Jama* 309 (21), 2232–2239. doi:10.1001/jama.2013.5827
170. Peng, S. C., Hu, X., Wei, L. Q., and Li, Z. H. (2013). The Correlation of Helper T Lymphocyte 1/helper T Lymphocyte 2 with Clinical and Image Features in Patients with Idiopathic Pulmonary Fibrosis. *Zhonghua Nei Ke Za Zhi* 52 (6), 489–493.
171. Phan, T. H. G., Paliogiannis, P., Nasrallah, G. K., Giordo, R., Eid, A. H., Fois, A. G., et al. (2021). Emerging Cellular and Molecular Determinants of Idiopathic Pulmonary Fibrosis. *Cell. Mol. Life Sci.* 78 (5), 2031–2057. doi:10.1007/s00018- 020-03693-7
172. Pilling, D., Vakil, V., Cox, N., and Gomer, R. H. (2015). TNF-α-stimulated Fibroblasts Secrete Lumican to Promote Fibrocyte Differentiation. *Proc. Natl. Acad. Sci. U. S. A.* 112 (38), 11929–11934. doi:10.1073/pnas.1507387112
173. Popescu, I., Mannem, H., Winters, S. A., Hoji, A., Silveira, F., McNally, E., et al. (2019). Impaired cytomegalovirus immunity in idiopathic pulmonary fibrosis lung transplant recipients with short telomeres. *Am. J. Respir. Crit. Care Med.* 199 (3), 362–376. doi:10.1164/rccm.201805-0825OC
174. Povedano, J. M., Martinez, P., Flores, J. M., Mulero, F., and Blasco, M. A. (2015). Mice with pulmonary fibrosis driven by telomere dysfunction. *Cell. Rep.* 12 (2), 286–299. doi:10.1016/j.celrep.2015.06.028
175. Prasse, A., Pechkovsky, D. V., Toews, G. B., Jungraithmayr, W., Kollert, F., Goldmann, T., et al. (2006). A Vicious Circle of Alveolar Macrophages and Fibroblasts Perpetuates Pulmonary Fibrosis via CCL18. *Am. J. Respir. Crit. Care Med.* 173 (7), 781–792. doi:10.1164/rccm.200509-1518OC
176. Raghu, G., Brown, K. K., Costabel, U., Cottin, V., du Bois, R. M., Lasky, J. A., et al. (2008). Treatment of Idiopathic Pulmonary Fibrosis with Etanercept: An Exploratory, Placebo-Controlled Trial. *Am. J. Respir. Crit. Care Med.* 178 (9), 948–955. doi:10.1164/rccm.200709-1446OC
177. Raghu, G., Remy-Jardin, M., Myers, J. L., Richeldi, L., Ryerson, C. J., Lederer, D. J., et al. (2018). Diagnosis of idiopathic pulmonary fibrosis. An official ATS/ERS/ JRS/ALAT clinical practice guideline. *Am. J. Respir. Crit. Care Med.* 198 (5), e44–e68. doi:10.1164/rccm.201807-1255ST
178. Raghu, G., Raghu, G., Anstrom, K. J., Jr., King, T. E., Lasky, J. A., and Martinez, F. J. (2012). Prednisone, Azathioprine, and N-Acetylcysteine for Pulmonary Fibrosis. *N. Engl. J. Med.* 366 (21), 1968–1977. doi:10.1056/NEJMoa1113354

179. Rahaman, S. O., Grove, L. M., Paruchuri, S., Southern, B. D., Abraham, S., Niese, K. A., et al. (2014). TRPV4 Mediates Myofibroblast Differentiation and Pulmonary Fibrosis in Mice. *J. Clin. Investig.* 124 (12), 5225–5238. doi:10.1172/jci75331

180. Rana, T., Jiang, C., Liu, G., Miyata, T., Antony, V., Thannickal, V. J., et al. (2020). PAI-1 regulation of TGF-B1-Induced alveolar type II cell senescence, SASP secretion, and SASP-Mediated activation of alveolar macrophages. *Am. J. Respir. Cell. Mol. Biol.* 62 (3), 319–330. doi:10.1165/rcmb.2019-0071OC

181. Ricard-Blum, S., and Salza, R. (2014). Matricryptins and Matrikines: Biologically Active Fragments of the Extracellular Matrix. *Exp. Dermatol* 23 (7), 457–463. doi:10.1111/exd.12435

182. Ricard-Blum, S., and Vallet, S. D. (2019). Fragments Generated upon Extracellular Matrix Remodeling: Biological Regulators and Potential Drugs. *Matrix Biol.* 75- 76, 170–189. doi:10.1016/j.matbio.2017.11.005

183. Richter, A. G., McKeown, S., Rathinam, S., Harper, L., Rajesh, P., McAuley, D. F., et al. (2009). Soluble Endostatin Is a Novel Inhibitor of Epithelial Repair in Idiopathic Pulmonary Fibrosis. *Thorax* 64 (2), 156–161. doi:10.1136/thx.2008. 102814

184. Riha, R. L., Yang, I. A., Rabnott, G. C., Tunnicliffe, A. M., Fong, K. M., and Zimmerman, P. V. (2004). Cytokine Gene Polymorphisms in Idiopathic Pulmonary Fibrosis. *Intern Med. J.* 34 (3), 126–129. doi:10.1111/j.1444-0903.2004.00503.x

185. Rock, J. R., Barkauskas, C. E., Cronce, M. J., Xue, Y., Harris, J. R., Liang, J., et al. (2011). Multiple Stromal Populations Contribute to Pulmonary Fibrosis without Evidence for Epithelial to Mesenchymal Transition. *Proc. Natl. Acad. Sci. U. S. A.* 108 (52), E1475–E1483. doi:10.1073/pnas.1117988108

186. Rohani, M. G., McMahan, R. S., Razumova, M. V., Hertz, A. L., Cieslewicz, M., Pun, S. H., et al. (2015). MMP-10 regulates collagenolytic activity of alternatively activated resident macrophages. *J. Investig. Dermatol* 135 (10), 2377–2384. doi:10.1038/jid.2015.167

187. Romagnani, S. (2000). T-Cell Subsets (Th1 versus Th2). *Ann. Allergy Asthma Immunol.* 85 (1), 9–21. quiz 18, 21. doi:10.1016/s1081-1206(10)62426-x

188. Ruffin, M., Thompson, K. E., Corvol, H., and Guillot, L. (2020). Two-hybrid Screening of FAM13A Protein Partners in Lung Epithelial Cells. *BMC Res. Notes* 12 (1), 804. doi:10.1186/s13104-019-4840-9

189. Sabeh, F., Li, X. Y., Saunders, T. L., Rowe, R. G., and Weiss, S. J. (2009). Secreted versus Membrane-Anchored Collagenases: Relative Roles in Fibroblast- dependent Collagenolysis and Invasion. *J. Biol. Chem.* 284 (34), 23001–23011. doi:10.1074/jbc.M109.002808

190. Saito, S., Zhuang, Y., Shan, B., Danchuk, S., Luo, F., Korfei, M., et al. (2017). Tubastatin Ameliorates Pulmonary Fibrosis by Targeting the TGFβ-Pi3k-Akt Pathway. *PLoS One* 12 (10), e0186615. doi:10.1371/journal.pone.0186615

191. Salton, F., Ruaro, B., Confalonieri, P., and Confalonieri, M. (2020). Epithelial-mesenchymal transition: A major pathogenic driver in idiopathic pulmonary fibrosis? *Med. Kaunas.* 56 (11), 608. doi:10.3390/medicina56110608

192. Salton, F., Volpe, M. C., and Confalonieri, M. (2019). Epithelial Mesenchymal transition in the pathogenesis of idiopathic pulmonary fibrosis. *Med. Kaunas.* 55 (4), 83. doi:10.3390/medicina55040083

193. Sanders, Y. Y., Ambalavanan, N., Halloran, B., Zhang, X., Liu, H., Crossman, D. K., et al. (2012). Altered DNA Methylation Profile in Idiopathic Pulmonary Fibrosis. *Am. J. Respir. Crit. Care Med.* 186 (6), 525–535. doi:10.1164/rccm.201201-0077OC

194. Sanders, Y. Y., Tollefsbol, T. O., Varisco, B. M., and Hagood, J. S. (2011). Epigenetic Regulation of Thy-1 by Histone Deacetylase Inhibitor in Rat Lung Fibroblasts. *Am. J. Respir. Cell. Mol. Biol.* 45 (1), 16–23. doi:10.1165/rcmb.2010-0154OC

195. Schafer, M. J., White, T. A., Iijima, K., Haak, A. J., Ligresti, G., Atkinson, E. J., et al. (2017). Cellular Senescence Mediates Fibrotic Pulmonary Disease. *Nat. Commun.* 8, 14532. doi:10.1038/ncomms14532

196. Selman, M., and Pardo, A. (2014). Revealing the Pathogenic and Aging-Related Mechanisms of the Enigmatic Idiopathic Pulmonary Fibrosis. An Integral Model. *Am. J. Respir. Crit. Care Med.* 189 (10), 1161–1172. doi:10.1164/rccm.201312-2221PP

197. Selman, M., and Pardo, A. (2020). The Leading Role of Epithelial Cells in the Pathogenesis of Idiopathic Pulmonary Fibrosis. *Cell. Signal* 66, 109482. doi:10. 1016/j.cellsig.2019.109482

198. Selman, M., Ruiz, V., Cabrera, S., Segura, L., Ramírez, R., Barrios, R., et al. (2000). TIMP-1, -2, -3, and -4 in Idiopathic Pulmonary Fibrosis. A Prevailing Nondegradative Lung Microenvironment? *Am. J. Physiol. Lung Cell. Mol. Physiol.* 279 (3), L562–L574. doi:10.1152/ajplung.2000.279.3.L562

199. Sgalla, G., Iovene, B., Calvello, M., Ori, M., Varone, F., and Richeldi, L. (2018). Idiopathic Pulmonary Fibrosis: Pathogenesis and Management. *Respir. Res.* 19 (1), 32. doi:10.1186/s12931-018-0730-2

200. She, Y. X., Yu, Q. Y., and Tang, X. X. (2021). Role of Interleukins in the Pathogenesis of Pulmonary Fibrosis. *Cell. Death Discov.* 7 (1), 52. doi:10.1038/s41420-021-00437-9

201. Shi-Wen, X., Chen, Y., Denton, C. P., Eastwood, M., Renzoni, E. A., Bou-Gharios, G., et al. (2004). Endothelin-1 Promotes Myofibroblast Induction through the ETA Receptor via a Rac/phosphoinositide 3-kinase/Akt-dependent Pathway and Is Essential for the Enhanced Contractile Phenotype of Fibrotic Fibroblasts. *Mol. Biol. Cell.* 15 (6), 2707–2719. doi:10.1091/mbc.e03-12-0902

202. Shifeng, L., Hong, X., Xue, Y., Siyu, N., Qiaodan, Z., Dingjie, X., et al. (2019). Ac- SDKP Increases α-TAT 1 and Promotes the Apoptosis in Lung Fibroblasts and Epithelial Cells Double-Stimulated with TGF-B1 and Silica. *Toxicol. Appl. Pharmacol.* 369, 17–29. doi:10.1016/j.taap.2019.02.015

203. Shukla, S., Jeong, H. C., Sturgeon, C. M., Parker, R., and Batista, L. F. Z. (2020). Chemical Inhibition of PAPD5/7 Rescues Telomerase Function and Hematopoiesis in Dyskeratosis Congenita. *Blood Adv.* 4 (12), 2717–2722. doi:10.1182/bloodadvances.2020001848

204. Shulenin, S., Nogee, L. M., Annilo, T., Wert, S. E., Whitsett, J. A., and Dean, M. (2004). ABCA3 Gene Mutations in Newborns with Fatal Surfactant Deficiency. *N. Engl. J. Med.* 350 (13), 1296–1303. doi:10.1056/NEJMoa032178

205. Silhan, L. L., Shah, P. D., Chambers, D. C., Snyder, L. D., Riise, G. C., Wagner, C. L., et al. (2014). Lung Transplantation in Telomerase Mutation Carriers with Pulmonary Fibrosis. *Eur. Respir. J.* 44 (1), 178–187. doi:10.1183/09031936.00060014

206. Smaldone, G. C. (2018). Repurposing of Gamma Interferon via Inhalation Delivery. *Adv. Drug Deliv. Rev.* 133, 87–92. doi:10.1016/j.addr.2018.06.004

207. Snetselaar, R., van Batenburg, A. A., van Oosterhout, M. F. M., Kazemier, K. M., Roothaan, S. M., Peeters, T., et al. (2017). Short Telomere Length in IPF Lung Associates with Fibrotic Lesions and Predicts Survival. *PLoS One* 12 (12), e0189467. doi:10.1371/journal.pone.0189467

208. Snetselaar, R., van Moorsel, C. H. M., Kazemier, K. M., van der Vis, J. J., Zanen, P., van Oosterhout, M. F. M., et al. (2015). Telomere Length in Interstitial Lung Diseases. *Chest* 148 (4), 1011–1018. doi:10.1378/chest.14-3078

209. Snijder, J., Peraza, J., Padilla, M., Capaccione, K., and Salvatore, M. M. (2019). Pulmonary Fibrosis: A Disease of Alveolar Collapse and Collagen Deposition. *Expert Rev. Respir. Med.* 13 (7), 615–619. doi:10.1080/17476348.2019.1623028

210. Sosulski, M. L., Gongora, R., Feghali-Bostwick, C., Lasky, J. A., and Sanchez, C. G. (2017). Sirtuin 3 deregulation promotes pulmonary fibrosis. *J. Gerontol. A Biol. Sci. Med. Sci.* 72 (5), 595–602. doi:10.1093/gerona/glw151

211. Spagnolo, P., Kropski, J. A., Jones, M. G., Lee, J. S., Rossi, G., Karampitsakos, T., et al. (2021). Idiopathic Pulmonary Fibrosis: Disease Mechanisms and Drug Development. *Pharmacol. Ther.* 222, 107798. doi:10.1016/j.pharmthera.2020. 107798

212. Spagnolo, P., Tzouvelekis, A., and Bonella, F. (2018). The management of patients with idiopathic pulmonary fibrosis. *Front. Med. (Lausanne)* 5, 148. doi:10.3389/fmed.2018.00148

213. Stanley, S. E., Gable, D. L., Wagner, C. L., Carlile, T. M., Hanumanthu, V. S., Podlevsky, J. D., et al. (2016a). Loss-of-function Mutations in the RNA Biogenesis Factor NAF1 Predispose to Pulmonary Fibrosis-Emphysema. *Sci. Transl. Med.* 8 (351), 351ra107. doi:10.1126/scitranslmed. aaf7837

214. Stanley, S. E., Merck, S. J., and Armanios, M. (2016b). Telomerase and the genetics of emphysema susceptibility. Implications for pathogenesis paradigms and patient care. *Ann. Am. Thorac. Soc.* 13 Suppl 5 (Suppl. 5), S447–s451. doi:10. 1513/AnnalsATS.201609-718AW

215. Stuart, B. D., Choi, J., Zaidi, S., Xing, C., Holohan, B., Chen, R., et al. (2015). Exome Sequencing Links Mutations in PARN and RTEL1 with Familial Pulmonary Fibrosis and Telomere Shortening. *Nat. Genet.* 47 (5), 512–517. doi:10.1038/ng. 3278

216. Stuart, B. D., Lee, J. S., Kozlitina, J., Noth, I., Devine, M. S., Glazer, C. S., et al. (2014). Effect of Telomere Length on Survival in Patients with Idiopathic Pulmonary Fibrosis: An Observational Cohort Study with Independent Validation. *Lancet Respir. Med.* 2 (7), 557–565. doi:10.1016/s2213-2600(14)70124-9

217. Suga, M., Iyonaga, K., Ichiyasu, H., Saita, N., Yamasaki, H., and Ando, M. (1999). Clinical Significance of MCP-1 Levels in BALF and Serum in Patients with Interstitial Lung Diseases. *Eur. Respir. J.* 14 (2), 376–382. doi:10.1034/j.1399-3003.1999.14b23.x

218. Sumida, A., Hasegawa, Y., Okamoto, M., Hashimoto, N., Imaizumi, K., Yatsuya, H., et al. (2008). TH1/TH2 Immune Response in Lung Fibroblasts in Interstitial Lung Disease. *Arch. Med. Res.* 39 (5), 503–510. doi:10.1016/j.arcmed.2008. 02.005

219. Suryadevara, V., Ramchandran, R., Kamp, D. W., and Natarajan, V. (2020). Lipid mediators regulate pulmonary fibrosis: Potential mechanisms and signaling pathways. *Int. J. Mol. Sci.* 21 (12), 4257. doi:10.3390/ijms21124257

220. Swaminathan, A. C., Neely, M. L., Frankel, C. W., Kelly, F. L., Petrovski, S., Durheim, M. T., et al. (2019). Lung transplant outcomes in patients with pulmonary fibrosis with telomere-related gene variants. *Chest* 156 (3), 477–485. doi:10.1016/j.chest.2019.03.030

221. Tager, A. M., LaCamera, P., Shea, B. S., Campanella, G. S., Selman, M., Zhao, Z., et al. (2008). The Lysophosphatidic Acid Receptor LPA1 Links Pulmonary Fibrosis to Lung Injury by Mediating Fibroblast Recruitment and Vascular Leak. *Nat. Med.* 14 (1), 45–54. doi:10.1038/nm1685

222. Taillé, C., Grootenboer-Mignot, S., Boursier, C., Michel, L., Debray, M. P., Fagart, J., et al. (2011). Identification of Periplakin as a New Target for Autoreactivity in Idiopathic Pulmonary Fibrosis. *Am. J. Respir. Crit. Care Med.* 183 (6), 759–766. doi:10.1164/rccm.201001-0076OC

223. Tanino, Y., Wang, X., Nikaido, T., Misa, K., Sato, Y., Togawa, R., et al. (2019). Syndecan-4 inhibits the development of pulmonary fibrosis by attenuating TGF-β signaling. *Int. J. Mol. Sci.* 20 (20), 4989. doi:10. 3390/ijms20204989

224. Taskar, V. S., and Coultas, D. B. (2006). Is Idiopathic Pulmonary Fibrosis an Environmental Disease? *Proc. Am. Thorac. Soc.* 3 (4), 293–298. doi:10.1513/pats.200512-131TK

225. Tokman, S., Singer, J. P., Devine, M. S., Westall, G. P., Aubert, J. D., Tamm, M., et al. (2015). Clinical Outcomes of Lung Transplant Recipients with Telomerase Mutations. *J. Heart Lung Transpl.* 34 (10), 1318–1324. doi:10.1016/j.healun. 2015.05.002

226. Townsley, D. M., Dumitriu, B., Liu, D., Biancotto, A., Weinstein, B., Chen, C., et al. (2016a). Danazol Treatment for Telomere Diseases. *N. Engl. J. Med.* 374 (20), 1922–1931. doi:10.1056/NEJMoa1515319

227. Townsley, D. M., Dumitriu, B., and Young, N. S. (2016b). Danazol Treatment for Telomere Diseases. *N. Engl. J. Med.* 375 (11), 1095–1096. doi:10.1056/NEJMc1607752

228. Upagupta, C., Shimbori, C., Alsilmi, R., and Kolb, M. (2018). Matrix Abnormalities in Pulmonary Fibrosis. *Eur. Respir. Rev.* 27 (148), 180033. doi:10.1183/ 16000617.0033-2018

229. Utz, J. P., Limper, A. H., Kalra, S., Specks, U., Scott, J. P., Vuk-Pavlovic, Z., et al. (2003). Etanercept for the Treatment of Stage II and III Progressive Pulmonary Sarcoidosis. *Chest* 124 (1), 177–185. doi:10.1378/chest.124.1.177

230. van Moorsel, C. H. M. (2018). Trade-offs in Aging Lung Diseases: A Review on Shared but Opposite Genetic Risk Variants in Idiopathic Pulmonary Fibrosis, Lung Cancer and Chronic Obstructive Pulmonary Disease. *Curr. Opin. Pulm. Med.* 24 (3), 309–317. doi:10.1097/mcp. 0000000000000476

231. Vasakova, M., Sterclova, M., Matej, R., Olejar, T., Kolesar, L., Skibova, J., et al. (2013). IL-4 Polymorphisms, HRCT Score and Lung Tissue Markers in Idiopathic Pulmonary Fibrosis. *Hum. Immunol.* 74 (1), 1346–51. doi:10. 1016/j.humimm.2013.07.011

232. Vasakova, M., Striz, I., Slavcev, A., Jandova, S., Kolesar, L., and Sulc, J. (2006). Th1/ Th2 Cytokine Gene Polymorphisms in Patients with Idiopathic Pulmonary Fibrosis. *Tissue Antigens* 67 (3), 229–232. doi:10.1111/j.1399-0039.2006. 00560.x

233. Venosa, A., Tomer, Y., Jamil, S., and Beers, M. (2017). Expression of A pulmonary fibrosis associated surfactant protein C mutant, SP-C^{i73t}, in alveolar type 2 cells induces lung inflammation and aberrant parenchymal remodeling. *Physiology* 31, 694.5–694.5. doi:10.1096/fasebj.31.1_supplement.694.5

234. Villavicencio, M. A., Axtell, A. L., Osho, A., Astor, T., Roy, N., Melnitchouk, S., et al. (2018). Single- versus double-lung transplantation in pulmonary fibrosis: Impact of age and pulmonary hypertension. *Ann. Thorac. Surg.* 106 (3), 856–863. doi:10.1016/j.athoracsur.2018.04.060

235. Wambach, J. A., Casey, A. M., Fishman, M. P., Wegner, D. J., Wert, S. E., Cole, F. S., et al. (2014). Genotype-phenotype Correlations for Infants and Children with ABCA3 Deficiency. *Am. J. Respir. Crit. Care Med.* 189 (12), 1538–1543. doi:10. 1164/rccm.201402-0342OC

236. Wang, H., and Dymock, B. W. (2009). New Patented Histone Deacetylase Inhibitors. *Expert Opin. Ther. Pat.* 19 (12), 1727–1757. doi:10.1517/13543770903393789

237. Wang, L., Chen, R., Li, G., Wang, Z., Liu, J., Liang, Y., et al. (2020). FBW7 mediates senescence and pulmonary fibrosis through telomere uncapping. *Cell. Metab.* 32 (5), 860–e9. e869. doi:10.1016/j.cmet.2020.10.004

238. Wang, Q., Xie, Z. L., Wu, Q., Jin, Z. X., Yang, C., and Feng, J. (2021). Role of Various Imbalances Centered on Alveolar Epithelial Cell/fibroblast Apoptosis Imbalance in the Pathogenesis of Idiopathic Pulmonary Fibrosis. *Chin. Med. J. Engl.* 134 (3), 261–274. doi:10.1097/cm9.0000000000001288

239. Wang, T., Feng, Y., Sun, H., Zhang, L., Hao, L., Shi, C., et al. (2012). miR-21 Regulates Skin Wound Healing by Targeting Multiple Aspects of the Healing Process. *Am. J. Pathol.* 181 (6), 1911–1920. doi:10.1016/j.ajpath.2012.08.022

240. Wang, W., Yu, Y., Xiao, J., Gao, Y., Sang, L., Lian, Y., et al. (2018). A novel variant of desmoplakin is potentially associated with silicosis risk. *DNA Cell. Biol.* 37 (11), 925–931. doi:10.1089/dna.2018.4370

241. Wang, Y., Kuan, P. J., Xing, C., Cronkhite, J. T., Torres, F., Rosenblatt, R. L., et al. (2009a). Genetic Defects in Surfactant Protein A2 Are Associated with Pulmonary Fibrosis and Lung Cancer. *Am. J. Hum. Genet.* 84 (1), 52–59. doi:10.1016/j.ajhg.2008.11.010

242. Wang, Z., Chen, C., Finger, S. N., Kwajah, S., Jung, M., Schwarz, H., et al. (2009b). Suberoylanilide Hydroxamic Acid: A Potential Epigenetic Therapeutic Agent for Lung Fibrosis? *Eur. Respir. J.* 34 (1), 145–155. doi:10.1183/09031936. 00084808

243. Wawrocki, S., Druszczynska, M., Kowalewicz-Kulbat, M., and Rudnicka, W. (2016). Interleukin 18 (IL-18) as a Target for Immune Intervention. *Acta Biochim. Pol.* 63 (1), 59–63. doi:10.18388/abp.2015_1153

244. Weichert, N., Kaltenborn, E., Hector, A., Woischnik, M., Schams, A., Holzinger, A., et al. (2011). Some ABCA3 Mutations Elevate ER Stress and Initiate Apoptosis of Lung Epithelial Cells. *Respir. Res.* 12 (1), 4. doi:10.1186/1465-9921-12-4

245. Whyte, M., Hubbard, R., Meliconi, R., Whidborne, M., Eaton, V., Bingle, C., et al. (2000). Increased Risk of Fibrosing Alveolitis Associated with Interleukin-1 Receptor Antagonist and Tumor Necrosis Factor-Alpha Gene Polymorphisms. *Am. J. Respir. Crit. Care Med.* 162 (2 Pt 1), 755–758. doi:10.1164/ajrccm.162.2. 9909053

246. Wolters, P. J., Collard, H. R., and Jones, K. D. (2014). Pathogenesis of Idiopathic Pulmonary Fibrosis. *Annu. Rev. Pathol.* 9, 157–179. doi:10.1146/annurev-pathol-012513-104706

247. Wu, B., Crampton, S. P., and Hughes, C. C. (2007). Wnt Signaling Induces Matrix Metalloproteinase Expression and Regulates T Cell Transmigration. *Immunity* 26 (2), 227–239. doi:10.1016/j.immuni.2006.12.007

248. Wu, M., Assassi, S., Salazar, G. A., Pedroza, C., Gorlova, O. Y., Chen, W. V., et al. (2016). Genetic Susceptibility Loci of Idiopathic Interstitial Pneumonia Do Not Represent Risk for Systemic Sclerosis: A Case Control Study in caucasian Patients. *Arthritis Res. Ther.* 18, 20. doi:10.1186/s13075-016-0923-3

249. Wu, M., Huang, Q., Xie, Y., Wu, X., Ma, H., Zhang, Y., et al. (2022). Improvement of the Anticancer Efficacy of PD-1/pd-L1 Blockade via Combination Therapy and PD-L1 Regulation. *J. Hematol. Oncol.* 15 (1), 24. doi:10.1186/s13045-022-01242-2

250. Wujak, L., Didiasova, M., Zakrzewicz, D., Frey, H., Schaefer, L., and Wygrecka, M. (2015). Heparan Sulfate Proteoglycans Mediate Factor XIIa Binding to the Cell Surface. *J. Biol. Chem.* 290 (11), 7027–7039. doi:10.1074/jbc.M114.606343

251. Wuyts, W. A., Dahlqvist, C., Slabbynck, H., Schlesser, M., Gusbin, N., Compere, C., et al. (2018). Baseline Clinical Characteristics, Comorbidities and Prescribed Medication in a Real-World Population of Patients with Idiopathic Pulmonary Fibrosis: The PROOF Registry. *BMJ Open Respir. Res.* 5 (1), e000331. doi:10. 1136/bmjresp-2018-000331

252. Xia, Y., Xu, F., Xiong, M., Yang, H., Lin, W., Xie, Y., et al. (2021). Repurposing of Antipsychotic Trifluoperazine for Treating Brain Metastasis, Lung Metastasis and Bone Metastasis of Melanoma by Disrupting Autophagy Flux. *Pharmacol. Res.* 163, 105295. doi:10.1016/j.phrs.2020.105295

253. Xiao, X., Senavirathna, L. K., Gou, X., Huang, C., Liang, Y., and Liu, L. (2016). EZH2 Enhances the Differentiation of Fibroblasts into Myofibroblasts in Idiopathic Pulmonary Fibrosis. *Physiol. Rep.* 4 (17), e12915. doi:10.14814/phy2.12915

254. Xiong, Y., Zhang, J., Shi, L., Ning, Y., Zhu, Y., Chen, S., et al. (2017). NOGO-B Promotes EMT in Lung Fibrosis via MMP14 Mediates Free TGF-Beta1 Formation. *Oncotarget* 8 (41), 71024–71037. doi:10.18632/oncotarget.20297

255. Xue, J., Gochuico, B. R., Alawad, A. S., Feghali-Bostwick, C. A., Noth, I., Nathan, S. D., et al. (2011). The HLA Class II Allele DRB1*1501 Is Over-represented in Patients with Idiopathic Pulmonary Fibrosis. *PLoS One* 6 (2), e14715. doi:10. 1371/journal.pone.0014715

256. Xue, T., Qiu, X., Liu, H., Gan, C., Tan, Z., Xie, Y., et al. (2021). Epigenetic Regulation in Fibrosis Progress. *Pharmacol. Res.* 173, 105910. doi:10.1016/j.phrs.2021.105910

257. Yagihashi, K., Huckleberry, J., Colby, T. V., Tazelaar, H. D., Zach, J., Sundaram, B., et al. (2016). Radiologic-pathologic Discordance in Biopsy-Proven Usual Interstitial Pneumonia. *Eur. Respir. J.* 47 (4), 1189–1197. doi:10.1183/13993003.01680-2015

258. Yamakawa, H., Oba, T., Ohta, H., Tsukahara, Y., Kida, G., Tsumiyama, E., et al. (2019). Nintedanib Allows Retreatment with Atezolizumab of Combined Non- small Cell Lung Cancer/idiopathic Pulmonary Fibrosis after Atezolizumab- Induced Pneumonitis: A Case Report. *BMC Pulm. Med.* 19 (1), 156. doi:10. 1186/s12890-019-0920-9

259. Yamashita, C. M., Dolgonos, L., Zemans, R. L., Young, S. K., Robertson, J., Briones, N., et al. (2011). Matrix Metalloproteinase 3 Is a Mediator of Pulmonary Fibrosis. *Am. J. Pathol.* 179 (4), 1733–1745. doi:10.1016/j.ajpath.2011.06.041

260. Yang, L., Herrera, J., Gilbertsen, A., Xia, H., Smith, K., Benyumov, A., et al. (2018). IL-8 Mediates Idiopathic Pulmonary Fibrosis Mesenchymal Progenitor Cell Fibrogenicity. *Am. J. Physiol. Lung Cell. Mol. Physiol.* 314 (1), L127–l136. doi:10.1152/ajplung.00200.2017
261. Yao, L., Conforti, F., Hill, C., Bell, J., Drawater, L., Li, J., et al. (2019). Paracrine Signalling during ZEB1-Mediated Epithelial-Mesenchymal Transition Augments Local Myofibroblast Differentiation in Lung Fibrosis. *Cell. Death Differ.* 26 (5), 943–957. doi:10.1038/s41418-018-0175-7
262. Yu, G., Kovkarova-Naumovski, E., Jara, P., Parwani, A., Kass, D., Ruiz, V., et al. (2012). Matrix Metalloproteinase-19 Is a Key Regulat or of Lung Fibrosis in Mice and Humans. *Am. J. Respir. Crit. Care Med.* 186 (8), 752–762. doi:10.1164/rccm.201202-0302OC
263. Yue, L., Shi, Y., Su, X., Ouyang, L., Wang, G., and Ye, T. (2021). Matrix Metalloproteinases Inhibitors in Idiopathic Pulmonary Fibrosis: Medicinal Chemistry Perspectives. *Eur. J. Med. Chem.* 224, 113714. doi:10.1016/j.ejmech.2021.113714
264. Zhang, H. P., Zou, J., Xie, P., Gao, F., and Mu, H. J. (2015). Association of HLA and Cytokine Gene Polymorphisms with Idiopathic Pulmonary Fibrosis. *Kaohsiung J. Med. Sci.* 31 (12), 613–620. doi:10.1016/j.kjms.2015.10.007
265. Zhang, K., Xu, L., and Cong, Y.-S. (2021). Telomere dysfunction in idiopathic pulmonary fibrosis. *Front. Med.* 8, 739810. doi:10.3389/fmed.2021.739810 Zhang, L., Wang, Y., Wu, G., Xiong, W., Gu, W., and Wang, C. Y. (2018).
266. Macrophages: Friend or Foe in Idiopathic Pulmonary Fibrosis? *Respir. Res.* 19 (1), 170. doi:10.1186/s12931-018-0864-2
267. Zhang, Q., Tu, W., Tian, K., Han, L., Wang, Q., Chen, P., et al. (2019). Sirtuin 6 Inhibits Myofibroblast Differentiation via Inactivating Transforming Growth Factor-β1/Smad2 and Nuclear Factor-Kb Signaling Pathways in Human Fetal Lung Fibroblasts. *J. Cell. Biochem.* 120 (1), 93–104. doi:10.1002/jcb.27128
268. Zhou, S., Wang, X., Gao, H., and Zeng, Y. (2020). DNA methylation in pulmonary fibrosis. *Adv. Exp. Med. Biol.* 1255, 51–62. doi:10.1007/978-981-15-4494-1_4
269. Zhou, W., and Wang, Y. (2016). Candidate Genes of Idiopathic Pulmonary Fibrosis: Current Evidence and Research. *Appl. Clin. Genet.* 9, 5–13. doi:10.2147/tacg.S61999
270. Zhou, W., Zhuang, Y., Sun, J., Wang, X., Zhao, Q., Xu, L., et al. (2017). Variants of the ABCA3 Gene Might Contribute to Susceptibility to Interstitial Lung Diseases in the Chinese Population. *Sci. Rep.* 7 (1), 4097. doi:10.1038/s41598-017-04486-y
271. Ziegenhagen, M. W., Zabel, P., Zissel, G., Schlaak, M., and Müller-Quernheim, J. (1998). Serum Level of Interleukin 8 Is Elevated in Idiopathic Pulmonary Fibrosis and Indicates Disease Activity. *Am. J. Respir. Crit. Care Med.* 157 (3 Pt 1), 762–768. doi:10.1164/ajrccm.157.3.9705014
272. Zolak, J. S., and de Andrade, J. A. (2012). Idiopathic Pulmonary Fibrosis. *Immunol. Allergy Clin. North Am.* 32 (4), 473–485. doi:10.1016/j.iac.2012.08.006

16

Autotaxin in Pathophysiology and Pulmonary Fibrosis

Ioanna Ninou[†], *Christiana Magkrioti*[†] *and Vassilis Aidinis*[*]

Division of Immunology, Alexander Fleming Biomedical Sciences Research Center, Athens, Greece

Correspondence:
Vassilis Aidinis
v.aidinis@fleming.gr

[†]*These authors have contributed equally to this work.*

Lysophospholipid signaling is emerging as a druggable regulator of pathophysiological responses, and especially fibrosis, exemplified by the relative ongoing clinical trials in idiopathic pulmonary fibrosis (IPF) patients. In this review, we focus on ectonucleotide pyrophosphatase-phosphodiesterase 2 (ENPP2), or as more widely known Autotaxin (ATX), a secreted lysophospholipase D (lysoPLD) largely responsible for extracellular lysophosphatidic acid (LPA) production. In turn, LPA is a bioactive phospholipid autacoid, forming locally upon increased ATX levels and acting also locally through its receptors, likely guided by ATX's structural conformation and cell surface associations. Increased ATX activity levels have been detected in many inflammatory and fibroproliferative conditions, while genetic and pharmacologic studies have confirmed a pleiotropic participation of ATX/LPA in different processes and disorders. In pulmonary fibrosis, ATX levels rise in the broncheoalveolar fluid (BALF) and stimulate LPA production. LPA engagement of its receptors activate multiple G-protein mediated signal transduction pathways leading to different responses from pulmonary cells including the production of pro-inflammatory signals from stressed epithelial cells, the modulation of endothelial physiology, the activation of TGF signaling and the stimulation of fibroblast accumulation. Genetic or pharmacologic targeting of the ATX/LPA axis attenuated disease development in animal models, thus providing the proof of principle for therapeutic interventions.

Keywords: autotaxin (ATX), lysophosphatidic acid (LPA), lysophosphatidic acid receptor (LPAR), g-proteins, pulmonary fibrosis

INTRODUCTION

ATX was first identified as an autocrine motility-stimulating factor, isolated from the supernatant of highly metastatic melanoma cells (1). Its cDNA cloning revealed that ATX was homologous to ectonucleotide pyrophosphatase-phosphodiesterase 1 (ENPP1), possessing phosphodiesterase activity *in vitro* (2); ATX was thus classified as ENPP2 in the ENPP (1–7) protein family, being the only secreted and not transmembrane member (3). In addition, several years later it was discovered that ATX is identical to the long elusive plasma lysoPLD (4, 5), and is now considered responsible for the synthesis of the majority of extracellular LPA (**Figure 1**).

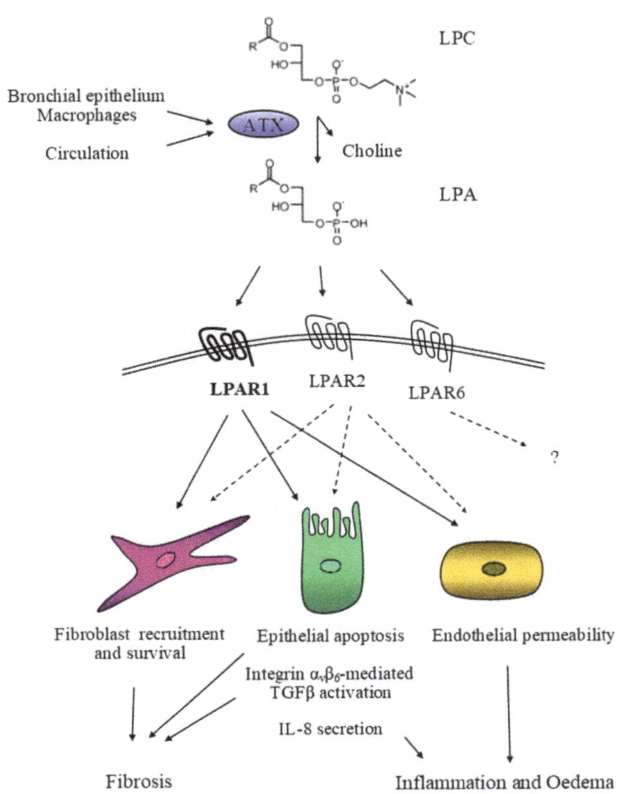

FIGURE 1 | Schematic representation of ATX's mode of action in pulmonary fibrosis. ATX, derived from the bronchial epithelium and alveolar macrophages or extravasated from the circulation, catalyses the hydrolysis of LPC and the local production of LPA. In turn, LPA activates its cognate receptors LPAR1, possibly LPAR2, and hypothetically LPAR6, activating the corresponding G-protein-mediated signal transduction cascades. As a result, LPA induces epithelial apoptosis, the initiating pathogenetic event in modeled pulmonary fibrosis and possibly IPF. LPA also induces IL-8 secretion from epithelial cells, promoting inflammation, while it also stimulates endothelial permeability, thus promoting pulmonary oedema. Moreover, LPA stimulate the $\alpha_V\beta_6$-mediated TGFβ activation leading to the activation and trans-differentiation of pulmonary fibroblasts, for which LPA is additionally a pro-survival and chemotactic factor.

THE *ENPP2/Enpp2* GENE; EXPRESSION AND REGULATION

ENPP2 consists of 27 exons and resides in the human chromosomal region 8q24 (6, 7), a region with frequent somatic copy number alterations in cancer patients, containing potential susceptibility loci for various types of cancers (8, 9). The 8q24 locus has been suggested to regulate the expression of the proto-oncogene *MYC,* also residing in the region (10). *In silico* analysis of publicly available genomic data at The Cancer Genome Atlas (11) indicated genetic alterations, mostly amplifications, of *ENPP2* in cancer patients, with the highest rates observed in ovarian (33%), breast (20%), liver (20%), and lung (11%) carcinomas (12). Moreover, a number of single nucleotide polymorphisms (SNPs) that associate with cancer susceptibility have been detected in or around *ENPP2* (9). Promoter regions of *ENPP2* were found hyper-methylated in primary invasive breast carcinomas (13), while inhibition of histone deacetylases 3 and 7 with trichostatin A also attenuated *ENPP2* expression in colon cancer cells (14), suggesting that *ENPP2* expression can be also amenable to epigenetic regulation. In mice, the highly (93%) homologous *Enpp2* gene is located in chromosome 15 and has a similar structure (15, 16).

A variety of cell types and/or tissues have been reported to express *ENPP2/Enpp2;* the highest mRNA levels in healthy conditions have been observed in adipose tissue, brain, and spinal cord, testis and ovary, followed by lung, kidney, and pancreas (15, 17–19), suggesting that ATX/LPA may participate in the homeostasis of these tissues. In disease states, increased mRNA expression has been reported in a large variety of cancer types and cell lines, as well as in different cell types in chronic inflammatory disorders (20).

Several transcription factors have been suggested to control *ENPP2/Enpp2* transcription in different cell types and pathophysiological states: Hoxa13 and Hoxd13 in mouse embryonic fibroblasts (21), v-jun in chick embryo fibroblasts (22), c-jun in soft tissue sarcomas (23), Stat3 in breast cancer cells (24), AP-1 in keratinocytes and neuroblastoma cells (25, 26), NFAT1 in melanoma and carcinoma cells (27, 28), as well as NF-kB in keratinocytes and hepatocytes (26, 29, 30). *Enpp2* mRNA stability has been reported to be controlled by the RNA-binding Proteins HuR and AUF1 (31), adding an extra level of regulation.

Several extracellular, mainly pro-inflammatory, factors have been suggested to stimulate *ENPP2/Enpp2* expression, many through the transcription factors indicated above: TNF in synovial fibroblasts, hepatocytes, hepatoma cell lines, and thyroid cancer cells (32–35), IL-1β in thyroid cancer cells (34), IL-6 in dermal fibroblasts (36), as well as galectin 3 in melanoma cells (27). Different TLR ligands, including LPS, CpG oligonucleotides and poly(I:C), were shown to stimulate *ENPP2* expression in THP-1 monocytic cells, likely involving an IFN autocrine-paracrine loop (37, 38). Lysophatidylcholine (LPC), a major component of cell membranes and oxidized lipoproteins as well as the enzymatic substrate of ATX, is a potent inducer of *Enpp2* expression in hepatocytes (32). On the other hand, the enzymatic product of ATX, LPA, as well as sphingosine 1 phosphate (S1P), have been suggested to create a negative feedback loop on *Enpp2* expression or activity, under certain conditions (34, 39).

ATX ISOFORMS, STRUCTURE, AND ENZYMATIC ACTIVITY

Alternative splicing of *ENPP2/Enpp2* exons 12 and 21 leads to five, all catalytically active, protein isoforms, named α to ε (15, 40). Isoform β is the most abundant one, likely accounting for the majority of ATX/LPA reported pathophysiological effects. Isoform δ is also abundant, lacking an exon 19 encoded tetrapeptide of unknown function, also missing in isoform ε. Isoform γ is brain specific, and contains an exon 21 encoded 25 aa insert of unknown function (20). Isoforms α and ε are much less abundant, while they contain a 52 aa polybasic insert, encoded by exon 12, that has been shown to bind to heparin and heparin sulfate proteoglycans (41). Proteolytic cleavage of a N-terminal hydrophobic sequence that functions as a signal peptide (42, 43) and glycosylation at asparagine residues (42–45), are necessary for secretion and optimal enzymatic activity.

ATX can be found catalytically active in most biological fluids, such as serum/plasma, bronchoalveolar lavage fluid (BALF), blister fluid, cerebrospinal fluid, synovial fluid, peritoneal fluid, and urine (20). The major source of serum ATX is likely the adipose tissue, as conditional genetic deletion of *Enpp2* in adipocytes resulted in a 38% decrease of plasma LPA (17), whereas ubiquitous heterozygous deletion results in a 50% reduction (46–48). Moreover, ATX has been shown to be secreted, in healthy conditions, from bronchial epithelial cells (49) and high endothelial venules (19), as well as choroid plexus epithelium cells (43), activated astrocytes and oligodendrocytes in the brain (50). Intriguingly, ATX has been also detected in exosomes (51), cell derived vesicles that have been suggested to mediate intercellular or cross-tissue signaling.

ATX consists of two N-terminal somatomedin B-like (SMB) domains, a central phosphodiesterase (PDE) domain and a nuclease-like domain (NUC) in its C-terminus (16, 52, 53). The SMB domains, stabilized by four pairs of disulphide bonds, likely mediate ATX binding to integrins, thus localizing LPA production to the cell surface (19, 52, 54–56). The PDE domain, which interacts with both SMB and NUC domains, contains the active catalytic site consisted of a threonine residue (Thr209/210, for mouse and human, respectively) and two zinc ions coordinated by conserved aspartate and histidine residues. It contains a hydrophobic lipid-binding pocket that can accommodate various LPC and LPA species and an open tunnel that could serve as an exit to LPA (53).

LPC, the enzymatic substrate of ATX, is highly abundant in the circulation, predominantly associated with albumin and lipoproteins (57). LPC is synthesized through the hydrolysis of phosphatidylcholine (PC) by phospholipases (PLA2, PLA1) and lecithin cholesterol acyltransferase (LCAT) enzymes (58). ATX has a preference for shorter and unsaturated fatty acid chains, depending on divalent cations such as Co^{2+} or Mn^{2+} (20, 53). Although ATX can also hydrolyze sphingosylphosphorylcholine (SPC, the precursor of S1P) and nucleotides *in vitro*, genetic and pharmacologic studies in mice established that the main enzymatic activity of ATX *in vivo* is LPC hydrolysis and the production of extracellular LPA (20, 53).

LPA, RECEPTORS, AND SIGNALING

LPA consists of a glycerol backbone, a single fatty acyl chain of varying length and saturation, and a free phosphate group as a polar head. It can be found in most biological fluids, mostly following the expression profile of ATX (57, 59). LPA levels in serum are much higher than those in plasma, due to the release of LPC and other phospholipids from activated platelets during coagulation and their hydrolysis by ATX (60, 61). Moreover, the LPA concentration in plasma (~0.7 μM) is significantly lower than LPC's (~200 μM), while the predominant LPA species (18:2 > 20:4 > 18:1) are not analogous to the corresponding LPC ones (16:0 > 18:1/18:0 > 20:4); similar observations were made in BALFs (62). This can be likely explained by the slow release of LPA from ATX, due to its high affinity for LPA (39, 63), as well by the rapid turnover of LPA, as shown after the pharmacological inhibition of ATX *in vivo* (64, 65). Although there are other biosynthetic routes for LPA production, any increases in the extracellular LPA content of biological fluids and local sites can be attributed to the lysoPLD activity of ATX (58). On the other hand, a group of membrane-associated lipid-phosphate phosphatases (LPPs) have been suggested as negative regulators of LPA levels, adding an extra layer of regulation of its effects (66, 67).

LPA signals through at least six type I rhodopsin-like receptors (LPARs) that exhibit widespread, but differential, tissue distribution, as well as overlapping specificities (68). The orphan GPR87 and P2Y10 receptors (69, 70), as well as the receptor for advanced glycation end products (RAGE) (71) and the intracellular peroxisome proliferator-activated receptor γ (PPARγ) (72), have also been suggested to mediate LPA signaling. Little is known on LPARs functional conformation and possible associations; LPAR1 has been detected in lipid rafts (73, 74) and suggested to heterodimerize with CD14 (74) and CD97 (75).

LPARs couple with G-proteins, crucial molecular switches activating numerous signal transduction pathways (76). G-protein coupled receptors (GPCRs) is the largest family of cell-surface molecules involved in signal transduction, and their aberrant function has been linked with various human diseases, thus representing almost 50% of current therapeutic targets (77). Many *in vitro* studies, extensively reviewed elsewhere (20, 57, 61), have shown that LPA: stimulates the mitogenic Ras-Raf-MEK-ERK pathway and the PI3K pathway promoting cell survival through $G_{\alpha i}$; induces RhoA-mediated cytoskeletal remodeling, as well as cell migration and invasion through $G_{\alpha 12/13}$ in cooperation with the $G_{\alpha i}$-mediated Rac activation pathway; activates phospholipase C, through $G_{\alpha q}$, with consequent production of second messengers. Of note, most *in vitro* effects of LPA were reported at concentrations much higher than the physiological concentrations, as found in healthy biological fluids, suggesting that they likely concern pathophysiological situations with increased levels of LPA. Overall, any LPA effect in each cell type will depend on its local concentration, regulated by ATX and LPPs, the levels of possible agonists and antagonists and the relative abundance of the different receptor subtypes.

ATX/LPA IN PATHOPHYSIOLOGY

Ubiquitous genetic deletion of ATX and abrogation of LPA production resulted to embryonic lethality in mice due to malformations of the vascular and neural systems (46–48, 78), indicating a major role for ATX in **development**; reviewed in Moolenaar et al. (79). Of note, the embryonic phenotype of ATX knock out mice did not resemble the phenotype of any of the individual LPA receptors knock out mice (68), suggesting that coordinated LPA signaling through various receptors is necessary for the observed ATX effects in embryonic development; non-catalytic effects of ATX in development are also possible especially in the neural system (50, 80). Accordingly, elevated

ATX levels have been detected in human pregnancy, further modulated in pregnancy-related pathophysiological conditions (81–86).

Notwithstanding the necessity for ATX in embryonic life, induced genetic deletion or long-term pharmaceutical targeting of ATX in adult mice was shown to be well tolerated (18), indicating that the majority of ATX/LPA (>80%) is dispensable in **adult healthy life**. The remaining ATX-mediated LPA levels, together possibly with LPA produced via other routes (58) are likely adequate to maintain a healthy tissue homeostasis. Given the importance of ATX in embryonic development but not in adult life, the overexpression of ATX in a pathophysiological condition suggests ATX/LPA as a developmental pathway aberrantly re-expressed in pathophysiological situations.

One of the main features of the embryonic lethal phenotype of ATX knock out mice was the aberrant vascular system, as also seen upon ATX knockdown in zebrafish (87) and in line with the suggested role of LPA in **vascular homeostasis** (88, 89). A similar phenotype was also seen in the embryos of transgenic mice overexpressing ATX (90) and LPP3 knock out mice (91, 92) that sustain much higher levels of LPA than wt mice, suggesting that LPA levels should be tightly regulated during development. Of note, $G_{a13}{}^{-/-}$ embryos display similar impairments in the vasculature as the *Enpp2*$^{-/-}$ embryos (46, 93), suggesting G_{a13} as the predominant G-protein mediating ATX/LPA effects in the vasculature. In adult life, LPA has been suggested to modulate endothelial cell physiology, through the stimulation of the expression of angiogenesis related genes and the modulation of their permeability (88, 89, 91). Beyond endothelial cells, LPA has a plethora of effects on other cells of the vessel wall, as well as on blood cells including platelets. Moreover, LPA is generated during mild oxidation of LDL, while its levels accumulate in atherosclerotic plaques, suggesting a role for ATX/LPA in **atherosclerosis** (94, 95).

The possible involvement of ATX/LPA in atherosclerosis is further underscored by the fact that the adipose tissue is a major source of systemic ATX, while its effects, through LPA, can classify ATX as an adipokine. Although the effects of ATX/LPA in adiposity are not clear (17, 96, 97), the ATX-LPA pathway has been suggested to participate in **obesity** related **insulin resistance** and the regulation of **glucose homeostasis** (98), with many implications for the pathogenesis of different metabolic disorders. However, the autocrine and/or paracrine effects of ATX/LPA in metabolism and the consequent effects in disease pathogenesis have not yet been fully explored.

ATX was first isolated due to its ability to promote the motility of melanoma cells (1). Accordingly, many xenograft studies have shown that ATX knock down in melanoma cells, as well as pharmacological inhibition of ATX and LPAR antagonism, attenuate the metastasis of melanoma cells in the lungs of mice, well establishing a role for ATX/LPA in **metastasis**; reviewed in Leblanc and Peyruchaud (99). Beyond melanomas, interaction of ATX with integrin $\alpha_V\beta_3$ on tumor cells, has been reported to control the metastasis of breast cancer to the bone [reviewed in (56, 100)].

Transgenic over-expression of *Enpp2*, as well as *Lpar 1, 2,* or *3*, in the mammary gland resulted in spontaneous breast cancer development (101), indicating a role for the ATX/LPA axis in **breast cancer**. However, spontaneous carcinogenesis was only observed in aged mice, suggesting that ATX/LPA act synergistically with oncogenic age-related signals. Notwithstanding the conflicting reports on ATX levels in breast cancer, the source of ATX in breast cancer was suggested to be the adjacent mammary fat pads, rather than the cancer cells themselves (102), suggesting that ATX can have paracrine effects in cancer development. In the liver, genetic deletion of *Enpp2* from hepatocytes attenuated **hepatocellular carcinoma** (HCC) development, revealing ATX/LPA autocrine effects in hepatocyte metabolism (32, 103). Increased ATX expression has been reported in many other types of cancer, including thyroid and ovarian (20, 104).

Increased ATX levels have been also reported in neuroblastomas and glioblastomas (50) and given the abundant expression of the brain specific isoform ATXγ as well the neuronal defects of the *Enpp2*$^{-/-}$ mice, a role for ATX/LPA in brain cancer seems likely, but it remains yet unexplored. However, another major role for ATX/LPA was revealed in the brain, as it was shown that PLA2/ATX-dependent LPA/LPAR1 signaling is crucial for the initiation of neuropathic pain (105, 106). Moreover, ATX was shown to modulate oligodendrocyte physiology and differentiation via catalytic and non-catalytic functions (50, 107). In this context, increased ATX and LPA levels have been reported in the sera and cerebrospinal fluid (CSF) of **multiple sclerosis** patients (108–110), while pharmacologic inhibition of ATX attenuated the development of experimental autoimmune encephalomyelitis (111).

Besides multiple sclerosis, ATX/LPA were shown to have a role in the pathogenesis of other chronic inflammatory diseases. Conditional genetic deletion of ATX from synovial fibroblasts or pharmacologic inhibition attenuated the development of inflammatory **arthritis** in animal models (33, 112), suggesting a major role for ATX/LPA in rheumatoid arthritis (113, 114). TNF-induced ATX secretion from synovial fibroblasts was shown to result in increased production of LPA which in turn stimulated, in an autocrine mode, cytoskeletal re-organization, proliferation, and migration of synovial fibroblasts (33), the main effector cells in disease pathogenesis. Moreover, increased ATX staining was noted in lymphoid aggregates, in line with the suggestion that ATX can be an adhesive substrate for homing lymphocytes, facilitating their transmigration across endothelial layers in different modes (19, 115–118). Further to the possible regulation of immune responses by ATX/LPA, LPA was recently shown to convert monocytes to macrophages (119).

Chronic inflammation of the liver, due to cytotoxic, viral or metabolic stimuli, was shown to stimulate ATX secretion from hepatocytes, while LPA was shown to activate hepatic stellate cells and to amplify pro-fibrotic signals (32). Conditional genetic deletion of *Enpp2* from hepatocytes or pharmacological inhibition of ATX, attenuated the development of fibrosis in a cytotoxic model (32). Increased ATX expression has been reported in patients with chronic liver diseases of different etiologies, suggesting ATX as a diagnostic marker of different forms of **liver fibrosis** (32, 120). ATX/LPA have been also implicated in the fibrosis of other tissues, such as renal fibrosis (121) and skin fibrosis (36, 122).

ATX/LPA IN PULMONARY FIBROSIS

Enpp2 has been suggested, using genome-wide linkage analysis coupled with expression profiling, as a candidate gene controlling lung function, development and remodeling (123). Accordingly, *Enpp2*$^{-/-}$ mice were found to be embryonically lethal (46–48, 78), while *Lpar1*$^{-/-}$ mice were shown to have reduced alveolar septal formation during development (124). In adult life, ATX is constitutively expressed by bronchial epithelial cells, in both humans, and mice, and can be detected in BALFs (49, 125). However, a 50% reduction of systemic ATX levels in the heterozygous *Enpp2*$^{+/-}$ mice or genetic abrogation of bronchial *Enpp2* expression had no major phenotypic effect in the lungs of mice, suggesting that tissue homeostasis in health does not require large amounts of LPA (49, 126). On the other hand, transgenic overexpression of *Enpp2* from the bronchial epithelium or from the liver resulting to 200% increases of ATX systemic levels, had no gross phenotypic effect in the lung either, suggesting that ATX/LPA are not sufficient to induce lung damage *per se* (126).

Subsegmental allergic challenge of asthma patients induced ATX/LPA levels in their BALFs (127, 128), while pharmacologic inhibition of ATX resulted in a marked attenuation of Th2 cytokines and allergic lung inflammation in a triple-allergen mouse asthma model (128); conflicting reports have suggested both pro-inflammatory and anti-inflammatory roles for LPAR2 (128–130). Therefore, a role for ATX/LPA in asthma seems likely and consistent with early reports on LPA effects in the proliferation and contraction of airway smooth muscle cells (131, 132).

Increased ATX staining has been detected in lung tissue samples from IPF and fibrotic non-specific interstitial pneumonia (fNSIP) patients, compared to other interstitial diseases and especially control samples (49). ATX localized mainly within the hyperplastic bronchiolar epithelium, but it was also detected weakly on alveolar epithelium around fibroblastic foci, interstitial macrophages, and fibroblast like cells. On the contrary, ATX was minimally localized within both the inflammatory components of cellular NSIP lung samples and in areas of loose connective tissue, called Masson bodies, representing the pathogenic hallmark of cryptogenic organizing pneumonia. These two latter forms of idiopathic interstitial pneumonias have a propitious prognosis and an excellent treatment response to corticosteroids, indicating that ATX up-regulation is closely associated with more progressive and irreversible forms of pulmonary fibrosis, such as IPF/UIP and fNSIP (49). Of note, as ATX has been suggested to bind to integrins at the surface of platelets and cancer cells (52, 54, 56), it cannot be excluded that ATX can bind to the surface of lung cells via integrins, thus avoiding clearance while exerting locally-produced LPA effects. In turn, the levels of specific LPA species have been found moderately increased in BALFs and exhaled breath condensates collected from IPF patients (133, 134); however, larger studies are needed.

A similar ATX staining profile was observed in the lungs of mice treated with bleomycin (BLM) (49), the most widely used animal model of pulmonary inflammation and fibrosis (135, 136), while increased ATX levels were detected in the corresponding BALFs (49, 62). Conditional genetic deletion of *Enpp2* from bronchial epithelial cells (CC10^{+}) and macrophages (LysM^{+}), the main pulmonary cells expressing ATX, reduced BALF ATX levels and disease severity thus confirming the pulmonary ATX sources as well as establishing a pathogenic role for ATX. However, BALF ATX levels remained relatively high, while the modeled disease was not completely attenuated, suggesting additional, extrapulmonary sources of ATX. ATX levels in BALF correlated with total protein and albumin measurements, pointing to a possible extravasation of ATX from the circulation; paradoxically, no major effects in BLM-induced fibrosis development were noted in genetically modified mice with increased or decreased serum and systemic levels of ATX (49). Nevertheless, systemic pharmacologic inhibition of ATX, both with small molecules and DNA aptamers, decreased LPA levels, and attenuated pulmonary fibrosis (49, 137, 138). It should be noted that ATX inhibition with PAT-048 (Bristol Myers Squibb; WO2012024620) was reported to have no effects in BLM-induced pulmonary fibrosis (62), most likely due to experimental settings and compound characteristics. However, the therapeutic potential of targeting the ATX/LPA axis was recently re-evaluated, where yet another ATX inhibitor was shown to prevent BLM-induced pulmonary fibrosis (139). Many more small molecule ATX inhibitors have been reported (140, 141), however they are still not tested in animal models of pulmonary fibrosis. Intriguingly, the bile salt tauroursodeoxycholate (TUDCA) was recently reported to be a partial non-competitive inhibitor of ATX (142), suggesting that the previously reported therapeutic effects of TUDCA in BLM-induced fibrosis (143), could be due to ATX inhibition.

Moreover, an autocrine pathway linking ATX, LPA signaling and b-catenin was recently reported to contribute to fibrosis progression in lung allografts, one of the primary causes of long-term graft failure after organ transplantation (144). Pharmacologic ATX inhibition or LPAR1 antagonism decreased allograft fibrosis (144), further extending the therapeutic potential of targeting the ATX/LPA axis in lung fibroproliferative disorders.

In agreement with a pathogenic role of ATX/LPA in pulmonary fibrosis, ubiquitous genetic deletion of either *Lpar1* or *Lpar2* also abrogated BLM-induced disease development (133, 145). Pharmacologic antagonism of LPAR1 was shown to be beneficial for the treatment of BLM-treated mice (146), thus stimulating the respective on-going clinical trial (NCT 02068053). Moreover, simultaneous ATX inhibition and LPAR1 antagonism has been reported to have some additive effect in melanoma metastasis (147), warranting further investigation and/or optimization. Beyond LPAR1&2, LPAR6 is the highest expressing LPAR in the lung (not published data), but its possible role in pulmonary pathophysiology and fibrosis has not been explored yet (**Figure 1**).

Reduced numbers of TUNEL$^+$ cells were noted in the alveolar and bronchial epithelium of BLM-treated *Lpar1*$^{-/-}$ and *Lpar2*$^{-/-}$ mice, suggesting that LPA, through LPAR1 and/or 2, promotes epithelial apoptosis (145, 148), the initiating pathogenetic event in this model (135) and, likely, in human patients (149). Interestingly, apoptosing epithelial cells post BLM were shown to express TNF that has a major contribution in the pathogenesis of the modeled disease (150), while TNF has been reported to stimulate ATX expression in other cell types (33, 35). Many other LPA possible effects in pulmonary epithelial cells *in vitro* have been reported and are detailed elsewhere (151), including the induction of IL-8 secretion resulting to neutrophil influx (152, 153).

LPA stimulation of normal human bronchial epithelial cells has been shown to increase stress fiber formation, and to reorganize integrin $\alpha_v\beta_6$ at their ends leading to TGF-β activation (154). Integrin $\alpha_v\beta_6$ has been shown previously to bind and activate TGF-β, a mechanism suggested to regulate pulmonary inflammation and fibrosis (155). TGF-β is the prototype pro-fibrotic factor with a well-documented involvement in the pathogenesis of both the human and the modeled disease, with effects on alveolar epithelial cell injury, myofibroblast differentiation, epithelial-to-mesenchymal transition, and ECM deposition and remodeling (156). TGF-β is produced by different cell types, including alveolar macrophages, while LPA was shown to induce TGF-β expression in pulmonary fibroblasts *in vitro* (145). Therefore, TGF-β activation and possibly expression is another important mechanism through which LPA promotes pulmonary fibrosis.

BALF isolated from BLM-treated mice stimulates the chemotaxis of pulmonary fibroblasts, which was found attenuated by more than 50% in the absence of *Lpar1* expression, indicating that LPA is a major fibroblast chemoattractant (133). The structural organization of LPAR2 has been suggested to govern gradient sensing and the directional migration of fibroblasts in response to LPA (157), while LPA-induced mTORC2-mediated PKC-δ phosphorylation was shown to be critically important for fibroblast migration and pulmonary fibrosis development (158). LPA has been reported to promote, through GPCR-mediated pathways, the cytoskeletal reorganization and proliferation of lung fibroblasts (151), mediated likely from LPAR2 (145) but not from LPAR1 (133). Moreover, LPA signaling, specifically through LPAR1, has been found to suppress, under certain conditions, the apoptosis of primary mouse lung fibroblasts induced by serum deprivation (148). Similar anti-apoptotic effects of LPA have been reported in many cell lines (151), further supporting a role for ATX/LPA in mediating pathologic fibroblast accumulation, the main pathogenetic event in IPF.

Calcium second messenger signals are essential for many critical cellular functions (159). In fibroblasts, calcium homeostasis and ionic mechanisms have been proposed to orchestrate many of their functions, including proliferation, secretion of extracellular matrix components, as well as TGF-β production and differentiation to myofibroblasts (160). In this context, transient receptor potential vanilloid 4 (TRPV4) Ca^{2+} channels have been shown to get activated in response to matrix stiffness, as found in fibrotic lungs (161), and to mediate fibroblast activation and differentiation (162). Interestingly, LPA is well known to stimulate Ca^{2+} influx and/or mobilization in many cells (163), while it was recently shown to directly activate a TRPV1 ion channel (164). Although, the activation was intracellular (164), transbilayer LPA movement has been suggested before in the activation of the nuclear PPARγ receptor (72). Therefore, LPA-induced alterations in calcium homeostasis can have dominant effects in the physiology of fibroblasts, as well as many other cell types.

One of the hallmarks of the observed protection from BLM-induced fibrosis in *Lpar1*$^{-/-}$ mice was the attenuation of BLM-induced vascular leak, indicating a major role of LPA in promoting endothelial permeability upon damage (133). Accordingly, transgenic overexpression of ATX from the liver resulting to elevated circulating LPA levels induced a bleeding diathesis (55). However, the effects of LPA on endothelial permeability remain controversial, while different LPA receptors have been proposed to mediate different effects on endothelial physiology (23, 151, 164). Endothelial dysfunction mainly characterizes the development of atherosclerosis and cardiovascular diseases, however, interstitial lung diseases have all been reported to have a lung vascular disease component (165).

Therefore, ATX-mediated LPA production promotes pleiotropic effects in pulmonary cells stimulating the development of pulmonary fibrosis (**Figure 1**). Accordingly, ATX inhibition was shown to attenuate BLM-induced pulmonary fibrosis (49, 137, 138), thus providing the proof of principle for therapeutic interventions and stimulating the on-going clinical trial. In a phase 1 study, GLPG1690, a potent and orally bioavailable ATX inhibitor exhibiting a good PK/PD profile (137), was shown to be safe and well tolerated (166), as previously shown with another compound and genetic interventions in mice (18). An exploratory phase 2a study in IPF patients (FLORA; NCT 02738801) was just completed with promising results (expected to be published soon), leading to phase IIb, currently recruiting.

AUTHOR CONTRIBUTIONS

IN and CM drafted the paper. VA edited it.

ACKNOWLEDGMENTS

This review is dedicated to the memory of Andrew Tager, a pioneer in the field of the review.

REFERENCES

1. Stracke ML, Krutzsch HC, Unsworth EJ, Arestad A, Cioce V, Schiffmann E, et al. Identification, purification, and partial sequence analysis of autotaxin, a novel motility-stimulating protein. *J Biol Chem.* (1992) 267:2524–9.
2. Murata J, Lee HY, Clair T, Krutzsch HC, Arestad AA, Sobel ME, et al. cDNA cloning of the human tumor motility-stimulating protein, autotaxin, reveals a homology with phosphodiesterases. *J Biol Chem.* (1994) 269:30479–84.
3. Stefan C, Jansen S, Bollen M. NPP-type ectophosphodiesterases: unity in diversity. *Trends Biochem Sci.* (2005) 30:542–50. doi: 10.1016/j.tibs.2005.08.005
4. Tokumura A, Majima E, Kariya Y, Tominaga K, Kogure K, Yasuda K, et al. Identification of human plasma lysophospholipase D, a lysophosphatidic acid-producing enzyme, as autotaxin, a multifunctional phosphodiesterase. *J Biol Chem.* (2002) 277:39436–42. doi: 10.1074/jbc.M205623200
5. Umezu-Goto M, Kishi Y, Taira A, Hama K, Dohmae N, Takio K, et al. Autotaxin has lysophospholipase D activity leading to tumor cell growth and motility by lysophosphatidic acid production. *J Cell Biol.* (2002) 158:227–33. doi: 10.1083/jcb.200204026
6. Kawagoe H, Soma O, Goji J, Nishimura N, Narita M, Inazawa J, et al. Molecular cloning and chromosomal assignment of the human brain-type phosphodiesterase I/nucleotide pyrophosphatase gene (PDNP2). *Genomics* (1995) 30:380–4. doi: 10.1006/geno.1995.0036
7. Lee HY, Murata J, Clair T, Polymeropoulos MH, Torres R, Manrow RE, et al. Cloning, chromosomal localization, and tissue expression of autotaxin from human teratocarcinoma cells. *Biochem Biophys Res Commun.* (1996) 218:714–9. doi: 10.1006/bbrc.1996.0127
8. Ciriello G, Miller ML, Aksoy BA, Senbabaoglu Y, Schultz N, Sander C. Emerging landscape of oncogenic signatures across human cancers. *Nat Genet.* (2013) 45:1127–33. doi: 10.1038/ng.2762
9. Brisbin AG, Asmann YW, Song H, Tsai YY, Aakre JA, Yang P, et al. Meta-analysis of 8q24 for seven cancers reveals a locus between NOV and ENPP2 associated with cancer development. *BMC Med Genet.* (2011) 12:156. doi: 10.1186/1471-2350-12-156
10. Grisanzio C, Freedman ML. Chromosome 8q24-Associated Cancers and MYC. *Genes Cancer.* (2010) 1:555–9. doi: 10.1177/1947601910381380
11. The Cancer Genome Atlas Research N. Comprehensive molecular profiling of lung adenocarcinoma. *Nature* (2014) 511:543–50. doi: 10.1038/nature13385
12. Federico L, Jeong KJ, Vellano CP, Mills GB. Autotaxin, a lysophospholipase D with pleomorphic effects in oncogenesis and cancer progression. *J Lipid Res.* (2015) 57:25–35. doi: 10.1194/jlr.R060020
13. Parris TZ, Kovacs A, Hajizadeh S, Nemes S, Semaan M, Levin M, et al. Frequent MYC coamplification and DNA hypomethylation of multiple genes on 8q in 8p11-p12-amplified breast carcinomas. *Oncogenesis* (2014) 3:e95. doi: 10.1038/oncsis.2014.8
14. Li S, Wang B, Xu Y, Zhang J. Autotaxin is induced by TSA through HDAC3 and HDAC7 inhibition and antagonizes the TSA-induced cell apoptosis. *Mol Cancer.* (2011) 10:18. doi: 10.1186/1476-4598-10-18
15. Giganti A, Rodriguez M, Fould B, Moulharat N, Coge F, Chomarat P, et al. Murine and human autotaxin alpha, beta, and gamma isoforms: gene organization, tissue distribution, and biochemical characterization. *J Biol Chem.* (2008) 283:7776–89. doi: 10.1074/jbc.M708705200
16. Nishimasu H, Okudaira S, Hama K, Mihara E, Dohmae N, Inoue A, et al. Crystal structure of autotaxin and insight into GPCR activation by lipid mediators. *Nat Struct Mol Biol.* (2011) 18:205–12. doi: 10.1038/nsmb.1998
17. Dusaulcy R, Rancoule C, Gres S, Wanecq E, Colom A, Guigne C, et al. Adipose-specific disruption of autotaxin enhances nutritional fattening and reduces plasma lysophosphatidic acid. *J Lipid Res.* (2011) 52:1247–55. doi: 10.1194/jlr.M014985
18. Katsifa A, Kaffe E, Nikolaidou-Katsaridou N, Economides AN, Newbigging S, McKerlie C, et al. The bulk of autotaxin activity is dispensable for adult mouse life. *PLoS ONE* (2015) 10:e0143083. doi: 10.1371/journal.pone.0143083
19. Kanda H, Newton R, Klein R, Morita Y, Gunn MD, Rosen SD. Autotaxin, an ectoenzyme that produces lysophosphatidic acid, promotes the entry of lymphocytes into secondary lymphoid organs. *Nat Immunol.* (2008) 9:415–23. doi: 10.1038/ni1573
20. Barbayianni E, Kaffe E, Aidinis V, Kokotos G. Autotaxin, a secreted lysophospholipase D, as a promising therapeutic target in chronic inflammation and cancer. *Prog Lipid Res.* (2015) 58:76–96. doi: 10.1016/j.plipres.2015.02.001
21. Williams TM, Williams ME, Kuick R, Misek D, McDonagh K, Hanash S, et al. Candidate downstream regulated genes of HOX group 13 transcription factors with and without monomeric DNA binding capability. *Dev Biol.* (2005) 279:462–80. doi: 10.1016/j.ydbio.2004.12.015
22. Black EJ, Clair T, Delrow J, Neiman P, Gillespie DA. Microarray analysis identifies Autotaxin, a tumour cell motility and angiogenic factor with lysophospholipase D activity, as a specific target of cell transformation by v-Jun. *Oncogene* (2004) 23:2357–66. doi: 10.1038/sj.onc.1207377
23. Sioletic S, Czaplinski J, Hu L, Fletcher JA, Fletcher CD, Wagner AJ, et al. c-Jun promotes cell migration and drives expression of the motility factor ENPP2 in soft tissue sarcomas. *J Pathol.* (2014) 234:190–202. doi: 10.1002/path.4379
24. Azare J, Doane A, Leslie K, Chang Q, Berishaj M, Nnoli J, et al. Stat3 mediates expression of autotaxin in breast cancer. *PLoS ONE* (2011) 6:e27851. doi: 10.1371/journal.pone.0027851
25. Farina AR, Cappabianca L, Ruggeri P, Di Ianni N, Ragone M, Merolle S, et al. Constitutive autotaxin transcription by Nmyc-amplified and non-amplified neuroblastoma cells is regulated by a novel AP-1 and SP-mediated mechanism and abrogated by curcumin. *FEBS Lett.* (2012) 586:3681–91. doi: 10.1016/j.febslet.2012.08.026
26. Ryborg AK, Johansen C, Iversen L, Kragballe K. Lysophosphatidylcholine induces keratinocyte differentiation and upregulation of AP-1- and NF-kappaB DNA-binding activity. *Acta Derm Venereol.* (2004) 84:433–8. doi: 10.1080/00015550410016930
27. Braeuer RR, Zigler M, Kamiya T, Dobroff AS, Huang L, Choi W, et al. Galectin-3 contributes to melanoma growth and metastasis via regulation of NFAT1 and autotaxin. *Cancer Res.* (2012) 72:5757–66. doi: 10.1158/0008-5472.CAN-12-2424
28. Chen M, O'Connor KL. Integrin alpha6beta4 promotes expression of autotaxin/ENPP2 autocrine motility factor in breast carcinoma cells. *Oncogene* (2005) 24:5125–30. doi: 10.1038/sj.onc.1208729
29. Lovas A, Weidemann A, Albrecht D, Wiechert L, Weih D, Weih F. p100 Deficiency is insufficient for full activation of the alternative NF-kappaB pathway: TNF cooperates with p52-RelB in target gene transcription. *PLoS ONE* (2012) 7:e42741. doi: 10.1371/journal.pone.0042741
30. Corcoran DL, Feingold E, Dominick J, Wright M, Harnaha J, Trucco M, et al. Footer: a quantitative comparative genomics method for efficient recognition of cis-regulatory elements. *Genome Res.* (2005) 15:840–7. doi: 10.1101/gr.2952005
31. Sun S, Zhang X, Lyu L, Li X, Yao S, Zhang J. Autotaxin expression is regulated at the post-transcriptional Level by the RNA-binding proteins HuR and AUF1. *J Biol Chem.* (2016) 291:25823–36. doi: 10.1074/jbc.M116.756908
32. Kaffe E, Katsifa A, Xylourgidis N, Ninou I, Zannikou M, Harokopos V, et al. Hepatocyte Autotaxin expression promotes liver fibrosis and cancer. *Hepatology* (2016) 65:1369–83. doi: 10.1002/hep.28973
33. Nikitopoulou I, Oikonomou N, Karouzakis E, Sevastou I, Nikolaidou-Katsaridou N, Zhao Z, et al. Autotaxin expression from synovial fibroblasts is essential for the pathogenesis of modeled arthritis. *J Exp Med.* (2012) 209:925–33. doi: 10.1084/jem.20112012
34. Benesch MG, Zhao YY, Curtis JM, McMullen TP, Brindley DN. Regulation of autotaxin expression and secretion by lysophosphatidate and sphingosine 1-phosphate. *J Lipid Res.* (2015) 56:1134–44. doi: 10.1194/jlr.M0 57661
35. Wu JM, Xu Y, Skill NJ, Sheng H, Zhao Z, Yu M, et al. Autotaxin expression and its connection with the TNF-alpha-NF-kappaB axis in human hepatocellular carcinoma. *Mol Cancer* (2010) 9:71. doi: 10.1186/1476-4598-9-71
36. Castelino FV, Bain G, Pace VA, Black KE, George L, Probst CK, et al. An Autotaxin/Lysophosphatidic Acid/Interleukin-6 Amplification Loop Drives Scleroderma Fibrosis. *Arthrit Rheumatol.* (2016) 68:2964–74. doi: 10.1002/art.39797
37. Li S, Xiong C, Zhang J. ATX and LPA receptor 3 are coordinately up-regulated in lipopolysaccharide-stimulated THP-1 cells through PKR and SPK1-mediated pathways. *FEBS Lett.* (2012) 586:792–7. doi: 10.1016/j.febslet.2012.01.044

38. Song J, Guan M, Zhao Z, Zhang J. Type I interferons function as autocrine and paracrine factors to induce autotaxin in response to TLR activation. *PLoS ONE* (2015) 10:e0136629. doi: 10.1371/journal.pone.0136629
39. van Meeteren LA, Ruurs P, Christodoulou E, Goding JW, Takakusa H, Kikuchi K, et al. Inhibition of autotaxin by lysophosphatidic acid and sphingosine 1-phosphate. *J Biol Chem.* (2005) 280:21155–61. doi: 10.1074/jbc.M413183200
40. Hashimoto T, Okudaira S, Igarashi K, Hama K, Yatomi Y, Aoki J. Identification and biochemical characterization of a novel autotaxin isoform, ATXdelta, with a four-amino acid deletion. *J Biochem.* (2012) 151:89–97. doi: 10.1093/jb/mvr126
41. Houben AJ, van Wijk XM, van Meeteren LA, van Zeijl L, van de Westerlo EM, Hausmann J, et al. The polybasic insertion in autotaxin alpha confers specific binding to heparin and cell surface heparan sulfate proteoglycans. *J Biol Chem.* (2013) 288:510–9. doi: 10.1074/jbc.M112.358416
42. Jansen S, Stefan C, Creemers JW, Waelkens E, Van Eynde A, Stalmans W, et al. Proteolytic maturation and activation of autotaxin (NPP2), a secreted metastasis-enhancing lysophospholipase D. *J Cell Sci.* (2005) 118(Pt 14):3081–9. doi: 10.1242/jcs.02438
43. Koike S, Keino-Masu K, Ohto T, Masu M. The N-terminal hydrophobic sequence of autotaxin (ENPP2) functions as a signal peptide. *Genes Cells* (2006) 11:133–42. doi: 10.1111/j.1365-2443.2006.00924.x
44. Jansen S, Callewaert N, Dewerte I, Andries M, Ceulemans H, Bollen M. An essential oligomannosidic glycan chain in the catalytic domain of autotaxin, a secreted lysophospholipase-D. *J Biol Chem.* (2007) 282:11084–91. doi: 10.1074/jbc.M611503200
45. Pradere JP, Tarnus E, Gres S, Valet P, Saulnier-Blache JS. Secretion and lysophospholipase D activity of autotaxin by adipocytes are controlled by N-glycosylation and signal peptidase. *Biochim Biophys Acta* (2007) 1771:93–102. doi: 10.1016/j.bbalip.2006.11.010
46. Fotopoulou S, Oikonomou N, Grigorieva E, Nikitopoulou I, Paparountas T, Thanassopoulou A, et al. ATX expression and LPA signalling are vital for the development of the nervous system. *Dev Biol.* (2010) 339:451–64. doi: 10.1016/j.ydbio.2010.01.007
47. van Meeteren LA, Ruurs P, Stortelers C, Bouwman P, van Rooijen MA, Pradere JP, et al. Autotaxin, a secreted lysophospholipase D, is essential for blood vessel formation during development. *Mol Cell Biol.* (2006) 26:5015–22. doi: 10.1128/MCB.02419-05
48. Tanaka M, Okudaira S, Kishi Y, Ohkawa R, Iseki S, Ota M, et al. Autotaxin stabilizes blood vessels and is required for embryonic vasculature by producing lysophosphatidic acid. *J Biol Chem.* (2006) 281:25822–30. doi: 10.1074/jbc.M605142200
49. Oikonomou N, Mouratis MA, Tzouvelekis A, Kaffe E, Valavanis C, Vilaras G, et al. Pulmonary autotaxin expression contributes to the pathogenesis of pulmonary fibrosis. *Am J Respir Cell Mol Biol.* (2012) 47:566–74. doi: 10.1165/rcmb.2012-0004OC
50. Yuelling LM, Fuss B. Autotaxin (ATX): A multi-functional and multi-modular protein possessing enzymatic lysoPLD activity and matricellular properties. *Biochim Biophys Acta.* (2008) 1781:525–30. doi: 10.1016/j.bbalip.2008.04.009
51. Jethwa SA, Leah EJ, Zhang Q, Bright NA, Oxley D, Bootman MD, et al. Exosomes bind autotaxin and act as a physiological delivery mechanism to stimulate LPA receptor signalling in cells. *J Cell Sci.* (2016) 129:3948–57doi: 10.1242/jcs.184424
52. Hausmann J, Kamtekar S, Christodoulou E, Day JE, Wu T, Fulkerson Z, et al. Structural basis of substrate discrimination and integrin binding by autotaxin. *Nat Struct Mol Biol.* (2011) 18:198–204. doi: 10.1038/nsmb.1980
53. Perrakis A, Moolenaar WH. Autotaxin: structure-function and signaling. *J Lipid Res.* (2014) 55:1010–8. doi: 10.1194/jlr.R046391
54. Fulkerson Z, Wu T, Sunkara M, Kooi CV, Morris AJ, Smyth SS. Binding of autotaxin to integrins localizes lysophosphatidic acid production to platelets and mammalian cells. *J Biol Chem.* (2011) 286:34654–63. doi: 10.1074/jbc.M111.276725
55. Pamuklar Z, Federico L, Liu S, Umezu-Goto M, Dong A, Panchatcharam M, et al. Autotaxin/lysopholipase D and lysophosphatidic acid regulate murine hemostasis and thrombosis. *J Biol Chem.* (2009) 284:7385–94. doi: 10.1074/jbc.M807820200
56. Leblanc R, Lee SC, David M, Bordet JC, Norman DD, Patil R, et al. Interaction of platelet-derived autotaxin with tumor integrin alphaVbeta3 controls metastasis of breast cancer cells to bone. *Blood* (2014) 124:3141–50. doi: 10.1182/blood-2014-04-568683
57. Sevastou I, Kaffe E, Mouratis MA, Aidinis V. Lysoglycerophospholipids in chronic inflammatory disorders: the PLA/LPC and ATX/LPA axes. *Biochim Biophys Acta.* (2013) 1831:42–60. doi: 10.1016/j.bbalip.2012.07.019
58. Aoki J, Inoue A, Okudaira S. Two pathways for lysophosphatidic acid production. *Biochim Biophys Acta* (2008) 1781:513–8. doi: 10.1016/j.bbalip.2008.06.005
59. Aikawa S, Hashimoto T, Kano K, Aoki J. Lysophosphatidic acid as a lipid mediator with multiple biological actions. *J Biochem.* (2015) 157:81–9. doi: 10.1093/jb/mvu077
60. Aoki J. Mechanisms of lysophosphatidic acid production. *Semin Cell Dev Biol.* (2004) 15:477–89. doi: 10.1016/j.semcdb.2004.05.001
61. van Meeteren LA, Moolenaar WH. Regulation and biological activities of the autotaxin-LPA axis. *Prog Lipid Res.* (2007) 46:145–60. doi: 10.1016/j.plipres.2007.02.001
62. Black KE, Berdyshev E, Bain G, Castelino FV, Shea BS, Probst CK, et al. Autotaxin activity increases locally following lung injury, but is not required for pulmonary lysophosphatidic acid production or fibrosis. *Faseb J.* (2016) 30:2435–50. doi: 10.1096/fj.201500197R
63. Saunders LP, Cao W, Chang WC, Albright RA, Braddock DT, De La Cruz EM. Kinetic analysis of autotaxin reveals substrate-specific catalytic pathways and a mechanism for lysophosphatidic acid distribution. *J Biol Chem.* (2011) 286:30130–41. doi: 10.1074/jbc.M111.246884
64. Gierse JK, Thorarensen A, Beltey K, Bradshaw-Pierce E, Cortes-Burgos L, Hall T, et al. A novel autotaxin inhibitor reduces lysophosphatidic acid levels in plasma and the site of inflammation. *J Pharmacol Exp Therapeut.* (2010) 334:310–7. doi: 10.1124/jpet.110.165845
65. Albers HM, Dong A, van Meeteren LA, Egan DA, Sunkara M, van Tilburg EW, et al. Boronic acid-based inhibitor of autotaxin reveals rapid turnover of LPA in the circulation. *Proc Natl Acad Sci USA.* (2010) 107:7257–62. doi: 10.1073/pnas.1001529107
66. Tang X, Benesch MG, Brindley DN. Lipid phosphate phosphatases and their roles in mammalian physiology and pathology. *J Lipid Res.* (2015) 56:2048–60. doi: 10.1194/jlr.R058362
67. Benesch MG, Tang X, Venkatraman G, Bekele RT, Brindley DN. Recent advances in targeting the autotaxin-lysophosphatidate-lipid phosphate phosphatase axis *in vivo*. *J Biomed Res.* (2016) 30:272–84. doi: 10.7555/JBR.30.20150058
68. Yung YC, Stoddard NC, Chun J. LPA receptor signaling: pharmacology, physiology, and pathophysiology. *J Lipid Res.* (2014) 55:1192–214. doi: 10.1194/jlr.R046458
69. Tabata K, Baba K, Shiraishi A, Ito M, Fujita N. The orphan GPCR GPR87 was deorphanized and shown to be a lysophosphatidic acid receptor. *Biochem Biophys Res Commun.* (2007) 363:861–6. doi: 10.1016/j.bbrc.2007.09.063
70. Murakami M, Shiraishi A, Tabata K, Fujita N. Identification of the orphan GPCR, P2Y(10) receptor as the sphingosine-1-phosphate and lysophosphatidic acid receptor. *Biochem Biophys Res Commun.* (2008) 371:707–12. doi: 10.1016/j.bbrc.2008.04.145
71. Rai V, Toure F, Chitayat S, Pei R, Song F, Li Q, et al. Lysophosphatidic acid targets vascular and oncogenic pathways via RAGE signaling. *J Exp Med.* (2012) 209:2339–50. doi: 10.1084/jem.20120873
72. McIntyre TM, Pontsler AV, Silva AR, St Hilaire A, Xu Y, Hinshaw JC, et al. Identification of an intracellular receptor for lysophosphatidic acid (LPA): LPA is a transcellular PPARgamma agonist. *Proc Natl Acad Sci USA.* (2003) 100:131–6. doi: 10.1073/pnas.0135855100
73. Gobeil F, Jr., Bernier SG, Vazquez-Tello A, Brault S, Beauchamp MH, Quiniou C, et al. Modulation of pro-inflammatory gene expression by nuclear lysophosphatidic acid receptor type-1. *J Biol Chem.* (2003) 278:38875–83. doi: 10.1074/jbc.M212481200
74. Zhao J, He D, Su Y, Berdyshev E, Chun J, Natarajan V, et al. Lysophosphatidic acid receptor 1 modulates lipopolysaccharide-induced inflammation in alveolar epithelial cells and murine lungs. *Am J Physiol Lung Cell Mol Physiol.* (2011) 301:L547–56. doi: 10.1152/ajplung.00058.2011

75. Ward Y, Lake R, Yin JJ, Heger CD, Raffeld M, Goldsmith PK, et al. LPA receptor heterodimerizes with CD97 to amplify LPA-initiated RHO-dependent signaling and invasion in prostate cancer cells. *Cancer Res.* (2011) 71:7301–11. doi: 10.1158/0008-5472.CAN-11-2381
76. Oldham WM, Hamm HE. Heterotrimeric G protein activation by G-protein-coupled receptors. *Nat Rev Mol Cell Biol.* (2008) 9:60–71. doi: 10.1038/nrm2299
77. Dorsam RT, Gutkind JS. G-protein-coupled receptors and cancer. *Nat Rev Cancer* (2007) 7:79–94. doi: 10.1038/nrc2069
78. Ferry G, Giganti A, Cogé F, Bertaux F, Thiam K, Boutin JA. Functional invalidation of the autotaxin gene by a single amino acid mutation in mouse is lethal. *FEBS Lett.* (2007) 581:3572–8. doi: 10.1016/j.febslet.2007.06.064
79. Moolenaar WH, Houben AJ, Lee SJ, van Meeteren LA. Autotaxin in embryonic development. *Biochim Biophys Acta* (2012) 1831:13–9. doi: 10.1016/j.bbalip.2012.09.013
80. Greenman R, Gorelik A, Sapir T, Baumgart J, Zamor V, Segal-Salto M, et al. Non-cell autonomous and non-catalytic activities of ATX in the developing brain. *Front Neurosci.* (2015) 9:53. doi: 10.3389/fnins.2015.00053
81. Kremer AE, Bolier R, Dixon PH, Geenes V, Chambers J, Tolenaars D, et al. Autotaxin activity has a high accuracy to diagnose intrahepatic cholestasis of pregnancy. *J Hepatol.* (2015) 62:897–904. doi: 10.1016/j.jhep.2014.10.041
82. Masuda A, Fujii T, Iwasawa Y, Nakamura K, Ohkawa R, Igarashi K, et al. Serum autotaxin measurements in pregnant women: application for the differentiation of normal pregnancy and pregnancy-induced hypertension. *Clin Chim Acta* (2011) 412:1944–50. doi: 10.1016/j.cca.2011.06.039
83. Sozen I, Aslan Cetin B, Gezer A, Ekmekci H, Kaya B, Tuten A, et al. Placental autotaxin expression is diminished in women with pre-eclampsia. *Hypert Preg.* (2015) 41:1406–11. doi: 10.1111/jog.12742
84. Erenel H, Yilmaz N, Cift T, Bulut B, Sozen I, Aslan Cetin B, et al. Maternal serum autotaxin levels in early- and late-onset preeclampsia. *Hypert Preg.* (2017) 36:310–4. doi: 10.1080/10641955.2017.1388389
85. Tokumura A, Kanaya Y, Miyake M, Yamano S, Irahara M, Fukuzawa K. Increased production of bioactive lysophosphatidic acid by serum lysophospholipase D in human pregnancy. *Biol Reprod.* (2002) 67:1386–92. doi: 10.1095/biolreprod.102.004051
86. Tokumura A, Kume T, Taira S, Yasuda K, Kanzaki H. Altered activity of lysophospholipase D, which produces bioactive lysophosphatidic acid and choline, in serum from women with pathological pregnancy. *Mol Human Reproduct.* (2009) 15:301–10. doi: 10.1093/molehr/gap017
87. Yukiura H, Hama K, Nakanaga K, Tanaka M, Asaoka Y, Okudaira S, et al. Autotaxin regulates vascular development via multiple lysophosphatidic acid (LPA) receptors in zebrafish. *J Biol Chem.* (2011) 286:43972–83. doi: 10.1074/jbc.M111.301093
88. Kazlauskas A. Lysophosphatidic acid contributes to angiogenic homeostasis. *Exp Cell Res.* (2015) 333:166–70. doi: 10.1016/j.yexcr.2014.11.012
89. Chen Y, Ramakrishnan DP, Ren B. Regulation of angiogenesis by phospholipid lysophosphatidic Acid. *Front Biosci.* (2013) 18:852–61. doi: 10.2741/4148
90. Yukiura H, Kano K, Kise R, Inoue A, Aoki J. Autotaxin overexpression causes embryonic lethality and vascular defects. *PLoS ONE* (2015) 10:e0126734. doi: 10.1371/journal.pone.0126734
91. Ren H, Panchatcharam M, Mueller P, Escalante-Alcalde D, Morris AJ, Smyth SS. Lipid phosphate phosphatase (LPP3) and vascular development. *Biochim Biophys Acta* (2013) 1831:126–32. doi: 10.1016/j.bbalip.2012.07.012
92. Escalante-Alcalde D, Hernandez L, Le Stunff H, Maeda R, Lee HS, Jr Gang C, et al. The lipid phosphatase LPP3 regulates extra-embryonic vasculogenesis and axis patterning. *Development* (2003) 130:4623–37. doi: 10.1242/dev.00635
93. Offermanns S, Mancino V, Revel JP, Simon MI. Vascular system defects and impaired cell chemokinesis as a result of Galpha13 deficiency. *Science* (1997) 275:533–6. doi: 10.1126/science.275.5299.533
94. Schober A, Siess W. Lysophosphatidic acid in atherosclerotic diseases. *Br J Pharmacol.* (2012) 167:465–82. doi: 10.1111/j.1476-5381.2012.02021.x
95. Abdel-Latif A, Heron PM, Morris AJ, Smyth SS. Lysophospholipids in coronary artery and chronic ischemic heart disease. *Curr Opin Lipidol.* (2015) 26:432–7. doi: 10.1097/MOL.0000000000000226
96. Nishimura S, Nagasaki M, Okudaira S, Aoki J, Ohmori T, Ohkawa R, et al. ENPP2 contributes to adipose tissue expansion in diet-induced obesity. *Diabetes* (2014) 63:4154–64. doi: 10.2337/db13-1694
97. Federico L, Ren H, Mueller PA, Wu T, Liu S, Popovic J, et al. Autotaxin and its product lysophosphatidic acid suppress brown adipose differentiation and promote diet-induced obesity in mice. *Mol Endocrinol.* (2012) 26:786–97. doi: 10.1210/me.2011-1229
98. Rancoule C, Dusaulcy R, Treguer K, Gres S, Attane C, Saulnier-Blache JS. Involvement of autotaxin/lysophosphatidic acid signaling in obesity and impaired glucose homeostasis. *Biochimie* (2013) 96:140–3. doi: 10.1016/j.biochi.2013.04.010
99. Leblanc R, Peyruchaud O. New insights in the autotaxin/LPA axis in cancer development and metastasis. *Exp Cell Res.* (2014) 333:183–9. doi: 10.1016/j.yexcr.2014.11.010
100. Peyruchaud O, Leblanc R, David M. Pleiotropic activity of lysophosphatidic acid in bone metastasis. *Biochim Biophys Acta* (2013) 1831:99–104. doi: 10.1016/j.bbalip.2012.06.004
101. Liu S, Umezu-Goto M, Murph M, Lu Y, Liu W, Zhang F, et al. Expression of autotaxin and lysophosphatidic acid receptors increases mammary tumorigenesis, invasion, and metastases. *Cancer Cell* (2009) 15:539–50. doi: 10.1016/j.ccr.2009.03.027
102. Benesch MG, Tang X, Dewald J, Dong WF, Mackey JR, Hemmings DG, et al. Tumor-induced inflammation in mammary adipose tissue stimulates a vicious cycle of autotaxin expression and breast cancer progression. *FASEB J.* (2015) 29:3990–4000. doi: 10.1096/fj.15-274480
103. Kime C, Sakaki-Yumoto M, Goodrich L, Hayashi Y, Sami S, Derynck R, et al. Autotaxin-mediated lipid signaling intersects with LIF and BMP signaling to promote the naive pluripotency transcription factor program. *Proc Natl Acad Sci USA.* (2016) 113:12478–83. doi: 10.1073/pnas.1608564113
104. Benesch MGK, Yang Z, Tang X, Meng G, Brindley DN. Lysophosphatidate signaling: the tumor microenvironment's new nemesis. *Trends Cancer.* (2017) 3:748–52. doi: 10.1016/j.trecan.2017.09.004
105. Bickelhaupt S, Erbel C, Timke C, Wirkner U, Dadrich M, Flechsig P, et al. Effects of CTGF blockade on attenuation and reversal of radiation-induced pulmonary fibrosis. *J Natl Cancer Inst.* (2017) 109. doi: 10.1093/jnci/djw339
106. Sakai N, Chun J, Duffield JS, Lagares D, Wada T, Luster AD, et al. Lysophosphatidic acid signaling through its receptor initiates profibrotic epithelial cell fibroblast communication mediated by epithelial cell derived connective tissue growth factor. *Kidney Int.* (2017) 91:628–41. doi: 10.1016/j.kint.2016.09.030
107. Wheeler NA, Lister JA, Fuss B. The autotaxin-lysophosphatidic acid axis modulates histone acetylation and gene expression during oligodendrocyte differentiation. *J Neurosci.* (2015) 35:11399–414. doi: 10.1523/JNEUROSCI.0345-15.2015
108. Kim SE, Choo J, Yoon J, Chu JR, Bae YJ, Lee S, et al. Genome-wide analysis identifies colonic genes differentially associated with serum leptin and insulin concentrations in C57BL/6J mice fed a high-fat diet. *PLoS ONE* (2017) 12:e0171664. doi: 10.1371/journal.pone.0171664
109. Hino K, Horigome K, Nishio M, Komura S, Nagata S, Zhao C, et al. Activin-A enhances mTOR signaling to promote aberrant chondrogenesis in fibrodysplasia ossificans progressiva. *J Clin Invest.* (2017) 127:3339–52. doi: 10.1172/JCI93521
110. Schmitz K, Brunkhorst R, de Bruin N, Mayer CA, Haussler A, Ferreiros N, et al. Dysregulation of lysophosphatidic acids in multiple sclerosis and autoimmune encephalomyelitis. *Acta Neuropathol Commun.* (2017) 5:42. doi: 10.1186/s40478-017-0446-4
111. Sakai N, Nakamura M, Lipson KE, Miyake T, Kamikawa Y, Sagara A, et al. Inhibition of CTGF ameliorates peritoneal fibrosis through suppression of fibroblast and myofibroblast accumulation and angiogenesis. *Sci Rep.* (2017) 7:5392. doi: 10.1038/s41598-017-05624-2
112. Nikitopoulou I, Kaffe E, Sevastou I, Sirioti I, Samiotaki M, Madan D, et al. A metabolically-stabilized phosphonate analog of lysophosphatidic acid attenuates collagen-induced arthritis. *PLoS ONE* (2013) 8:e70941. doi: 10.1371/journal.pone.0070941
113. Bourgoin SG, Zhao C. Autotaxin and lysophospholipids in rheumatoid arthritis. *Curr Opin Investig Drugs.* (2010) 11:515–26.

114. Orosa B, Garcia S, Conde C. The Autotaxin-Lysophosphatidic acid pathway in pathogenesis of rheumatoid arthritis. *Eur J Pharmacol.* (2015) 765:228–33. doi: 10.1016/j.ejphar.2015.08.028
115. Nakasaki T, Tanaka T, Okudaira S, Hirosawa M, Umemoto E, Otani K, et al. Involvement of the lysophosphatidic acid-generating enzyme autotaxin in lymphocyte-endothelial cell interactions. *Am J Pathol.* (2008) 173:1566–76. doi: 10.2353/ajpath.2008.071153
116. Zhang Y, Chen YC, Krummel MF, Rosen SD. Autotaxin through lysophosphatidic acid stimulates polarization, motility, and transendothelial migration of naive t cells. *J Immunol.* (2012) 189:3914–24. doi: 10.4049/jimmunol.1201604
117. Bai Z, Cai L, Umemoto E, Takeda A, Tohya K, Komai Y, et al. Constitutive lymphocyte transmigration across the basal lamina of high endothelial venules is regulated by the autotaxin/lysophosphatidic acid axis. *J Immunol.* (2013) 190:2036–48. doi: 10.4049/jimmunol.1202025
118. Knowlden S, Georas SN. The Autotaxin-LPA Axis Emerges as a Novel Regulator of Lymphocyte Homing and Inflammation. *J Immunol.* (2014) 192:851–7. doi: 10.4049/jimmunol.1302831
119. Sun S, Wang R, Song J, Guan M, Li N, Zhang X, et al. Blocking gp130 signaling suppresses autotaxin expression in adipocytes and improves insulin sensitivity in diet-induced obesity. (2017) 58:2102–13. doi: 10.1194/jlr.M075655
120. Ikeda H, Yatomi Y. Autotaxin in liver fibrosis. *Clin Chim Acta* (2012) 413:1817–21. doi: 10.1016/j.cca.2012.07.014
121. Pradere JP, Gonzalez J, Klein J, Valet P, Gres S, Salant D, et al. Lysophosphatidic acid and renal fibrosis. *Biochim Biophys Acta.* (2008) 1781:582–7. doi: 10.1016/j.bbalip.2008.04.001
122. Zheng H, Högberg J, Stenius U. ATM-activated autotaxin (ATX) propagates inflammation and DNA damage in lung epithelial cells: a new mode of action for silica-induced DNA damage? *Carcinogenesis* (2017) 38:1196–206. doi: 10.1093/carcin/bgx100
123. Ganguly K, Stoeger T, Wesselkamper SC, Reinhard C, Sartor MA, Medvedovic M, et al. Candidate genes controlling pulmonary function in mice: transcript profiling and predicted protein structure. *Physiol Genomics* (2007) 31:410–21. doi: 10.1152/physiolgenomics.00260.2006
124. Funke M, Knudsen L, Lagares D, Ebener S, Probst CK, Fontaine BA, et al. Lysophosphatidic acid signaling through the lysophosphatidic acid-1 receptor is required for alveolarization. *Am J Res Cell Mol Biol.* (2016) 55:105–16. doi: 10.1165/rcmb.2015-0152OC
125. Yang Y, Mou L, Liu N, Tsao MS. Autotaxin expression in non-small-cell lung cancer. *Am J Res Cell Mol Biol.* (1999) 21:216–22. doi: 10.1165/ajrcmb.21.2.3667
126. Mouratis MA, Magkrioti C, Oikonomou N, Katsifa A, Prestwich GD, Kaffe E, et al. Autotaxin and endotoxin-induced acute lung injury. *PLoS ONE.* (2015) 10:e0133619. doi: 10.1371/journal.pone.0133619
127. Georas SN, Berdyshev E, Hubbard W, Gorshkova IA, Usatyuk PV, Saatian B, et al. Lysophosphatidic acid is detectable in human bronchoalveolar lavage fluids at baseline and increased after segmental allergen challenge. *Clin Exp Allergy* (2007) 37:311–22. doi: 10.1111/j.1365-2222.2006.02626.x
128. Park GY, Lee YG, Berdyshev E, Nyenhuis S, Du J, Fu P, et al. Autotaxin production of lysophosphatidic acid mediates allergic asthmatic inflammation. *Am J Res Crit Care Med.* (2013) 188:928–40. doi: 10.1164/rccm.201306-1014OC
129. Zhao Y, Tong J, He D, Pendyala S, Evgeny B, Chun J, et al. Role of lysophosphatidic acid receptor LPA2 in the development of allergic airway inflammation in a murine model of asthma. *Respir Res.* (2009) 10:114. doi: 10.1186/1465-9921-10-114
130. Emo J, Meednu N, Chapman TJ, Rezaee F, Balys M, Randall T, et al. Lpa2 is a negative regulator of both dendritic cell activation and murine models of allergic lung inflammation. *J Immunol.* (2012) 188:3784–90. doi: 10.4049/jimmunol.1102956
131. Cerutis DR, Nogami M, Anderson JL, Churchill JD, Romberger DJ, Rennard SI, et al. Lysophosphatidic acid and EGF stimulate mitogenesis in human airway smooth muscle cells. *Am J Physiol.* (1997) 273(1 Pt 1):L10–5. doi: 10.1152/ajplung.2002.282.1.L91
132. Toews ML, Ustinova EE, Schultz HD. Lysophosphatidic acid enhances contractility of isolated airway smooth muscle. *J Appl Physiol.* (1997) 83:1216–22. doi: 10.1152/jappl.1997.83.4.1216
133. Tager AM, LaCamera P, Shea BS, Campanella GS, Selman M, Zhao Z, et al. The lysophosphatidic acid receptor LPA1 links pulmonary fibrosis to lung injury by mediating fibroblast recruitment and vascular leak. *Nat Med.* (2008) 14:45–54. doi: 10.1038/nm1685
134. Martinez FJ, Collard HR, Pardo A, Raghu G, Richeldi L, Selman M, et al. Idiopathic pulmonary fibrosis. *Nat Rev Dis Prim.* (2017) 3:17074. doi: 10.1038/nrdp.2017.74
135. Valdes-Rives SA, Gonzalez-Arenas A. Autotaxin-Lysophosphatidic acid: from inflammation to cancer development. *Med Inflamm.* (2017) 2017:15. doi: 10.1155/2017/9173090
136. Baader M, Bretschneider T, Broermann A, Rippmann JF, Stierstorfer B, Kuttruff CA, et al. Characterisation of the properties of a selective, orally bioavailable autotaxin inhibitor in preclinical models of advanced stages of liver fibrosis. *Br J Pharmacol.* (2017) 175:693–707. doi: 10.1111/bph.14118
137. Desroy N, Housseman C, Bock X, Joncour A, Bienvenu N, Cherel L, et al. Discovery of 2-[[2-Ethyl-6-[4-[2-(3-hydroxyazetidin-1-yl)-2-oxoethyl]piperazin-1-yl]-8-methyli midazo[1,2-a]pyridin-3-yl]methylamino]-4-(4-fluorophenyl)thiazole-5-carbonitrile (GLPG1690), a first-in-class autotaxin inhibitor undergoing clinical evaluation for the treatment of idiopathic pulmonary fibrosis. *J Med Chem.* (2017) 60:3580–90. doi: 10.1021/acs.jmedchem.7b00032
138. Kato K, Ikeda H, Miyakawa S, Futakawa S, Nonaka Y, Fujiwara M, et al. Structural basis for specific inhibition of Autotaxin by a DNA aptamer. *Nat Struct Mol Biol.* (2016) 23:395–401. doi: 10.1038/nsmb.3200
139. Nikolaou A, Ninou I, Kokotou MG, Kaffe E, Afantitis A, Aidinis V, et al. Hydroxamic acids constitute a novel class of autotaxin inhibitors that exhibit *in vivo* efficacy in a pulmonary fibrosis model. *J Med Chem.* (2018) 61:3697–711. doi: 10.1021/acs.jmedchem.8b00232
140. Barbayianni E, Magrioti V, Moutevelis-Minakakis P, Kokotos G. Autotaxin inhibitors: a patent review. *Expert Opin Ther Pat.* (2013) 23:1123–32. doi: 10.1517/13543776.2013.796364
141. Nikolaou A, Kokotou MG, Limnios D, Psarra A, Kokotos G. Autotaxin inhibitors: a patent review (2012-2016). *Expert Opin Ther Pat.* (2017) 27:815–29. doi: 10.1080/13543776.2017.1323331
142. Keune WJ, Hausmann J, Bolier R, Tolenaars D, Kremer A, Heidebrecht T, et al. Steroid binding to Autotaxin links bile salts and lysophosphatidic acid signalling. *Nat Commun.* (2016) 7:11248. doi: 10.1038/ncomms11248
143. Tanaka Y, Ishitsuka Y, Hayasaka M, Yamada Y, Miyata K, Endo M, et al. The exacerbating roles of CCAAT/enhancer-binding protein homologous protein (CHOP) in the development of bleomycin-induced pulmonary fibrosis and the preventive effects of tauroursodeoxycholic acid (TUDCA) against pulmonary fibrosis in mice. *Pharmacol Res.* (2015) 99:52–62. doi: 10.1016/j.phrs.2015.05.004
144. Cao P, Aoki Y, Badri L, Walker NM, Manning CM, Lagstein A, et al. Autocrine lysophosphatidic acid signaling activates beta-catenin and promotes lung allograft fibrosis. *J Clin Inv.* (2017) 127:1517–30. doi: 10.1172/JCI88896
145. Huang LS, Fu P, Patel P, Harijith A, Sun T, Zhao Y, et al. Lysophosphatidic acid receptor-2 deficiency confers protection against bleomycin-induced lung injury and fibrosis in mice. *Am J Res Cell Mol Biol.* (2013) 49:912–22. doi: 10.1165/rcmb.2013-0070OC
146. Swaney JS, Chapman C, Correa LD, Stebbins KJ, Bundey RA, Prodanovich PC, et al. A novel, orally active LPA receptor antagonist inhibits lung fibrosis in the mouse bleomycin model. *Br J Pharmacol.* (2010) 160:1699–713. doi: 10.1111/j.1476-5381.2010.00828.x
147. Lee SC, Fujiwara Y, Liu J, Yue J, Shimizu Y, Norman DD, et al. Autotaxin, LPA receptors (1 and 5) exert disparate functions in tumor cells versus the host tissue microenvironment in melanoma invasion and metastasis. *Mol Cancer Res.* (2014) 13:174–85. doi: 10.1158/1541-7786.MCR-14-0263
148. Funke M, Zhao Z, Xu Y, Chun J, Tager AM. The lysophosphatidic acid receptor LPA1 promotes epithelial cell apoptosis after lung injury. *Am J Res Cell Mol Biol.* (2012) 46:355–64. doi: 10.1165/rcmb.2010-0155OC
149. Wynn TA. Integrating mechanisms of pulmonary fibrosis. *J Exp Med.* (2011) 208:1339–50. doi: 10.1084/jem.20110551
150. Oikonomou N, Harokopos V, Zalevsky J, Valavanis C, Kotanidou A, Szymkowski DE, et al. Soluble TNF mediates the transition from pulmonary inflammation to fibrosis. *PLoS ONE* (2006) 1:e108. doi: 10.1371/journal.pone.0000108

151. Magkrioti C, Aidinis V. ATX and LPA signalling in lung pathophysiology. *World J Respirol.* (2013) 3:77–103. doi: 10.5320/wjr.v3.i3.77
152. Cummings R, Zhao Y, Jacoby D, Spannhake EW, Ohba M, Garcia JG, et al. Protein kinase Cdelta mediates lysophosphatidic acid-induced NF-kappaB activation and interleukin-8 secretion in human bronchial epithelial cells. *J Biol Chem.* (2004) 279:41085–94. doi: 10.1074/jbc.M404045200
153. Saatian B, Zhao Y, He D, Georas SN, Watkins T, Spannhake EW, et al. Transcriptional regulation of lysophosphatidic acid-induced interleukin-8 expression and secretion by p38 MAPK and JNK in human bronchial epithelial cells. *Biochem J.* (2006) 393(Pt 3):657–68. doi: 10.1042/BJ20050791
154. Xu MY, Porte J, Knox AJ, Weinreb PH, Maher TM, Violette SM, et al. Lysophosphatidic acid induces alphavbeta6 integrin-mediated TGF-beta activation via the LPA2 receptor and the small G protein G alpha(q). *Am J Pathol.* (2009) 174:1264–79. doi: 10.2353/ajpath.2009.080160
155. Munger JS, Huang X, Kawakatsu H, Griffiths MJ, Dalton SL, Wu J, et al. The integrin alpha v beta 6 binds and activates latent TGF beta 1: a mechanism for regulating pulmonary inflammation and fibrosis. *Cell* (1999) 96:319–28. doi: 10.1016/S0092-8674(00)80545-0
156. Fernandez IE, Eickelberg O. The impact of TGF-beta on lung fibrosis: from targeting to biomarkers. *Proc Am Thorac Soc.* (2012) 9:111–6. doi: 10.1513/pats.201203-023AW
157. Ren A, Moon C, Zhang W, Sinha C, Yarlagadda S, Arora K, et al. Asymmetrical macromolecular complex formation of lysophosphatidic acid receptor 2 (LPA2) mediates gradient sensing in fibroblasts. *J Biol Chem.* (2014) 289:35757–69. doi: 10.1074/jbc.M114.595512
158. Gan X, Wang J, Wang C, Sommer E, Kozasa T, Srinivasula S, et al. PRR5L degradation promotes mTORC2-mediated PKC-delta phosphorylation and cell migration downstream of Galpha12. *Nat Cell Biol.* (2012) 14:686–96. doi: 10.1038/ncb2507
159. Berridge MJ, Bootman MD, Roderick HL. Calcium signalling: dynamics, homeostasis and remodelling. *Nat Rev Mol Cell Biol.* (2003) 4:517–29. doi: 10.1038/nrm1155
160. Janssen LJ, Mukherjee S, Ask K. Calcium homeostasis and ionic mechanisms in pulmonary fibroblasts. *Am J Res Cell Mol Biol.* (2015) 53:135–48. doi: 10.1165/rcmb.2014-0269TR
161. Kulkarni T, O'Reilly P, Antony VB, Gaggar A, Thannickal VJ. Matrix remodeling in pulmonary fibrosis and emphysema. *Am J Res Cell Mol Biol.* (2016) 54:751–60. doi: 10.1165/rcmb.2015-0166PS
162. Rahaman SO, Grove LM, Paruchuri S, Southern BD, Abraham S, Niese KA, et al. TRPV4 mediates myofibroblast differentiation and pulmonary fibrosis in mice. *J Clin Invest.* (2014) 124: 5225–38. doi: 10.1172/JCI75331
163. Meyer Zu Heringdorf D. Lysophospholipid receptor-dependent and -independent calcium signaling. *J Cell Biochem.* (2004) 92:937–48. doi: 10.1002/jcb.20107
164. Nieto-Posadas A, Picazo-Juarez G, Llorente I, Jara-Oseguera A, Morales-Lazaro S, Escalante-Alcalde D, et al. Lysophosphatidic acid directly activates TRPV1 through a C-terminal binding site. *Nat Chem Biol.* (2011) 8:78–85. doi: 10.1038/nchembio.712
165. Farkas L, Kolb M. Pulmonary microcirculation in interstitial lung disease. *Proc Am Thorac Soc.* (2011) 8:516–21. doi: 10.1513/pats.201101-007MW
166. Van Der Aar EM, Fagard L, Desrivot J, Dupont S, Heckmann B, Blanque R, et al. Favorable human safety, pharmacokinetics and pharmacodynamics of the autotaxin inhibitor GLPG1690, a potential new treatment in idiopathic pulmonary fibrosis. A103 IPF: More about therapy and outcomes. In: *American Thoracic Society International Conference Abstracts: American Thoracic Society*, San Francisco, CA (2016). p. A2701.

17

Myeloid Fbxw7 Prevents Pulmonary Fibrosis by Suppressing TGF-β Production

Jia He[1,2†], *Yue Du*[1,2†], *Gaopeng Li*[1,2†], *Peng Xiao*[1,2], *Xingzheng Sun*[1,2], *Wenjun Song*[1,2], *Lihua Lai*[1,2], *Meng Xia*[1,2], *Jianhua Zhang*[3*] and *Qingqing Wang*[1,2*]

[1] Institute of Immunology, Zhejiang University School of Medicine, Hangzhou, China, [2] The Key Laboratory for Immunity and Inflammatory Diseases of Zhejiang Province, Hangzhou, China, [3] Department of Medical Laboratory, School of Medicine, Shaoxing University, Shaoxing, China

***Correspondence:**
Qingqing Wang
wqq@zju.edu.cn
Jianhua Zhang
sxzjh1018@126.com

[†]These authors have contributed equally to this work and share first authorship

Idiopathic pulmonary fibrosis (IPF) is a group of chronic interstitial pulmonary diseases characterized by an inexorable decline in lung function with limited treatment options. The abnormal expression of transforming growth factor-β (TGF-β) in profibrotic macrophages is linked to severe pulmonary fibrosis, but the regulation mechanisms of TGF-β expression are incompletely understood. We found that decreased expression of E3 ubiquitin ligase *Fbxw7* in peripheral blood mononuclear cells (PBMCs) was significantly related to the severity of pulmonary fibrosis in IPF patients. Fbxw7 is identified to be a crucial suppressing factor for pulmonary fibrosis development and progression in a mouse model induced by intratracheal bleomycin treatment. Myeloid cell-specific *Fbxw7* deletion increases pulmonary monocyte-macrophages accumulation in lung tissue, and eventually promotes bleomycin-induced collagen deposition and progressive pulmonary fibrosis. Notably, the expression of TGF-β in profibrotic macrophages was significantly upregulated in myeloid cell-specific *Fbxw7* deletion mice after bleomycin treatment. C-Jun has long been regarded as a critical transcription factor of *Tgfb1*, we clarified that Fbxw7 inhibits the expression of TGF-β in profibrotic macrophages by interacting with c-Jun and mediating its K48-linked ubiquitination and degradation. These findings provide insight into the role of Fbxw7 in the regulation of macrophages during the pathogenesis of pulmonary fibrosis.

Keywords: IPF - idiopathic pulmonary fibrosis, TGF-β, Fbxw7, macrophage, c-Jun

INTRODUCTION

Idiopathic pulmonary fibrosis (IPF) is a lung disease characterized by fibroblast hyperproliferation and extracellular matrix (ECM) deposition (1), which can cause pulmonary fibrosis and eventually lead to respiratory failure. However, the etiology of IPF remains unclear. Transforming growth factor-β (TGF-β) is one of the best-characterized pro-fibrotic factors (2). In mammals, there are three isoforms of TGF-β (TGF-β1, TGF-β2, and TGF-β3), of which TGF-β1 most closely related to the development of IPF (2). Disturbances of the pulmonary microenvironment induced by TGF-β are critical to promote the recruitment of circulating fibrocytes and bone marrow–derived progenitor cells to the lung (3), and enhance the pro-fibrotic capacities of these cells or induce their differentiation into activated myofibroblasts (4), eventually leading to the typical IPF symptoms like ECM deposition and abnormal collagen accumulation (5). Moreover, TGF-β1 induces macrophage recruitment and stimulates the expression of several pro-inflammatory and profibrogenic cytokines in macrophages, such as TNF-α and IL-1β (5). IPF patients have much higher TGF-β1 mRNA expression in profibrotic macrophages compared to normal volunteers (6, 7). Previous studies have reported that TGF-β1 expression can be induced by cytokines, such as IL-1β, TNF-α (8), IL-13 (9, 10) and IL-24 (11), the increased generation of ROS also induces TGF-β1 production (12). Moreover, the activation of TGF-β1 in fibrotic disorders can be induced by multiple factors, such as matrix metalloproteinases (MMP) 3 and MMP9 (13), thrombospodin-1 (14) and integrins $\alpha_V\beta_6$ (15). TGF-β1 signaling pathways and their downstream signal transduction mechanisms have been extensively studied, but there are few reports involved in the regulation mechanism of TGF-β1 expression.

Pulmonary macrophages derived from blood monocytes and classified into $CD64^+SiglecF^+$ alveolar macrophages (AMs) and $CD11b^+CD206^+$ interstitial macrophages (IMs) based on the different anatomical locations (16), both of those macrophage subsets derived from blood monocytes have been known to play a crucial role in IPF pathogenesis. Pulmonary macrophages polarized into alternatively activated anti-inflammatory phenotypes to promote tissue repair and fibrosis after lung injury (17). Aberrant immune function of anti-inflammatory macrophages present profibrogenic phenotypes, which induce the dysfunction of wound repair and accumulate in fibrotic lung, further support fibrogenesis of lung by generating reactive oxygen species (ROS) (6), contributing to collagen synthesis and ECM remodeling. Increased accumulation of profibrotic AMs have been detected in lung of IPF patients (6). During lung fibrogenesis, profibrotic macrophages release soluble factors to create and sustain the profibrotic lung microenvironment (18–20), such as TGF-β1, CCL8 (21), IGF-I (22), PDGF (23), and arginase 1 (24). In contrast, loss of profibrotic macrophages promotes the resolution of established pulmonary fibrosis (25) and the reduction of lung collagen deposition (26). Importantly, in rodents with bleomycin-induced lung fibrosis, pulmonary macrophages have been demonstrated to be the predominant source of profibrogenic mediator TGF-β (27). However, the specific mechanism of TGF-β1 secreted by macrophages in the pathogenesis of IPF is remain poorly understood.

F-box and WD repeat domain–containing 7 (Fbxw7) is a member of the F-box protein family, which is a component of the SKP1-cullin-F-box-protein (SCF) ubiquitin ligase complex. Many studies have shown that Fbxw7 is a tumor suppressor by targeting c-Myc, Notch, MCL1 and c-Jun (28). Fbxw7 mutation was detected in squamous cell carcinoma developed on IPF (29). Fbxw7 also participates in the regulation of Parkinson's disease (30) and circadian rhythm (31). Moreover, Fbxw7 controls neural stem cell differentiation (32) and myelination (33). Fbxw7 has immunoregulatory capacities, it controls effector T cell polyfunctionality and survival in tumor environment by inhibiting Notch activation (34). Our previous studies have shown that Fbxw7 enhances antiviral innate immune response (35) and aggravate intestinal inflammation (36). These observations implicate that Fbxw7 may act as a transducer of tissue microenvironment, regulating the plastic function of macrophages. In this work, we further investigated the function of Fbxw7 in pulmonary macrophages during the pathogenesis of IPF. Our findings demonstrate that *Fbxw7* expression decreased significantly in peripheral blood mononuclear cells (PBMCs) of IPF patients and lung tissues of the mice model of bleomycin-induced fibrosis. *Fbxw7* deletion in myeloid cells increased the release of fibrogenic factors and the recruitment of monocytes into lung tissues. In terms of the mechanism, the *Fbxw7* deletion promoted the TGF-β expression in macrophages through reducing c-Jun ubiquitination, thereby aggravating the severity of pulmonary fibrosis.

MATERIALS AND METHODS

Mice Information

$Fbxw7^{fl/fl}$ mice (C57BL/6J background) were obtained from Jackson Laboratories. *LysM-Cre* mice C57BL/6J were kindly provided by Dr. Ximei Wu (Zhejiang University School of Medicine, Hangzhou, China). $LysM^+Fbxw7^{fl/fl}$ mice were generated by crossing $Fbxw7^{f/f}$ mice with *LysM-Cre* transgenic mice as previously described (36). All mice were bred at the laboratory animal center of Zhejiang University under specific pathogen-free conditions. In all experiments, age-matched (8-12 week) mice were randomized into the experimental or control groups. All animal experiments were performed according to the protocol approved by the Animal Ethics Committee of Zhejiang University and were in compliance with institutional guidelines.

Cell Culture and DNA Transfection

Bone marrow cells were isolated by flushing femurs and tibias of 6- to 8-week-old mice with PBS and differentiated into BMDMs in RPMI-1640 medium with 10% (vol/vol) FCS and 10 ng/ml recombinant mouse M-CSF (R&D, 416-ML). To induce M2 macrophages, BMDMs were stimulated by adding the recombinant mouse IL-4 (30 ng/ml, PeproTech, 214-14). Proteasome inhibitors MG132 (M8699), protein synthesis inhibitor CHX (C4859), and JNK inhibitor SP600125 (420119) were from Sigma-Aldrich. TGF-β neutralizing antibody (MAB1835) and mouse IgG1 isotype control (MAB002) were from R&D systems.

Mouse embryonic fibroblast cell line (MEF) was obtained from American Type Culture Collection (ATCC) and maintained in Dulbecco's modified Eagle medium (DMEM) with 10% fetal bovine serum (FBS; BI). Murine macrophage-like RAW264.7 cells were cultured in RPMI 1640 medium with 10% fetal bovine serum (FBS; BI), 100 U/ml penicillin and 100 mg/ml streptomycin in an atmosphere of humidified 5% CO_2 at 37°C.

Recombinant vectors encoding mouse c-Jun (NM_010591) were cloned into pcDNA3.1-c-Myc eukaryotic expression vector. The RAW264.7 cells (3×10^5 cells/well, in 24-well plate) were incubated with NATE™ (*In vivo*gen, lyec-nate) for 30 min to enhance the transfection efficiency and transient expression of target plasmid. Then RAW264.7 cells were transfected with c-Jun plasmid (Roche, FuGENE HD Reagent) and treated with IL-4 for the indicated time.

Co-Culture Experiments

MEF cells (2×10^5) were cultured in the lower chamber and macrophages (5×10^5) were added to the upper chamber of a 12-well transwell apparatus (0.4 mm pore size, Costar, Cambridge, MA). The MEF were subjected to the further analysis at 48 h after co-culturing.

Induction of Pulmonary Fibrosis

An experimental pulmonary fibrosis model was established using the direct endotracheal injection of bleomycin (37). Briefly, 6- to 8-week-old C57BL/6 mice were anesthetized with pentobarbital by intraperitoneal injections. Neck area of mice was sterilized using povidone-iodine swabs after depilation of hairs, and 1 cm midline incision was made with sterile scissors. Intratracheal administration of 3.5 mg/kg bleomycin hydrochloride (Hisun-Pfizer Pharmaceuticals, Taizhou, China) in sterile PBS, an equal volume of sterile PBS for controls by using 1 ml syringe fitted with a 26 G needle (carefully insert the needle into the visualized trachea and rapidly inject the bleomycin solution during a single inspiration). The incision was closed with surgical sutures after withdrawing the needle. The mice were placed on warmer pads and monitored until fully awake. Mouse lung tissues were sacrificed at 14 days and 21 days post-bleomycin injection for subsequent experiments.

LPS induced pulmonary injury model (38, 39) were established using the direct endotracheal injection of 5 mg/kg LPS (Sigma-Aldrich, St. Louis, Missouri, USA). Mouse lung tissues were sacrificed at 10 days post-LPS injection for subsequent experiments.

Flow Cytometry

Cells were stained with fluorochrome-labeled mAbs and analyzed with an LSRII flow cytometer (BD). Flow cytometric analysis was performed using FlowJo software. The following fluorochrome-labeled mAbs were purchased from Biolegend, Inc. and used according to the manufacturers' protocols: anti-CD11b-FITC (101205, RRID: AB_312788), anti-CD206-APC (141707, RRID: AB_10896057), anti-Ly6C-APC-Cy7 (128026, RRID: AB_10640120), anti-Ly6G-PE (127608, RRID: AB_1186099), anti-F4/80-Brilliant Violet 421 (123132, RRID: AB_11203717), anti-CD64-PE (139303, RRID: AB_10613467), and anti-Siglec-F-APC (155507, RRID: AB_2750236).

Immunoprecipitation and Immunoblot Analysis

Immunoprecipitation, SDS-PAGE and immunoblot analysis were performed according to a standard protocol as described previously (35). The following antibodies were used according to the manufacturers' protocols: anti-Fbxw7 (Abcam, ab12292, RRID: AB_442966), anti-Lys48-specific linked polyubiquitin (MilliporeSigma, 05-1307, RRID: AB_1587578), anti-c-Jun (CST, #9165S, RRID: AB_2130165), anti-p65 (CST, #8242, RRID: AB_10859369), anti-p-p65 (CST, #3036, RRID: AB_331281), Collagen-I(Abcam, ab34710, RRID: AB_731684), Collagen-III (Abcam, ab7778, RRID: AB_306066), EGR-1 (CST, #4154S, RRID: AB_2097035). The PVDF membranes were incubated with corresponding primary antibodies followed by horseradish peroxidase-linked secondary antibodies. The images were developed and captured using Chemiluminescence imaging system (ChemiScope 3000 Mini, Clinx Science Instruments Co., Ltd). Relative quantities of target protein were determined comparing to β-actin expression using densitometric analysis (ImageJ 1.52v). The standard deviation was calculated for biological duplicates.

Lung Histology

Lungs from bleomycin-treated or control mice were dissected, fixed in 10% phosphate-buffered formalin, and embedded into paraffin. Tissue sections were stained with H&E for morphological analysis and with Masson's trichrome for the detection of collagen fibers according to the manufacturers' instructions (Nanjing Jiancheng, Nanjing, China). The Szapiel's score was used to evaluate the severity of fibrosis using the following criteria (40): none (0), no evidence of fibrosis; mild (1), <20% of the lung affected; moderate (2), 20%–50% affected; severe (3), >50% affected.

Hydroxyproline Assay

To assess collagen synthesis in the lung, pulmonic hydroxyproline levels were determined using a hydroxyproline assay kit obtained from Jiancheng Bioengineering Institute (Nanjing, China), according to manufacturer's instructions. Hydroxyproline content was expressed as μg/mg lung wet weight.

Quantitative RT-PCR

Total RNA was extracted from tissues or cells using RNAiso Plus (TakaRa), and then reversely transcribed to cDNA using the PrimeScript RT reagent kit (TaKaRa) with random primers according to the manufacturer's instructions. Quantitative PCR was performed using KAPA SYBR Green (SYBR Green Fast qPCR Master Mix) on CFX96 Touch™ Real-Time PCR Detection System (BioRad). Expression data were normalized to the mRNA levels of the β-actin gene and calculated using the $2^{-\Delta\Delta Ct}$ method (41). The sequences for primers were listed in **Supplementary Table 1**.

ELISA

The levels of mouse TGF-β in bronchoalveolar lavage fluid (BALF) or culture supernatants were measured with ELISA kits (Invitrogen, 88-8350-88) according to the manufacturer's instructions.

Statistical Analysis

Statistical analysis was performed with GraphPad Prism 7.0. All data are shown as mean ± SD. The comparisons of two experimental groups were determined using an unpaired, 2-tailed student's t-test. Multiple comparisons were assessed by one-way ANOVA with Tukey's multiple comparisons test. P-values less than 0.05 were considered significant.

RESULTS

Decreased Expression of *Fbxw7* Is Related to IPF

We first investigated whether Fbxw7 was related to the development of IPF, the expression level of *Fbxw7* from IPF patients was analyzed in the data from Gene Expression Omnibus (GEO) database (GSE70867) (42). The result showed that *Fbxw7* mRNA expression in bronchoalveolar lavage (BAL) cells of IPF patients was significantly lower than that in healthy controls (**Figure 1A**). In another database of microarray expression profiling of PBMCs from IPF patients in the training cohort (GSE132607) (43), *Fbxw7* mRNA expression level in 12-months IPF patients was significantly lower than that in baseline, 4-months, and 8-months IPF patients (**Figure 1B**). We then used the bleomycin-induced mouse model of pulmonary fibrosis to observe the expression of *Fbxw7* in lung tissues (**Figure 1C**) and peripheral blood monocytes (**Figure 1D**). qRT-PCR results showed that the expression level of *Fbxw7* was significantly reduced after 21 days of intratracheal bleomycin administration compared to the PBS controls. Moreover, the expression of *Fbxw7* in the macrophages in mice pulmonary fibrosis tissue was markedly decreased compared with those in healthy control subjects detected by immunofluorescence staining (**Figure 1E**). These results suggest that the decreased expression of Fbxw7 is associated with the formation of pulmonary fibrosis.

Myeloid Deficiency of *Fbxw7* Aggravates Bleomycin-Induced Collagen Deposition in Lung Tissue

Augmented collagen deposition within the interstitium (44, 45) and the remodeling of ECM (46) are recognized as one of the primordial pathophysiological events of IPF. To investigate the role of Fbxw7 in macrophages in the pathogenesis of IPF, we generated LysM-Cre^{+}Fbxw7$^{fl/fl}$ (*LysM*$^{+}$*Fbxw7*$^{fl/fl}$) mice (**Supplementary Figure 1A**) and confirmed that myeloid

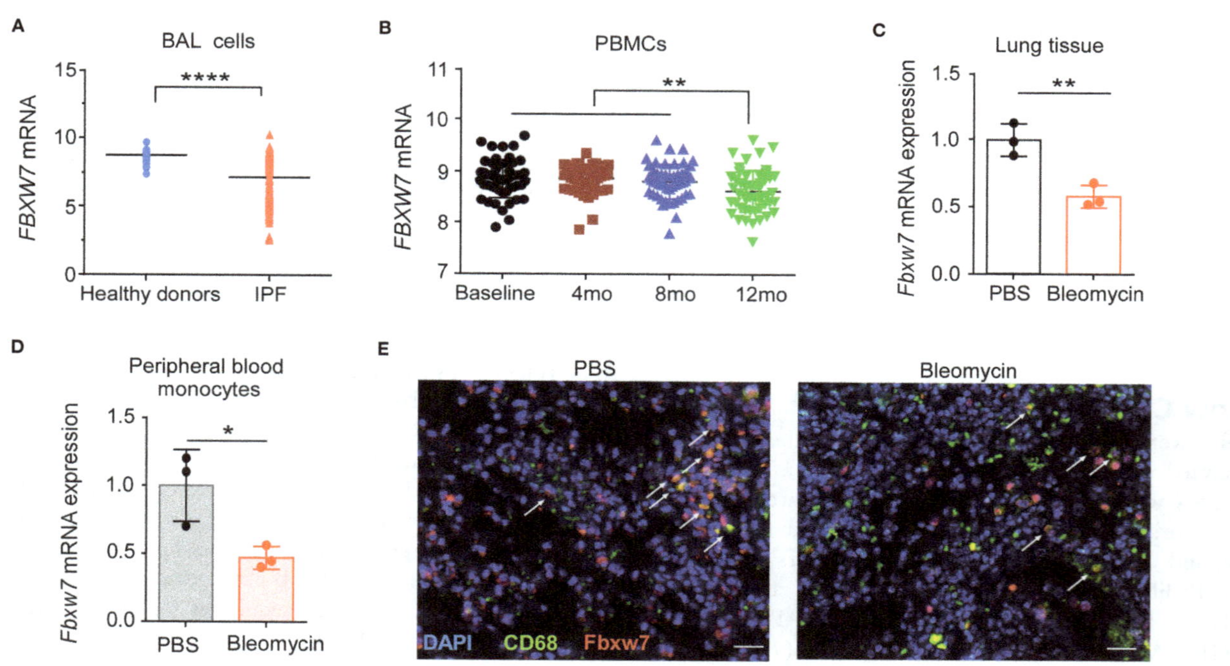

FIGURE 1 | Decreased Fbxw7 expression is related to pulmonary fibrosis. **(A)** Fbxw7 mRNA expression in bronchoalveolar lavage (BAL) cells from healthy donors (n=48) and from IPF patients (n=176), the data were collected from GEO database (GSE70867), P value was obtained using two-tailed Student's t test, ****P < 0.0001. **(B)** *Fbxw7* mRNA expression in PBMCs from baseline (n=74), 4 months (4 mo, n=74), 8 months (8 mo, n=68) and 12 months (12 mo, n=60) IPF patients, the data were collected from the GEO database (GSE132607). Statistical significance was assessed by one-way ANOVA with Tukey's multiple comparisons test, **P < 0.01. qRT-PCR analysis of lung tissues **(C)** and peripheral blood monocytes **(D)** obtained from mice after 21 days of bleomycin-induced lung injury and healthy controls. Data are expressed as mean ± SD of biological duplicates (n=3) and are representative of three independent experiments. P value was obtained using two-tailed Student's t test, *P < 0.05, **P < 0.01. **(E)** Immunofluorescence staining for FBXW7 (red), CD68 (green), and DAPI for nuclei (blue) in lung tissues obtained from mice after 21 days of bleomycin-induced lung injury and healthy control mice. Scale bars: 20 μm. Data shown are the representative of three independent experiments.

specific deletion of *Fbxw7* does not affect the differentiation and development of myeloid cells (**Supplementary Figures 1B-F**).

*LysM⁺Fbxw7^fl/fl^* mice and their *Fbxw7^fl/fl^* littermates were subjected to establish experimental pulmonary fibrosis model. Masson staining of lung tissues showed that collagen deposition was significantly increased in *LysM⁺Fbxw7^fl/fl^* mice 14 days after bleomycin administration, compared with *Fbxw7^fl/fl^ mice* (**Supplemental Figure 2A**), and further increased after 21 days (**Figure 2A**). Szapiel scores also showed that Fbxw7 knockout exacerbated the degree of fibrosis (**Supplemental Figure 2B** and **Figure 2B**). The expression of collagen III and α-SMA observed by immune-histochemical staining was also significantly higher in the fibrotic lung tissue of *LysM⁺Fbxw7^fl/fl^* mice compared with *Fbxw7^fl/fl^* littermates (**Figure 2C**). Furthermore, *LysM⁺Fbxw7^fl/fl^* mice had significantly higher levels of hydroxyproline in lung tissues compared with *Fbxw7^fl/fl^* mice (**Figure 2D**).

Moreover, we examined the mRNA expression levels of collagen-related genes in the lung tissues after bleomycin administration. Fibronectin 1 (Fn1), a pro-fibrotic marker, is an important member of the fibronectin family (47). Col1α1 and

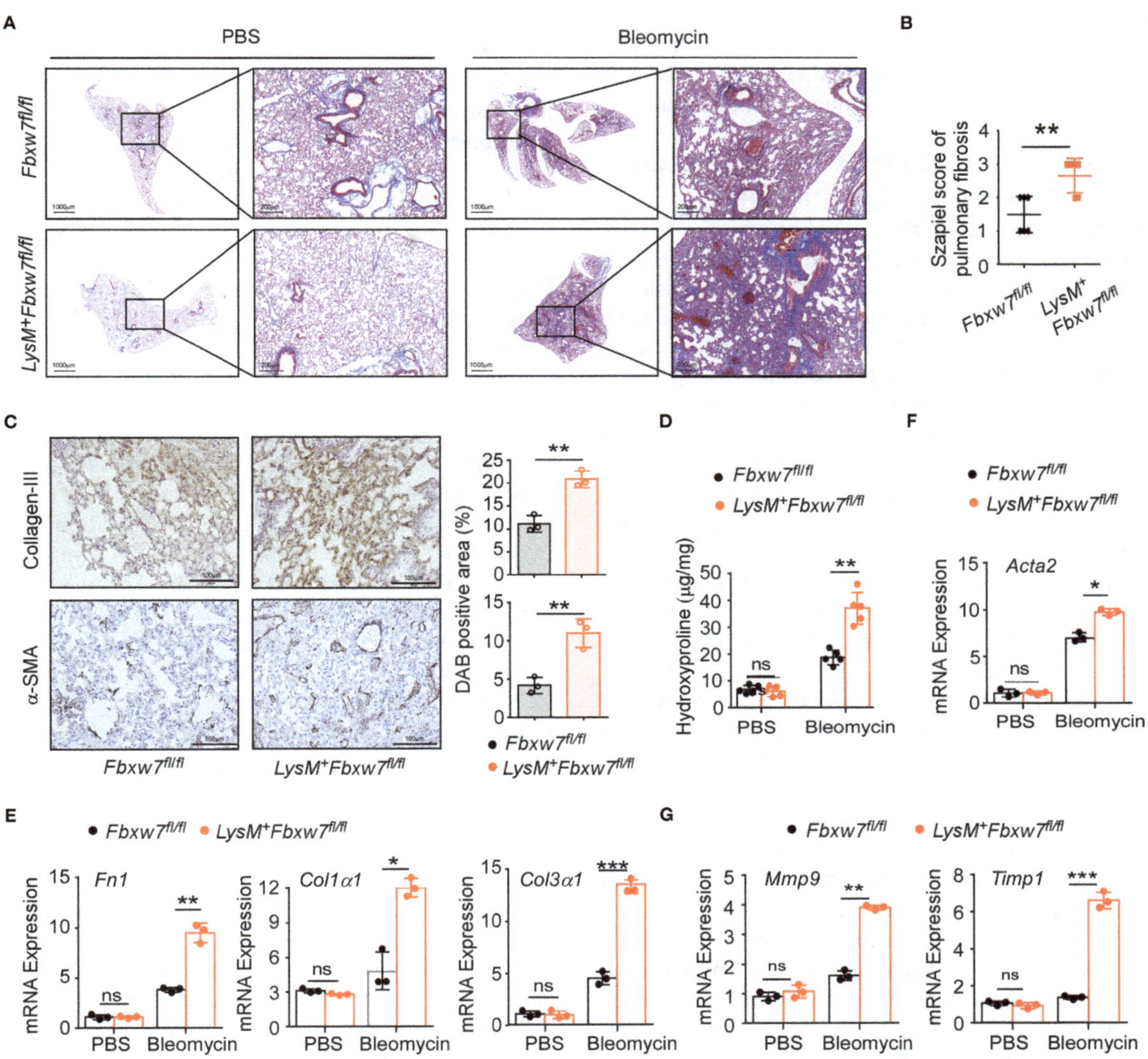

FIGURE 2 | *LysM⁺Fbxw7^fl/fl^* mice show aggravated pulmonary fibrosis. *Fbxw7^fl/fl^* and *LysM⁺Fbxw7^fl/fl^* mice were administered bleomycin by direct endotracheal injection to induce pulmonary fibrosis. Three weeks later, lung tissues were isolated for Masson staining and RT-PCR analysis. **(A)** Masson staining of collagen fiber, scale bars 1000 μm (whole pulmonary section), and 200 μm (detail) and sapiel score of pulmonary tissue **(B)** obtained from *Fbxw7^fl/fl^* and *LysM⁺Fbxw7^fl/fl^* mice. **(C)** Representative collagen III and α-SMA immunohistochemical staining of lung tissues obtained from *Fbxw7^fl/fl^* and *LysM⁺Fbxw7^fl/fl^* mice after 21 days of bleomycin-induced lung injury, scale bars 100 μm. Comparison of DAB staining intensity (Image J) among the groups is shown. Quantification of hydroxyproline contents **(D)** and relative mRNA expression of collagen genes **(E)**, Acta2 gene (α-SMA) **(F)**, and matrix metalloproteinases **(G)** in the lungs from *Fbxw7^fl/fl^* and *LysM⁺Fbxw7^fl/fl^* mice after bleomycin treatment for 21 days. Data are expressed as mean ± SD of biological duplicates (n≥3) and are the representative of three independent experiments. P values were obtained using two-tailed Student's *t* test. *$P < 0.05$, **$P < 0.01$, ***$P < 0.001$, ns, not significant.

Col3α1 is component of the ECM in IPF. qRT-PCR results showed that the expression of *Fn1* and *Col3α1* increased significantly in *LysM⁺Fbxw7^fl/fl^* mice (**Supplemental Figure 2C** and **Figure 2E**). Furthermore, as a surface molecular marker of myofibroblasts, the mRNA expression of α-smooth muscle actin (*α-SMA* or *Acta2*) was also significantly increased in $LysM^+Fbxw7^{fl/fl}$ mice (**Supplemental Figure 2D** and **Figure 2F**). Matrix metalloproteinases (MMPs) and their specific inhibitors (tissue inhibitors of metalloproteinases, TIMPs) participate in the formation and degradation of ECM, and the imbalance between MMPs and TIMPs plays a pivotal role in pulmonary fibrosis pathogenesis. qRT-PCR results demonstrated that *Fbxw7* deletion significantly increased the expression of *Mmp9* and *Timp1* (**Figure 2G**). These results suggest that the myeloid cell specific *Fbxw7* knockout mice have increased collagen deposition in their lung tissue that may aggravate the degree of fibrosis induced by bleomycin.

Myeloid Deficiency of *Fbxw7* Aggravates Bleomycin-Induced Lung Injury and Monocytes Recruitment

Tissue damage and inflammation are important triggers for pulmonary fibrosis (48). To determine whether *Fbxw7* deletion in myeloid cells aggravates lung injury and inflammation, we evaluated the morphological characteristics in mouse lung tissues. The H & E staining results showed that the lung tissues of $Lysm^+Fbxw7^{fl/fl}$ mice were more severely damaged 14 days (**Supplemental Figure 3A**) and 21 days (**Figure 3A**) after bleomycin administration. Lung tissues of $LysM^+Fbxw7^{fl/fl}$ mice appeared to be denser, congestion and edema, as well as loss of alveolar structures compared with $Fbxw7^{fl/fl}$ mice. Moreover, we examined the mRNA expression of surfactant protein-D (*Sftpd*) and qRT-PCR results showed that myeloid deficiency of *Fbxw7* resulted in higher levels of *Sftpd* in fibrotic lung tissues (**Supplemental Figure 3B** and **Figure 3B**).

Furthermore, $LysM^+Fbxw7^{fl/fl}$ mice had higher degree of inflammatory cell infiltration in the alveolar space observed by H & E staining (**Figure 3A**). Flow cytometric analysis was used to investigate the changes in mononuclear phagocyte subpopulations in bronchoalveolar lavage fluid (BALF) and lung tissue during pulmonary fibrosis development. After 21 days of bleomycin-induced pulmonary fibrosis in mice, *Fbxw7* knockout did not increase $CD64^+SiglecF^+$ AMs accumulation (**Supplemental Figure 3C**), but significantly increased $CD11b^+Ly6C^+$ monocytes recruitment (**Figure 3C**) in BALF. Moreover, a single-cell suspension was prepared by digesting lung tissues and analyzed by flow cytometry. Compared with the PBS group, the percentages of $CD11b^+CD206^+$ IMs (**Figure 3D**) and $CD11b^+Ly6C^+$ monocytes (**Figure 3E**) in lung tissues of mice treated with bleomycin were increased. Importantly, $LysM^+Fbxw7^{fl/fl}$ mice showed an obviously increased accumulation of IM and monocyte cell populations compared with $Fbxw7^{fl/fl}$ littermates (**Figures 3D, E**). These results suggest that the deletion of *Fbxw7* exacerbates injury-induced lung fibrosis by promoting the recruitment and accumulation of mononuclear phagocytes.

Fbxw7 Deficiency Upregulates TGF-β Expression in Macrophages

Macrophages are the major source of multiple profibrotic mediators in pulmonary fibrosis (49). We next investigated whether myeloid *Fbxw7* deletion altered the cytokine profile in fibrotic lung tissues. The qRT-PCR results showed that the mRNA expressions of *Tnf-α*, and *Il1β* in lung tissues of $LysM^+Fbxw7^{fl/fl}$ mice was significantly higher than that of $Fbxw7^{fl/fl}$ mice 14 days after bleomycin administration, but the expression of *Il6* and *Il10* was not significantly different (**Supplemental Figure 4A**). In contrast, $LysM^+Fbxw7^{fl/fl}$ mice had significantly higher levels of *Il6* and *Il1β*, but not *Tnf-α* and *Il10*, compared with $Fbxw7^{fl/fl}$ mice 21 days after administration of bleomycin (**Supplemental Figure 4B**). Furthermore, we evaluated cytokines expression in alveolar macrophages and found that the mRNA expressions of *Il1β*, *Tnf-α*, *Il6* and *Il10* were significantly increased after bleomycin administration, however, there were no significant differences in the expression level between $LysM^+Fbxw7^{fl/fl}$ mice and $Fbxw7^{fl/fl}$ littermates (**Figure 4A**). Interestingly, mRNA expression of *Tgfb1*, the macrophage-derived fibrogenic cytokine, was significantly increased in lung tissues and alveolar macrophages in $LysM^+Fbxw7^{fl/fl}$ mice compared to $Fbxw7^{fl/fl}$ littermates (**Figure 4B**). ELISA further confirmed that the concentration of TGF-β protein in BALF from $LysM^+Fbxw7^{fl/fl}$ mice was significantly higher than that from $Fbxw7^{fl/fl}$ littermates (**Figure 4C**). In lung injury model established by LPS, more severe lung injury, fibrosis associated collagen deposition as well as higher expression of *Tgfb1* were found in lung tissue and BAL cells from $LysM^+Fbxw7^{fl/fl}$ mice compared to $Fbxw7^{fl/fl}$ littermates (**Supplemental Figures 4C, D** and **Figure 4D**). The significantly elevated concentration of TGF-β protein in BALF and serum from $LysM^+Fbxw7^{fl/fl}$ mice was observed by ELISA compared with that from $Fbxw7^{fl/fl}$ littermates (**Figure 4E**). These data suggest that deficiency of *Fbxw7* in macrophages exacerbates pulmonary fibrosis, which may be related to the up-regulation of TGF-β expression.

IL-4, as a Th2 cytokine, was reported to induce TGF-β expression in profibrotic macrophage to activate fibroblasts and promotes extensive tissue fibrosis (50, 51). qRT-PCR confirmed that the expression of *Il4* was abundant in fibrotic lung tissues, but the level of *Il4* was similar between $LysM^+Fbxw7^{fl/fl}$ mice and their $Fbxw7^{fl/fl}$ littermates (**Supplemental Figure 4E**). Next, we performed a Transwell co-culture assay to evaluate the profibrogenic capability of macrophages from $LysM^+Fbxw7^{fl/fl}$ mice and $Fbxw7^{fl/fl}$ littermates after IL-4 treatment *in vitro* (**Figure 4F**), the results consistently showed that myeloid *Fbxw7* deficiency resulted in higher secretion levels of TGF-β in co-cultured macrophages after IL-4 treatment (**Figure 4G**), *Fbxw7* deficient macrophages treated with IL-4 mediates a higher activation of co-cultured fibroblasts by the examination of the expression levels of collagen-I and collagen-III through western blot (**Figure 4H**). To further confirm that the enhanced profibrogenic capability of macrophages from $LysM^+Fbxw7^{fl/fl}$ mice is TGF-β-dependent, transwell co-culture assay was performed after IL-4 treatment with or without TGF-β neutralizing antibody. Neutralization of TGF-β abrogated the

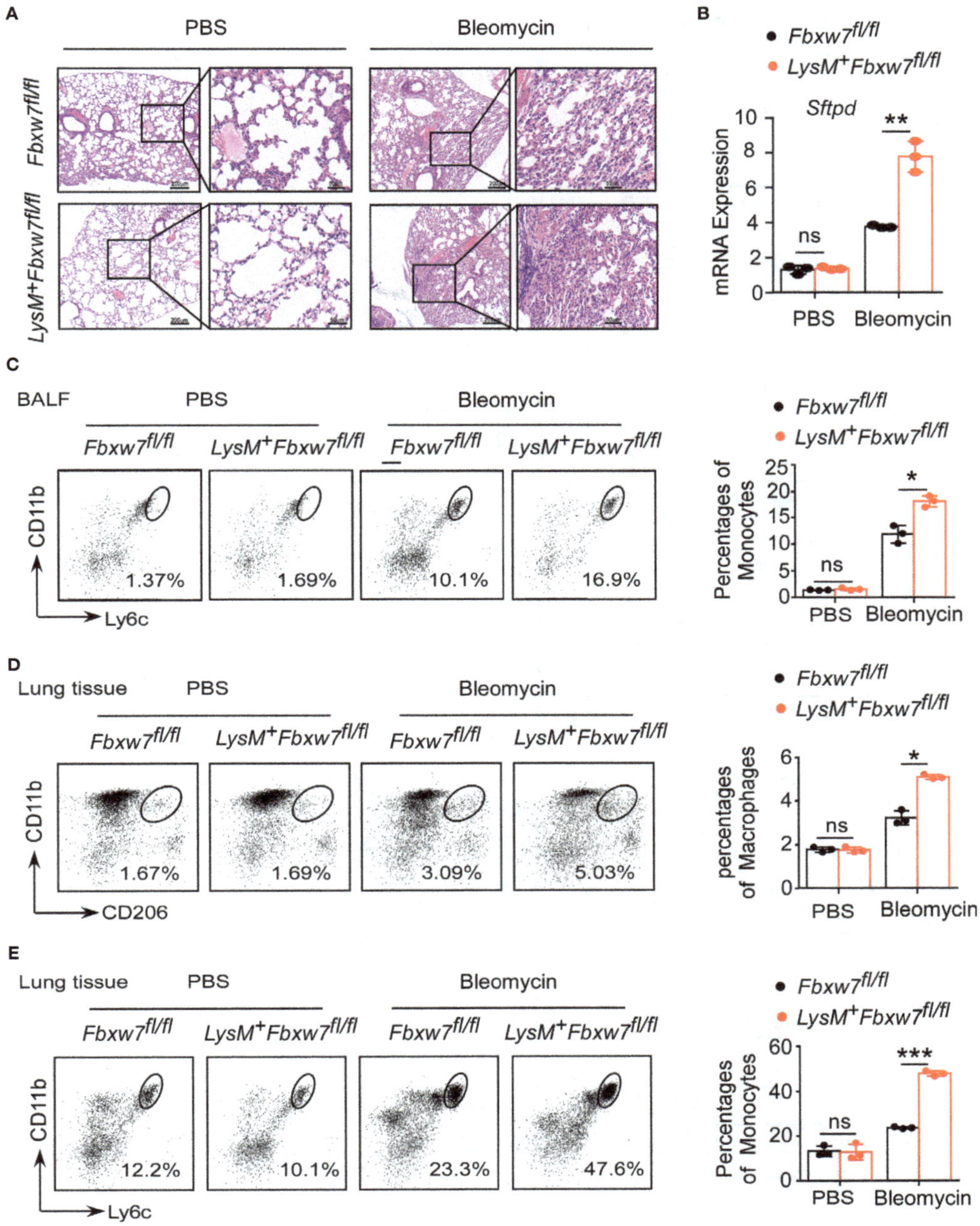

FIGURE 3 | *Fbxw7* deficiency increases recruitment of monocytes and macrophages after bleomycin-induced lung injury. *Fbxw7$^{fl/fl}$* and *LysM^{+}Fbxw7$^{fl/fl}$* mice were administered PBS or bleomycin for 21 days to induce pulmonary fibrosis. **(A)** H&E staining of lung sections, scale bars 200 μm (whole pulmonary section), and 50 μm (detail). **(B)** qRT-PCR analysis of relative expression of *Sftpd* in lung tissue. Flow cytometry and statistical analysis of the percentage of CD11b^{+}Ly6C^{+} monocytes in bronchoalveolar lavage fluid (BALF) **(C)**, CD11b^{+}CD206^{+} IMs **(D)** and CD11b^{+}Ly6C^{+} monocytes **(E)** in lung tissues, data are expressed as mean ± SD of biological duplicates (n=3) and are the representative of three independent experiments. P values were obtained using two-tailed Student's *t* test. $^{*}P < 0.05$, $^{**}P < 0.01$, $^{***}P < 0.001$, ns, not significant.

difference of profibrogenic ability between *LysM^{+}Fbxw7$^{fl/fl}$* macrophages and *Fbxw7$^{fl/fl}$* macrophages (**Figure 4I**). Collectively, these data further support that *Fbxw7* deletion in myeloid cells can exacerbate bleomycin-induced production of TGF-β and promote the development of pulmonary fibrosis.

Fbxw7 Regulates TGF-β Expression by Mediating the Ubiquitination and Degradation of c-Jun

Transcription factors including early growth response protein 1 (EGR-1) (52, 53) and NF-κB (54) have been reported to be

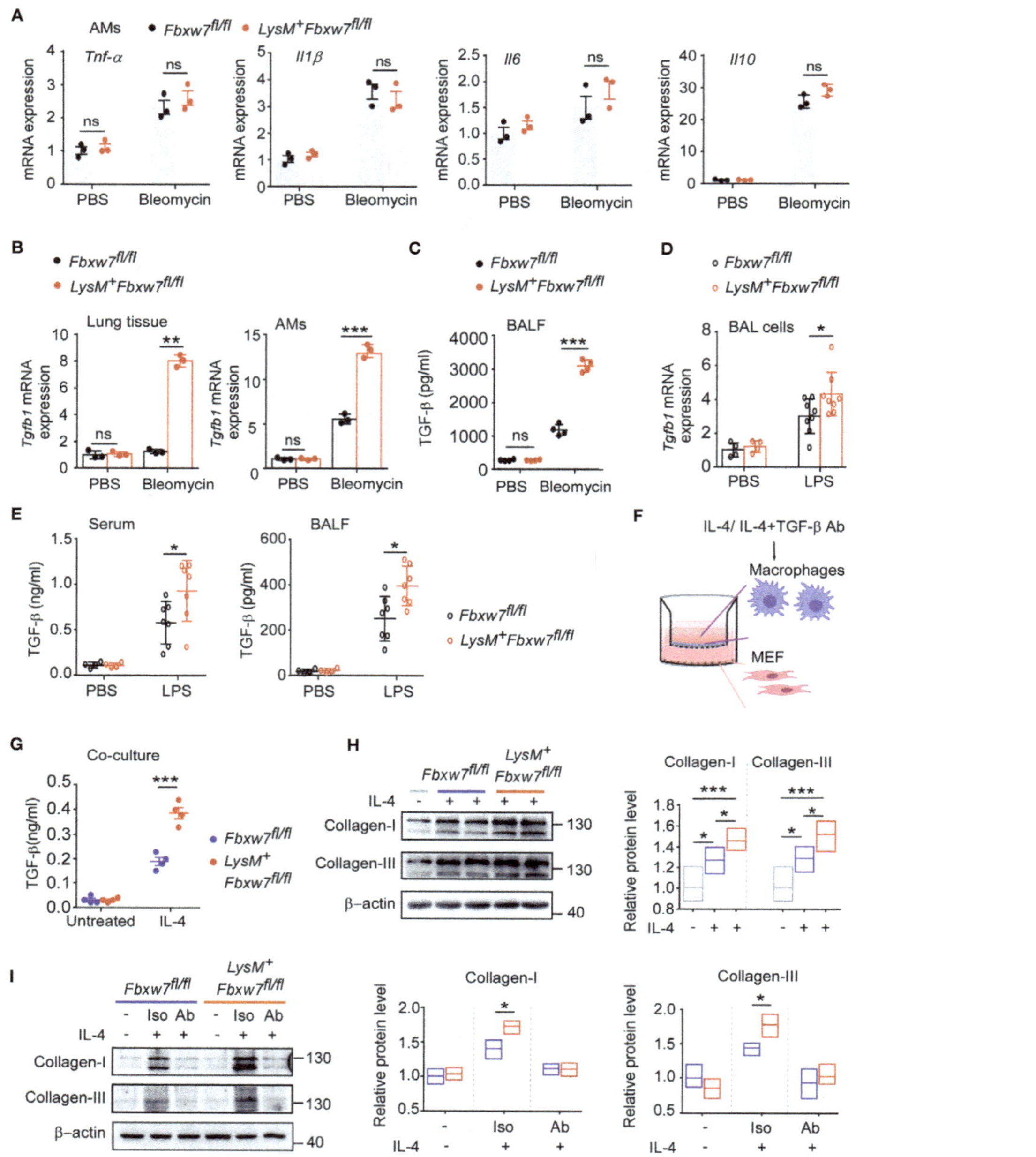

FIGURE 4 | *Fbxw7* deletion upregulates TGF-β expression in lung fibrosis model induced by bleomycin. qRT-PCR analysis of *Tnf-α*, *Il1β*, *Il6*, and *Il10* relative mRNA expression of AMs **(A)** after $Fbxw7^{fl/fl}$ and $LysM^{+}Fbxw7^{fl/fl}$ mice were administered PBS or bleomycin for 21 days to induce pulmonary fibrosis. After a 21d period of bleomycin-induced lung injure, qRT-PCR analysis of *Tgfb1* relative mRNA expression in lung tissue and AMs **(B)**, TGF-β content in BALF was detected by ELISA **(C)**. *Tgfb1* relative mRNA expression in BAL cells was analyzed by qRT-PCR **(D)**, TGF-β content in serum and BALF was detected by ELISA **(E)** after 10 days of LPS-induced lung injury. Macrophages from $Fbxw7^{fl/fl}$ and $LysM^{+}Fbxw7^{fl/fl}$ mice were stimulated with IL-4 (30 ng/ml) and treated with or without TGF-β neutralizing antibody for 12 h, then co-cultured with MEF for another 48 h. **(F)** The schematics of the approach. **(G)** TGF-β in the media of the macrophage co-culture system. Data are expressed as mean ± SD of biological duplicates (n≥3) and are the representative of three independent experiments. P values were obtained using two-tailed Student's *t* test, $^{*}P < 0.05$, $^{**}P < 0.01$, $^{***}P < 0.001$, ns, not significant. **(H)** Representative images of western blot analysis of collagen-I and collagen-III in co-cultured MEF after IL-4 treatment. Densitometric fold change of target proteins based on IL-4 untreated group was calculated. **(I)** Representative images of western blot analysis of collagen-I and collagen-III in co-cultured MEF after IL-4 with TGF-β neutralizing antibody (Ab) treatment (3 μg/ml). Iso: Isotype. Relative protein levels were presented by densitometric fold change quantified by ImageJ based on $Fbxw7^{fl/f}$ untreated group, the floating bars indicate the min, mean and max value of biological duplicates (n=3), which are the representative of three independent experiments. P values were obtained using One-way ANOVA with Tukey's Multiple Comparison test **(H)** or two-tailed Student's *t* test **(I)**. $^{*}P < 0.05$, $^{**}P < 0.01$, $^{***}P < 0.001$.

involved in the pathogenesis of fibrosis *via* enhancing TGF-β dependent signaling. To further elucidate the mechanisms how Fbxw7 regulates TGF-β production in profibrotic macrophages, we investigated the effect of *Fbxw7* deletion on the protein levels of EGR-1 and NF-κB by western blot. The protein levels of EGR1 and NF-κB in alveolar macrophages after bleomycin stimulation were not significantly changed between *Fbxw7*$^{fl/fl}$ and *LysM*$^{+}$*Fbxw7*$^{fl/fl}$ mice, but the level of c-Jun was significantly higher in *LysM*$^{+}$*Fbxw7*$^{fl/fl}$ mice than that in *Fbxw7*$^{fl/fl}$ mice (**Figure 5A**). Subsequently, we found significantly higher protein expression of c-Jun in IL-4-stimulated BMDMs after *Fbxw7* deletion (**Figure 5B**). We then overexpressed c-Jun in RAW264.7 cells (**Supplemental Figure 5A**) and analyzed the expression of TGF-β by qRT-PCR and ELISA, the results showed that the expression level of TGF-β was significantly increased after c-Jun overexpression (**Supplemental Figure 5B**), indicating

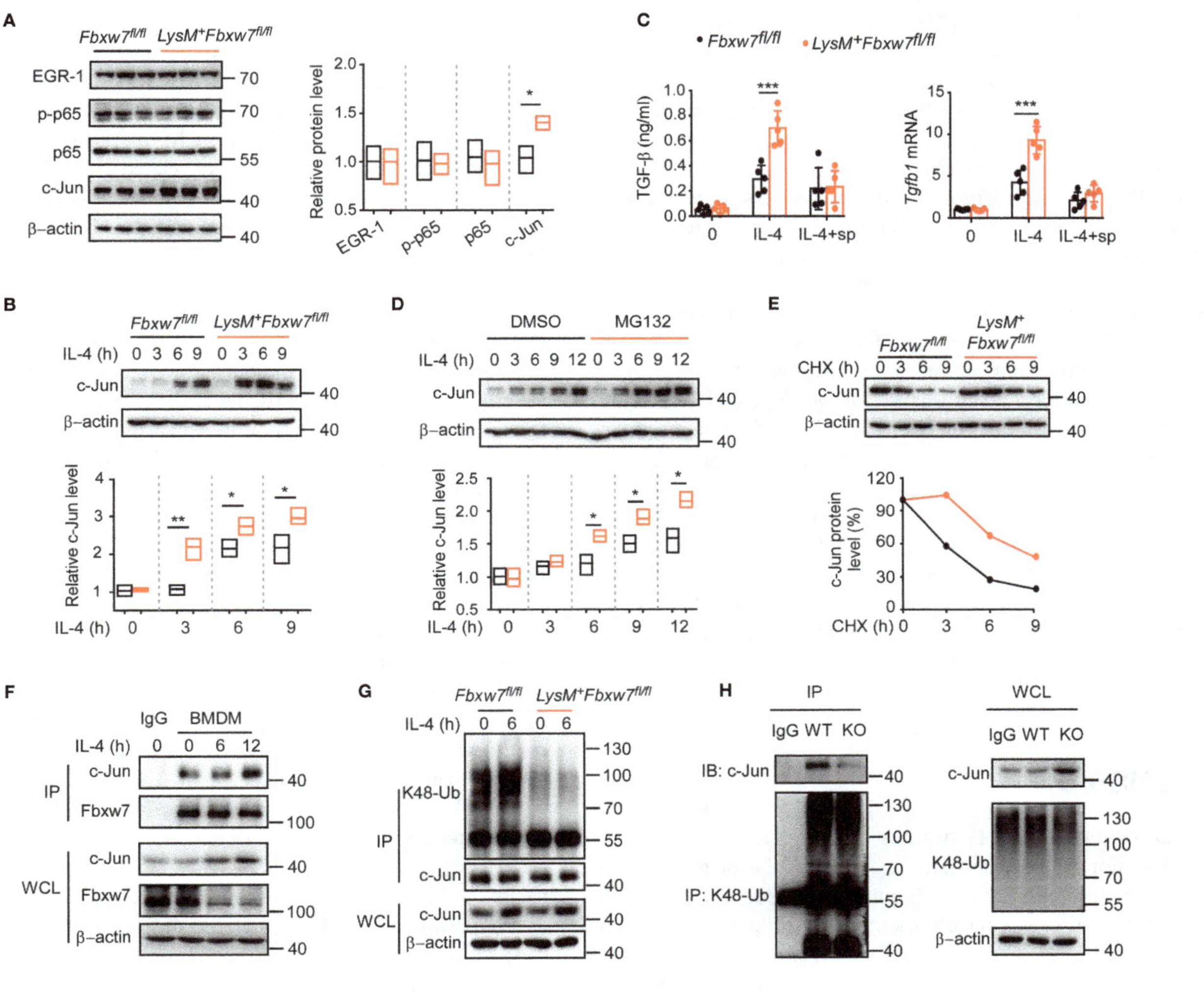

FIGURE 5 | Fbxw7 regulates TGF-β expression *via* mediating the ubiquitination of c-Jun. **(A)** Immunoblot analysis of phosphorylated and/or total proteins in lysates of lung tissues obtained from bleomycin-treated *Fbxw7*$^{fl/fl}$ and *LysM*$^{+}$*Fbxw7*$^{fl/fl}$ mice. Densitometric fold change of target proteins based on *Fbxw7*$^{fl/fl}$ group was calculated. **(B)** Immunoblot analysis of c-Jun protein levels in lysates of IL-4 (30 ng/ml) stimulated BMDMs from *Fbxw7*$^{fl/fl}$ and *LysM*$^{+}$*Fbxw7*$^{fl/fl}$ mice. Densitometric fold change for the relative c-Jun level based on *Fbxw7*$^{fl/fl}$ untreated group was calculated. **(C)** *Fbxw7*$^{fl/fl}$ and *LysM*$^{+}$ *Fbxw7*$^{fl/fl}$ BMDMs stimulated with IL-4 and treated or not with SP600125 (15 μM), qRT-PCR analysis for *Tgfb1* relative mRNA expression and ELISA for TGF-β protein expression. Data are expressed as mean ± SD of biological duplicates (n=5) and are the representative of three independent experiments. P values were obtained using two-tailed Student's *t* test, ***$P <$ 0.001. **(D)** Immunoblot analysis of c-Jun expression in BMDMs treated or not with MG132 (20 μM) for 8 hours and stimulated with IL-4 for the indicated durations. Densitometric fold change of c-Jun based on IL-4, MG132 untreated group was calculated. **(E)** Immunoblot analysis and relative protein levels of c-Jun in lysates of *Fbxw7*$^{fl/fl}$ and *LysM*$^{+}$*Fbxw7*$^{fl/fl}$ BMDMs treated with CHX (40 μg/ml) for indicated hours after stimulation with IL-4 for 6 h. **(F)** Coimmunoprecipitation and immunoblot of BMDMs stimulated with IL-4 for indicated hours. **(G)** Immunoblot analysis of the K48 ubiquitination of c-Jun in *Fbxw7*$^{fl/fl}$ and *LysM*$^{+}$*Fbxw7*$^{fl/fl}$ BMDMs stimulated with IL-4 for 6 h. **(H)** Peritoneal macrophages from *LysM*$^{+}$*Fbxw7*$^{fl/fl}$ (WT) and *Fbxw7*$^{fl/fl}$ (KO) mice were stimulated with IL-4 for 6 h, coimmunoprecipitation was performed with K48-Ub to pull-down ubiquitylated proteins, followed by IB with c-Jun. Relative protein levels were presented by densitometric fold change quantified by ImageJ, the floating bars indicate the min, mean and max value of biological duplicates and are the representative of three independent experiments. P values were obtained using two-tailed Student's *t* test. *$P < 0.05$, **$P < 0.01$, ***$P < 0.001$.

that c-Jun expression is sufficient for TGF-β in macrophages. SP600125 is a specific JNK inhibitor that competes with ATP to inhibit the phosphorylation of c-Jun (55). qRT-PCR analysis and ELISA results showed that the mRNA and protein expression of TGF-β increased significantly after the deletion of *Fbxw7* (**Figures 4C, D**), but this effect was abrogated after inhibition of c-Jun phosphorylation by SP600125 (**Figure 5C**). The MEF cells, co-cultured with peritoneal macrophage from *LysM*$^{+}$*Fbxw7*$^{fl/fl}$ mice or *Fbxw7*$^{fl/fl}$ littermates after inhibiting the phosphorylation of c-Jun, showed similar protein levels of collagen-I and collagen-III, which were detected by western blot (**Supplemental Figures 5C, D**). Taken together, *Fbxw7* deletion leads to the upregulation of TGF-β expression and severity of pulmonary fibrosis through the regulation of c-Jun.

It has been demonstrated that the transcription factor c-Jun can be degraded by the ubiquitin-proteasome system as a substrate for Fbxw7 (56). As expected, western blot analysis showed that the degradation of c-Jun protein could be inhibited by protease inhibitor MG132 (**Figure 5D**). A cycloheximide chase assay showed that *Fbxw7* deletion extended the half-life of endogenous c-Jun protein in BMDMs (**Figure 5E**). Immunoprecipitation assay results showed that Fbxw7 can physically bind to c-Jun protein (**Figure 5F**) and induce K48-linked polyubiquitination of c-Jun (**Figure 5G**). Moreover, immunoprecipitation assay was performed by using K48-Ub to pull-down c-Jun and the peritoneal macrophages from *LysM*$^{+}$*Fbxw7*$^{f/f}$ mice showed weaker ability of mediating c-Jun ubiquitination and proteasomal degradation compared with cells from *Fbxw7*$^{f/f}$ littermates (**Figure 5H**). This result further revealed that the myeloid *Fbxw7* deficiency leads to a significantly accumulation of c-Jun by abolishing its K48 ubiquitination. Collectively, these data confirmed that Fbxw7 promotes TGF-β expression by inducing K48-linked polyubiquitination and proteasome degradation of c-Jun in macrophages.

DISCUSSION

The E3 ubiquitin ligase Fbxw7 has been well characterized as a critical tumor suppressor that can mediate the degradation of various oncoproteins by the ubiquitin-proteasome system (57). Our studies and others have presented compelling evidence that Fbxw7 plays a crucial role in inflammation and antivirus immune response through regulating the function of macrophages (35, 36, 58). In this study, we demonstrated that the deletion of *Fbxw7* in the myeloid lineages aggravates bleomycin-induced lung injury, collagen deposition, and monocyte recruitment, and eventually leads to the exacerbation of pulmonary fibrosis in mice. We revealed its underlying mechanism that *Fbxw7* deletion will upregulate TGF-β expression by inhibiting the degradation of c-Jun in macrophages. These findings will be beneficial for understanding the role of innate immune response in the pathogenesis of IPF.

Macrophages are the most abundant immune cell population in the lung environment and are involved in tissue repair and lung fibrosis progression, it has also been recognized to play a significant role in driving the fibrogenesis and matrix remodeling. Given the high plasticity of lung macrophages, the relative roles of tissue-resident alveolar macrophages, interstitial macrophages and monocyte-derived infiltrating macrophages in pulmonary fibrosis is complicated (59). High numbers of both interstitial and alveolar macrophages were detected in pulmonary fibrosis (24), the depletion of macrophages, including alveolar and infiltrating macrophage, reduces fibrogenesis (25, 60). Experimental fibrosis leads to the recruitment of bone marrow-derived AMs that are more profibrogenic than their disrupted resident counterparts (61). Selectively targeting alveolar macrophage differentiation without affecting global monocytes or tissue-resident alveolar macrophage may ameliorate fibrosis depletion, while the depletion of tissue-resident AMs cannot alter fibrosis severity (61). In addition, IMs are also thought to arise from monocytes, and highly expression of monocyte-related genes, such as *Cd14*, *Cd163*, and *Csfr1* (62), activated IMs have been reported to induce myofibroblastic activation and ECM production (24). Furthermore, those more profibrogenic macrophages which play a vital role in airway remodeling in pulmonary fibrosis biases alternatively activated macrophages, so we used IL-4-stimulated BMDMs for *in vitro* experiments to mimic profibrogenic macrophages *in vivo*. Our data showed that more monocytes are recruited into the lung tissues and BALF of *Fbxw7*-KO mice, these monocytes further differentiate into profibrogenic macrophages and then participate in the development of pulmonary fibrosis.

The abundant expression of *Fbxw7* mRNA and protein can be detected in most human and mice tissues. The decreased level of *Fbxw7* mRNA in IPF may be regulated by many factors, including DNA or RNA silencing. The expression of microRNA-155 (miR-155) has been reported to be correlated to the damage degree of IPF (63), and miR-155 reduces the levels of *Fbxw7* mRNA (64). The *Fbxw7* promoter can be regulated through epigenetic mechanism during lung fibrosis, including histone modifications. Aberrant elevation of DNA methyltransferase 1 (Dnmt1) can mediate the hypermethylation of *Fbxw7* promoter and result in decreased gene level of *Fbxw7* (65), subsequently contributes significantly to the development of pulmonary fibrosis (66). Moreover, the expression of enhancer of zeste homolog 2 (Ezh2) is increased in IPF patients, increased Ezh2 recruitment and hypermethylated H3K27 at the promoter of fibrotic related genes have been demonstrated, such as *Cox-2* (67) and *Cxcl10* (68). We speculate the function of Ezh2 in inducing the increase of H3K27me3 at *Fbxw7* promotor and silencing of *Fbxw7* gene (34) might also be involved in regulating pulmonary fibrosis. IL-4 has been shown to induce TGF-β expression in profibrotic macrophage to activate fibroblasts and promotes extensive tissue fibrosis (50). In our study, we found IL-4 was highly expressed in lung fibrosis tissue of bleomycin-induced mice, and the expression of Fbxw7 was significantly decreased in bleomycin-induced mice lung issue and in BMDMs after IL-4 stimulation as shown in **Figures 1**, **S4B** and **5G**. These findings suggest that IL-4 in the profibrotic microenvironment might downregulate Fbxw7 expression and block c-Jun degradation.

TGF-β can be produced by a wide variety of cell types, including lung macrophages, alveolar epithelial cells, endothelial cells, fibroblasts and myofibroblasts. However, lung macrophages are revealed to be the main source of TGF-β (6, 69). In bleomycin induced pulmonary fibrosis, macrophages induce fibroblast differentiation and proliferation by producing TGF-β, thereby exacerbating pulmonary fibrosis (70, 71). The widespread accumulation of collagen in lungs, which was observed in WT mice, disappeared in the myeloid *TGF-β* deficient mice, which showed similar lung architecture to saline controls (6). Several factors have previously been implicated in the transcriptional induction of *Tgfb1*, bacterial induction of *Tgfb1* mRNA expression in human intestinal epithelial cells is butyrate and SP1-dependent (72). P38/MAPK signal, MEK-1 and JNK are involved in *Tgfb1* transcription (73). The higher mRNA expression of *Tgfb1* was detected in *Egr-1* overexpressed mesangial cell compared with control cells (74). Moreover, p65 and c-Jun were recruited to the promoter of *Tgfb1* in A549 cells upon IL-1β stimulation, this result suggesting the role of NF-κB and AP-1 in regulating *Tgfb1* expression (75).

C-Jun protein is a component of the dimeric transcription factor activator protein 1 (AP-1) (76), it has been shown to play essential roles in most fibrotic conditions, which can activate multiple signaling pathways, resulting in the expression of many fibrogenesis-associated genes (77). C-Jun N-terminal kinase JNK1 has been reported to promote fibrosis in the lung (78), inhibition of c-Jun phosphorylation *in vivo* reduced fibrosis and mRNA levels of *Tgfb1* in the unilateral ischemia reperfusion injury model (79). C-Jun expression in non-parenchymal liver cells (NPLCs) promotes the fibrogenesis and was particularly correlated with liver fibrosis during non-alcoholic steatohepatitis (80). Moreover, studies have shown that c-Jun can be degraded by the ubiquitin-proteasome system as the substrate of Fbxw7 (81, 82), which was also confirmed by our study. Our data show that deletion of *Fbxw7* in macrophages does not affect the levels of P65, EGR-1 and their phosphorylation, but significantly increases the level of AP-1 transcription factor subunit c-Jun.

Notably, the published data from Wang et al. (83) showed that FBXW7 deficiency prevents fibrogenesis by increasing telomere capping, which is contrary to the conclusion of our finding. Several potential possibilities exist for this discrepancy. Wang et al. used a mouse model of Fbw7 conditional knockout in pulmonary alveolar epithelial type 2 (AEC2) stem cells, while we used a model of *Fbxw7* conditional knockout in myeloid cells. Those reverse effects of Fbxw7 in AEC2 stem cells and myeloid cells in regulating lung fibrosis indicated that the pathogenesis of IPF is complicated, it involves the abnormal repair of lung tissue injury by alveolar epithelial cells, the disordered differentiation and proliferation of fibroblasts, or the hyperactivated recruitment and activation of innate immune cells. The dysfunction in any cell type can lead to different outcomes of IPF. Moreover, subtle genetic background differences in the strains of the mice used and microbiome differences between the mouse colonies may also contribute to these discrepancies.

In conclusion, our study revealed that Fbxw7 plays a crucial role in regulating pulmonary fibrosis progression. Myeloid-specific deletion of *Fbxw7* exacerbates pulmonary fibrosis by inhibiting c-Jun degradation and upregulating TGF-β expression in macrophages.

ETHICS STATEMENT

The animal study was reviewed and approved by Medical Experimental Animal Care Commission of Zhejiang University.

AUTHOR CONTRIBUTIONS

QW, JZ, and JH designed the research. JH, YD, GL, XS, WS, LL, and MX performed experiments and acquired and analyzed data. JZ, JH, and PX drafted the manuscript. QW revised the manuscript. All authors read and approved the submitted version.

ACKNOWLEDGMENTS

We would like to thank Prof. Ximei Wu for providing the Lysm-Cre mice. We thank the Core Facilities, Zhejiang University School of Medicine for technical support.

REFERENCES

1. Wolters PJ, Blackwell TS, Eickelberg O, Loyd JE, Kaminski N, Jenkins G, et al. Time for a Change: Is Idiopathic Pulmonary Fibrosis Still Idiopathic and Only Fibrotic? *Lancet Respir Med* (2018) 2:154–60. doi: 10.1016/s2213-2600(18)30007-9
2. Xaubet A, Marin-Arguedas A, Lario S, Ancochea J, Morell F, Ruiz-Manzano J, et al. Transforming Growth Factor-Beta1 Gene Polymorphisms Are Associated With Disease Progression in Idiopathic Pulmonary Fibrosis. *Am J Respir Crit Care Med* (2003) 4:431–5. doi: 10.1164/rccm.200210-1165OC
3. Mura M, Porretta MA, Bargagli E, Sergiacomi G, Zompatori M, Sverzellati N, et al. Predicting Survival in Newly Diagnosed Idiopathic Pulmonary Fibrosis: A 3-Year Prospective Study. *Eur Respir J* (2012) 1:101–9. doi: 10.1183/09031936.00106011
4. King TEJr., Tooze JA, Schwarz MI, Brown KR, Cherniack RM. Predicting Survival in Idiopathic Pulmonary Fibrosis: Scoring System and Survival Model. *Am J Respir Crit Care Med* (2001) 7:1171–81. doi: 10.1164/ajrccm.164.7.2003140
5. Fernandez IE, Eickelberg O. The Impact of Tgf-Beta on Lung Fibrosis: From Targeting to Biomarkers. *Proc Am Thorac Soc* (2012) 3:111–6. doi: 10.1513/pats.201203-023AW
6. Larson-Casey JL, Deshane JS, Ryan AJ, Thannickal VJ, Carter AB. Macrophage Akt1 Kinase-Mediated Mitophagy Modulates Apoptosis Resistance and Pulmonary Fibrosis. *Immunity* (2016) 3:582–96. doi: 10.1016/j.immuni.2016.01.001
7. Yu X, Buttgereit A, Lelios I, Utz SG, Cansever D, Becher B, et al. The Cytokine Tgf-Beta Promotes the Development and Homeostasis of Alveolar Macrophages. *Immunity* (2017) 5:903–12 e4. doi: 10.1016/j.immuni.2017.10.007
8. Phillips AO, Topley N, Steadman R, Morrisey K, Williams JD. Induction of Tgf-Beta 1 Synthesis in D-Glucose Primed Human Proximal Tubular Cells by Il-1 Beta and Tnf Alpha. *Kidney Int* (1996) 5:1546–54. doi: 10.1038/ki.1996.470
9. Zhu Z, Homer RJ, Wang Z, Chen Q, Geba GP, Wang J, et al. Pulmonary Expression of Interleukin-13 Causes Inflammation, Mucus Hypersecretion, Subepithelial Fibrosis, Physiologic Abnormalities, and Eotaxin Production. *J Clin Invest* (1999) 6:779–88. doi: 10.1172/JCI5909

10. Lee CG, Homer RJ, Zhu Z, Lanone S, Wang X, Koteliansky V, et al. Interleukin-13 Induces Tissue Fibrosis by Selectively Stimulating and Activating Transforming Growth Factor Beta(1). *J Exp Med* (2001) 6:809–21. doi: 10.1084/jem.194.6.809
11. Rao LZ, Wang Y, Zhang L, Wu G, Zhang L, Wang FX, et al. Il-24 Deficiency Protects Mice Against Bleomycin-Induced Pulmonary Fibrosis by Repressing Il-4-Induced M2 Program in Macrophages. *Cell Death Differ* (2021) 4:1270–83. doi: 10.1038/s41418-020-00650-6
12. Sunaga H, Matsui H, Ueno M, Maeno T, Iso T, Syamsunarno MR, et al. Deranged Fatty Acid Composition Causes Pulmonary Fibrosis in Elovl6-Deficient Mice. *Nat Commun* (2013) 4:2563. doi: 10.1038/ncomms3563
13. Mahalanobish S, Saha S, Dutta S, Sil PC. Matrix Metalloproteinase: An Upcoming Therapeutic Approach for Idiopathic Pulmonary Fibrosis. *Pharmacol Res* (2020) 152:104591. doi: 10.1016/j.phrs.2019.104591
14. Murphy-Ullrich JE, Suto MJ. Thrombospondin-1 Regulation of Latent Tgf-Beta Activation: A Therapeutic Target for Fibrotic Disease. *Matrix Biol* (2018) 68-69:28–43. doi: 10.1016/j.matbio.2017.12.009
15. Dong X, Zhao B, Iacob RE, Zhu J, Koksal AC, Lu C, et al. Force Interacts With Macromolecular Structure in Activation of Tgf-Beta. *Nature* (2017) 7639:55–9. doi: 10.1038/nature21035
16. Byrne AJ, Maher TM, Lloyd CM. Pulmonary Macrophages: A New Therapeutic Pathway in Fibrosing Lung Disease? *Trends Mol Med* (2016) 4:303–16. doi: 10.1016/j.molmed.2016.02.004
17. Laskin DL, Malaviya R, Laskin JD. Role of Macrophages in Acute Lung Injury and Chronic Fibrosis Induced by Pulmonary Toxicants. *Toxicol Sci* (2019) 2:287–301. doi: 10.1093/toxsci/kfy309
18. Gibbons MA, MacKinnon AC, Ramachandran P, Dhaliwal K, Duffin R, Phythian-Adams AT, et al. Ly6chi Monocytes Direct Alternatively Activated Profibrotic Macrophage Regulation of Lung Fibrosis. *Am J Respir Crit Care Med* (2011) 5:569–81. doi: 10.1164/rccm.201010-1719OC
19. Fernandez IE, Eickelberg O. New Cellular and Molecular Mechanisms of Lung Injury and Fibrosis in Idiopathic Pulmonary Fibrosis. *Lancet* (2012) 9842:680–8. doi: 10.1016/S0140-6736(12)61144-1
20. Zhang L, Wang Y, Wu G, Xiong W, Gu W, Wang CY. Macrophages: Friend or Foe in Idiopathic Pulmonary Fibrosis? *Respir Res* (2018) 1:170. doi: 10.1186/s12931-018-0864-2
21. Prasse A, Pechkovsky DV, Toews GB, Jungraithmayr W, Kollert F, Goldmann T, et al. A Vicious Circle of Alveolar Macrophages and Fibroblasts Perpetuates Pulmonary Fibrosis *via* Ccl18. *Am J Respir Crit Care Med* (2006) 7:781–92. doi: 10.1164/rccm.200509-1518OC
22. Wynes MW, Frankel SK, Riches DW. Il-4-Induced Macrophage-Derived Igf-I Protects Myofibroblasts From Apoptosis Following Growth Factor Withdrawal. *J Leukoc Biol* (2004) 5:1019–27. doi: 10.1189/jlb.0504288
23. Nagaoka I, Trapnell BC, Crystal RG. Upregulation of Platelet-Derived Growth Factor-A and -B Gene Expression in Alveolar Macrophages of Individuals With Idiopathic Pulmonary Fibrosis. *J Clin Invest* (1990) 6:2023–7. doi: 10.1172/JCI114669
24. Meziani L, Mondini M, Petit B, Boissonnas A, Thomas de Montpreville V, Mercier O, et al. Csf1r Inhibition Prevents Radiation Pulmonary Fibrosis by Depletion of Interstitial Macrophages. *Eur Respir J* (2018) 3:1702120. doi: 10.1183/13993003.02120-2017
25. Redente EF, Keith RC, Janssen W, Henson PM, Ortiz LA, Downey GP, et al. Tumor Necrosis Factor-Alpha Accelerates the Resolution of Established Pulmonary Fibrosis in Mice by Targeting Profibrotic Lung Macrophages. *Am J Respir Cell Mol Biol* (2014) 4:825–37. doi: 10.1165/rcmb.2013-0386OC
26. Murray LA, Chen Q, Kramer MS, Hesson DP, Argentieri RL, Peng X, et al. Tgf-Beta Driven Lung Fibrosis Is Macrophage Dependent and Blocked by Serum Amyloid P. *Int J Biochem Cell Biol* (2011) 1:154–62. doi: 10.1016/j.biocel.2010.10.013
27. Khalil N, Bereznay O, Sporn M, Greenberg AH. Macrophage Production of Transforming Growth Factor Beta and Fibroblast Collagen Synthesis in Chronic Pulmonary Inflammation. *J Exp Med* (1989) 3:727–37. doi: 10.1084/jem.170.3.727
28. Sailo BL, Banik K, Girisa S, Bordoloi D, Fan L, Halim CE, et al. Fbxw7 in Cancer: What Has Been Unraveled Thus Far? *Cancers (Basel)* (2019) 2:246. doi: 10.3390/cancers11020246
29. Guyard A, Danel C, Theou-Anton N, Debray MP, Gibault L, Mordant P, et al. Morphologic and Molecular Study of Lung Cancers Associated With Idiopathic Pulmonary Fibrosis and Other Pulmonary Fibroses. *Respir Res* (2017) 1:120. doi: 10.1186/s12931-017-0605-y
30. Ekholm-Reed S, Goldberg MS, Schlossmacher MG, Reed SI. Parkin-Dependent Degradation of the F-Box Protein Fbw7beta Promotes Neuronal Survival in Response to Oxidative Stress by Stabilizing Mcl-1. *Mol Cell Biol* (2013) 18:3627–43. doi: 10.1128/MCB.00535-13
31. Zhao X, Hirota T, Han X, Cho H, Chong LW, Lamia K, et al. Circadian Amplitude Regulation *via* Fbxw7-Targeted Rev-Erbalpha Degradation. *Cell* (2016) 7:1644–57. doi: 10.1016/j.cell.2016.05.012
32. Hoeck JD, Jandke A, Blake SM, Nye E, Spencer-Dene B, Brandner S, et al. Fbw7 Controls Neural Stem Cell Differentiation and Progenitor Apoptosis *via* Notch and C-Jun. *Nat Neurosci* (2010) 11:1365–72. doi: 10.1038/nn.2644
33. Kearns CA, Ravanelli AM, Cooper K, Appel B. Fbxw7 Limits Myelination by Inhibiting Mtor Signaling. *J Neurosci* (2015) 44:14861–71. doi: 10.1523/JNEUROSCI.4968-14.2015
34. Zhao E, Maj T, Kryczek I, Li W, Wu K, Zhao L, et al. Cancer Mediates Effector T Cell Dysfunction by Targeting Micrornas and Ezh2 *via* Glycolysis Restriction. *Nat Immunol* (2016) 1:95–103. doi: 10.1038/ni.3313
35. Song Y, Lai L, Chong Z, He J, Zhang Y, Xue Y, et al. E3 Ligase Fbxw7 Is Critical for Rig-I Stabilization During Antiviral Responses. *Nat Commun* (2017) 8:14654. doi: 10.1038/ncomms14654
36. He J, Song Y, Li G, Xiao P, Liu Y, Xue Y, et al. Fbxw7 Increases Ccl2/7 in Cx3cr1hi Macrophages to Promote Intestinal Inflammation. *J Clin Invest* (2019) 129:3877–93. doi: 10.1172/JCI123374
37. Liu T, De Los Santos FG, Phan SH. The Bleomycin Model of Pulmonary Fibrosis. *Methods Mol Biol* (2017) 1627:27–42. doi: 10.1007/978-1-4939-7113-8_2
38. Li Y, Li H, Liu S, Pan P, Su X, Tan H, et al. Pirfenidone Ameliorates Lipopolysaccharide-Induced Pulmonary Inflammation and Fibrosis by Blocking Nlrp3 Inflammasome Activation. *Mol Immunol* (2018) 99:134–44. doi: 10.1016/j.molimm.2018.05.003
39. Liu YY, Shi Y, Liu Y, Pan XH, Zhang KX. Telomere Shortening Activates Tgf-Beta/Smads Signaling in Lungs and Enhances Both Lipopolysaccharide and Bleomycin-Induced Pulmonary Fibrosis. *Acta Pharmacol Sin* (2018) 11:1735–45. doi: 10.1038/s41401-018-0007-9
40. Szapiel SV, Elson NA, Fulmer JD, Hunninghake GW, Crystal RG. Bleomycin-Induced Interstitial Pulmonary Disease in the Nude, Athymic Mouse. *Am Rev Respir Dis* (1979) 4:893–9. doi: 10.1164/arrd.1979.120.4.893
41. Schmittgen TD, Livak KJ. Analyzing Real-Time Pcr Data by the Comparative C(T) Method. *Nat Protoc* (2008) 6:1101–8. doi: 10.1038/nprot.2008.73
42. Prasse A, Binder H, Schupp JC, Kayser G, Bargagli E, Jaeger B, et al. Data From: BAL Cell Gene Expression is Predictive of Mortality in Idiopathic Pulmonary Fibrosis and Enriched for Genes of Airway Basal Cells. *Gene Expression Omnibus* (2018), GSE70867.
43. Huang Y, Oldham JM, Ma S, Martinez FJ, Noth I. Data From: Longitudinal Blood Transcriptomic Changes Predict Lung Function Decline in Idiopathic Pulmonary Fibrosis. *Gene Expression Omnibus* (2019), GSE132607.
44. Desogere P, Tapias LF, Hariri LP, Rotile NJ, Rietz TA, Probst CK, et al. Type I Collagen-Targeted Pet Probe for Pulmonary Fibrosis Detection and Staging in Preclinical Models. *Sci Transl Med* (2017) 384:eaaf4696. doi: 10.1126/scitranslmed.aaf4696
45. Tsukui T, Sun KH, Wetter JB, Wilson-Kanamori JR, Hazelwood LA, Henderson NC, et al. Collagen-Producing Lung Cell Atlas Identifies Multiple Subsets With Distinct Localization and Relevance to Fibrosis. *Nat Commun* (2020) 1:1920. doi: 10.1038/s41467-020-15647-5
46. Tschumperlin DJ. Matrix, Mesenchyme, and Mechanotransduction. *Ann Am Thorac Soc* (2015) 12:S24–9. doi: 10.1513/AnnalsATS.201407-320MG
47. Ryu C, Sun H, Gulati M, Herazo-Maya JD, Chen Y, Osafo-Addo A, et al. Extracellular Mitochondrial DNA Is Generated by Fibroblasts and Predicts Death in Idiopathic Pulmonary Fibrosis. *Am J Respir Crit Care Med* (2017) 12:1571–81. doi: 10.1164/rccm.201612-2480OC
48. Dong J, Ma Q. Type 2 Immune Mechanisms in Carbon Nanotube-Induced Lung Fibrosis. *Front Immunol* (2018) 9:1120. doi: 10.3389/fimmu.2018.01120
49. He C, Murthy S, McCormick ML, Spitz DR, Ryan AJ, Carter AB. Mitochondrial Cu,Zn-Superoxide Dismutase Mediates Pulmonary Fibrosis by Augmenting H2o2 Generation. *J Biol Chem* (2011) 17:15597–607. doi: 10.1074/jbc.M110.187377
50. Su S, Zhao Q, He C, Huang D, Liu J, Chen F, et al. Mir-142-5p and Mir-130a-3p Are Regulated by Il-4 and Il-13 and Control Profibrogenic Macrophage Program. *Nat Commun* (2015) 6:8523. doi: 10.1038/ncomms9523

51. Zhu L, Fu X, Chen X, Han X, Dong P. M2 Macrophages Induce Emt Through the Tgf-Beta/Smad2 Signaling Pathway. *Cell Biol Int* (2017) 9:960–68. doi: 10.1002/cbin.10788
52. Lee CG, Cho SJ, Kang MJ, Chapoval SP, Lee PJ, Noble PW, et al. Early Growth Response Gene 1-Mediated Apoptosis Is Essential for Transforming Growth Factor Beta1-Induced Pulmonary Fibrosis. *J Exp Med* (2004) 3:377–89. doi: 10.1084/jem.20040104
53. Ghosh AK, Bhattacharyya S, Lafyatis R, Farina G, Yu J, Thimmapaya B, et al. P300 Is Elevated in Systemic Sclerosis and Its Expression Is Positively Regulated by Tgf-Beta: Epigenetic Feed-Forward Amplification of Fibrosis. *J Invest Dermatol* (2013) 5:1302–10. doi: 10.1038/jid.2012.479
54. Freudlsperger C, Bian Y, Contag Wise S, Burnett J, Coupar J, Yang X, et al. Tgf-Beta and Nf-Kappab Signal Pathway Cross-Talk Is Mediated Through Tak1 and Smad7 in a Subset of Head and Neck Cancers. *Oncogene* (2013) 12:1549–59. doi: 10.1038/onc.2012.171
55. Zhang S, Che D, Yang F, Chi C, Meng H, Shen J, et al. Tumor-Associated Macrophages Promote Tumor Metastasis *via* the Tgf-Beta/Sox9 Axis in Non-Small Cell Lung Cancer. *Oncotarget* (2017) 59:99801–15. doi: 10.18632/oncotarget.21068
56. Babaei-Jadidi R, Li N, Saadeddin A, Spencer-Dene B, Jandke A, Muhammad B, et al. Fbxw7 Influences Murine Intestinal Homeostasis and Cancer, Targeting Notch, Jun, and Dek for Degradation. *J Exp Med* (2011) 2:295–312. doi: 10.1084/jem.20100830
57. Yeh CH, Bellon M, Nicot C. Fbxw7: A Critical Tumor Suppressor of Human Cancers. *Mol Cancer* (2018) 1:115. doi: 10.1186/s12943-018-0857-2
58. Zhang C, Chen F, Feng L, Shan Q, Zheng GH, Wang YJ, et al. Fbxw7 Suppresses Hmgb1-Mediated Innate Immune Signaling to Attenuate Hepatic Inflammation and Insulin Resistance in a Mouse Model of Nonalcoholic Fatty Liver Disease. *Mol Med* (2019) 1:29. doi: 10.1186/s10020-019-0099-9
59. Guilliams M, Scott CL. Does Niche Competition Determine the Origin of Tissue-Resident Macrophages? *Nat Rev Immunol* (2017) 7:451–60. doi: 10.1038/nri.2017.42
60. Osterholzer JJ, Olszewski MA, Murdock BJ, Chen GH, Erb-Downward JR, Subbotina N, et al. Implicating Exudate Macrophages and Ly-6c(High) Monocytes in Ccr2-Dependent Lung Fibrosis Following Gene-Targeted Alveolar Injury. *J Immunol* (2013) 7:3447–57. doi: 10.4049/jimmunol.1200604
61. Misharin AV, Morales-Nebreda L, Reyfman PA, Cuda CM, Walter JM, McQuattie-Pimentel AC, et al. Monocyte-Derived Alveolar Macrophages Drive Lung Fibrosis and Persist in the Lung Over the Life Span. *J Exp Med* (2017) 8:2387–404. doi: 10.1084/jem.20162152
62. Gibbings SL, Thomas SM, Atif SM, McCubbrey AL, Desch AN, Danhorn T, et al. Three Unique Interstitial Macrophages in the Murine Lung at Steady State. *Am J Respir Cell Mol Biol* (2017) 1:66–76. doi: 10.1165/rcmb.2016-0361OC
63. Li P, Zhao GQ, Chen TF, Chang JX, Wang HQ, Chen SS, et al. Serum Mir-21 and Mir-155 Expression in Idiopathic Pulmonary Fibrosis. *J Asthma* (2013) 9:960–4. doi: 10.3109/02770903.2013.822080
64. Cao S, Wang Y, Li J, Lv M, Niu H, Tian Y. Tumor-Suppressive Function of Long Noncoding Rna Malat1 in Glioma Cells by Suppressing Mir-155 Expression and Activating Fbxw7 Function. *Am J Cancer Res* (2016) 11:2561–74.
65. Kitade S, Onoyama I, Kobayashi H, Yagi H, Yoshida S, Kato M, et al. Fbxw7 Is Involved in the Acquisition of the Malignant Phenotype in Epithelial Ovarian Tumors. *Cancer Sci* (2016) 10:1399–405. doi: 10.1111/cas.13026
66. Wei A, Gao Q, Chen F, Zhu X, Chen X, Zhang L, et al. Inhibition of DNA Methylation Derepresses Ppargamma and Attenuates Pulmonary Fibrosis. *Br J Pharmacol* (2021). doi: 10.1111/bph.15655
67. Coward WR, Feghali-Bostwick CA, Jenkins G, Knox AJ, Pang L. A Central Role for G9a and Ezh2 in the Epigenetic Silencing of Cyclooxygenase-2 in Idiopathic Pulmonary Fibrosis. *FASEB J* (2014) 7:3183–96. doi: 10.1096/fj.13-241760
68. Coward WR, Brand OJ, Pasini A, Jenkins G, Knox AJ, Pang L. Interplay Between Ezh2 and G9a Regulates Cxcl10 Gene Repression in Idiopathic Pulmonary Fibrosis. *Am J Respir Cell Mol Biol* (2018) 4:449–60. doi: 10.1165/rcmb.2017-0286OC
69. Broekelmann TJ, Limper AH, Colby TV, McDonald JA. Transforming Growth Factor Beta 1 Is Present at Sites of Extracellular Matrix Gene Expression in Human Pulmonary Fibrosis. *Proc Natl Acad Sci USA* (1991) 15:6642–6. doi: 10.1073/pnas.88.15.6642
70. Toossi Z, Hirsch CS, Hamilton BD, Knuth CK, Friedlander MA, Rich EA. Decreased Production of Tgf-Beta 1 by Human Alveolar Macrophages Compared With Blood Monocytes. *J Immunol* (1996) 9:3461–8.
71. Young LR, Gulleman PM, Short CW, Tanjore H, Sherrill T, Qi A, et al. Epithelial-Macrophage Interactions Determine Pulmonary Fibrosis Susceptibility in Hermansky-Pudlak Syndrome. *JCI Insight* (2016) 17: e88947. doi: 10.1172/jci.insight.88947
72. Martin-Gallausiaux C, Beguet-Crespel F, Marinelli L, Jamet A, Ledue F, Blottiere HM, et al. Butyrate Produced by Gut Commensal Bacteria Activates Tgf-Beta1 Expression Through the Transcription Factor Sp1 in Human Intestinal Epithelial Cells. *Sci Rep* (2018) 1:9742. doi: 10.1038/s41598-018-28048-y
73. Xiao Y, Freire-de-Lima C, Schiemann W, Bratton D, Vandivier R, Henson P, et al. Transcriptional and Translational Regulation of Tgf-Beta Production in Response to Apoptotic Cells. *J Immunol* (2008) 5:3575–85. doi: 10.4049/jimmunol.181.5.3575
74. Peng W, Huang S, Shen L, Tang Y, Li H, Shi Y. Long Noncoding Rna Nonhsag053901 Promotes Diabetic Nephropathy *via* Stimulating Egr-1/Tgf-Beta-Mediated Renal Inflammation. *J Cell Physiol* (2019) 10:18492–503. doi: 10.1002/jcp.28485
75. Lee KY, Ito K, Hayashi R, Jazrawi EP, Barnes PJ, Adcock IM. Nf-Kappab and Activator Protein 1 Response Elements and the Role of Histone Modifications in Il-1beta-Induced Tgf-Beta1 Gene Transcription. *J Immunol* (2006) 1:603–15. doi: 10.4049/jimmunol.176.1.603
76. Eferl R, Wagner EF. Ap-1: A Double-Edged Sword in Tumorigenesis. *Nat Rev Cancer* (2003) 11:859–68. doi: 10.1038/nrc1209
77. Wernig G, Chen SY, Cui L, Van Neste C, Tsai JM, Kambham N, et al. Unifying Mechanism for Different Fibrotic Diseases. *Proc Natl Acad Sci USA* (2017) 18:4757–62. doi: 10.1073/pnas.1621375114
78. Velden JL, Alcorn JF, Guala AS, Badura EC. And Janssen-Heininger Y M. C-Jun N-Terminal Kinase 1 Promotes Transforming Growth Factor-Beta1-Induced Epithelial-To-Mesenchymal Transition *via* Control of Linker Phosphorylation and Transcriptional Activity of Smad3. *Am J Respir Cell Mol Biol* (2011) 4:571–81. doi: 10.1165/rcmb.2009-0282OC
79. Yang L, Besschetnova TY, Brooks CR, Shah JV, Bonventre JV. Epithelial Cell Cycle Arrest in G2/M Mediates Kidney Fibrosis After Injury. *Nat Med* (2010) 5:535–43. doi: 10.1038/nm.2144
80. Schulien I, Hockenjos B, Schmitt-Graeff A, Perdekamp MG, Follo M, Thimme R, et al. The Transcription Factor C-Jun/Ap-1 Promotes Liver Fibrosis During Non-Alcoholic Steatohepatitis by Regulating Osteopontin Expression. *Cell Death Differ* (2019) 9:1688–99. doi: 10.1038/s41418-018-0239-8
81. Nateri AS, Riera-Sans L, Da Costa C, Behrens A. The Ubiquitin Ligase Scffbw7 Antagonizes Apoptotic Jnk Signaling. *Science* (2004) 5662:1374–8. doi: 10.1126/science.1092880
82. Kravchick DO, Karpova A, Hrdinka M, Lopez-Rojas J, Iacobas S, Carbonell AU, et al. Synaptonuclear Messenger Prr7 Inhibits C-Jun Ubiquitination and Regulates Nmda-Mediated Excitotoxicity. *EMBO J* (2016) 17:1923–34. doi: 10.15252/embj.201593070
83. Wang L, Chen R, Li G, Wang Z, Liu J, Liang Y, et al. Fbw7 Mediates Senescence and Pulmonary Fibrosis Through Telomere Uncapping. *Cell Metab* (2020) 5:860–77 e9. doi: 10.1016/j.cmet.2020.10.004

18

Hyperoside Attenuates Bleomycin-Induced Pulmonary Fibrosis Development in Mice

*Jizhen Huang[1], Xiang Tong[1], Li Zhang[1], Yuan Zhang[2], Lei Wang[1], Dongguang Wang[1], Shijie Zhang[1] and Hong Fan[1]**

[1] Department of Respiratory and Critical Care Medicine, West China Hospital/West China School of Medicine, Sichuan University, Chengdu, China, [2] Department of Ophthalmology, Renmin Hospital of Wuhan University, Wuhan, China

***Correspondence:**
Hong Fan
fanhongfan@qq.com

Idiopathic pulmonary fibrosis (IPF) is a progressive, lethal, and chronic lung disease. There are no effective drug therapies for IPF. Hyperoside, a flavonoid glycoside, has been proven to have anti-inflammatory, anti-fibrosis, antioxidant, and anti-cancer effects. The aim of this study was to explore the role of hyperoside in bleomycin-induced pulmonary fibrosis development in mice. We established the pulmonary fibrosis model by a single intratracheal aerosol injection of bleomycin. Seven days after the bleomycin treatment, the mice were intraperitoneally administered with hyperoside for 14 days. We found that hyperoside treatment ameliorated fibrotic pathological changes and collagen deposition in the lungs of mice with bleomycin-induced pulmonary fibrosis. Hyperoside treatment also reduced the levels of MDA, TNF-α, and IL-6 and increased the activity of SOD. In addition, hyperoside might inhibit the epithelial-mesenchymal transition (EMT) *via* the AKT/GSK3β pathway. Based on these findings, hyperoside attenuated pulmonary fibrosis development by inhibiting oxidative stress, inflammation, and EMT in the lung tissues of mice with pulmonary fibrosis. Therefore, hyperoside might be a promising candidate drug for the treatment of pulmonary fibrosis.

Keywords: hyperoside, pulmonary fibrosis, epithelial-mesenchymal transition, oxidative stress, inflammation

INTRODUCTION

Idiopathic pulmonary fibrosis (IPF) is a progressive, lethal, and chronic lung disease (Kim et al., 2015). IPF patients have poor long-term survival (Scotton and Chambers, 2007). The incidence of IPF is increasing over time throughout the world (Hutchinson et al., 2015). IPF is characterized by aberrant alveolar epithelial cells, uncontrolled myofibroblast proliferation, and abnormal extracellular matrix (ECM) deposition (Richeldi et al., 2017). EMT plays an important role in many respiratory diseases, including pulmonary fibrosis (Marmai et al., 2011), chronic obstructive pulmonary disease (Xu et al., 2017), and lung cancer (Yin et al., 2020). This transition includes the loss of epithelial markers and the acquisition of mesenchymal markers, which leads to functional changes, including cell migration, invasion, and cell cycle arrest (Willis and Borok, 2007; Lovisa et al., 2015; Yang et al., 2020). Although pirfenidone and nintedanib, which have been approved by the FDA for treating IPF patients, may be able to alleviate the development of IPF, they provide only limited help and entail adverse side effects such as diarrhea and nausea (Canestaro et al., 2016; Galli et al., 2017).

Although the pathogenesis of pulmonary fibrosis is unclear, studies have shown that the transforming growth factor β (TGF-β) plays an important role in the development of pulmonary fibrosis (Yan et al., 2014). TGF-β1 can lead to the phenotypic transition of fibroblasts to myofibroblasts (Wei et al., 2019). TGF-β1 also can induce EMT through smad-dependent pathways or non-smad-dependent pathways, including the phosphoinositide 3 kinase/protein kinase B(PI3K/AKT) pathway and the mitogen-activated protein kinase (MAPK) pathway (Willis and Borok, 2007). The EMT induced by TGF-β1 contributes to the development of pulmonary fibrosis (Willis and Borok, 2007; Zhang C. et al., 2019). The AKT pathway is aberrantly activated in pulmonary fibrosis cellular and animal models (Qu et al., 2019; Ma Z. et al., 2020). The AKT/FOXO3a pathway promotes the proliferation of human pulmonary fibroblasts and the production of collagen (Ma Z. et al., 2020). Other studies have shown that the AKT pathway participates in EMT (Qu et al., 2019). It has been revealed that bleomycin (Blm) can activate the AKT/glycogen synthase kinase 3β (GSK3β) pathway in Blm-induced bronchial epithelial cell injury (Ma et al., 2009). Moreover, the AKT/GSK3β pathway is associated with EMT induced by cigarette smoke extract (Agraval and Yadav, 2019).

Oxidative stress is another significant pathogenesis in the development of pulmonary fibrosis (Cameli et al., 2020). Oxidative stress can contribute to the differentiation of fibroblasts into myofibroblasts (Bai et al., 2018), the apoptosis of alveolar epithelial cells (Liu et al., 2010), and the EMT (Felton et al., 2009). One study found that the level of antioxidants, including superoxide dismutase (SOD) is reduced, and the level of oxidants, including methane dicarboxylic aldehyde (MDA) is increased in the lungs and serum of a rat pulmonary fibrosis model (Bai et al., 2018).

Hyperoside (Hyp) is extracted from Rhododendron brachycarpum G. Don (Ye et al., 2017). Studies have shown that Hyp has numerous biological effects, such as anti-inflammatory (Ye et al., 2017), antioxidant (Ye et al., 2017), anti-fibrosis (Zou et al., 2017), and anti-cancer (Yang et al., 2017) effects. Hyp has been revealed to alleviate allergic airway inflammation through the activation of the Nf-E2 related factor 2 (Nrf2) pathway (Ye et al., 2017). Additionally, Hyp was found to have a protective effect on chronic liver fibrosis induced through carbon tetrachloride (Zou et al., 2017). Moreover, Hyp could protect against cardiac remodeling induced by pressure overload through the inhibition of AKT signaling (Wang et al., 2018). In the present study, we explored the protective effects of Hyp on Blm-induced pulmonary fibrosis in a C57BL/6 mice model.

MATERIALS AND METHODS

Materials

Hyp (purity over 98%, B20631) was bought from the Yuanye Biotechnology Co., Ltd. (Shanghai, China). Bleomycin sulfate (S1214) was obtained from Selleck (Shanghai, China). Primary antibodies used in our project were as follows: anti-p-AKT Ser473(Cell Signaling Technology, 4060, dilution 1:2000), anti-AKT(Cell Signaling Technology, 4691, dilution 1:1000), anti-GSK-3β (Cell Signaling Technology, 12456, dilution 1:1000), anti-p-GSK-3β Ser9 (Cell Signaling Technology, 9323, dilution 1:1000), anti-TGF-β1 (Proteintech, 21898-1-AP, dilution 1:1000), anti-SNAIL1 (Proteintech, 13099-1-AP, dilution 1:1000), anti-E-cadherin (Proteintech, 20874-1-AP, dilution 1:1000), anti-a-SMA (Proteintech, 14395-1-AP, dilution 1:1000), anti-vimentin (Cell Signaling Technology, 5741, dilution 1:1000), anti-fibronectin (Proteintech, 15613-1-AP, dilution 1:1000), anti-TWIST1 (Proteintech, 25465-1-AP, dilution 1:1000), anti-N-cadherin (Proteintech, 22018-1-AP, dilution 1:1000), anti-GAPDH (Servicebio Biotechnology Co., Ltd., GB12002, dilution 1:1000), and anti-collagen I (Abcam, ab34710, dilution 1:1000).

Mouse Models and Treatment

A single intratracheal aerosol injection of Blm (2 mg/kg) dissolved in saline was administered to induce pulmonary fibrosis in C57BL/6 mice (Li et al., 2018). A total of 10 mg of Hyp was dissolved in 20 ul of dimethyl sulfoxide, and then diluted with saline. Hyp was intraperitoneally administered to mice at a dose of 50 mg/kg/d on the basis of a previous study (Jin et al., 2016). The C57BL/6 male mice were procured from the GemPharmatech Co., Ltd. (Jiangsu, China). A total of 32 mice were randomly divided into four groups with eight mice per group: control group, Hyp group, Blm group, Blm plus Hyp group. The control group and Hyp group mice were intratracheally aerosol injected with the same dose of saline. The pulmonary fibrosis mice model was constructed on day 0. Seven days after Blm treatment, the Hyp group and the Blm plus Hyp group mice were intraperitoneally administered with Hyp for 14 days. The control group and Blm group were intraperitoneally administered with a vehicle solution at the same time. Afterwards, the lungs were harvested and weighed on the 21st day. The lung tissues were stored at −80°C and fixed with 10% buffered formalin. The lung index was determined as follows: lung index = lung weight (mg)/body weight (g). The animal experimental procedures were approved by the animal ethics committee of West China Hospital, Sichuan University, and consistent with the National Institutes of Health Guide for Care and Use of Laboratory Animals.

Histopathological Analysis and Immunohistochemical Analysis

After the lung tissues were fixed with 10% buffered formalin over 24 h, the lung tissues were embedded in paraffin and cut at 4 μm. Then, the sections underwent hematoxylin-eosin (HE) staining, Masson trichrome staining, and Sirius Red staining. The fibrosis levels were evaluated through the Ashcroft scoring system (Ashcroft et al., 1988). Immunohistochemistry was used to research the level of E-cadherin and a-SMA in the lung tissues. After the sections were dewaxed and rehydrated, they were treated with 3% H_2O_2 to inactivate the endogenous peroxidase activity. Then, the sections were blocked through 5% bull serum albumin and incubated with primary antibodies against E-cadherin and a-SMA at a 1:400 dilution. Next, the sections were incubated with secondary antibodies, developed with diaminobenzidine, and stained with hematoxylin.

Determination of Hydroxyproline, Oxidative Stress, and Inflammatory Cytokine in Lung Tissues

The hydroxyproline, SOD (A001-3,Nanjing Jiancheng, Nanjing, China), and MDA (A003-1,Nanjing Jiancheng, Nanjing, China) contents in the mice lung tissues were detected according to the manufacturer's instructions. The inflammatory cytokine levels, including tumor necrosis factor-alpha (TNF-α) (E-EL-M0049c, Elabscience, Wuhan, China) and interleukin 6 (IL-6) (E-EL-M0044c, Elabscience, Wuhan, China), were determined by using an ELISA kit as per the manufacturer's instructions.

Real-Time PCR Analysis

Total RNA was isolated from the four groups of homogenized mice lung tissues using the TRIzol reagent (Invitrogen, USA) and then were reverse transcribed into cDNA using a PrimeScript™ RT reagent kit (Takara, Japan) as per the kit's instructions. Real-time PCR (RT-PCR) was performed with a SYBR Green Kit (Takara, Japan) to determine the mRNA levels of E-cadherin, a-SMA, collagen I, vimentin, twist1, fibronectin, snail1, and N-cadherin, and the $2^{-\Delta\Delta Ct}$ method was used to analyze the data. The primer information of GAPDH, E-cadherin, a-SMA, collagen I, vimentin, twist1, fibronectin, snail1, and N-cadherin are presented as follows. GAPDH-F 5′-CCTCGTCC CGTAGACAAAATG-3′, GAPDH-R 5′-TGAGGTCAATGAA GGGGTCGT-3′;E-cadherin-F 5′-CGACCGGAAGTGACTC GAAAT-3′, E-cadherin-R 5′-TCAGAACCACTGCCCT CGTAAT-3′;a-SMA-F 5′-TCAGGGAGTAATGGTTGGAATG-3′, a-SMA- R 5′-CCAGAGTCCAGCACAATACCAG-3′; collagen I-F 5′-AAGAAGCACGTCTGGTTTGGAG-3′, collagen I-R 5′-GGTCCATGTAGGCTACGCTGTT-3′, vimentin-F 5′-GCAGTATGAAAGCGTGGCTG-3′, vimentin-R 5′-CTCCAGGGACTCGTTAGTGC-3′; twist1-F 5′-CGG CCAGGTACATCGACTTC-3′, twist1-R 5′-TGCAGCTT GCCATCTTGGAG-3′; fibronectin-F 5′-ACACGGTTTCCCAT TACGCC-3′, fibronectin-R 5′-GGTCTTCCCATCGTC ATAGCAC-3′; snail1-F 5′-AAGCCATTCTCCTGCTCCCA-3′, snail1-R 5′-AGCCAGACTCTTGGTGCTTGTG-3′; N-cadherin -F 5′-CCCTGACTGAGGAGCCTATGAA-3′, N-cadherin –R 5′-GGTTGATAATGAAGATGCCCGTT-3′.

Western Blot Analysis

Frozen lung tissues were homogenized in RIPA lysis buffer (Beyotime, China). Then, the samples were placed on ice for 10 min and centrifuged for 15 min at 12,000 r/min. After adding 5× protein sample loading buffers (Epizyme, China), the supernatants of the samples were boiled for 10 min. Protein concentrations were detected with a BCA Protein Kit (Beyotime, China). The proteins were separated using 10% SDS-PAGE (Epizyme, China), then transferred onto polyvinylidene difluoride (PVDF) membranes (Millipore, USA) at a constant current of 200 mA. Next, after blocking with 5% non-fat milk for one hour, the membranes were incubated with different primary antibodies against p-AKT, AKT, GSK-3β, p-GSK-3β, TGF-β1, SNAIL1, E-cadherin, vimentin, TWIST1, fibronectin, N-cadherin, a-SMA, collagen I, and GAPDH at 4°C overnight. Subsequently, the membranes were incubated with the appropriate secondary antibodies. The blot was analyzed using the Image J software.

Statistical Analysis

The experimental data were expressed as the mean ± standard deviation. The differences were analyzed by student's t tests or one-way ANOVA tests using SPSS 16.0, and the graphs were performed through GraphPad Prism 6.0. A p-value < 0.05 was regarded as statistically significant.

RESULTS

Hyp Attenuated Blm-Induced Pulmonary Fibrosis Development in Mice

After a single intratracheal aerosol injection of Blm, the Blm group showed a significant body weight loss and lung index increase compared to the control group, and it was dramatically reversed by Hyp intervention (**Figures 1A, B**). Meanwhile, as shown in **Figure 1C**, the Ashcroft scores, which reflect the fibrosis levels (Ashcroft et al., 1988), were also markedly increased in the Blm group. Compared with the Blm group, the Blm plus Hyp group had lower Ashcroft scores (**Figure 1C**). Compared to the control group, the Blm treatment contributed to the damaged lung tissue morphological structure, the thickened alveolar wall, and the excessive collagen deposition, as revealed *via* HE staining, Masson trichrome staining, and Sirius Red staining. These effects were dramatically alleviated by Hyp intervention (**Figures 1D–F**).

Hydroxyproline Content, Oxidative Stress, and Inflammatory Cytokine in the Mice Lung Tissues

As shown in **Figure 2A**, the mouse lung hydroxyproline content (a main ingredient of collagen) was elevated after Blm treatment compared to the control group. However, intervention with Hyp remarkably alleviated the mice's lung hydroxyproline content. The study found that oxidative stress also plays a significant role in the development of pulmonary fibrosis (Cameli et al., 2020). Hence, to further study the potential mechanisms of the protective effects of Hyp, we measured the oxidative stress in the mice lung tissues. As shown in **Figures 2B, C**, in the mice pulmonary fibrosis model, the activity of SOD, one kind of antioxidant, was dramatically decreased, while the content of MDA, another kind of oxidant, was dramatically increased. However, intervention with Hyp remarkably elevated the activity of SOD and remarkably reduced the content of MDA. In addition, the inflammatory cytokines, including IL-6 and TNF-α, were markedly elevated in the mice lung tissues of the pulmonary fibrosis model and were dramatically inhibited by Hyp (**Figures 2D, E**).

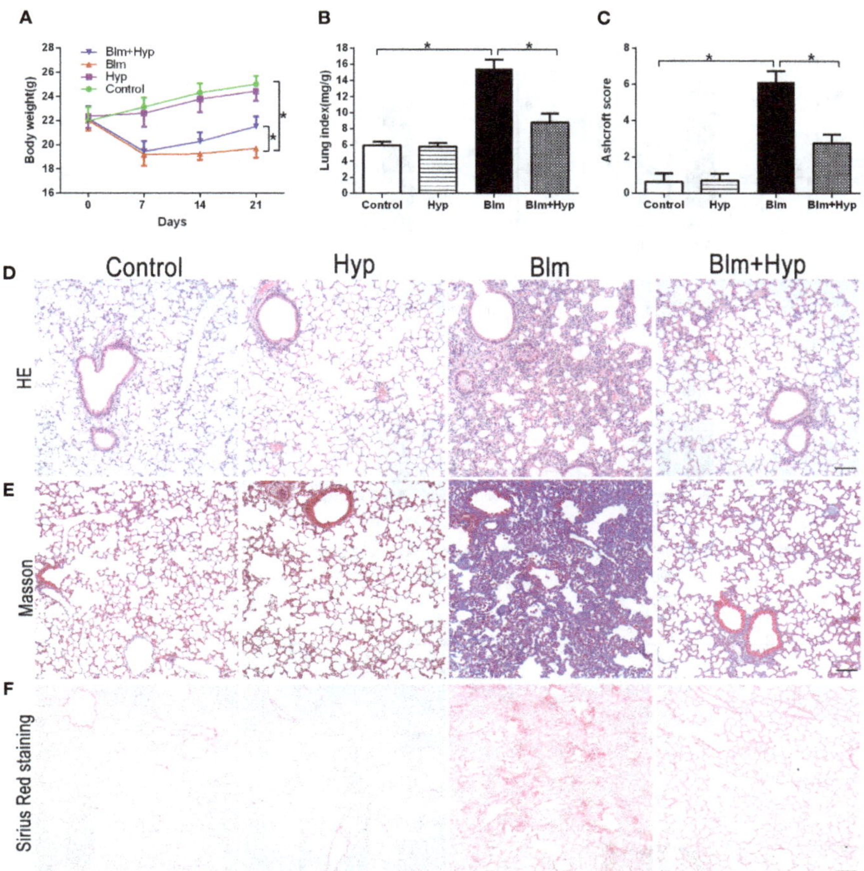

FIGURE 1 | Effect of Hyp on pulmonary fibrosis development induced by Blm in mice. **(A)** Mice body weights were measured (n=8). The pulmonary fibrosis mice model was established on day 0. **(B)** Mice lung index (lung weight/body weight) was calculated on the 21st day (n=8). **(C)** Ashcroft scores for the four groups were based on HE staining (n=4). Representative images of HE staining **(D)**, Masson trichrome staining **(E)**, and Sirius Red staining **(F)** for the four groups (scale bars =50 μm).*$P < 0.05$.

Hyp Inhibited EMT Induced by Blm *In Vivo*

As shown in **Figures 3A–E**, the Western blot and RT-PCR showed that the protein and gene levels of a-SMA and collagen I were up-regulated in the Blm group, and Hyp reduced the expression of a-SMA and collagen I. Hyp also inhibited the expression of TGF-β1 in the mice lung tissues treated with Blm (**Figures 3F, G**). Among the EMT-related markers, the Western blot showed that the protein levels of E-cadherin were down-regulated and the protein levels of fibronectin, N-cadherin, vimentin, TWIST1, and SNAIL1 were up-regulated in the Blm group, and the RT-PCR also showed that the gene levels of E-cadherin were down-regulated and the gene levels of fibronectin, N-cadherin, vimentin, twist1, and snail1 were up-regulated in the Blm group (**Figure 4**). However, compared to the Blm group, the EMT was markedly reversed by the intervention of Hyp. As shown in **Figure 5**, the immunohistochemical staining demonstrated that Blm treatment dramatically reduced the expression of E-cadherin and elevated the expression of a-SMA in mice lungs, and it was also reversed by the intervention of Hyp.

Hyp Inhibited the AKT/GSK3β Signaling Pathway *In Vivo*

To study the potential molecular mechanism of Hyp on pulmonary fibrosis, we detected the effects of Hyp on the AKT signaling pathway. The phosphorylation of AKT and GSK-3β were significantly increased in pulmonary fibrosis mice, and were dramatically inhibited by Hyp (**Figure 6**). GSK-3β is constitutively active and can be inactivated by phosphorylation of Ser9 in an AKT-dependent manner (Grimes and Jope, 2001). Therefore, Hyp intervention blocked activation of AKT and the inactivation of GSK-3β by AKT, and could inhibit the AKT/GSK3β signaling pathway *in vivo*.

DISCUSSION

Pulmonary fibrosis, the end stage of several diffuse parenchymal lung diseases, is a progressive disease, which leads to eventual death (Wuyts et al., 2013). Although the FDA has approved

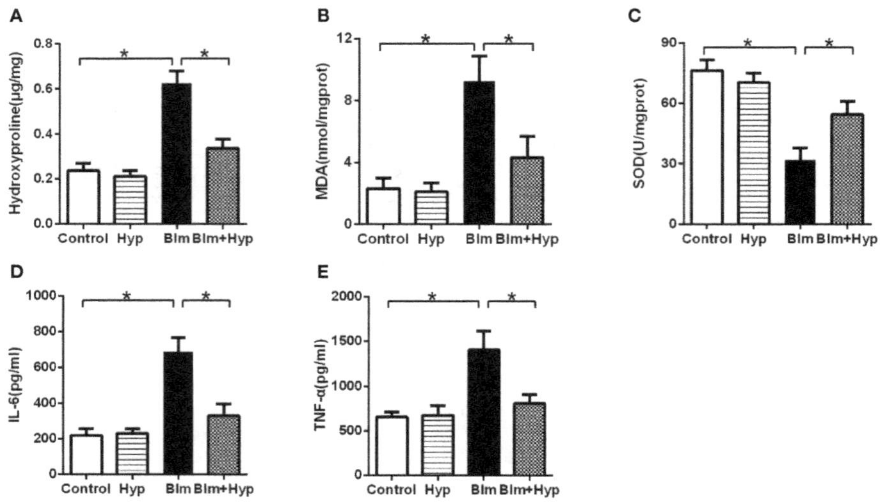

FIGURE 2 | Effect of Hyp on hydroxyproline, oxidative stress, and inflammatory cytokine in pulmonary fibrosis mice induced by Blm. The hydroxyproline content **(A)**, the MDA content **(B)**, the SOD activity **(C)**, the IL-6 level **(D)**, and the TNF-α level **(E)** were determined in the mice lung tissues (n=5). *P < 0.05.

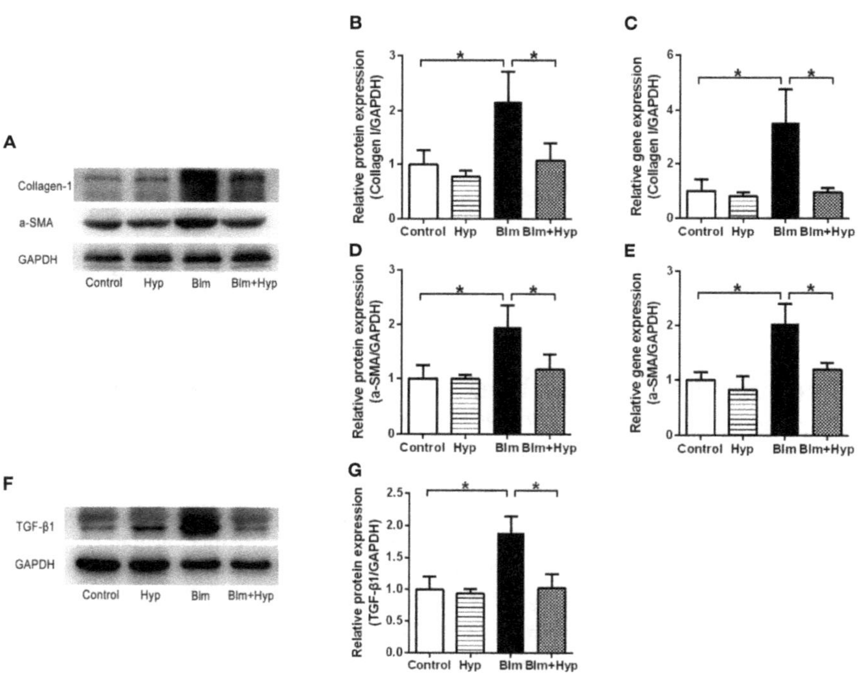

FIGURE 3 | Effect of Hyp on the fibrosis proteins in Blm-induced pulmonary fibrosis in mice. The protein expression of collagen I **(A, B)**, a-SMA **(D)**, TGF-β1 **(F, G)** was determined in each group *via* Western blot analysis (n=3). The gene expression of collagen I **(C)** and a-SMA **(E)** was determined in each group *via* RT-PCR analysis (n=3). *P < 0.05.

pirfenidone and nintedanib to treat IPF, none of these markedly decreases patients' mortality (Canestaro et al., 2016; Galli et al., 2017). Furthermore, few effective drugs can reverse human pulmonary fibrosis and prevent chronic progression to respiratory failure (Li and Kan, 2017). Therefore, it is very meaningful to seek new effective and targeted therapies for pulmonary fibrosis. Recent studies have revealed that the active ingredients from traditional Chinese medicine have anti-fibrotic effects (Li and Kan, 2017). Hyp is an active ingredient extracted from Rhododendron brachycarpum G. Don (Ye et al.,

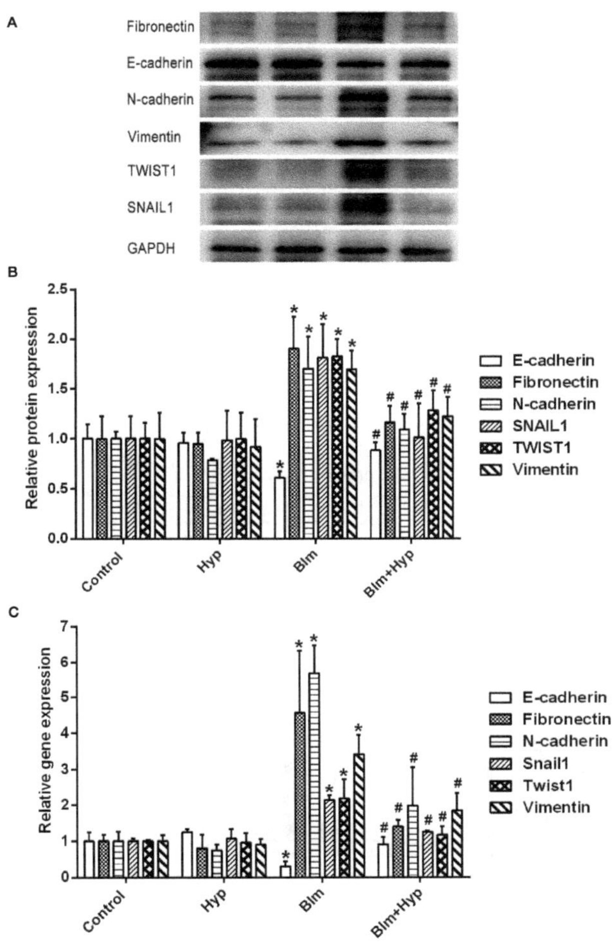

FIGURE 4 | Hyp inhibited EMT induced by Blm *in vivo*. The protein expression of fibronectin, E-cadherin, N-cadherin, vimentin, TWIST1, and SNAIL1 **(A, B)** was determined in each group *via* Western blot analysis (n=3). The gene expression of fibronectin, E-cadherin, N-cadherin, vimentin, twist1 and snail1 **(C)** was determined in each group *via* RT-PCR analysis (n=3). *P < 0.05 compared with the control group; #P < 0.05 compared with the Blm model group.

2017). Hyp is known to exert many pharmacological actions, including antioxidant and anti-fibrosis effects (Ye et al., 2017; Zou et al., 2017). Studies have shown that Hyp protects against oxidative damage and cytotoxicity induced by oxalic acid in human kidney-2 cells (Chen et al., 2018). Hyp has also been revealed to prevent heart failure-induced liver fibrosis (Guo et al., 2019). In this study, we revealed that Hyp attenuated Blm-induced pulmonary fibrosis development in mice *via* inhibiting oxidative stress, inflammation, and EMT.

After treatment with Blm, the mouse lung weight dramatically increased due to many factors, including inflammatory cell infiltration, cell swelling, and capillary congestion, and body weight was decreased (Xin et al., 2019). So, the lung index increased in the pulmonary fibrosis model and reflected the degree of pulmonary fibrosis (Xin et al., 2019). As expected, our results showed that the lung index was remarkably increased in the Blm group compared to the control group. After treatment with Hyp, the lung index was decreased.

The main characteristics of pulmonary fibrosis are the activation of myofibroblasts, the deposition of ECM, and the destruction of normal lung structure (Wuyts et al., 2013). Myofibroblasts, transformed from epithelial cells *via* EMT, produce ECM and contribute to the progression of pulmonary fibrosis (Scotton and Chambers, 2007; Zhang L. M. et al., 2019). However, some researchers took the opposite view. Rock et al. thought that epithelial cells were not the origin of myofibroblasts in pulmonary fibrosis (Rock et al., 2011). The origin of myofibroblasts is still controversial. Although it seemed to be a fact that EMT might contribute to pulmonary fibrosis (Willis and Borok, 2007; Zhang C. et al., 2019). We observed Blm-induced pathological changes in mice lung tissues *via* HE staining, Masson trichrome staining, and Sirius Red staining. As expected, the damaged lung tissue's morphological structure, the thickened alveolar walls, and the excessive collagen deposition were found in the Blm group. Moreover, the Ashcroft scores in the Blm model were significantly higher than in the control group. On the contrary, after treatment with Hyp, these pathological changes were dramatically alleviated. Lung hydroxyproline content, a main ingredient of collagen, was also remarkably reduced by Hyp treatment.

Oxidative stress, an imbalance between oxidants and antioxidants, and inflammation also play important roles in the development and progression of pulmonary fibrosis (Cameli et al., 2020; Otoupalova et al., 2020). One study found that the levels of T-SOD, catalase (CAT), and glutathione (GSH) were significantly decreased, and the expressions of MDA were significantly increased in rat lung and serum after Blm treatment (Bai et al., 2018). The inflammatory cytokines, such as TNF-α and IL-6, were also significantly increased after Blm administration (Ma W. H. et al., 2020). Furthermore, the inhibition of oxidative stress and inflammation might ameliorate pulmonary fibrosis in mice models (Ma W. H. et al., 2020). In our investigation, when compared with the control group, the levels of MDA, TNF-α, and IL-6 were dramatically increased and SOD was dramatically reduced in Blm-treated pulmonary fibrosis mice lung tissues. Meanwhile, Hyp markedly inhibited Blm-induced oxidative stress and inflammation in the lung tissues of mice.

TGF-β, one kind of multifunctional cytokine, regulates cell proliferation, cell differentiation, cell apoptosis, and cell migration and favors ECM production (Dennler et al., 2002). The TGF-β signaling pathway is implicated in many diseases, such as cancer, fibrosis, and autoimmune diseases (Dennler et al., 2002). TGF-β1 is an important profibrogenic cytokine in pulmonary fibrosis (Wei et al., 2019). During the progression of pulmonary fibrosis, TGF-β1 induces the differentiation of lung fibroblasts to myofibroblasts and increases the production of collagen (Wei et al., 2019). As expected, our results showed that TGF-β1 was remarkably increased in Blm-treated pulmonary fibrosis mice, and this effect was inhibited by Hyp. Likewise, the

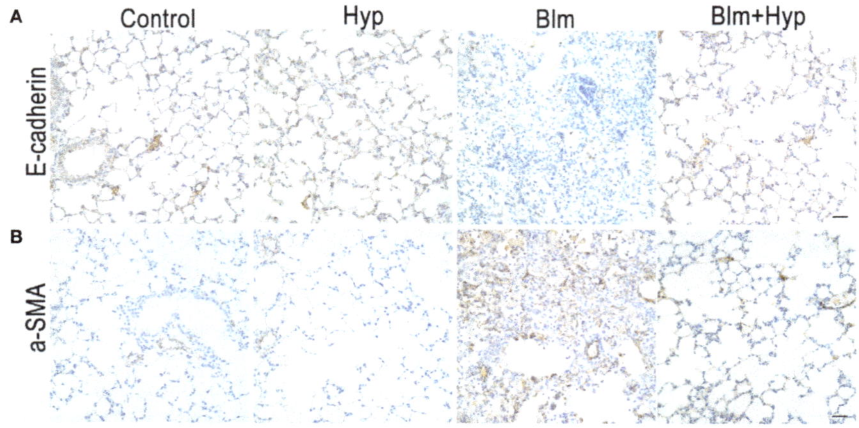

FIGURE 5 | The immunohistochemical analysis of E-cadherin **(A)** and a-SMA **(B)** in mice lung tissues (scale bars =20 μm).

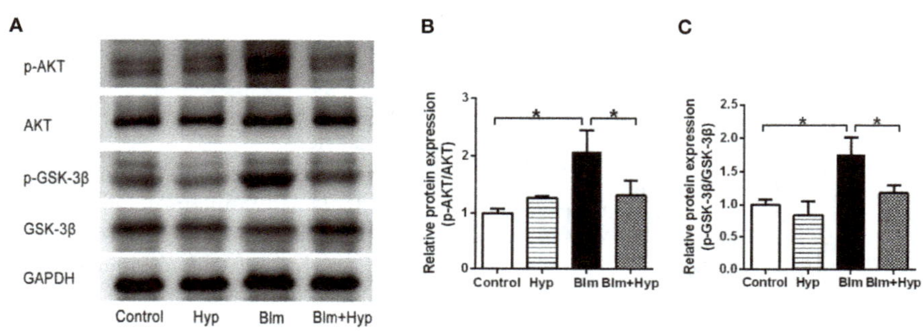

FIGURE 6 | Effect of Hyp on the AKT/GSK-3β signaling pathway in pulmonary fibrosis in mice induced by Blm. The protein expression of p-AKT and p-GSK-3β **(A–C)** was determined in each group *via* Western blot analysis (n=3). *P < 0.05.

levels of a-SMA and collagen I were raised in the Blm group, and Hyp could inhibit the increase of a-SMA and collagen I. Moreover, our study also found that Hyp inhibited the protein and gene levels of fibronectin, N-cadherin, vimentin, TWIST1, and SNAIL1 and increased the protein and gene levels of E-cadherin. However, there was no strong evidence to confirm the contribution of epithelial cells to fibroblasts in our study. Further studies would be needed to confirm the roles of epithelial cells in EMT and pulmonary fibrosis, including lineage tracing studies and cell studies.

The activation of several non-smad-dependent pathways, including the PI3K/AKT pathway and the MAPK pathway, are involved in TGF-β1-induced EMT (Willis and Borok, 2007). The PI3K/AKT pathway plays an important role in cell growth and cell proliferation (Yan et al., 2014). Recent studies have shown that the activation of the AKT pathway plays a considerable role in pulmonary fibrosis (Qu et al., 2019; Ma Z. et al., 2020).

GSK-3β, a serine threonine kinase, is a key downstream target of AKT that is involved in many cellular processes (Grimes and Jope, 2001). GSK-3β is constitutively active and can be inactivated by phosphorylation of Ser9 in an AKT-dependent manner (Grimes and Jope, 2001). One study found that the phosphorylation of AKT was increased in human pulmonary fibroblasts during Blm-induced fibrotic processes (Ma Z. et al., 2020). The phosphorylation of AKT was also increased in radiation-induced pulmonary fibrosis (Qu et al., 2019). Furthermore, during the Blm-induced toxic lung injury, the phosphorylation of AKT at Ser473 and GSK-3β at Ser9 were increased in human bronchial epithelial cells, and the increasing phosphorylation of GSK-3β at Ser9 could inhibit the activity of GSK-3β (Ma et al., 2009). However, the phosphorylation of GSK-3β was decreased after the human bronchial epithelial cells were pretreated with LY294002 (Ma et al., 2009). Cigarette smoke extract induced EMT in airway epithelial cells by the AKT/GSK3β pathway (Agraval and Yadav, 2019). One study found that during the development of Blm-induced pulmonary fibrosis, the up-regulation of SNAIL1 contributed to EMT (Zhang L. M. et al., 2019). Multi-walled carbon nanotubes could prompt the secretion of

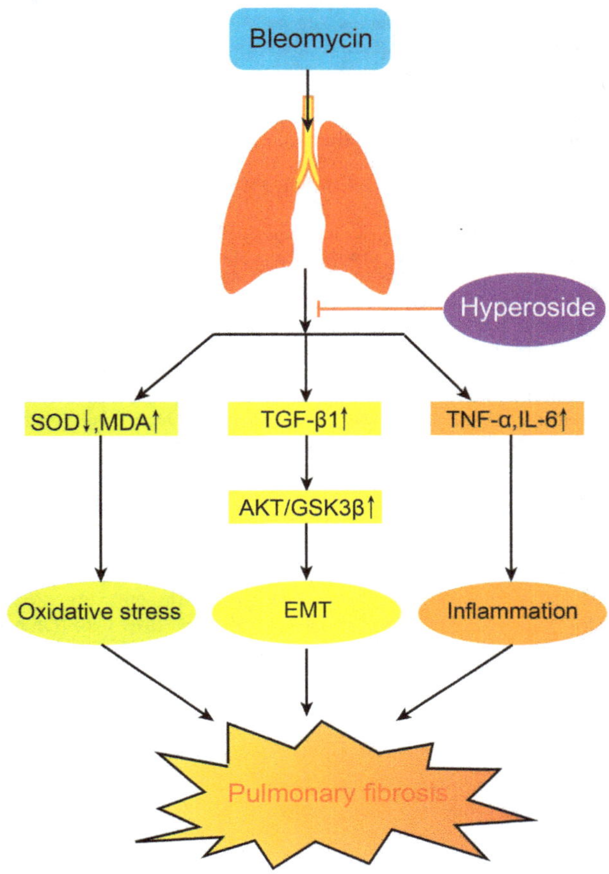

FIGURE 7 | The potential mechanism of Hyp on pulmonary fibrosis mice induced by Blm.

TGF-β, the activation of AKT, the inhibition of GSK-3β, and the up-regulation of SNAIL1 in human bronchial epithelial cells (Polimeni et al., 2016). This study demonstrated that multi-walled carbon nanotubes could induce EMT by the AKT/GSK-3β/SNAIL1 signaling pathway (Polimeni et al., 2016). Thus, we studied the changes of the AKT/GSK3β signaling pathway in Blm-induced pulmonary fibrosis. In the present study, the p-AKT and p-GSK-3β were significantly elevated in pulmonary fibrosis mice, and these increased expressions were reversed after Hyp treatment. Therefore, Hyp might inhibit EMT *via* the AKT/GSK3β pathway in pulmonary fibrosis. The precise mechanisms between EMT and the AKT/GSK3β pathway need further cell studies.

CONCLUSIONS

In summary, we revealed that Hyp attenuated pulmonary fibrosis development in mice, and the potential mechanism might be due to inhibiting the Blm-induced inflammation, oxidative stress, and EMT *via* the AKT/GSK3β pathway (**Figure 7**). Hyp might offer a promising candidate drug for the treatment of pulmonary fibrosis.

ETHICS STATEMENT

The animal study was reviewed and approved by the animal ethics committee of West China Hospital, Sichuan University.

AUTHOR CONTRIBUTIONS

JH and HF conceived the study. JH, XT,and LZ conducted the experiments. JH wrote the manuscript. JH and YZ conducted the statistical analysis and revised the manuscript. DW and SZ were involved in conducting the experiments. All authors contributed to the article and approved the submitted version.

REFERENCES

1. Agraval, H., and Yadav, U. C. S. (2019). MMP-2 and MMP-9 mediate cigarette smoke extract-induced epithelial-mesenchymal transition in airway epithelial cells via EGFR/Akt/GSK3**b**/**b**-catenin pathway: Amelioration by fisetin. *Chem. Biol. Interact.* 314, 108846. doi: 10.1016/j.cbi.2019.108846
2. Ashcroft, T., Simpson, J. M., and Timbrell, V. (1988). Simple method of estimating severity of pulmonary fibrosis on a numerical scale. *J. Clin. Pathol.* 41, 467–470. doi: 10.1136/jcp.41.4.467
3. Bai, Y., Li, J., Zhao, P., Li, Y., Li, M., Feng, S., et al. (2018). A Chinese herbal formula ameliorates pulmonary fibrosis by inhibiting oxidative stress via upregulating Nrf2. *Front. Pharmacol.* 9, 628. doi: 10.3389/fphar.2018.00628
4. Cameli, P., Carleo, A., Bergantini, L., Landi, C., Prasse, A., and Bargagli, E. (2020). Oxidant/antioxidant disequilibrium in idiopathic pulmonary fibrosis pathogenesis. *Inflammation* 43, 1–7. doi: 10.1007/s10753-019-01059-1
5. Canestaro, W. J., Forrester, S. H., Raghu, G., Ho, L., and Devine, B. E. (2016). Drug treatment of idiopathic pulmonary fibrosis: Systematic review and network meta-analysis. *Chest* 149, 756–766. doi: 10.1016/j.chest.2015.11.013
6. Chen, Y., Ye, L., Li, W., Li, D., and Li, F. (2018). Hyperoside protects human kidney-2 cells against oxidative damage induced by oxalic acid. *Mol. Med. Rep.* 18, 486–494. doi: 10.3892/mmr.2018.8948
7. Dennler, S., Goumans, M. J., and ten Dijke, P. (2002). Transforming growth factor beta signal transduction. *J. Leukoc. Biol.* 71, 731–740.
8. Felton, V. M., Borok, Z., and Willis, B. C. (2009). N-acetylcysteine inhibits alveolar epithelial-mesenchymal transition. *Am. J. Physiol. Lung Cell Mol. Physiol.* 297, L805–L812. doi: 10.1152/ajplung.00009.2009
9. Galli, J. A., Pandya, A., Vega-Olivo, M., Dass, C., Zhao, H., and Criner, G. J. (2017). Pirfenidone and nintedanib for pulmonary fibrosis in clinical practice: Tolerability and adverse drug reactions. *Respirology* 22, 1171–1178. doi: 10.1111/resp.13024
10. Grimes, C. A., and Jope, R. S. (2001). The multifaceted roles of glycogen synthase kinase 3beta in cellular signaling. *Prog. Neurobiol.* 65, 391–426. doi: 10.1016/ s0301-0082(01)00011-9
11. Guo, X., Zhu, C., Liu, X., Ge, Y., Jiang, X., and Zhao, W. (2019). Hyperoside protects against heart failure-induced liver fibrosis in rats. *Acta Histochem.* 121, 804–811. doi: 10.1016/j.acthis.2019.07.005
12. Hutchinson, J., Fogarty, A., Hubbard, R., and McKeever, T. (2015). Global incidence and mortality of idiopathic pulmonary fibrosis: A systematic review. *Eur. Respir. J.* 46, 795–806. doi: 10.1183/09031936.00185114
13. Jin, X. N., Yan, E. Z., Wang, H. M., Sui, H. J., Liu, Z., Gao, W., et al. (2016). Hyperoside exerts anti-inflammatory and anti-arthritic effects in LPS-stimulated human fibroblast-like synoviocytes in vitro and in mice with collagen-induced arthritis. *Acta Pharmacol. Sin.* 37, 674 686. doi: 10.1038/aps.2016.7

14. Kim, H. J., Perlman, D., and Tomic, R. (2015). Natural history of idiopathic pulmonary fibrosis. *Respir. Med.* 109, 661–670. doi: 10.1016/j.rmed.2015.02.002
15. Li, L. C., and Kan, L. D. (2017). Traditional Chinese medicine for pulmonary fibrosis therapy: Progress and future prospects. *J. Ethnopharmacol.* 198, 45–63. doi: 10.1016/j.jep.2016.12.042
16. Li, B., Huang, X., Liu, Z., Xiu, X., Xiao, H., Zhang, X., et al. (2018). Ouabain ameliorates bleomycin induced pulmonary fibrosis by inhibiting proliferation and promoting apoptosis of lung fibroblasts. *Am. J. Transl. Res.* 10, 2967–2974.
17. Liu, G., Beri, R., Mueller, A., and Kamp, D. W. (2010). Molecular mechanisms of asbestos-induced lung epithelial cell apoptosis. *Chem. Biol. Interact.* 188, 309–318. doi: 10.1016/j.cbi.2010.03.047
18. Lovisa, S., LeBleu, V. S., Tampe, B., Sugimoto, H., Vadnagara, K., Carstens, J. L., et al. (2015). Epithelial-to-mesenchymal transition induces cell cycle arrest and parenchymal damage in renal fibrosis. *Nat. Med.* 21, 998–1009. doi: 10.1038/ nm.3902
19. Ma, Y., Wang, M., Li, N., Wu, R., and Wang, X. (2009). Bleomycin-induced nuclear factor-kappaB activation in human bronchial epithelial cells involves the phosphorylation of glycogen synthase kinase 3beta. *Toxicol. Lett.* 187, 194– 200. doi: 10.1016/j.toxlet.2009.02.023
20. Ma, W. H., Li, M., Ma, H. F., Li, W., Liu, L., Yin, Y., et al. (2020). Protecti ve effects of GHK-Cu in bleomycin-induced pulmonary fibrosis via anti-oxidative stress and anti-inflammation pathways. *Life Sci.* 241:117139. doi: 10.1016/j.lfs.2019.117139
21. Ma, Z., Yu, R., Zhu, Q., Sun, L., Jian, L., Wang, X., et al. (2020). CXCL16/ CXCR6 axis promotes bleomycin-induced fibrotic process in MRC-5 cells via the PI3K/ AKT/FOXO3a pathway. *Int. Immunopharmacol.* 81, 106035. doi: 10.1016/ j.intimp.2019.106035
22. Marmai, C., Sutherland, R. E., Kim, K. K., Dolganov, G. M., Fang, X., Kim, S. S., et al. (2011). Alveolar epithelial cells express mesenchymal proteins in patients with idiopathic pulmonary fibrosis. *Am. J. Physiol. Lung Cell Mol. Physiol.* 301, L71–L78. doi: 10.1152/ajplung.00212.2010
23. Otoupalova, E., Smith, S., Cheng, G., and Thannickal, V. J. (2020). Oxidative stress in pulmonary fibrosis. *Compr. Physiol.* 10, 509–547. doi: 10.1002/cphy.c190017
24. Polimeni, M., Gulino, G. R., Gazzano, E., Kopecka, J., Marucco, A., Fenoglio, I., et al. (2016). Multi-walled carbon nanotubes directly induce epithelial-mesenchymal transition in human bronchial epithelial cells via the TGF-**b**-mediated Akt/GSK-3**b**/SNAIL-1 signaling pathway. *Part Fibre Toxicol.* 13, 27.doi: 10.1186/s12989-016-0138-4
25. Qu, H., Liu, L., Liu, Z., Qin, H., Liao, Z., Xia, P., et al. (2019). Blocking TBK1 alleviated radiation-induced pulmonary fibrosis and epithelial-mesenchymal transition through Akt-Erk inactivation. *Exp. Mol. Med.* 51, 1–17. doi: 10.1038/ s12276-019-0240-4
26. Richeldi, L., Collard, H. R., and Jones, M. G. (2017). Idiopathic pulmonary fibrosis. *Lancet* 389, 1941–1952. doi: 10.1016/s0140-6736(17)30866-8
27. Rock, J. R., Barkauskas, C. E., Cronce, M. J., Xue, Y., Harris, J. R., Liang, J., et al. (2011). Multiple stromal populations contribute to pulmonary fibrosis without evidence for epithelial to mesenchymal transition. *Proc. Natl. Acad. Sci. U. S. A.* 108, E1475–E1483. doi: 10.1073/pnas.1117988108
28. Scotton, C. J., and Chambers, R. C. (2007). Molecular targets in pulmonary fibrosis: The myofibroblast in focus. *Chest* 132, 1311–1321. doi: 10.1378/ chest.06-2568
29. Wang, X., Liu, Y., Xiao, L., Li, L., Zhao, X., Yang, L., et al. (2018). Hyperoside protects against pressure overload-induced cardiac remodeling via the AKT signaling pathway. *Cell. Physiol. Biochem.* 51, 827–841. doi: 10.1159/000495368
30. Wei, P., Xie, Y., Abel, P. W., Huang, Y., Ma, Q., Li, L., et al. (2019). Transforming growth factor (TGF)-**b**1-induced miR-133a inhibits myofibroblast differentiation and pulmonary fibrosis. *Cell Death Dis.* 10, 670. doi: 10.1038/ s41419-019-1873-x
31. Willis, B. C., and Borok, Z. (2007). TGF-beta-induced EMT: Mechanisms and implications for fibrotic lung disease. *Am. J. Physiol. Lung Cell Mol. Physiol.* 293, L525–L534. doi: 10.1152/ajplung.00163.2007
32. Wuyts, W. A., Agostini , C., Antoniou, K. M., Bouros, D., Chambers, R. C., Cottin, V., et al. (2013). The pathogenesis of pulmonary fibrosis: A moving target. *Eur. Respir. J.* 41, 1207–1218. doi: 10.1183/09031936.00073012
33. Xin, X., Yao, D., Zhang, K., Han, S., Liu, D., Wang, H., et al. (2019). Protective effects of Rosavin on bleomycin-induced pulmonary fibrosis via suppressing fibrotic and inflammatory signaling pathways in mice. *Biomed. Pharmacother.* 115, 108870. doi: 10.1016/j.biopha.2019.108870
34. Xu, F., Liu, X. C., Li, L., Ma, C. N., and Zhang, Y. J. (2017). Effects of TRPC1 on epithelial mesenchymal transition in human airway in chronic obstructive pulmonary disease. *Medicine* 96, e8166. doi: 10.1097/md.0000000000008166
35. Yan, Z., Kui, Z., and Ping, Z. (2014). Reviews and prospectives of signaling pathway analysis in idiopathic pulmonary fibrosis. *Autoimmun. Rev.* 13, 1020– 1025. doi: 10.1016/j.autrev.2014.08.028
36. Yang, Y., Tantai, J., Sun, Y., Zhong, C., and Li, Z. (2017). Effect of Hyperoside on the apoptosis of A549 human non-small cell lung cancer cells and the underlying mechanism. *Mol. Med. Rep.* 16, 6483–6488. doi: 10.3892/ mmr.2017.7453
37. Yang, J., Antin, P., Berx, G., Blanpain, C., Brabletz, T., Bronner, M., et al. (2020). Guidelines and definitions for research on epithelial-mesenchymal transition. *Nat. Rev. Mol. Cell Biol.* 21, 341–352. doi: 10.1038/s41580-020-0237-9
38. Ye, P., Yang, X. L., Chen, X., and Shi, C. (2017). Hyperoside attenuates OVA-induced allerg ic airway inflammation by activating Nrf2. *Int. Immunopharmacol.* 44, 168–173. doi: 10.1016/j.intimp.2017.01.003
39. Yin, C., Lin, X., Wang, Y., Liu, X., Xiao, Y., Liu, J., et al. (2020). FAM83D promotes epithelial-mesenchymal transition, invasion and cisplatin resistance through regulating the AKT/mTOR pathway in non-small-cell lung cancer. *Cell Oncol.* 43, 395–407. doi: 10.1007/s13402-020-00494-9
40. Zhang, C., Zhu, X., Hua, Y., Zhao, Q., Wang, K., Zhen, L., et al. (2019). YY1 mediates TGF-**b**1-induced EMT and pro-fibrogenesis in alveolar epithelial cells. *Respir. Res.* 20, 249. doi: 10.1186/s12931-019-1223-7
41. Zhang, L. M., Zhang, Y., Fei, C., Zhang, J., Wang, L., Yi, Z. W., et al. (2019). Neutralization of IL-18 by IL-18 binding protein ameliorates bleomycin-induced pulmonary fibrosis via inhibition of epithelial-mesenchymal transition. *Biochem. Biophys. Res. Commun.* 508, 660–666. doi: 10.1016/ j.bbrc.2018.11.129
42. Zou, L., Chen, S., Li, L., and Wu, T. (2017). The protective effect of Hyperoside on carbon tetrachloride-induced chronic liver fibrosis in mice via upregulation of Nrf2. *Exp. Toxicol. Pathol.* 69, 451–460. doi: 10.1016/j.etp.2017.04.001

19

Potential Mechanism Prediction of Herbal Medicine for Pulmonary Fibrosis Associated with SARS-CoV-2 Infection Based on Network Analysis and Molecular Docking

De Jin[1†], Xuedong An[1†], Yuqing Zhang[1†], Shenghui Zhao[2], Liyun Duan[1], Yingying Duan[2], Fengmei Lian[1] and Xiaolin Tong[1*]*

[1]Guang'anmen Hospital, China Academy of Chinese Medical Sciences, Beijing, China, [2]Graduate School, Beijing University of Chinese Medicine, Beijing, China

***Correspondence:**
Fengmei Lian
694397644@qq.com
Xiaolin Tong
tongxiaolin66@sina.com

[†]These authors have contributed equally to this work

Background: Coronavirus Disease 2019 (COVID-19) is still a relevant global problem. Although some patients have recovered from COVID-19, the sequalae to the SARS-CoV-2 infection may include pulmonary fibrosis, which may contribute to considerable economic burden and health-care challenges. Convalescent Chinese Prescription (CCP) has been widely used during the COVID-19 recovery period for patients who were at high risk of pulmonary fibrosis and is recommended by the Diagnosis and Treatment Protocol for COVID-19 (Trial Version sixth, seventh). However, its underlying mechanism is still unclear.

Methods: In this study, an integrated pharmacology approach was implemented, which involved evaluation of absorption, distribution, metabolism and excretion of CCP, data mining of the disease targets, protein-protein interaction (PPI) network construction, and analysis, enrichment analysis, and molecular docking simulation, to predict the bioactive components, potential targets, and molecular mechanism of CCP for pulmonary fibrosis associated with SARS-CoV-2 infection.

Results: The active compound of CCP and the candidate targets, including pulmonary fibrosis targets, were obtained through database mining. The Drug-Disease network was constructed. Sixty-five key targets were identified by topological analysis. The findings of Gene Ontology (GO) terms and Kyoto Encyclopedia of Genes and Genomes (KEGG) pathway annotation suggested that the VEGF, Toll-like 4 receptor, MAPK signaling pathway, and TGF-β1 signaling pathways may be involved in pulmonary fibrosis. In the molecular docking analyses, VEGF, TNF-α, IL-6, MMP9 exhibited good binding activity. Findings from our study indicated that CCP could inhibit the expression of *VEGF, TNF-α, IL-6, MMP9, TGF-β1* via the VEGF, Toll-like 4 receptor, MAPK, and TGF-β1 signaling pathways.

Conclusion: Potential mechanisms involved in CCP treatment for COVID-19 pulmonary fibrosis associated with SARS-CoV-2 infection involves multiple components and multiple target points as well as multiple pathways. These findings may offer a profile for further investigations of the anti-fibrotic mechanism of CCP.

Keywords: network pharmacology, molecular mechanisms, pulmonary fibrosis, SARS-CoV-2, Chinese herbal medicine

INTRODUCTION

Severe acute respiratory syndrome coronavirus 2 (SARS-CoV-2) is a newly discovered coronavirus responsible for COVID-19, which causes atypical pneumonia progressing to acute respiratory distress syndrome (ARDS) and acute lung injury (Marini and Gattinoni, 2020). After SARS-CoV-2 infection, patients who have experienced and survived the COVID-19 outbreak may face a greater risk of developing pulmonary fibrosis (PF), which is a chronic, severe, and progressive interstitial lung disease (George et al., 2020). A meta-analysis demonstrated that there was a clear association between the development of PF and respiratory viral infection (Hutchinson et al., 2015). A well-known mechanism is that SARS-CoV-2 invades host cells and interacts with ACE2, which is highly expressed in pneumocytes type II cells and is directly involved in the initiation and progression of inflammation and fibrosis (Ksiazek et al., 2003; Li et al., 2003; Xu et al., 2020). Importantly, PF not only forms as a sequelae to chronic inflammation but is also is genetically influenced by an age-related fibroproliferative process such as idiopathic PF. Further, PF is a well-recognized sequela of ARDS (Burnham et al., 2014). Existing data show that about 40% of COVID-19 patients may develop ARDS, which accounts for a high percentage of COVID-19 patients (Wu et al., 2020). Although in most patients, the virus in patients recovering from COVID-19 has been eradicated, this does not prevent the development of PF. Given these observations, PF after recovery from COVID-19 may result in a substantial medical burden and health-care challenges. Therefore, preventing PF in patients recovering from SARS-CoV-2 infection is an urgent issue that needs to be addressed.

Currently, there are few anti-fibrotic drugs available with clinically positive results, and a limited number of such agents are under investigation (Canestaro et al., 2016). Although the antifibrotic medicines, such as pirfenidone and nintedanib approved by FDA, could delay the decline in lung function, these drugs may not improve the quality of life (QoL) or reduce early mortality (Rochwerg et al., 2016; Brown et al., 2020). More importantly, these drugs may not be prescribed for severe or critical cases with COVID-19 on mechanical ventilation due to oral use only. Moreover, pirfenidone and nintedanib are associated with a high incidence of drug-related side effects such as abnormal liver function and uncomfortable clinical manifestations such as gastrointestinal disturbances and skin reactions (King et al., 2014; Kim and Keating, 2015; Noble et al., 2016; Hanta et al., 2019), which have restricted their clinical application. Thus, the development of an effective therapeutic strategy for PF is urgent.

Traditional Chinese medicines (TCM) have been widely used to treat lung diseases. Recently, several meta-analyses have shown that TCM exerted positive effects on PF, such as delaying the decline of pulmonary function and improving the QoL, with a good safety profile (Liu et al., 2018; Ji et al., 2020). In addition, several pharmacological studies are investigating TCM as an anti-PF treatment. Some studies have revealed that TCM could effectively resist oxidative lesion, histopathological damage (Sun et al., 2018), and reverse extracellular matrix (ECM) as well as Lox2 proliferation by modulating MAPK activation and suppressing the TGF-β/Smad pathway (Tao et al., 2017). A convalescent Chinese prescription (CCP) was widely used for patients with COVID-19 who were in the recovery period and were at high-risk of pulmonary fibrosis, as recommended by the Diagnosis and Treatment Protocol for COVID-19 (Trial Version sixth, seventh) published by the National Health Commission of the People's Republic of China (National Health Commission of the People's Republic of China, 2020a; National Health Commission of the People's Republic of China, 2020b).

Although clear clinical benefits exist, very little has been elucidated about the potential molecular mechanism involved. Network pharmacology is a branch of pharmacology that uses network methods to analyze the synergistic relationship among drugs and diseases and targets via "multi-component, multi-target, multi-pathway" analyses, and can build a multi-dimensional network model of "drug–component–target–disease" to explore the relationship between drugs and diseases (Missiuro et al., 2009; von Mering et al., 2003). This study was based on network pharmacology and systematically analyzed the effective ingredients, potential targets, pathways, and biological processes of CCP used during the recovery period of COVID-19. The study screened the main active ingredients of CCP via a molecular docking approach to explore the potential molecular mechanisms of action involved in CCP interference with PF associated with SARS-CoV-2 infection. The flowchart of the whole study design is illustrated in **Figure 1**.

MATERIALS AND METHODS

Active Components Database

CCP contains 18 types of Chinese herbal medicine (**Table 1**). All ingredients related to CCP were screened by the Traditional Chinese Medicine Systems Pharmacology database and Analysis Platform (TCMSP), PubChem database (http://pubchem.ncbi.nlm.nih.gov), China Knowledge Network, PubMed and BATMAN-TCM) and Shanghai Institute of Organic Chemistry of CAS. Chemistry Database [DB/OL].

Screening of Active Ingredients

The critical parameters of oral bioavailability (OB), drug-likeness (DL), and drug half-life (HL) were used to screen the active components of CCP. OB is an essential indicator for objective

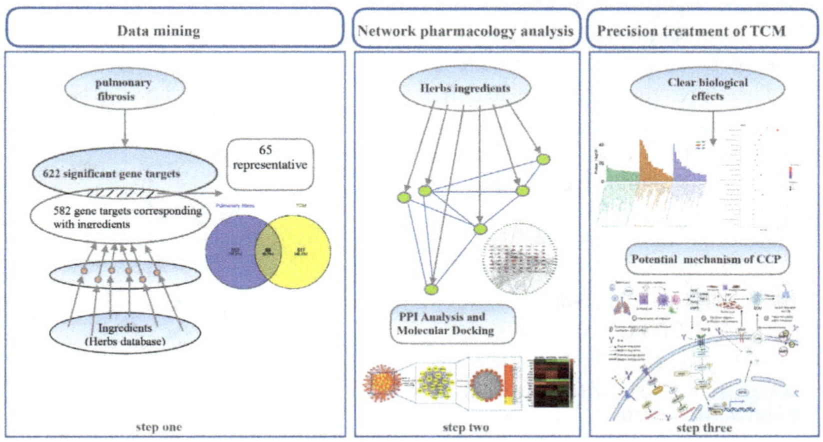

FIGURE 1 | Schematic diagram of the integrated pharmacology strategy approach that combines quantitative analysis of components, network analysis, and molecular docking to investigate the mechanisms of Convalescent Chinese prescription (CCP) treatment against pulmonary fibrosis.

TABLE 1 | Composition of herbs in Convalescent Chinese prescription (CCP).

Latin name	English name	Chinese name	Abbreviation
Radix astragali seu hedysari	Milkvetch root	Huang qi	HQ
Radix codonopsis	Tangshen	Dang sheng	DS
Rhizoma atractylodis Macrocephalae	Largehead atractylodes rhizome	Bai zhu	BZ
Radix adenophorae	Fourleaf ladybell root	Nan sha shen	NSS
Radix glehniae	Coastal glehnia root	Bei sha shen	BSS
Pericarpium citri reticulatae	Dried tangerine peel	Chen pi	CP
Poria	Lndian bread	Fu ling	FL
Radix ophiopogonis	Dwarf lilyturf tuber	Mai dong	MD
Radix salviae miltiorrhizae	Radix salviae miltiorrhizae	Dan shen	DSH
Bulbus fritillariae thunbergii	Thunberbg fritillary bulb	Zhe bei mu	ZBM
Hirudo	Leech	Shui zhi	SZ
Fructus crataegi	Hawthorn fruit	Chao Shan zha	CSZ
Massa medicata fermentata	Medicated leaven	Shen qu	SQ
Fructus hordei germinatus	Germinated barley	Mai ya	MY
Rhizoma dioscoreae	Common yam rhizome	Shan yao	SY
Eupolyphaga seu steleophaga	Ground beetle	Tu bie chong	TBC
Liquorice root	Radix glycyrrhizae	Gan cao	GC
Rhizoma pinelliae	Pinellia tuber	Ban xia	BX

evaluation of the internal quality of drugs. OB defines the percentage of an orally administered dose of unchanged drug that reaches the systemic circulation and represents the convergence of the absorption, distribution, metabolism, and excretion (ADME) process. High OB is often a key indicator to determine the "drug-like" properties of bioactive molecules as therapeutic agents. Molecules with OB >30% were considered to have good OB in the present study (Xu et al., 2012). DL is a qualitative concept used in drug design to estimate the drug-like properties of a prospective compound and helps to optimize pharmacokinetics and pharmaceutical properties, such as solubility and chemical stability. The "drug-like" level of the compounds was set at 0.18, which is used as a selection criterion for the "drug-like" compounds for traditional Chinese herbs (Tao et al., 2013); thus, ingredients with DL > 0.18 were selected. The HL (t1/2) means that the time it takes to reduce the number of compounds in the body by half, is arguably the most important property of an active ingredient as it dictates the timescale over which the compound may elicit therapeutic activity (Ma et al., 2018). HL values > 4 h were selected.

Drug and Disease Target Fishing

We screened for potential targets of the herbs constituting CCP in the TCMSP database. If there was no corresponding drug target in the database, we determined the molecular structural formula based on available chemical formulas from the literature and predicted their potential targets based on the spatial structure of the molecular structure formula in the Swiss-target prediction. The final potential targets of these herbs were obtained by screening the corresponding drug targets for constituents and removing duplicates. The qualitative targets were matched to the UniProt database for normalization (Missiuro et al., 2009). In this study, PF was considered a phenotype in a convalescent patient with SARS-CoV-2 infection. Therefore, the targets related to pulmonary fibrosis were explored based on the OMIM database, drug bank database, and the DisGeNET database. We merged all queried targets and eliminated duplicated results. Finally, standardized names were implemented via the UniProt database.

Network Construction and Analysis

To further explore the mechanisms of CCP's treatment effects on PF of patients with COVID-19 during the rehabilitation stage, we established a network drug-disease map to show the association between the active components in the CCP and its potential targets using Cytoscape v3.7.1. The components and targets were represented by triangles and circles, respectively, and the interaction between the two was shown by a connecting line. Overlapping portions between drug targets and disease targets are represented by Wayne's diagram. To explain the interaction between target proteins, overlapping target proteins between CCP and PF were uploaded to STRING to obtain information on protein-protein interaction (PPI) (Mering et al., 2003). We selected a medium confidence data threshold of >0.4. The obtained protein-protein interaction data were submitted to Cytoscape 3.7.1 to build a PPI network. Additionally, the Significant Gene Ontology (GO) Pathway and the Kyoto Encyclopedia of Genes and Genomes (KEGG) Pathway were screened by the DAVID database.

Molecular Docking

The above-mentioned PPI analysis generated potential hub genes active in PF treatment. Binding activity between the active drug components and the hub genes were evaluated by flexible molecular docking using Surflex-Dock software (Jain, 2007). Surflex-Dock uses an idealized active site ligand called a prototype molecule as a target for generating a hypothetical conformation of a molecule or a molecular fragment (Jain, 2007). These hypothetical conformations are all scored by the Hammerhead scoring function, which also serves as the objective function for the local optimization of the conformation (Welch et al., 1996). Through the crossover process, a large number of conformations are assembled from the complete molecule to achieve flexible docking. The crystal structure of the target proteins was obtained from the Protein Data Bank (Berman et al., 2003). The structural formula (MOL2 format) of the compounds were available at the TCMSP database and PubChem. If the structural formula was not available, we would manually draw the molecular structure with ChemDraw software. The protein targets were processed by removing water, adding hydrogen, and extracting the ligand structure accordingly and finally, Surflex-Dock v.2.1 was run to perform molecular docking (Lill and Danielson, 2011; Spitzer and Jain, 2012; Yuan et al., 2016). In order to examine the stability of molecular Docking, we also perform another molecular docking (dockthor, https://dockthor.lncc.br/v2/). A similar result occurs if molecular docking is relatively precise.

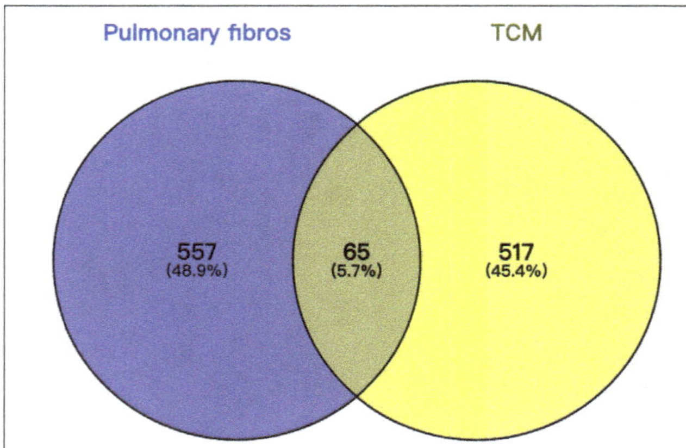

FIGURE 2 | Wayne diagram of commo gene targets of Convalescent Chinese prescription (CCP) drug therapy and pulmonary fibrosis.

RESULTS

Active Component Screening

The active components of CCP were retrieved from the TCMSP database based on three parameters (OB>30%; DL > 0.18; HL > 4). Ultimately, 308 related components were identified as active ingredients in the CCP. Milkvetch root (HQ, 16 ingredients), Tangshen (DS, 19 ingredients), Largehead atractylodes rhizome (BZ, 5 ingredients), Fourleaf ladybell root (NSS, 5 ingredients), Coastal glehnia root (BSS, 3 ingredients), Dried tangerine peel (CP, 5 ingredients), Indian bread (FL, 14 ingredients), Dwarf lilyturf tuber (MD, 4 ingredients), Radix Salviae Miltiorrhizae (DSH, 52 ingredients), Thunberbg fritillary bulb (ZBM, 4 ingredients), Leech (SZ, 32 ingredients), Hawthorn fruit (CSZ, 7 ingredients), Medicated leaven (SQ, 12 ingredients), Germinated barley (MY, 10 ingredients), Common yam rhizome (SY, 16 ingredients), Ground beetle (TBC, 17 ingredients), Radix glycyrrhiza (GC, 76 ingredients), and Pinellia tuber (BX, 11 ingredients). Leech and Ground beetle were obtained by literature mining via China National Knowledge Infrastructure (CNKI) (Guoqiang et al., 2018; Wu et al., 2018). The potential compounds of the CCP formulation and the respective ADME parameters are shown in detail in **Supplementary Material S1**.

Target Fishing for Drug Components and Disease and Establishing the Drug–Disease Target Network

Targets from 14 Chinese herbs were available in the TCMSP database. Targets from Leech (SZ) were available from a previous report (Guoqiang et al., 2018). Targets from Ground beetle (TBC) were available in Swiss-target Prediction software according to its components (Wu et al., 2018). Targets from Dwarf lilyturf tuber (MD) and Hawthorn fruit (CSZ) were available in the Chemistry Database. We matched the components of herbals with the corresponding targets. We obtained 307 targets of HQ, 102

TABLE 2 | Shared hub targets between Convalescent Chinese prescription (CCP) and pulmonary fibrosis.

Number	Gene name	Number	Gene name
1	ADORA2B	37	HTR2C
2	AKT1	38	ICAM1
3	CTSK	39	PLG
4	ELANE	40	SELE
5	F2	41	DNMT1
6	HTR2B	42	SETD2
7	MAPKAPK2	43	SRC
8	MMP1	44	RAC1
9	MMP13	45	TNF
10	MMP2	46	PLAU
11	MMP3	47	IL6
12	MMP9	48	IFNG
13	MTOR	49	CCL2
14	NOX4	50	IL1B
15	PIK3CA	51	F3
16	STAT3	52	SOD1
17	FADS1	53	TP53
18	FAP	54	COL1A1
19	HSP90AB1	55	EGF
20	LTB4R	56	TOP1
21	PARP1	57	COL3A1
22	TGFB1	58	PPARG
23	EGFR	59	PIK3CG
24	VEGFA	60	CHRM3
25	ACE	61	PLA2G4A
26	BRD2	62	CAT
27	BRD4	63	MMP12
28	DPP9	64	ARG1
29	HLA-A	65	GLB1
30	HMOX1		
31	PIN1		
32	PTGS2		
33	SIRT3		
34	CASP1		
35	ECE1		
36	FOS		

targets of DS, 19 targets of BZ, 39 targets of NSS, 181 targets of BSS, 30 targets of MD, 6 targets of CP, 59 targets of FL, 127 targets of BX, 129 targets of DSH, 33 targets of ZBM, 319 targets of SZ, 307 targets of GC, 73 targets of MY, 209 targets of CSZ, 32 targets of SQ, 96 targets of SY. In order to obtain the targets of TBC, we manually searched the literature to find the components (Wu et al., 2018), submitting components into SwissTargetPredict Tools. We obtained 251 targets of TBC. After eliminating duplicates, the final number of identified targets in CCP was 582. The potential targets in detail are shown in **Supplementary Material S2**. In total, 622 targets associated with PF were collected through the OMIM, Drugbank, and DisGeNET databases. Details on the targets associated with PF are shown in Supplementary Materials 3.

The intersection (65 common targets) between drug targets and disease targets is shown in **Figure 2**, and the details of the shared targets are shown in **Table 2**. Subsequently, we mapped the components of CCP based on these 65 targets to construct the drug (components)–disease (PF targets) network shown in **Figure 3**. Next, we submitted the 65 targets to the string tool to generate the PPI network. The PPI network was also visualized using Cytoscape 3.7.1 software. As shown in **Figure 4A**, 65 nodes and 683 edges were identified in the PPI network (Network Properties: Degree = 20, Betweenness = 21.65795, Closeness = 40.83333). Subsequently, a topological analysis of the PPI network was implemented using network properties values greater than the median values (Degree = 34, Betweenness = 65.59, Closeness = 50.25), as shown in **Figure 4B**. The identified targets (*AKT1, TNF, IL6, TP53, VEGFA, IL1B, MMP9, EGFR, CCL2, PTGS2, STAT3, EGF, SRC, MMP2, FOS, CAT, HMOX1, ICAM1, MMP1, TGFB1*) represented potential key targets for the therapeutic effects of CCP (**Figure 4C**).

Enrichment Analysis

Using the DAVID database, GO enrichment analysis yielded GO entries ($p < 0.05$) comprising 336 biological processes (BP), 30 cellular components (CC), and 27 molecular functions (MF). The top 20 entries were selected from BP, CC, and MF, respectively, in order of -lgP value (**Figure 5**). In the BP, the primary target in the extracellular region was the cytosol; for MF, the targets mainly involved enzyme binding, protein binding, and identity protein binding, and cytokine activity.

In total, 93 terms ($p < 0.05$) were obtained from the KEGG pathway enrichment analysis using DAVID data. The first 20 entries were selected according to the–lgP value to draw a bubble diagram (**Figure 6**). The main pathways included the VEGF, Toll-like 4 receptor, mitogen-activated protein kinase family (MAPK), NOD–like receptor signaling pathways. Targets involved in the signaling pathways were as follows: VEGF pathway (*PIK3CG, AKT1, PLA2G4A, PTGS2, VEGFA, RAC1, PIK3CA, MAPKAPK2, SRC*); Toll-like 4 receptor pathway (*PIK3CG, AKT1, FOS, IL6, TNF, RAC1, IL1B, PIK3CA*); MAPK pathway (*EGFR, AKT1, FOS, PLA2G4A, TNF, RAC1, TP53, IL1B, MAPKAPK2, EGF, TGFB1*); and in the NOD-like receptor pathway (*HSP90AB1, IL6, TNF, CCL2, IL1B, CASP1*).

Molecular Docking

The binding ability and of herbal components to core protein targets were validated by molecular simulations. Using molecular docking by Surflex-Dock modeling, a docking score greater than 3 was considered as a stable compound binding to the protein. In this respect, the top 20 nodes were selected from the drug-disease network (**Figure 3**) according to the degree value. They were as follows: TOP1 (PDB ID: 1K4t), MMP2 (PDB ID: 1cxw), MMP9 (PDB ID:1eak), IFNG (PDB ID: 1fyh), SELE (PDB ID: 1git), PLAU (PDB ID:1kdu), VEGFA (PDB ID: 1kmx), HMOX1 (PDB ID: 1ni6), F2 (PDB ID: 1nL1), TNF (PDB ID: 2e7a), TP53 (PDB ID: 2k8f), PPARG (PDB ID: 3e00), PIK3CG (PDB ID: 3I13), IL6 (PDB ID: 4cni), PTGS2 (PDB ID: 5f19), HSP90AB1 (PDB ID: 5ucj), EGFR (PDB ID: 5wb7), quercetin (MOL0000098), kaempferol (MOL000422), and luteolin (MOL000006). As shown in **Figure 7**, quercetin, kaempferol, and luteolin exhibited high binding activity to targets associated with PF. for example IL-6 (score = 3.0236, 3.6316, 3.7055, respectively), TNF-α (score = 3.2116, 3.9889, 5.9409, respectively), VEGF (score = 3.0175, 3.844, 3.1564, respectively), MMP9 (score = 5.7384, 3.079, 5.9618, respectively). Detailed blinding scores were shown in the Heat map in **Figure 7** and in the **Supplementary**

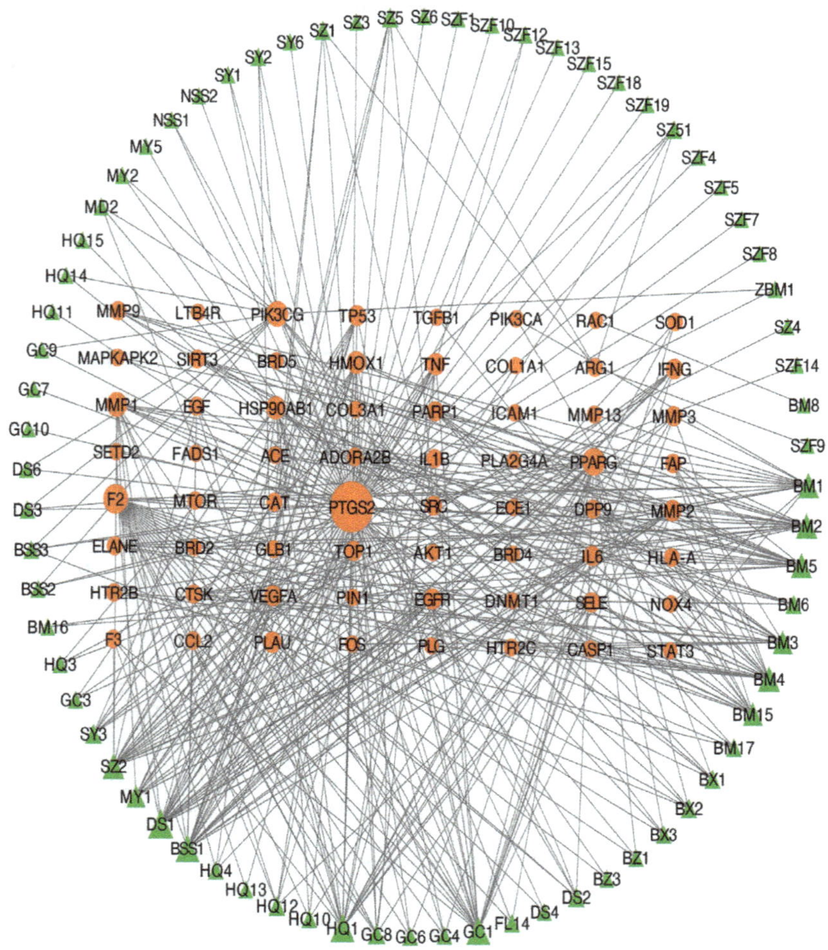

FIGURE 3 | Construction of the drug (herbal ingredients)–disease (pulmonary fibrosis targets) network. The nodes representing drug candidate compounds are shown as green triangles and the targets are indicated by orange circles.

Material S4. Moreover, another molecular docking presents a similar outcome by dockthor. The molecular docking gives higher reliability of obtained results in this work. Detailed blinding scores in dockthor were shown in **Supplementary Material S5**.

DISCUSSION

CCP has been described as a suitable treatment for the recovery phase of patients with COVID-19. In this study, a total of 116 active ingredients and 583 action targets of CCP were screened based on the network pharmacology approach. By further screening, 72 core compounds and 26 key action targets were obtained. Network pharmacology analysis embodies the holistic and correlative characteristics of the combined action of multiple components and targets of traditional Chinese medicine. According to the topological property analysis of the "drug-disease" network, the top 5 key compounds in CCP are quercetin, kaempferol, luteolin, TBC2, and TBC4. In addition, other the components were collected through multiple databases such as China Knowledge, PubMed, and BATMAN-TCM. The chemical constituents (TBC2, TBC4, TBC5) are not included in the TCMSP platform. The targets of these components need to be further studied. Quercetin is known to possess marked antioxidative, anti-inflammatory, and antifibrotic capacities. Dietary quercetin supplementation also decreases chronic systemic inflammation (Stewart et al., 2008). Quercetin can reduce the expression of transforming growth factor-β1 (*TGF-β1*), *α-smooth* muscle actin (*α-SMA*), and tumor necrosis factor-α (*TNF-α*), inhibit alveolar cell apoptosis and reduce lung tissue inflammation and fibrosis injury in rats, which can effectively improve lung fibrosis (Ma et al., 2018; Zhang et al., 2018; Wei et al., 2019). Kaempferol, a polyphenol with potent antioxidant activity, is an ester of caffeic acid and quinic acid (Nardini et al., 2002). Luteolin exhibits various pharmacological activities, including antioxidative, antiviral, antibacterial, anti-inflammatory, anti-endotoxin, antitumor, and liver-protective effects (Rohit and Mohan Rao, 2013; Tajik et al., 2017; Wei et al., 2017).

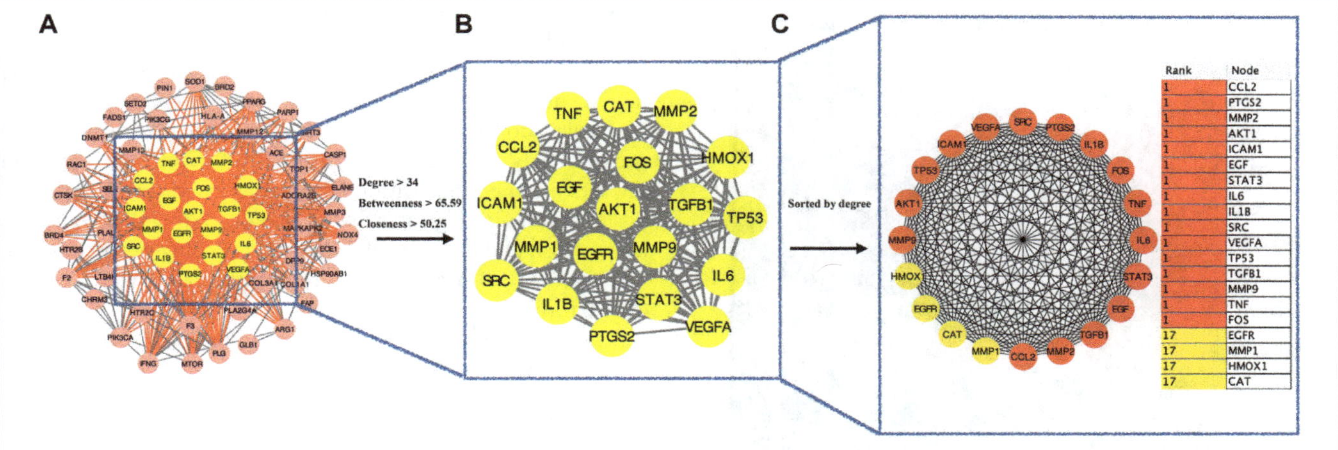

FIGURE 4 | Identification of candidate targets for Convalescent Chinese prescription (CCP) against pulmonary fibrosis via Protein–protein interaction Analysis. **(A)**. Protein–protein interaction (PPI) networks of shared targets between Convalescent Chinese prescription (CCP) and pulmonary fibrosis were analyzed by STRING 11.0. **(B)**. The most significant module identified by the topology selection (degree centrality >34, betweenness centrality >65.59, closeness centrality >50.2). **(C)**. The core 20 targets (hub targets) in the PPI network ranked by degree centrality using the cytoHubba plug-in.

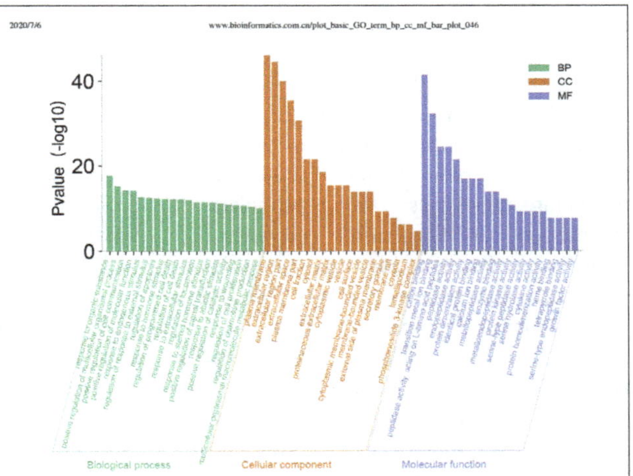

FIGURE 5 | Enrichment analysis of the potential targets of Convalescent Chinese prescription (CCP) against pulmonary fibrosis by R software 3.4.2 for the Gene Ontology database. Top 20 biological process (BP) terms, cellular component (CC) terms, and molecular function (MF) terms are shown as green bars, orange bars, and purple bars, respectively, according to "*p*-value (<0.05), Bonferroni correction."

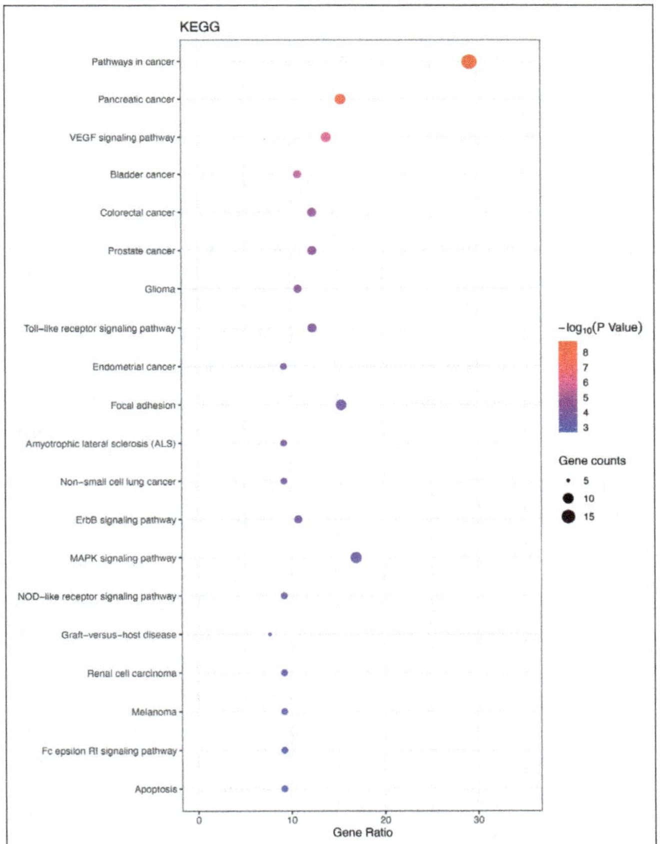

FIGURE 6 | Enrichment analysis for KEGG. Top 20 KEGG pathways listed by bubble chart according to the "*p*-value (<0.05), Bonferroni correction."

According to the results of the PPI network analysis and the topological property analysis of the "Drug–disease" network, the targets of action of CCP were the cytokine IL-6, members of the MAPK family, and PTGSE or prostaglandin G/H synthase. The results of GO functional enrichment analysis revealed that CCP components were mainly involved in the cell communication, endogenous stimulus regulation, apoptosis, programmed cell death, steroid hormone stimulus, signal transduction, regulation of catalytic activity, wounding regulation of cell

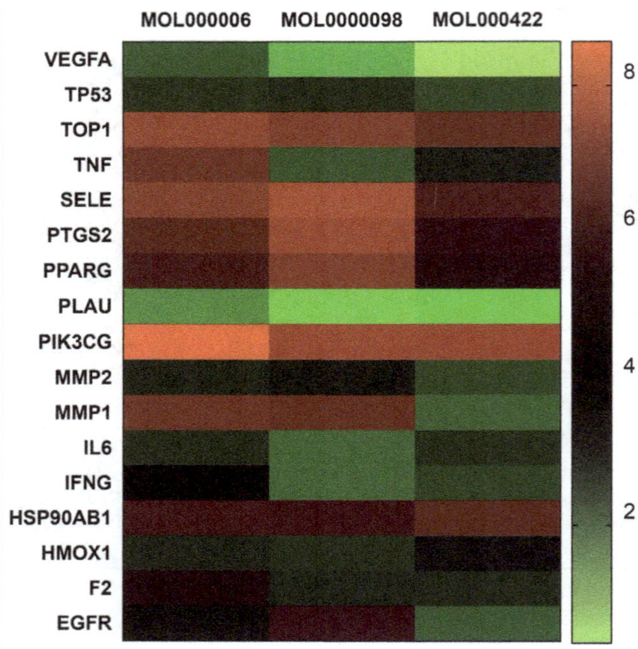

FIGURE 7 | Heat map of Molecular docking. Molecular models of the binding of quercetin (MOL0000098), kaempferol (MOL000422), luteolin (MOL000006) with TOP, MMP2, MMP9, IFNG, SELE, PLAU, VEGFA, HMOX1, F2, TNF, TP53, PPARG, PIK3CG, IL6, PTGS2, HSP90AB1, and EGFR, respectively.

proliferation, regulation of chemokine production and multicellular organismal macromolecule metabolic process. The KEGG pathway enrichment mainly involved Toll-like 4 receptor signaling and immune response pathways. Additionally, the NOD-like receptor signaling pathway and the Graft-versus-host disease pathway involved the *IL-6* gene. IL-6 is a complex ~25-kDa cytokine, acting in both pro- and anti-inflammatory capacities (Weidhase et al., 2019). Importantly, IL-6 trans-signaling via IL-6/soluble IL-6 receptor (sIL-6R) complexes, but not classic signaling via IL-6/membrane bound IL-6 receptor (IL-6R) complexes, has been shown to prevent the apoptosis of T cells and promote tissue damage (Sommer et al., 2014).

The results of this study suggested that CCP may have an interventional effect on viral infections and lung injury. The pleotropic cytokine, TNF-α, plays a significant role in the pathogens of chronic inflammatory diseases. The MAPK signaling pathway controls diverse cellular processes in response to a variety of extracellular stimuli (Kiss et al., 2019). Taken together, the results suggest that CCP may play a role in the recovery period of COVID-19 by exerting antiviral, bacteriostatic, anti-inflammatory, and immunomodulatory activity. Chinese medicine has always been known for its theoretical understanding and clinical practice of "preventing diseases before disease onset." COVID-19 has a relatively long disease duration, and the recovery period is characterized by a state of low immunity. This study revealed that CCP could regulate immune function through multiple pathways and multiple targets.

We then performed docking studies for TOP, MMP2, MMP9, IFNG, SELE, PLAU, VEGFA, HMOX1, F2, TNF, TP53, PPARG, PIK3CG, IL6, PTGS2, HSP90AB1, EGFR, using the critical ingredients quercetin, kaempferol, and luteolin as ligands. Molecular docking is used to evaluate whether ligands and proteins may bind thermodynamically. Overall, the scores of the active compounds with the key targets were for the majority positive with scores greater than 3, demonstrating that quercetin, kaempferol, and luteolin exhibited good binding properties with VEGFA, TNF, MMP9, and IL-6, respectively, all of which play an essential role in PF.

The pathological process of PF could be roughly divided into three stages. The first stage involves the diffuse damage of vascular endothelial cells and alveolar epithelial cells by pathogenic factors, which initiates the inflammatory immune response. Second, inflammatory cells release a variety of cytokines and inflammatory mediators, expanding tissue damage and causing interstitial hyperplasia. The third step involves the migration and proliferation of fibroblasts and endothelial cells and the metabolic disorders of collagen and other ECM components, which further aggravate inflammatory damage and proliferation in a positive feedback manner. Eventually, the process could lead to the replacement and reconstruction of normal lung tissue. These three processes exist simultaneously, which are interrelated and interact (Fernandez and Eickelberg, 2012; Todd et al., 2012; Kolahian et al., 2016).

VEGF-A is considered a critical factor in the pathogenesis of PF (Medford and Millar, 2006; Barratt et al., 2014). VEGFR is a functional receptor of VEGF and an important target for mediating angiogenesis, which stimulates the proliferation and aggregation of fibroblasts, promotes epithelial-mesenchymal transition, activates multiple abnormal signaling pathways, further induces the formation of fibroblast foci, and causes the activation of the MMP family members to destroy the alveolar structure, promote matrix deposition, and induce scar formation (Leung et al., 1989; Ferrara et al., 2003; Bates, 2010). This process generates other mediators involved in the inflammatory response, such as TNF-α and IL-6, which directly or indirectly promote the synthesis of the ECM through interaction with other cytokines (Le et al., 2014; Hou et al., 2018; Papiris et al., 2018). More importantly, several studies have robustly documented that silencing the expression of TGF-β1 reduces inflammation and slows the progression of PF (Baowen et al., 2010; Liu et al., 2013; Peng et al., 2013), which play a pivotal role in PF (Hu et al., 2018; Li et al., 2018). Findings from our study indicated that CCP could inhibit the expression of *VEGF, TNF-α, IL-6, MMP9*, and *TGF-β1* via the VEGF, Toll-like 4 receptor, MAPK, and TGF-β1 signaling pathways. The potential mechanisms involved in CCP activity are summarized in **Figure 8**.

CONCLUSION

The findings suggest that CCP treatment of COVID-19 PF associated with SARS-CoV-2 infection involves multiple components and multiple target points as well as multiple pathways. Such proteins should be interesting to future studies that provide a novel direction for the mechanisms of PF

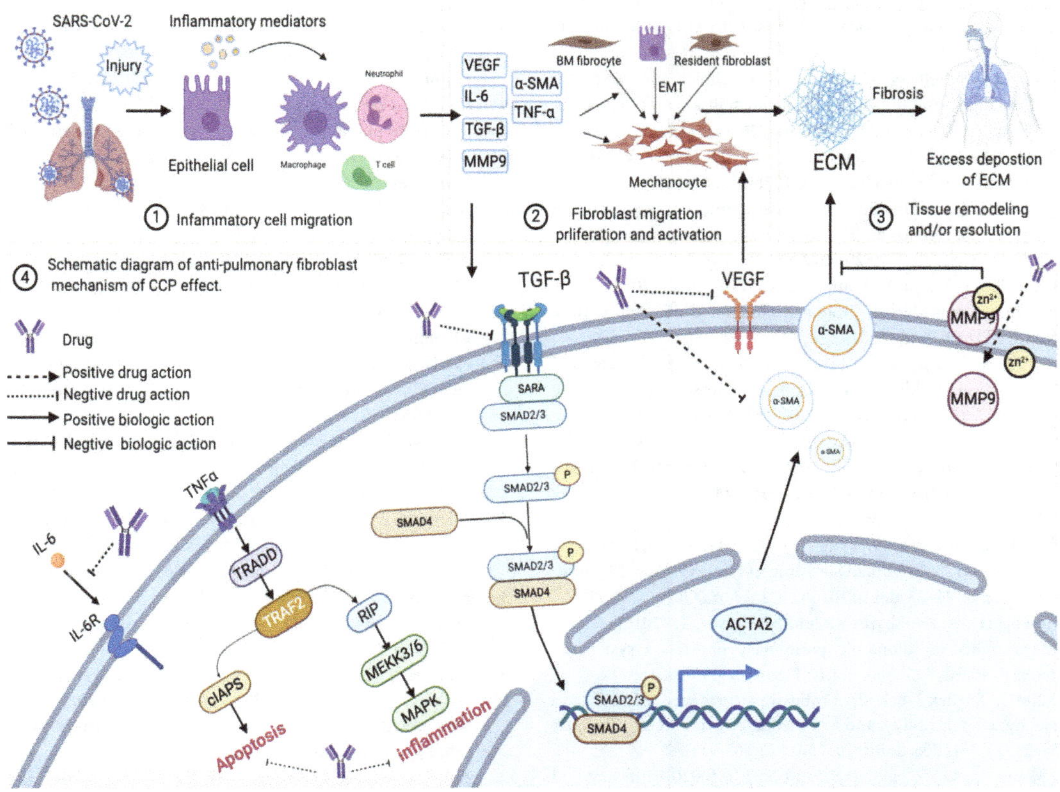

FIGURE 8 | The schematic diagram illustrating the proposed activity model of Convalescent Chinese prescription (CCP) in pulmonary fibrosis. Exposure to SARS-CoV-2 infection damages lung epithelial cell, resulting in injury or cell death and the release of inflammatory mediators into the extracellular space. This signal is recognized by Macrophages cell, T cell, Neutrophils cell. Activation of these cells leads to inflammatory responses in lung epithelial cell. Lung injury also induces fibroblast migration proliferation and activation. These processes result in tissue remodeling or resolution and excess deposition of extracellular matrix (ECM). Chronic, unresolved lung inflammation owing to the activation of various signaling pathways (such as TNFa, MAPK and TGFβ) eventually results in progressive lung fibrosis.

associated with SARS-CoV-2 infection development and a new intervention target for clinical investigations, covering these gaps in research to be able to draw more meaningful conclusions about the benefits of CCP. These findings may offer a rationale for further investigations of the anti-fibrotic mechanisms of CCP therapy.

AUTHOR CONTRIBUTIONS

DJ, XA, and YZ contributed to the drafting of the manuscript. FL and XT revised the manuscript. All authors agreed with the integrity of the study and gave their approval.

ACKNOWLEDGMENTS

We thank the National Administration of Traditional Chinese Medicine for supporting our work.

REFERENCES

1. Baowen, Q., Yulin, Z., Xin, W., Wenjing, X., Hao, Z., Zhizhi, C., et al. (2010). A further investigation concerning correlation between anti-fibrotic effect of liposomal quercetin and inflammatory cytokines in pulmonary fibrosis. *Eur. J. Pharmacol.* 642 (1-3), 134–139. doi:10.1016/j.ejphar.2010.05.019Epub 2010 May 26. PMID: 20510684
2. Barratt, S., Medford, A. R., and Millar, A. B. (2014). Vascular endothelial growth factor in acute lung injury and acute respiratory distress syndrome. *Respiration* 87 (4), 329–342. doi:10.1159/000356034
3. Bates, D. O. (2010). Vascular endothelial growth factors and vascular permeability. *Cardiovasc. Res.* 87 (2), 262–271. doi:10.1093/cvr/cvq105
4. Berman, H., Henrick, K., and Nakamura, H. (2003). Announcing the worldwide protein Data Bank. *Nat. Struct. Mol. Biol.* 10 (12), 980. doi:10.1038/nsb1203-980
5. Brown, K. K., Martinez, F. J., Walsh, S. L. F., Thannickal, V. J., Prasse, A., Schlenker-Herceg, R., et al. (2020). The natural history of progressive fibrosing interstitial lung diseases. *Eur. Respir. J.* 55 (6), 2000085. doi:10.1183/13993003.00085-2020
6. Burnham, E. L., Janssen, W. J., Riches, D. W. H., Moss, M., and Downey, G. P. (2014). The fibroproliferative response in acute respiratory distress syndrome: mechanisms and clinical significance. *Eur. Respir. J.* 43 (1), 276–285. doi:10. 1183/09031936.00196412

7. Canestaro, W. J., Forrester, S. H., Raghu, G., Ho, L., and Devine, B. E. (2016). Drug treatment of idiopathic pulmonary fibrosis. *Chest* 149 (3), 756–766. doi:10. 1016/j.chest.2015.11.013
8. Fernandez, I. E., and Eickelberg, O. (2012). New cellular and molecular mechanisms of lung injury and fibrosis in idiopathic pulmonary fibrosis. *The Lancet* 380 (9842), 680–688. doi:10.1016/s0140-6736(12)61144-1
9. Ferrara, N., Gerber, H.-P., and Lecouter, J. (2003). The biology of VEGF and its receptors. *Nat. Med.* 9 (6), 669–676. doi:10.1038/nm0603-669
10. George, P. M., Wells, A. U., and Jenkins, R. G. (2020). Pulmonary fibrosis and COVID-19: the potential role for antifibrotic therapy. *Lancet Respir. Med.* 8 (8), 807–815. doi:10.1016/S2213-2600(20)30225-3
11. Guoqiang, Li., Li, Y., Tao, Li., Li, Y., Wang, G., Wang, C., et al. (2018). Study on the chemical constituents of leech. *Tianjin Traditional Chin. Med.* 35 (09), 703–705. CNKI:SUN:TJZY.0.2018-09-017
12. Hanta, I., Cilli, A., and Sevinc, C. (2019). The effectiveness, safety, and tolerability of Pirfenidone in idiopathic pulmonary fibrosis: a retrospective study. *Adv. Ther.* 36 (5), 1126–1131. doi:10.1007/s12325-019-00928-3
13. Hou, J., Ma, T., Cao, H., Chen, Y., Wang, C., Chen, X., et al. (2018). TNF-α-induced NF-κB activation promotes myofibroblast differentiation of LR-MSCs and exacerbates bleomycin-induced pulmonary fibrosis. *J. Cel Physiol* 233 (3), 2409–2419. doi:10.1002/jcp.26112
14. Hu, H.-H., Chen, D.-Q., Wang, Y.-N., Feng, Y.-L., Cao, G., Vaziri, N. D., et al. (2018). New insights into TGF-β/Smad signaling in tissue fibrosis. *Chemico-Biological Interactions* 292, 76–83. doi:10.1016/j.cbi.2018.07.008
15. Hutchinson, J., Fogarty, A., Hubbard, R., and McKeever, T. (2015). Global incidence and mortality of idiopathic pulmonary fibrosis: a systematic review. *Eur. Respir. J.* 46 (3), 795–806. doi:10.1183/09031936.00185114
16. Jain, A. N. (2007). Surflex-Dock 2.1: robust performance from ligand energetic modeling, ring flexibility, and knowledge-based search. *J. Comput. Aided Mol. Des.* 21 (5), 281–306. doi:10.1007/s10822-007-9114-2
17. Ji, K., Ma, J., Wang, L., Li, N., Dong, S., and Shi, L. (2020). Efficacy and safety of traditional Chinese medicine in idiopathic pulmonary fibrosis: a meta-analysis. *Evidence-Based Complement. Altern. Med.* 2020, 1–11. doi:10.1155/2020/ 1752387
18. Kim, E. S., and Keating, G. M. (2015). Pirfenidone: a review of its use in idiopathic pulmonary fibrosis. *Drugs* 75 (2), 219–230. doi:10.1007/s40265-015-0350-9
19. King, T. E., Bradford, W. Z., Castro-Bernardini, S., Fagan, E. A., Glaspole, I., Glassberg, M. K., et al. (2014). A phase 3 trial of pirfenidone in patients with idiopathic pulmonary fibrosis. *N. Engl. J. Med.* 370 (22), 2083–2092. doi:10. 1056/NEJMoa1402582
20. Kiss, A., Koppel, A., Murphy, E., Sall, M., Barlas, M., Kissling, G., et al. (2019). Cell type-specific p38δ targeting reveals a context-, stage-, and sex-dependent regulation of skin carcinogenesis. *Int. J. Mol. Sci.* 20 (7), 1532–1535. doi:10. 3390/ijms20071532
21. Kolahian, S., Fernandez, I. E., Eickelberg, O., and Hartl, D. (2016). Immune mechanisms in pulmonary fibrosis. *Am. J. Respir. Cel Mol Biol* 55 (3), 309–322. doi:10.1165/rcmb.2016-0121TR
22. Ksiazek, T. G., Erdman, D., Goldsmith, C. S., Zaki, S. R., Peret, T., Emery, S., et al. (2003). A novel coronavirus associated with severe acute respiratory syndrome. *N. Engl. J. Med.* 348 (20), 1953–1966. doi:10.1056/nejmoa030781
23. Le, T.-T. T., Karmouty-Quintana, H., Melicoff, E., Le, T.-T. T., Weng, T., Chen, N.- Y., et al. (2014). Blockade of IL-6 trans signaling attenuates pulmonary fibrosis. *J. Immunol.* 193 (7), 3755–3768. doi:10.4049/jimmunol.1302470
24. Leung, D. W., Cachianes, G., Kuang, W. J., Goeddel, D. V., and Ferrara, N. (1989). Vascular endothelial growth factor is a secreted angiogenic mitogen. *Science* 246 (4935), 1306–1309. doi:10.1126/science.2479986
25. Li, W., Moore, M. J., Vasilieva, N., Sui, J., Wong, S. K., Berne, M. A., et al. (2003). Angiotensin-converting enzyme 2 is a functional receptor for the SARS coronavirus. *Nature* 426 (6965), 450–454. doi:10.1038/nature02145
26. Li, X., Lu, C., Liu, S., Shuaishuai Liu, S., Su, C., Xiao, T., et al. (2018). Synthesis and discovery of a drug candidate for treatment of idiopathic pulmonary fibrosis through inhibition of TGF-β1 pathway. *Eur. J. Med. Chem.* 157, 229–247. doi:10.1016/j.ejmech.2018.07.074
27. Lill, M. A., and Danielson, M. L. (2011). Computer-aided drug design platform using PyMOL. *J. Comput. Aided Mol. Des.* 25 (1), 13–19. doi:10.1007/s10822- 010-9395-8
28. Liu, H., Xue, J.-X., Li, X., Ao, R., and Lu, Y. (2013). Quercetin liposomes protect against radiation-induced pulmonary injury in a murine model. *Oncol. Lett.* 6 (2), 453 459. doi:10.3892/ol.2013.1365
29. Liu, M., Chen, M. H., Wei, C. L., and Zhao, Q. L. (2018). Treatment of idiopathic pulmonary fibrosis by traditional Chinese medicine:a systematic review and meta-analysis. *Tianjin J. Trad. Chin. Med.* 35 (3), 200–204. [Chinese]
30. Ma, N., Li, Y., and Fan, J. (2018). Research progress on pharmacological action of quercetin. *J. Liaoning Univ. Traditional Chin. Med.* 20, 221–224. doi:10.3969/j. issn.1001-6880.2003.02.023
31. Marini, J. J., and Gattinoni, L. (2020). Management of COVID-19 respiratory distress. *JAMA* 323 (22), 2329–2330. doi:10.1001/jama.2020.6825
32. Medford, A. R. L., and Millar, A. B. (2006). Vascular endothelial growth factor (VEGF) in acute lung injury (ALI) and acute respiratory distress syndrome (ARDS): paradox or paradigm?. *Thorax* 61 (7), 621–626. doi:10.1136/ thx.2005.040204
33. Mering, C. v., Huynen, M., Jaeggi, D., Schmidt, S., Bork, P., Snel, B., et al. (2003). STRING: a database of predicted functional associations between proteins. *Nucl. Acids Res.* 31 (1), 258–261. doi:10.1093/nar/gkg034
34. Missiuro, P. V., Liu, K., Zou, L., Ross, B. C., Zhao, G., Liu, J. S., et al. (2009). Information flow analysis of interactome networks. *Plos Comput. Biol.* 5 (4), e1000350. doi:10.1371/journal.pcbi.1000350
35. Nardini, M., Cirillo, E., Natella, F., and Scaccini, C. (2002). Absorption of phenolic acids in humans after coffee consumption. *J. Agric. Food Chem.* 50 (20), 5735–5741. doi:10.1021/jf0257547
36. National Health Commission of the People's Republic of China (2020a). *Diagnosis and treatment Protocol for COVID-19.* (Trial Version 7). http://www.nhc.gov. cn/yzygj/s7653p/202003/46c9294a7dfe4cef80dc7f5912eb1989. shtml [Accessed March 4, 2020)
37. National Health Commission of the People's Republic of China (2020b). *Diagnosis and treatment Protocol for COVID-19.* (Trial Version 6). http://www.nhc.gov. cn/yzygj/s7653p/202002/8334a8326dd94d329df351d7da8aefc2. shtml [Accessed February 19, 2020)
38. Noble, P. W., Albera, C., Bradford, W. Z., Costabel, U., du Bois, R. M., Fagan, E. A., et al. (2016). Pirfenidone for idiopathic pulmonary fibrosis: analysis of pooled data from three multinational phase 3 trials. *Eur. Respir. J.* 47 (1), 243–253. doi:10.1183/13993003.00026-2015
39. Papiris, S. A., Tomos, I. P., Karakatsani, A., Spathis, A., Korbila, I., Analitis, A., et al. (2018). High levels of IL-6 and IL-8 characterize early-on idiopathic pulmonary fibrosis acute exacerbations. *Cytokine* 102, 168–172. doi:10.1016/j. cyto.2017. 08.019
40. Peng, H., Liu, Y., Wang, J., Zhao, X., and Wang, X. (2013). Effect of quercetin on the expression of TGF-beta1 in human embryonic lung fibroblasts activated by the silicotic alveolar macrophages. *Wei Sheng Yan Jiu* 42, 99–102. doi:10.19813/ j.cnki.weishengyanjiu.2013.01.023
41. Rochwerg, B., Neupane, B., Zhang, Y., Garcia, C. C., Raghu, G., Richeldi, L., et al. (2016). Treatment of idiopathic pulmonary fibrosis: a network meta-analysis. *BMC Med.* 14 (1), 18. doi:10.1186/s12916-016-0558-x
42. Rohit, U., and Mohan Rao, L. J. (2013). An outlook on chlorogenic acids—occurrence, chemistry, technology, and biological activities. *Crit. Rev. Food Sci. Nutr.* 53 (9), 968–984. doi:10.1080/10408398.2011.576319
43. Sommer, J., Engelowski, E., Baran, P., Garbers, C., Floss, D. M., and Scheller, J. (2014). Interleukin-6, but not the interleukin-6 receptor plays a role in recovery from dextran sodium sulfate-induced colitis. *Int. J. Mol. Med.* 34 (3), 651–660. doi:10.3892/ijmm.2014.1825
44. Spitzer, R., and Jain, A. N. (2012). Surflex-Dock: docking benchmarks and real-world application. *J. Comput. Aided Mol. Des.* 26 (6), 687–699. doi:10.1007/ s10822-011-9533-y
45. Stewart, L. K., Soileau, J. L., Ribnicky, D., Wang, Z. Q., Raskin, I., Poulev, A., et al. (2008). Quercetin transiently increases energy expenditure but persistently decreases circulating markers of inflammation in C57BL/6J mice fed a high-fat diet. *Metabolism* 57, S39–S46. doi:10.1016/j.metabol.2008.03.003
46. Sun, L., Mao, M., Yan, Z., Zuo, C., and Zhang, X. (2018). A Chinese traditional therapy for bleomycin-induced pulmonary fibrosis in mice. *Can. Respir. J.* 2018, 1–8. doi:10.1155/2018/8491487

47. Tajik, N., Tajik, M., Mack, I., and Enck, P. (2017). The potential effects of chlorogenic acid, the main phenolic components in coffee, on health: a comprehensive review of the literature. *Eur. J. Nutr.* 56 (7), 2215–2244. doi:10.1007/s00394-017-1379-1
48. Tao, L., Cao, J., Wei, W., Xie, H., Zhang, M., and Zhang, C. (2017). Protective role of rhapontin in experimental pulmonary fibrosis *in vitro* and *in vivo*. *Int. Immunopharmacology* 47, 38–46. doi:10.1016/j.intimp.2017.03.020
49. Tao, W., Xu, X., Wang, X., Li, B., Wang, Y., Li, Y., et al. (2013). Network pharmacology-based prediction of the active ingredients and potential targets of Chinese herbal Radix Curcumae formula for application to cardiovascular disease. *J. Ethnopharmacol* 145, 1–10. doi:10.1016/j.jep.2012.09.051
50. Todd, N. W., Luzina, I. G., and Atamas, S. P. (2012). Molecular and cellular mechanisms of pulmonary fibrosis. *Fibrogenesis & Tissue Repair* 5, 1–24. doi:10. 1186/1755-1536-5-11
51. von Mering, C., Huynen, M., Jaeggi, D., Schmidt, S., Bork, P., and Snel, B. (2003). STRING: a database of predicted functional associations between proteins. *Nucleic Acids Res.* 31 (1), 258–261. doi:10.1093/nar/gkg034
52. Wei, F., Jiang, X., Gao, H.-Y., and Gao, S.-H. (2017). Liquiritin induces apoptosis and autophagy in cisplatin (DDP)-resistant gastric cancer cells *in vitro* and xenograft nude mice *in vivo*. *Int. J. Oncol.* 51 (5), 1383–1394. doi:10.3892/ijo.2017.4134
53. Wei, P., Chen, Z., and Wang, C. (2019). The protective effect of quercetin on rats with chronic obstructive pulmonary disease. *Chin. J. Immunol.* 35, 2570–2575. CNKI:SUN:ZMXZ.0.2019-21-004
54. Weidhase, L., Wellhöfer, D., Schulze, G., Kaiser, T., Drogies, T., Wurst, U., et al. (2019). Is Interleukin-6 a better predictor of successful antibiotic therapy than procalcitonin and C-reactive protein? A single center study in critically ill adults. *BMC Infect. Dis.* 19 (1), 150. doi:10.1186/s12879-019-3800-2
55. Welch, W., Ruppert, J., and Jain, A. N. (1996). Hammerhead: fast, fully automated docking of flexible ligands to protein binding sites. *Chem. Biol.* 3 (6), 449–462. doi:10.1016/s1074-5521(96)90093-9
56. Wu, C., Chen, X., Cai, Y., Xia, J. a., Zhou, X., Xu, S., et al. (2020). Risk factors associated with acute respiratory distress syndrome and death in patients with coronavirus disease 2019 pneumonia in wuhan, China. *JAMA Intern. Med.* 180 (7), 934–943. doi:10.1001/jamainternmed.2020.0994
57. Wu, F., Zhou, B., Dong, Q., Wang, H., Tan, J., Li, P., et al. (2018). The pharmacology, medicinal chemistry and clinical research progress of Eupolyphaga sinensis. *Specialty Res.* 3, 67–74. doi:10.16720/j.cnki.tcyj.2018.03.014
58. Xu, X., Zhang, W., Huang, C., Li, Y., Yu, H., Wang, Y., et al. (2012). A novel chemometric method for the prediction of human oral bioavailability. *Int. J. Mol. Sci.* 13 (6), 6964–6982. doi:10.3390/ijms13066964
59. Xu, X., Chen, P., Wang, J., Feng, J., Zhou, H., Li, X., et al. (2020). Evolution of the novel coronavirus from the ongoing Wuhan outbreak and modeling of its spike protein for risk of human transmission. *Sci. China Life Sci.* 63 (3), 457–460. doi:10.1007/s11427-020-1637-5
60. Yuan, S., Chan, H. C. S., Filipek, S., and Vogel, H. (2016). PyMOL and inkscape bridge the data and the data visualization. *Structure* 24 (12), 2041–2042. doi:10. 1016/j.str.2016.11.012
61. Zhang, X., Cai, Y., Zhang, W., and Chen, X. (2018). Quercetin ameliorates pulmonary fibrosis by inhibiting SphK1/S1P signaling. *Biochem. Cel Biol.* 96 (6), 742–751. doi:10.1139/bcb-2017-0302

20

Antifibrotic Mechanism of Cinobufagin in Bleomycin-Induced Pulmonary Fibrosis in Mice

Xiaohe Li[1,2†], Zhun Bi[1†], Shuaishuai Liu[1,2†], Shaoyan Gao[1,2], Yunyao Cui[1,2], Kai Huang[1,2], Mengying Huang[1,2], Jiahe Mao[1,2], Lixin Li[2], Jingjing Gao[2], Tao Sun[1,2], Honggang Zhou[1,2*] and Cheng Yang[1,2*]*

[1] State Key Laboratory of Medicinal Chemical Biology, College of Pharmacy and Tianjin Key Laboratory of Molecular Drug Research, Nankai University, Haihe Education Park, Tianjin, China, [2] Tianjin Key Laboratory of Molecular Drug Research, Tianjin International Joint Academy of Biomedicine, Tianjin, China

***Correspondence:**
Tao Sun
tao.sun@nankai.edu.cn
Honggang Zhou
honggang.zhou@nankai.edu.cn
Cheng Yang
cheng.yang@nankai.edu.cn

†These authors have contributed equally to this work

Idiopathic pulmonary fibrosis (IPF) is a progressive and usually fatal lung disease that is characterized by fibroblast proliferation and extracellular matrix remodeling, which result in irreversible distortion of the lung's architecture and the formation of focal fibrous hyperplasia. The molecular mechanism by which pulmonary fibrosis develops is not fully understood, and no satisfactory treatment currently exists. However, many studies consider that aberrant activation of TGF-β1 frequently promotes epithelial-mesenchymal transition (EMT) and fibroblast activation in pulmonary fibrosis. Cinobufagin (CBG), a traditional Chinese medicine, has been widely used for long-term pain relief, cardiac stimulation, and anti-inflammatory and local anesthetic treatments. However, its role in pulmonary fibrosis has not yet been established. We investigated the hypothesis that cinobufagin plays an inhibitory role on TGF-β1 signaling using a luciferase-reporter assay. We further explored the effect of cinobufagin on pulmonary fibrosis both *in vitro* and *in vivo*. The *in vitro* experiments showed that cinobufagin suppresses TGF-β1/Smad3 signaling in a dose-dependent manner, attenuates the activation and differentiation of lung fibroblasts and inhibits EMT induced by TGF-β1 in alveolar epithelial cells. The *in vivo* experiments indicated that cinobufagin significantly alleviates bleomycin-induced collagen deposition and improves pulmonary function. Further study showed that cinobufagin could attenuate bleomycin-induced inflammation and inhibit fibroblast activation and the EMT process *in vivo*. In summary, cinobufagin attenuates bleomycin-induced pulmonary fibrosis in mice *via* suppressing inflammation, fibroblast activation and epithelial–mesenchymal transition.

Keywords: cinobufagin, pulmonary fibrosis, fibroblasts, epithelial-mesenchymal transition, TGF-β1

INTRODUCTION

Pulmonary fibrosis (PF) is the final stage of various interstitial lung diseases and is characterized by excessive deposition of extracellular matrix and destruction of lung parenchyma. Idiopathic pulmonary fibrosis (IPF) is the most common and ultimately fatal respiratory disease, with a mean survival of 2.5 years after diagnosis (Borensztajn et al., 2013; Maher, 2013). IPF is characterized by diffuse alveolitis and alveolar structure disorder, the formation of honeycomb focal fibrous in the patient's lungs, and the occurrence of pulmonary interstitial fibrosis. The incidence and mortality of

IPF has risen annually, which increases the medical burden (King et al., 2014). At present, there are only two drugs available for the treatment of mild/moderate IPF, pirfenidone and nintedanib, but these two drugs cannot prolong the survival of patients (Ogura et al., 2015; Jo et al., 2016). Therefore, it is important to study the pathogenesis of the disease and develop new therapeutic drugs or methods.

Although the exact etiology and pathogenesis of IPF are still unclear, it is well known that the myofibroblasts are the primary effector cell in the process of pulmonary fibrosis (Wand and Kremer, 2015). Myofibroblasts are highly produced for collagen and α-smooth muscle actin stress fibers and exhibit higher proliferation rates and a contractile phenotype. Recent evidence suggests that myofibroblasts are mainly derived from the activation/proliferation of resident fibroblasts and epithelial–mesenchymal transition (EMT) (Willis et al., 2005; Kim et al., 2006). Emerging evidence has demonstrated that EMT plays an important role in pulmonary fibrosis, while transforming growth factor-β (TGF-β) plays an important role in the EMT process. TGF-β is a key fibrogenetic factor that can activate fibroblasts that differentiate into myofibroblasts, resulting in extracellular matrix deposition (Kim et al., 2006; Hisatomi et al., 2012). Consequently, targeting the trans differentiation of myofibroblasts and TGF-β signaling may be an effective strategy in the preservation of normal lung structure during pulmonary fibrosis.

In recent years, compounds isolated from natural plants, such as Chinese medicines, have attracted the attention of researchers for their anti-fibrotic biological activities (Zhou et al., 2014; Li et al., 2015). ChanSu is made from the post-auricular and skin glands of Bufo Gargarizans (Cui et al., 2014). The main component of Chansu is cinobufagin (CBG) (**Figure 1A**), a major bioactive component of the traditional Chinese medicine, and it has been reported to have potent pharmacological activity (Zhang et al., 2007). Bufo venom contains a large number of toad toxins, which have cardiotonic activity. They are chemical steroids, and substances with such a skeleton, bufadienolide, are the main active ingredients of toad serum and toad venom. Bufotalin, cinobufagin, cinobufotalin, and bufalin are the bufadienolides in toad venom. (Li et al., 2009; Cui et al., 2010; Wang et al., 2010). In recent years, research on the pharmacological effects and clinical application of cinobufagin has confirmed that cinobufagin has anti-tumor, anti-virus, anesthetic, and analgesic effects; promotes bone marrow hyperplasia; and enhances immunity (Waiwut et al., 2012). The anti-tumor mechanisms of cinobufagin mainly include inhibiting the proliferation of tumor cells, promoting tumor cell apoptosis, reversing multi-drug resistance, and inhibiting angiogenesis and inflammation (Zhai et al., 2014; Dai et al., 2018). In 2005, cinobufagin was approved by the Chinese State Food and Drug Administration (SFDA) and then widely accepted to treat cancer patients at oncologic clinics in China. (Qi et al., 2008; Zhang et al., 2015). The role of cinobufagin in pulmonary fibrosis has not yet been established. According to the official report, murine intratracheal bleomycin model is the best-characterized animal model available for preclinical experiments of pulmonary fibrosis (Jenkins et al., 2017). Therefore, we explored the activity of cinobufagin in bleomycin-induced pulmonary fibrosis model in this study.

METHODS

Cell Culture

Mouse fibroblast cells (NIH3T3, purchased from ATCC, passage number 32-37), $(CAGA)_{12}$-Lux reporter stably transfected NIH 3T3 cells (CAGA-NIH3T3, passage number 30-35) and mouse lung fibroblast cells (Mlg, purchased from ATCC, passage number 25-30) were grown in DMEM (KeyGEN BioTECH, Nan Jing, China) supplemented with 10% fetal bovine serum (FBS, ExCell Bio, Shanghai, China). A549 cells (purchased from ATCC, passage number 27-29) were grown in RPMI-1640 (KeyGEN BioTECH, Nan Jing, China) supplemented with 10% FBS. Cells were maintained at 37°C with 5% CO_2 in a humidified atmosphere.

Animals and Bleomycin Administration

All animal care and experimental procedures complied with guidelines approved by the Institutional Animal Care and Use Committee (IACUC) of Nankai University (Permit No. SYXK 2014-0003). Animal studies are reported in compliance with the ARRIVE guidelines (Kliment and Oury, 2010; McGrath and Lilley, 2015). Six- to eight-week-old male C57BL/6 mice were obtained from Laboratory Animal Center, Academy of Military Medical Sciences of People's Liberation Army (Beijing, China). In total, 24 mice weighing between 22 and 25 g were used in the experiments. Mice were housed under controlled temperature (22–26°C) and a 12 h light–dark cycle.

Intratracheal bleomycin administration was performed as described previously (Jiang et al., 2004). In brief, mice were anesthetized with an intraperitoneal injection of 10% chloral hydrate and then intratracheally injected with 2.5 U/kg bleomycin (Blenoxane, Nippon Kayaku Co Ltd) using a sterile insulin syringe. After injection, the mice were immediately erected and rotated left and right to make the drug solution evenly distributed in the lungs. In the sham operation group, the same amount of saline was injected intratracheally by the same method. For fibrosis model, 48 mice were divided into four groups, with 12 mice per group randomly: control group, BLM group, BLM+Pirfenidone group (200 $mg{\cdot}kg^{-1}$), and BLM+ CBG group (10 $mg{\cdot}kg^{-1}$). CBG was intragastrically administered daily for 1 week beginning 7 days after BLM injury, and Pirfenidone was used as the positive control. Control and model groups received an equal volume of vehicle (0.9% NaCl) using the same schedule and route of administration. Mice were sacrificed on the 14th day after bleomycin administration for the evaluation of pulmonary fibrosis. Six mice in each group were used for protein and mRNA analyses, and the rest of the 6 mice in each group underwent pathological analyses, with the left lung used for histology and the right lung for hydroxyproline content

Abbreviations: α-SMA, α-smooth muscle actin; BLM, bleomycin; Col1, collagen-1; CBG, Cinobufagin; ECM, extracellular matrix; EMT, epithelial-mesenchymal transition; Fn, fibronectin; PF, pulmonary fibrosis; IPF, idiopathic pulmonary fibrosis; TGF-β1, Transforming growth factor-β1.

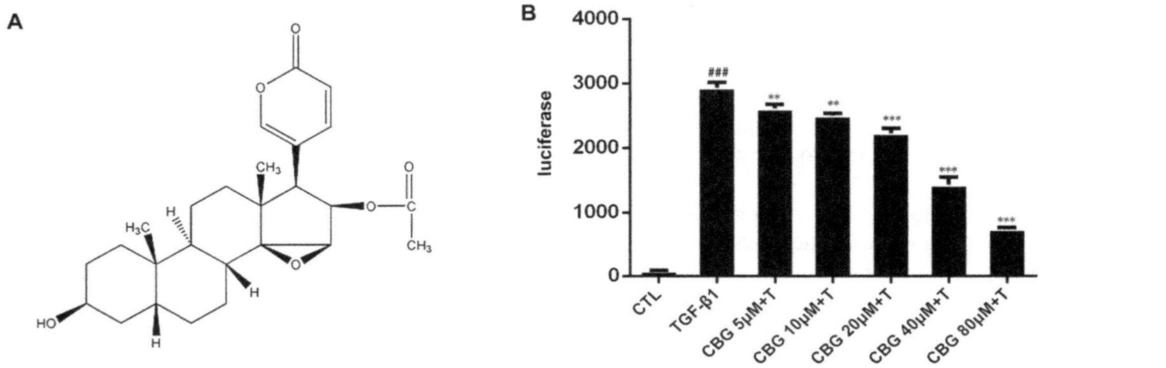

FIGURE 1 | Cinobufagin inhibits TGF-β1/Smad3 signaling in fibroblasts. **(A)** Chemical structure of cinobufagin. **(B)** Cinobufagin antagonized TGF-β1-induced reporter activity in a dose-dependent manner. As described in the Materials and methods section, CAGA-NIH3T3 cells were incubated with TGF-β1 (5 ng·ml^{-1}) with/without different doses of cinobufagin and then analyzed using a luciferase assay (n = 3 per group). Experiments were performed in triplicate, and statistical significance was obtained by one-way ANOVA. #represents a comparison with the blank control group, * represents a comparison with the TGF-β1 group. $^{\#}P < 0.05$; $^{\#\#}P < 0.01$; $^{\#\#\#}P < 0.001$; $P < 0.05$; $^{**}P < 0.01$; $^{***}P < 0.001$.

determination. For inflammation model, 24 mice were divided into four groups, with 6 mice per group randomly: control group, BLM group, BLM+Pirfenidone group (200 mg·kg^{-1}), and BLM+ CBG group (10 mg·kg^{-1}). CBG was intragastrically administered daily for 1 week beginning 1 day after BLM injury, and Pirfenidone was used as the positive control. Mice were sacrificed on the 8th day after bleomycin administration for the evaluation of inflammation.

Pulmonary Function Testing

Mice were anesthetized with 6% chloral hydrate in saline (360 mg·kg^{-1}, i.p.), tracheotomized below the larynx, and intubated with a Y-type tracheal cannula (2.5 mm inner diameter). After the surgery, the mice were placed in a supine position with their whole body inside the plethysmographic chamber (4,665 ml volume) to analyze pulmonary function using the Anires2005 system (Beijing Biolab, Beijing, China). One branch of the Y-type tracheal cannula was connected to a venthole on the chamber wall, and the venthole was connected to a ventilator from the outside of the chamber by polyethylene tubing (8 mm inner diameter, 10 cm length). Natural air was given to the animal through the ventilator, with a rate of 80 breaths/min. The other branch of the cannula was connected to the pressure-detecting channel of the Anires2005 system, and the peak inspiratory pressure was maintained at 10–16 cm H_2O. By detecting the ventilation-associated pressure change inside the chamber, the Anires2005 system automatically calculates and displays pulmonary function parameters, such as inspiratory resistance (Ri), expiratory resistance (Re), dynamic compliance (Cdyn), forced vital capacity (FVC) and forced expiratory volume in one second (FEV1).

Histopathological Examination

Left lungs were fixed in 10% formalin for 24 h and embedded in paraffin. Then, lung sections (4 μm) were prepared and stained with hematoxylin–eosin. Quantification of pulmonary fibrosis was performed as described previously (Jiang et al., 2004). In brief, images were photographed with an upright transmission fluorescence microscope (Olympus) and analyzed by Image-Pro Plus Version 6.0 (Media Cybernetics, Inc. American). The software selection tool can select the entire lung tissue area and automatically calculate the total pixel Pw of the region. It can then use the same method to calculate the total pixel Pf of the fibrosis region (fibrosis ratio = fibrosis area total pixel Pf/total lung total pixel Pw).

Hydroxyproline Content Determination

The right lungs of mice were isolated, placed in 5 ml ampoules, dried, acid hydrolyzed, adjusted to pH 6.5–8.0, filtered, and adjusted to a total volume of 10 ml with 1×PBS. Each tube was comprised of 350 μl H_2O, 50 μl sample, and 200 μl Chioramino-T. The samples were vortexed and incubated at room temperature for 20 min. Then, 200 μl perchloric acid was added, and the samples were vortexed and incubated at room temperature for 5 min. P-DMAB (200 μl) was added, and the samples were vortexed and incubated at 60°C in a water bath for 20 min. The samples were cooled, 200 μl of each sample was transferred to 96-well plates in triplicate, and the absorbance was measured at 577 nm.

Cell Viability Analysis

NIH3T3, Mlg and A549 cells were initially seeded in 96-well plates prior to incubation for 24 h at 37°C. The cell culture media was then replaced by complete media containing the indicated concentrations (0 to 80 μM) of cinobufagin prior to incubation for specific times (24 or 48 h). After incubation as indicated, 15 μl of Thiazolyl Blue Tetrazolium Bromide (MTT, 5 mg·ml^{-1}, KeyGENE BioTech, Nanjing, China) was administered to cells, followed by incubation for 4 h at 37°C following the manufacturer's instructions. Then, 120 μl DMSO was added per well, and the absorbance was read at 570 nm by a microplate reader. Cell viability (%) was evaluated as the ratio of cells that survived.

Luciferase Reporter Assay

For luciferase reporter assays, CAGA-NIH3T3 cells were plated in 96-well plates. When the cell density reached 80%, the DMEM containing 10% FBS was replaced with DMEM containing 1% FBS. After 24 h of incubation, cinobufagin was added, and cultures were incubated in the presence or absence of 5 ng·ml^{-1} TGF-β1 for 18 h. Cells were harvested in lysis buffer, and the luciferase activity was determined after adding the substrate.

Wound Healing Assay

NIH 3T3 cells were seeded in a six-well plate and treated with cinobufagin in the presence or absence of TGF-β1 (5 ng·ml^{-1}) for the indicated period. Three parallel lines were drawn on the underside of each well to demarcate the wound areas for analysis. Before inflicting the wound, the cells were fully confluent. A scratch was made in the center of the culture well using a sterile 200 μl micropipette tip. The wounds were observed using an inverted optical microscope, and multiple images were obtained at areas flanking the intersections of the wound and the marker lines after the scratch at 0, 6, and 24 h. Images were obtained for analysis using Image J software.

Quantitative Real-Time PCR (qRT-PCR)

We performed RNA isolation and qRT-PCR analysis as previously described (Geng et al., 2011). The total RNA was extracted from Mlg cells and tissue using TRIzol Reagent. The cDNA was obtained from the total RNA through reverse transcription. qRT-PCR was performed using SYBR GreenER qPCR SuperMix Universal (Invitrogen) according to the manufacturer's protocols. The relative quantification of gene expression was measured relative to the endogenous reference gene (human: β-glucuronidase; mouse: β-actin) using the comparative CT method. Sequences of the specific primer sets are as follows: α-SMA (NM_007392.2), 5-GCTGGTGATGATGCTCCCA-3 and 5-GCCCATTCCAACC ATTACTCC-3; *Col1a1* (NM_007742.3), 5-CCAAGAAGACAT CCCTGAAGTCA-3 and 5-TGCACGTCATCGCACACA-3; *Fn* (NM_010233.1), 5-GTGTAGCACAACTTCCAATTACGAA-3 and 5-GGAATTTCCGCCTCGAGTCT-3; *Vimentin* (NM_ 011701.4), 5-ATGACCGCTTTGCCAACTAC-3 and 5-GTGCCA GAGAAGCATTGTCA-3; *Cdh1 (E-cadherin)* (NM_000074.6), 5-CAGCCTTCTTTTCGGAAGACT-3 and 5-GGTAGACAGC TCCCTATGACTG-3; *IL-6* (NM_031168.2), 5'-TAGTCCTTCC TACCCCAATTTCC-3' and 5'-TTGGTCCTTAGCCACTCC TTC-3'; *IL-1β* (NM_008361.4), 5'-GTTCCCATTAGACAACTGC ACTACAG-3' and 5'-GTCGTTGCTTGGTTCTCCTTGTA-3'; β-actin (NM_007393.3), 5-AGGCCAACCGTGAAAAGATG-3 and 5-AGAG- CATAGCCCTCGTAGATGG-3; *CDH1 (E-CAD)* (NM_000016.10), 5-CACGGTAACCGATCAGAATG-3 and 5-ACC TCCATCACAGAGGTTCC-3; *CDH2 (N-CAD)* (NM_000018. 10), 5-AGCCAACCTTAACTGAGGAGT-3 and 5-GGCAAGTT GATTGGAGGGATG-3; *GUSB* (NM_000181.3), 5-CCAAACCA GCCTGACAACTT-3 and 5-TCTAGCATGCTCCACCACTG-3.

Western Blot

The proteins were extracted from cells or lung tissues following standard protocols, as described previously (Ning et al., 2004). All of the protein was extracted from lung tissue homogenates or cells using Radio-Immunoprecipitation Assay (RIPA) lysis buffer containing phenylmethylsulfonyl fluoride (PMSF) and sodium fluoride (NaF). After electrophoresis and membrane transfer, the immunoblots were probed with the following primary antibodies: Phospho-Smad3, Smad3, α-SMA, collagen I, Fibronectin, E-cadherin, Vimentin, β-catenin, TGF-β1, TβRI, TβRII, and GAPDH. The secondary antibodies were goat anti-rabbit or goat anti-mouse horseradish peroxidase-conjugated antibodies. Enhanced chemiluminescence reagent was used for detection, and blots were scanned using Alphaview SA software. Three cell lines were used to analyze the above proteins: CAGA-NIH3T3 (for P-Smad3, Smad3), Mlg (for α-SMA, Collagen-1, Fibronectin), and A549 (for E-cadherin, Vimentin, β-catenin). In addition, lung tissue was used to detect all of the above proteins.

Cell Transfection

Plasmid expressing constitutively active β-catenin (plasmid pcDNA3.1-3XHA-β-catenin) was purchased from Miao Ling Plasmid Company (China). The plasmid was transfected using Polyethylenimine, Linear (MW25000, Polysciences) according to manufacturer's instructions. Briefly, plasmid and Polyethylenimine were diluted separately in 1 ml Opti-MEM (Gibco, Shanghai, China). The complexes were then incubated at room temperature for 20 min and added to the A549 cells. Following incubating for 4 h, the cell medium was replaced by fresh 1,640 medium with 10% FBS and the cells were incubated for further 18 h, and then stimulated with TGF-β1 and cinobufagin for 24 h.

Immunofluorescence Staining

Cells were cultured in a 48-well chamber prior to immunofluorescence staining. After 24 h of treatment, the cells were fixed in 4% paraformaldehyde for 20 min at room temperature. After washing with PBS, cells were permeabilized with 0.2% Triton X-100 (Fluorochem) for 30 min and blocked with 5% BSA in phosphate-buffered saline (PBS) for 60 min in a humidified chamber. Mlg and A549 cells were incubated with α-SMA antibody (1:200 dilutions) and both E-cadherin (1:200 dilutions) and Vimentin (1:200 dilutions) overnight at 4°C, respectively. After washing with 1×PBS, cells were incubated with TRITC-conjugated or FITC-conjugated secondary antibody. Cell nuclei were counterstained with DAPI (Beyotime Biotechnology). Phase contrast and fluorescent microscopy was performed using an Olympus IX81 inverted research microscope.

Immunohistochemistry Staining

Paraffin-embedded lung tissue was dewaxed with xylene, and the sections were immersed in a microwave oven with antigen-fixing solution (0.01 M citrate buffer) and retrieved after 20 min. After cooling to room temperature and blocking with 5% bovine serum albumin (BSA) for 20 min, the primary antibody was incubated at 4°C overnight. The primary antibodies were as follows: mouse anti-α-SMA antibody (1:200 dilution), rabbit anti-collagen I antibody (1:100 dilution), and rabbit anti-p-Smad3 (1:50 dilution). After washing with TBST three times, the tissue sections were incubated with the secondary antibody at 4°C at room temperature for 1 h. Subsequently, tissue sections were rehydrated through a series of ethanol solutions, and sections of lung tissues were stained with hematoxylin to observe histological changes and target gene expression in lung tissues of mice under an optical microscope.

Bronchoalveolar Lavage

Mice were sacrificed with excessive of 10% chloral hydrate. Then, the left and right lungs were separated and underwent lavage through a blunt needle attached to a syringe, which worked as a trachea cannula in the airway. Bronchoalveolar lavage fluid (BALF) was collected by washing the lung through a tracheal intubation. The lungs were washed three times, and each time 1 ml 1XPBS was used. Total fluid recovery is about 80% per time. BALF centrifuged at 3,000 rpm for 10 min. The supernatant was kept at −80°C for following cytokine analysis, and sediment cells were resuspended with 1 ml red blood cell lysis buffer. Then the lysis buffer was centrifuged at room temperature at 3,000 rpm for 10 min, the supernatant removed and suspended again with 200 μl 1xPBS. Total cell count was performed by Countstar automatic cell counting instrument. Macrophages, neutrophils, and lymphocytes were counted under optical microscope, and 50 μl suspension was smeared and stained with HE staining.

ELISA Detection

BALF was prepared for ELISA. The concentration of inflammatory factors including IL-1β, IL-4, IL-6, and TNF-α was detected by ELISA kits following the manufacturer's protocol.

Data and Statistical Analysis

The data and statistical analysis complied with the recommendations on experimental design and analysis in pharmacology (Curtis et al., 2015). Data were processed with Sigma Plot 12.5 software and expressed as the means ± SD. Kolmogorov-Smirnov tests were used to test normal distribution, and two-tailed, unpaired Student's t tests were used to compare two groups with normal distribution. Significant differences among three or more groups were evaluated by one-way ANOVA. A value of $P < 0.05$ was considered statistically significant.

Materials

Cinobufagin (CBG) was purchased from Pusi Biotechnology Co. Ltd, and the purity of CBG was 99.21%. For each experiment, CBG was freshly prepared by dissolving in DMSO (Sigma, USA). Bleomycin (BLM) was acquired from Nippon Kayaku (Tokyo, Japan). TRIzol reagent was from Ambion Life Technology. DEPC TREATED H_2O, RNASE AWAY H_2O and SYBR Green Real-time PCR Master Mix were from Life Technologies. M-MLV Reverse Transcriptase was purchased from Promega, and PCR Buffer without $MgCl_2$ and $MgCl_2$ Stock Solution were acquired from Roche. In addition, Recombinant Ribonuclease Inhibitor, dATP, dTTP, dCTP, and dGTP were acquired from Takara. RIPA lysis buffer (middle) and the BCA kit were purchased from Beyotime Biotechnology. The primary antibodies described in the study include: anti-E-cadherin, anti-Vimentin, anti-fibronectin, and anti-collagen I (Affinity Biosciences, OH, USA) and anti-GAPDH, Smad3, P-Smad3, ERK, P-ERK, JNK, P-JNK, P38, P-P38 antibody (Cell Signaling Technology, Boston, United States); α-SMA and β-catenin antibody were from Santa Cruz Biotechnology (China) and Protein-Tech (China), respectively. The secondary antibodies anti-rabbit IgG (H+L) and anti-mouse IgG (H+L) were from Applygen (Beijing). Polyethylenimine, Linear purchased from Tianjin Hao Trading. β-catenin plasmid was purchased from MiaoLingPlasmid. ELISA kits were purchased from Beijing Suobao Technology.

Nomenclature of Targets and Ligands

Key protein targets and ligands in this article are hyperlinked to corresponding entries in http://www.guidetopharmacology.org, the common portal for data from the IUPHAR/BPS Guide to PHARMACOLOGY (Southan et al., 2016), and are permanently archived in the Concise Guide to PHARMACOLOGY 2015/16 (Alexander et al., 2015).

RESULTS

Cinobufagin Inhibits TGF-β1/Smad3 Signaling in Fibroblasts

As TGF-β1 is the main promoting factor of the activation, proliferation, and differentiation of myofibroblasts, we initially assessed whether cinobufagin could inhibit the classical TGF-β1 signaling pathway. We established an NIH3T3 fibroblast cell line stably transfected with $(CAGA)_{12}$-Lux-reporter, which encoded 12 copies of the canonical Smad3 DNA-binding sequence 5'-CAGA-3' (the SBE). This CAGA-NIH3T3 cell line was utilized to search for compounds that could effectively inhibit the TGF-β signaling pathway (Chen et al., 2013). After the administration of 5 $ng \cdot ml^{-1}$ TGF-β1, CAGA-NIH3T3 cells were stimulated with different concentrations of cinobufagin (5, 10, 20, 40, and 80 μM). After 18 h, the fluorescence value of each group was detected. The results showed that cinobufagin inhibited the TGF-β1/Smad3 signaling pathway in a concentration-dependent manner (**Figure 1B**). To further study the effect of cinobufagin on TGF-β1/Smad3 signaling and pulmonary fibrosis, we performed follow-up *in vitro* and *in vivo* experiments.

Effect of Cinobufagin on the Proliferation and Migration of TGF-β1-Activated Fibroblasts

The proliferation and migration of activated fibroblasts occur at the initial stage of tissue repair in response to injury and contribute to the development of lung fibrosis (Willis and Borok, 2007; Coward et al., 2010). To investigate the effects of cinobufagin on the proliferation and migration of fibroblasts/activated fibroblasts, NIH3T3 cells were cultured with or without 5 $ng \cdot ml^{-1}$ TGF-β1 and different doses of cinobufagin were administered for 24 and 48 h. We first explored whether cinobufagin affected the proliferation of NIH3T3 cells using the MTT assay. The results showed that cinobufagin did not significantly inhibit the proliferation of normal or activated fibroblasts, indicating that cinobufagin shows no cytotoxicity on fibroblasts *in vitro* (**Figures 2A, B**). Meanwhile, wound healing assays were evaluated to analyze the effects of cinobufagin on the migration of activated fibroblasts. The experimental results showed that cinobufagin inhibits the migration of activated fibroblasts (**Figures 2C, D**).

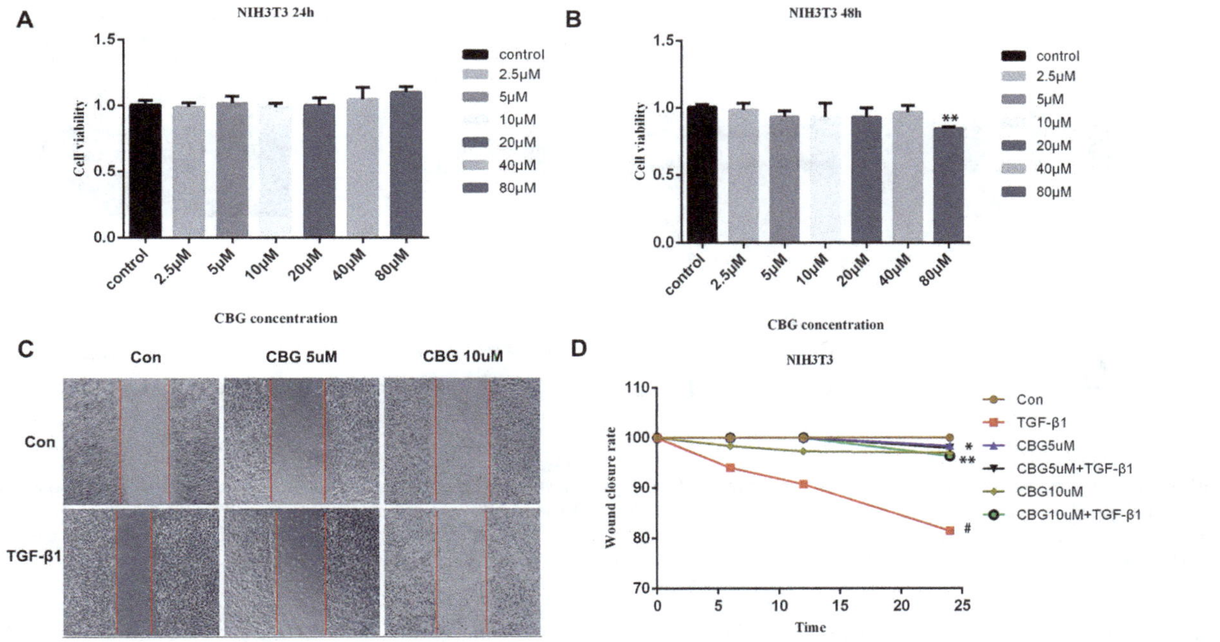

FIGURE 2 | Cinobufagin inhibits TGF-β1-induced migration of lung fibroblasts. **(A, B)** NIH3T3 cells were treated with TGF-β1 (5 ng·ml^{-1}) and different doses of cinobufagin for 24 h. Cells treated with DMSO served as controls. Cinobufagin was measured by MTT value-added assays at 24 and 48 h to determine the inhibitory effect of cinobufagin on fibroblast proliferation induced by TGF-β1 (n = 5 per group). **(C, D)** A wound healing assay was used to assess the effect of cinobufagin on fibroblast migration. The wound closure was photographed at 0, 12, and 24 h post-scratching (n = 3 per group). Experiments were performed in triplicate. *P < 0.05; **P < 0.01; #P < 0.05.

Cinobufagin Inhibits TGF-β1-Induced Fibroblast Differentiation and ECM Production *In Vitro*

To further investigate the inhibitory effect of cinobufagin on the TGF-β1-induced differentiation of lung fibroblasts, we treated mouse lung fibroblasts (Mlg) with TGF-β1 and different doses of cinobufagin to detect the expression of a typical activation marker: α-smooth muscle actin (α-SMA). The experimental results showed that administration of TGF-β1 substantially enhanced α-SMA mRNA expression compared with the control group, and cinobufagin (10 μM) treatment significantly down-regulated TGF-β1-induced α-SMA mRNA expression (**Figure 3A**). Western blotting analysis gave similar results, cinobufagin treatment significantly down-regulated TGF-β1-induced α-SMA protein expression, which indicated that cinobufagin could inhibit fibroblast differentiation into myofibroblasts (**Figures 3B, C**). We also performed immunofluorescence assays of α-SMA and obtained the same conclusion (**Figure 3D**). Extracellular matrix deposition is an important pathological feature of pulmonary fibrosis, mainly reflected in the overexpression of collagen I (Col1) and fibronectin (Fn). Not surprisingly, cinobufagin could also reduce the mRNA and protein expression levels of Col1a1 and Fn in TGF-β1-stimulated fibroblasts (**Figures 3E–G**).

In the TGF-β signaling pathway, transcription factor Smad3 plays an important regulatory role in IPF. Therefore, we examined the effect of cinobufagin on the expression and activation of Smad3. The results showed that cinobufagin could significantly reduce the phosphorylation level of Smad3 protein and had no influence on the expression of Smad3 (**Figure 3H**). Furthermore, TGF-β can also activate the MAPK pathway, in which a kinase cascade leads to the activation of ERK, JNK, and the p38 subunit. We also measured whether cinobufagin could suppress the TGF-β/MAPK signaling pathway. The results showed that cinobufagin significantly inhibited activation of ERK, JNK, and p38 without influencing the expression of MAPK (**Figure S1**). Also we found that cinobufagin had no effect on the total levels of TGF-β1 in the lungs of bleomycin treated mice and could not influence the expression levels of TGF-β receptor I and TGF-β receptor II (**Figure S2**), which indicated that cinobufagin may actualized the inhibitory role mainly through direct effect on TGF-β1 downstream signaling pathway. In summary, these data suggest that cinobufagin could inhibit fibroblast activation and reduce extracellular matrix deposition through inhibiting TGF-β1/Smad3 and TGF-β/MAPK signaling pathway.

Cinobufagin Inhibits TGF-β1-Induced EMT in Alveolar Epithelial Cells

EMT plays an important role in pulmonary fibrosisthor (Willis and Borok, 2007). To investigate whether cinobufagin exerts anti-lung fibrosis effects by inhibiting the EMT process, we used TGF-β1 to induce EMT in A549 cells and treated cells with different doses of cinobufagin. After 24 h, the morphology changes and expression of epithelial/mesenchymal phenotypic markers of A549 cells were detected. **Figure 4A** shows that TGF-β1 resulted in extended pseudopodia and fibroblast-like morphology changes in the A549 cells, while cinobufagin treatment reversed the features of EMT to different degrees. The qRT-PCR results showed that cinobufagin can reduce the induction of mesenchymal markers by TGF-β1, such as Vimentin and N-cadherin (N–Ca), and increase the expression of the

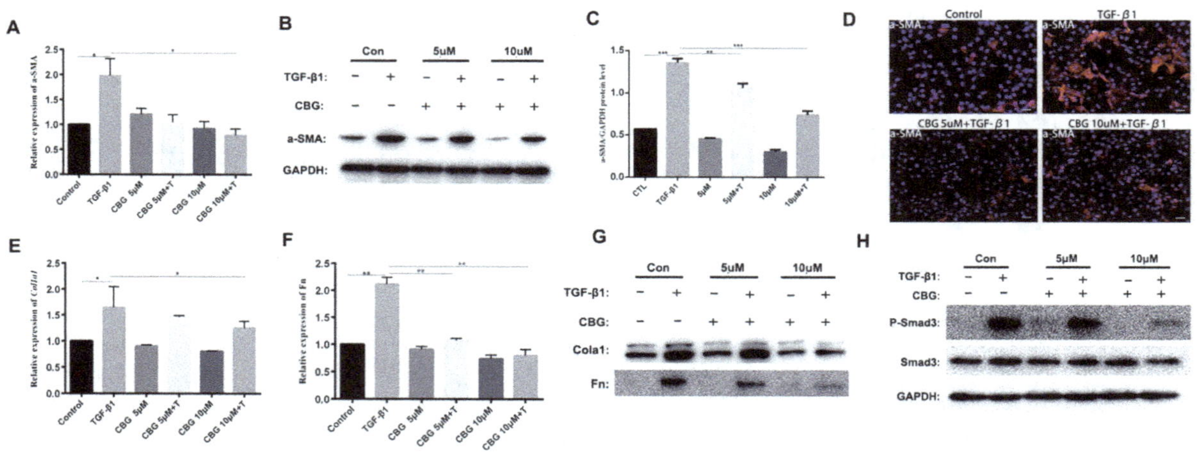

FIGURE 3 | Cinobufagin inhibits TGF-β1-induced expression of α-SMA, Col1 and Fn *in vitro*. Mlg cells were treated with TGF-β1 (5 ng·ml^{-1}) and cinobufagin (5 and 10 μM) for 24 h (n = 3 per group). The mRNA levels of α-SMA **(A)**, Col1a1 **(E)** and Fn **(F)** were analyzed by Real-time PCR. The protein levels of α-SMA **(B, C)**, Col1a1, Fn **(G)** and P-Smad3 **(H)** were analyzed by western blot. **(D)** Immunofluorescence staining for α-SMA (a marker of myofibroblast differentiation) was performed on Mlg cells treated with/without TGF-β1 (5 ng·ml^{-1}) and/or cinobufagin (5 and 10 μM) for 24 h. *P < 0.05; **P < 0.01; ***P < 0.001.

epithelial marker E-cadherin (E–Ca) (**Figures 4B–D**). Consistent with the qRT-PCR results, immunofluorescence assays showed that cinobufagin could up-regulate E–Ca expression and down-regulate Vim expression in TGF-β1-treated A549 cells (**Figures 4E, F**). Western blotting analysis showed a similar result (**Figures 4G–I**).

Since TGF-β1 signaling pathway plays an important role in the progression of EMT, and former studies showed that cinobufagin could suppressing TGF-β1/Smad3 and TGF-β/MAPK signaling pathway in the activation of fibroblasts, we further evaluated whether cinobufagin could regulated Smad3 and MAPK signaling in EMT process of A549 cells. As shown in **Figure S3**, cinobufagin could significantly inhibit TGF-β1-induced phosphorylation of Smad3 in A549 cells, but had no influence on TGF-β/MAPK signaling pathway. The results indicated different mechanisms under cinobufagin-regulated EMT and fibroblast differentiation.

Ample evidence links β-catenin activation with the induction of EMT (Kim et al., 2002; Moustakas and Heldin, 2007). Excitingly, cinobufagin also reduced the expression levels of β-catenin in TGF-β1-treated A549 cells (**Figures 4J, K**). In addition, we used the method of transfection β-catenin plasmid to verify that cinobufagin did affect EMT in pulmonary epithelial cells by regulating the expression of β-catenin. The results showed that when we overexpressed the β-catenin plasmid in A549 cells, the expression of E–Ca was down-regulated, while the expression of Vim was up-regulated. But the cinobufagin-treated group could resist the change of cells and decreased the overexpression of β-catenin (**Figure 4L**). Collectively, these data indicate that cinobufagin may inhibit the EMT process in alveolar epithelial cells by suppressing TGF-β1/Smad3 signaling and β-catenin expression.

Cinobufagin Alleviates Bleomycin-Induced Pulmonary Fibrosis in Mice

To evaluate the anti-fibrotic potential of cinobufagin *in vivo*, C57BL/6 mice were intratracheally instilled with bleomycin (BLM, 2.5U) to induce pulmonary fibrosis. On the seventh day after modeling, cinobufagin (10 mg·kg^{-1}) was intraperitoneally injected and continuously administered for 7 days. Pirfenidone, a listed drug for the treatment of IPF, was used as a positive control. The results showed that the cinobufagin-administered group alleviated bleomycin-induced weight loss compared with the model group (**Figure 5A**). Treatment of bleomycin-injured mice with cinobufagin significantly reduced the collagen content and percentage of fibrotic areas compared to mice treated with Pirfenidone (**Figures 5B, C**). At the same time, HE staining, Sirius red staining and Trichrome staining were carried out to examine the histological conditions of pulmonary tissue samples. HE staining suggested that enhanced pathologic reorganization and alveolar–capillary structure damage were induced by bleomycin, while they were ameliorated by cinobufagin administration (**Figure 5D**).

We further measured the changes in pulmonary function after cinobufagin treatment. As shown in **Figure 6**, the pulmonary function of cinobufagin-treated mice was significantly improved, as seen by increased forced vital capacity (FVC), increased forced expiratory volume in one second (FEV1) and forced expiratory volume in one second/forced expiratory volume (FEV1/FVC), decreased inspiratory resistance (Ri) and expiratory resistance (Re), and increased dynamic compliance (Cdyn) when compared with bleomycin-treated mice and the Pirfenidone group. Taken together, these data suggest that cinobufagin can attenuate pulmonary fibrosis induced by BLM in mice.

Cinobufagin Reduced the Inflammatory Response in Bleomycin-Treated Mice and Macrophage

Studies have shown that inflammation may occur in the early stage of IPF. Therefore, we used BLM intratracheal instillation to simulate the inflammatory response to mimic the early stage of IPF, and investigated whether cinobufagin could alleviate inflammatory response. HE staining of left lung pathological sections showed that cinobufagin could alleviate inflammatory

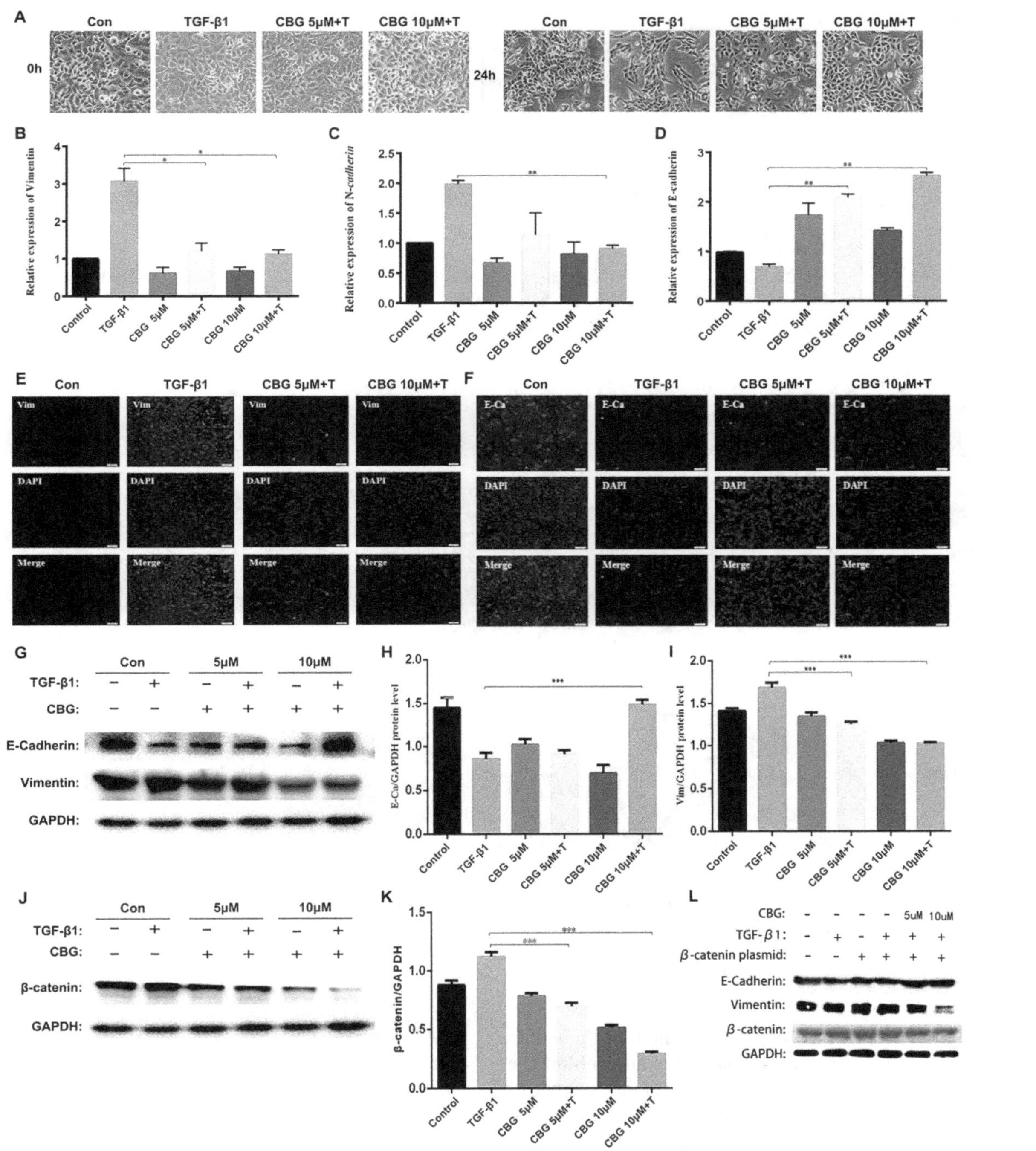

FIGURE 4 | Cinobufagin suppresses TGF-β1-induced EMT in alveolar epithelial cells. A549 cells were treated with TGF-β1 and different concentrations of cinobufagin (5 and 10 μM) for 24 h. Cells stimulated with DMSO served as controls (n = 3 per group). **(A)** Morphological changes of A549 cells. **(B-D)** mRNA levels of EMT makers, including Vimentin, N-cadherin, and E-cadherin. **(E–F)** Immunofluorescence analysis of Vimentin and E-cadherin in A549 cells. **(G–I)** Quantitative densitometry of different samples by western blot. Expression levels of E-cadherin and Vimentin were normalized to GAPDH. **(J–K)** Quantitative densitometry of different samples by western blot. Expression levels of β-catenin were normalized to GAPDH. **(L)** Detection of E-Ca, Vim and β-catenin protein expression after transfection of β-catenin plasmid by Western blot. *P < 0.05; **P < 0.01; ***P < 0.001.

cell infiltration in lung tissues, and the therapeutic effect was better than positive drug pirfenidone (**Figure 7A**). In addition, we detected the total number of cells, numbers of inflammatory cells and secretion of inflammatory cytokines including IL-1β, IL-4, IL-6, and TNF-α in BALF. It is no surprise that cinobufagin reduced the number of inflammatory cells and the expression of inflammatory factors in BALF, and the inhibitory effect was better than positive drug pirfenidone (**Figures 7B–D**). Furthermore,

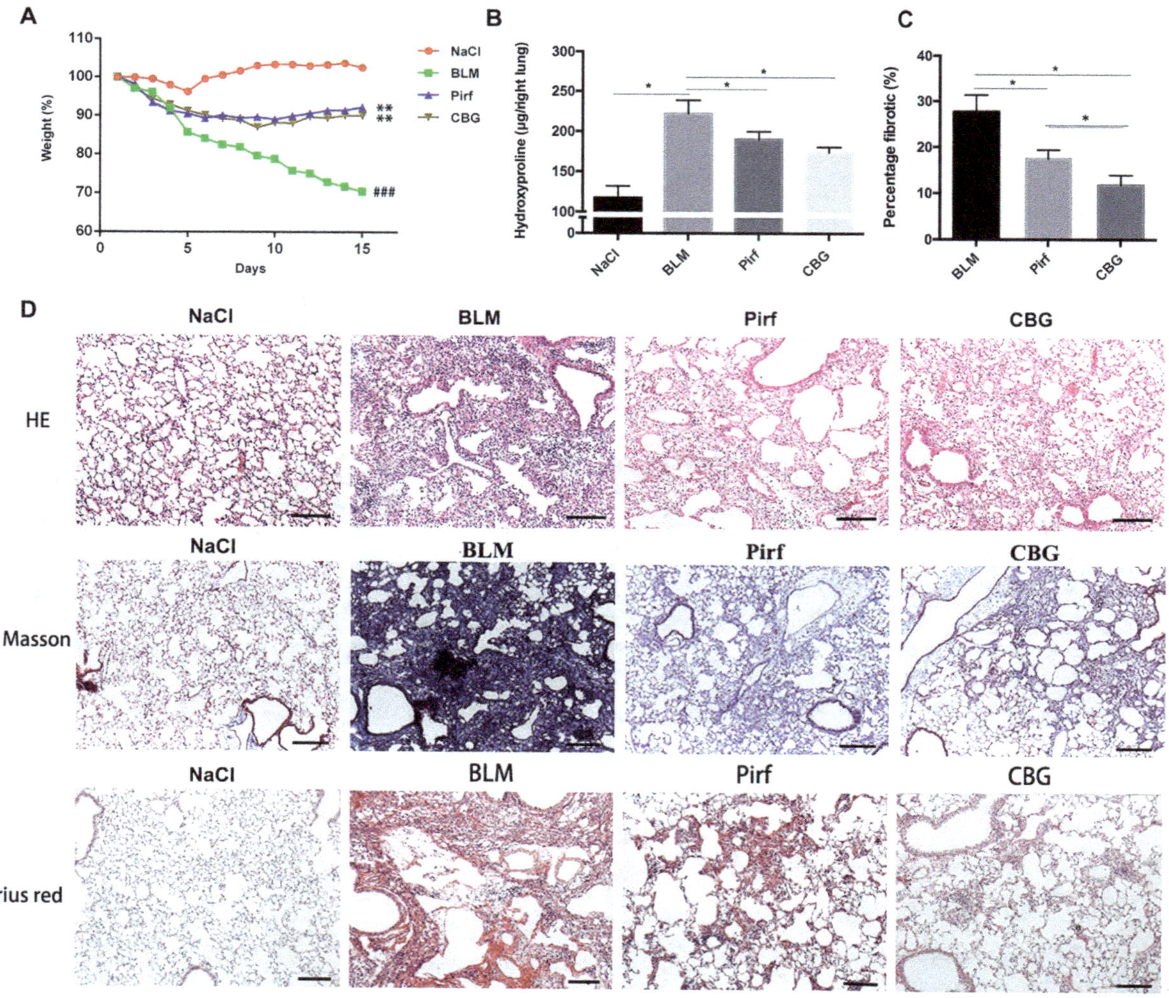

FIGURE 5 | Cinobufagin attenuates BLM-induced pulmonary fibrosis in mice. Mice were intratracheally injected with a single dose of BLM (2 mg·kg^{-1}). Cinobufagin (10 mg·kg^{-1}) and Pirfenidone (200 mg·kg^{-1}) were given from day 7 to day 14 (n = 6 per group). **(A)** Average body weight of mice in each group. **(B)** Determination of hydroxyproline content in lung tissues of each group. **(C)** Statistics of pulmonary fibrosis area in each group. **(D)** Photomicrographs of lung sections stained with hematoxylin–eosin (HE), Masson Trichrome staining and Sirius red staining. Data are presented as the means ± SD (n = 6), # represents a comparison with the NaCl control group, * represents a comparison with the BLM group. ###P < 0.001; *P < 0.05; **P < 0.01.

we detected the anti-inflammatory effect of cinobufagin *in vitro* and the results indicated that cinobufagin could inhibit the expression of IL-6 and IL-1β in LPS-treated bone marrow derived macrophages while had no effect on TGF-β1-induced expression of IL-6 and IL-1β in fibroblasts (**Figure S4**). These data indicated that cinobufagin could inhibit the inflammatory response in bleomycin-treated mice and had anti-inflammatory effect on the immune response of macrophage.

Cinobufagin Inhibits Fibrogenic Activation of Pulmonary Fibroblasts *In Vivo*

To further verify whether cinobufagin can attenuate the activation of pulmonary fibroblasts *in vivo*, we extracted protein and RNA from the lungs of C57BL/6 mice and analyzed the expression of α-SMA and Col1 by western blotting and real-time PCR. As expected, the protein levels of and Col1 in the tissue of cinobufagin-treated lungs were lower than the bleomycin model group (**Figures 8A–C**). Similarly, in the cinobufagin-treated group, the RNA expression levels of α-SMA and Col1a1 were also significantly lower than in the bleomycin model group (**Figures 8D, F**). Subsequently, we also performed immunohistochemical studies with murine lung sections. The results also confirmed the above observation (**Figures 8E, G**). In conclusion, cinobufagin down-regulates the expression of α-SMA and Col1 in lung tissues, thereby reducing extracellular matrix deposition and releasing bleomycin-induced lung fibrosis in mice.

Cinobufagin Prevents EMT Phenotype *In Vivo*

We further evaluated the role of cinobufagin in EMT progression during bleomycin-induced pulmonary fibrosis in C57BL/6 mice. Similar to our *in vitro* results, western blot assays showed that E-cadherin expression was increased and Vimentin expression decreased by cinobufagin treatment (**Figures 9A–C**). In addition,

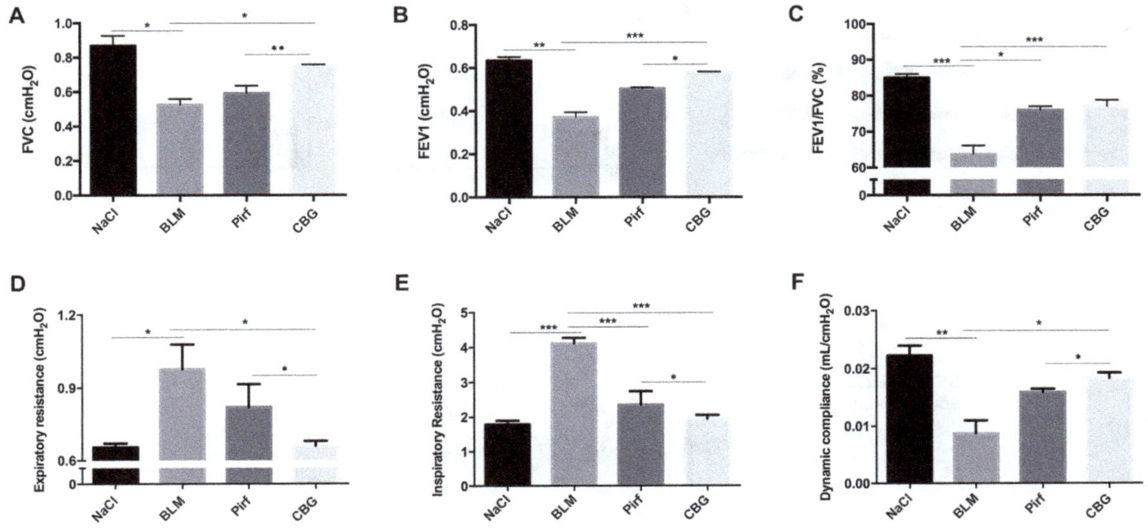

FIGURE 6 | Cinobufagin improves pulmonary function in BLM-treated mice. Two weeks after BLM administration, pulmonary function of mice was determined. Pulmonary function parameters, including **(A)** Forced vital capacity (FVC), **(B)** Forced expiratory volume in one second (FEV1), **(C)** Forced expiratory volume in one second/forced expiratory volume (FEV1/FVC), **(D)** Expiratory resistance (Re), **(E)** Inspiratory resistance (Ri) and **(F)** dynamic compliance (Cdyn), were compared among different groups. Data are presented as the means ± SD (n = 6). *P < 0.05; **P < 0.01; ***P < 0.001.

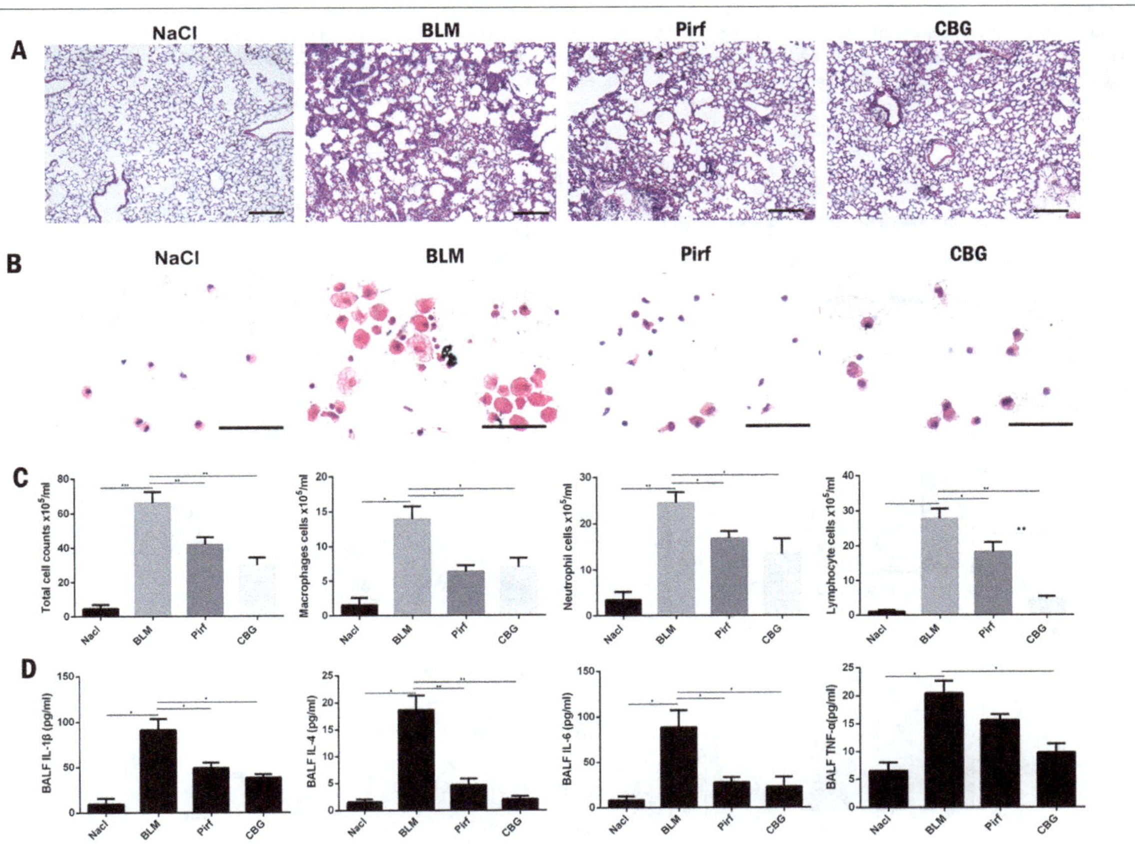

FIGURE 7 | Cinobufagin reduced the inflammatory response in bleomycin-treated mice. **(A)** HE staining of left lung tissues in each group. **(B)** HE staining of inflammatory cells in the BALF. Representative visual fields of HE staining from NaCl group, BLM group, Pirfenidone group and cinobufagin group, respectively. Cells were mainly macrophages, neutrophils and lymphocytes. Original magnification, ×200. **(C)** Total cell, macrophages, neutrophils and lymphocytes from BALF in each groups were counted on day 7. **(D)** The expression of inflammatory factors including IL-1β, IL-4, IL-6 and TNF-α in BALF were detected by ELISA kit. Data are presented as mean ± SD (n = 6).*P < 0.05; **P < 0.01; ***P < 0.001.

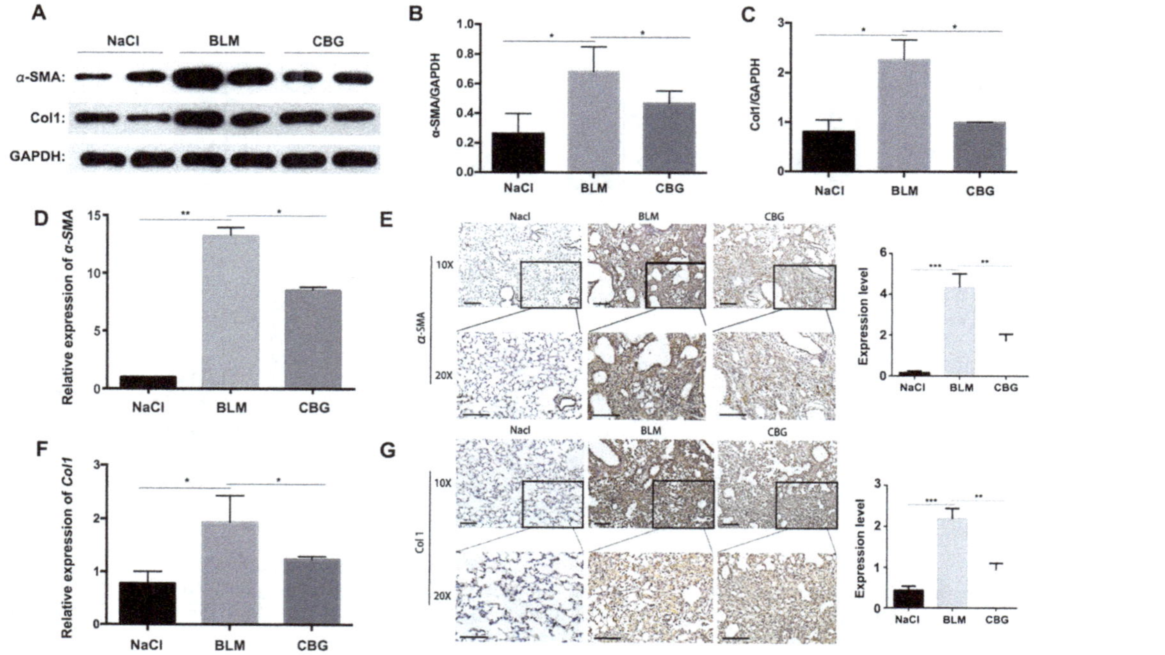

FIGURE 8 | Cinobufagin attenuates BLM-induced myofibroblast differentiation and ECM deposition *in vivo*. **(A)** Western blot analysis of the protein levels of α-SMA and Col1 in lung tissues. **(B, C)** Densitometric analysis of α-SMA and Col1a1 in the immunoblots, using GAPDH as the internal reference. **(D, F)** Real-time PCR was performed to detect the mRNA levels of α-SMA and Col1a1 in the pulmonary tissues derived from each group. **(E, G)** Immunohistochemical staining of α-SMA and Col1-positive cells in the lungs. Data are expressed as the means ± SD (n = 6), *$P < 0.05$; **$P < 0.01$; ***$P < 0.01$.

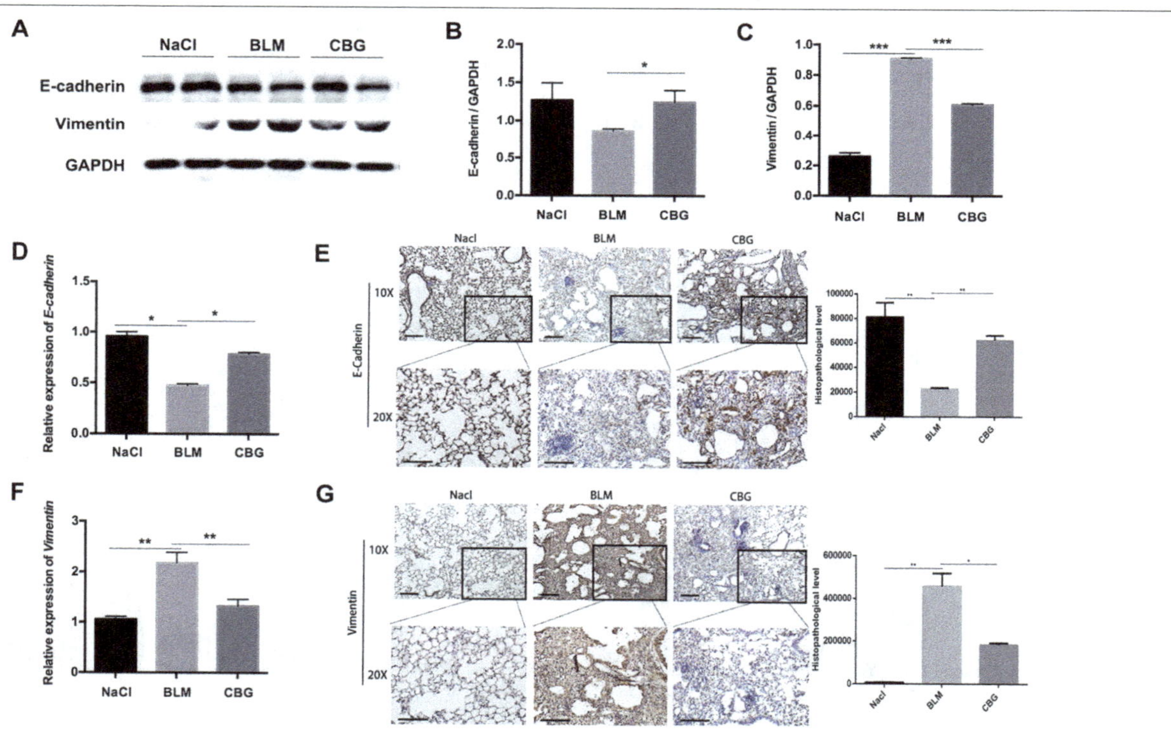

FIGURE 9 | Cinobufagin represses EMT *in vivo*. **(A)** Western blot was used to analyze the protein levels of E-cadherin and Vimentin in lung tissues. **(B, C)** Densitometric analysis of E-cadherin and Vimentin in immunoblots using GAPDH as the internal reference. **(D, F)** Real-time PCR was performed to detect the mRNA levels of E-cadherin and Vimentin in the pulmonary tissues derived from each group. **(E, G)** Immunohistochemical staining of E-cadherin and Vimentin-positive cells in the lungs. Data are expressed as the means ± SD (n = 6), *$P < 0.05$; **$P < 0.01$; ***$P < 0.01$.

qRT-PCR analysis of lungs showed that cinobufagin up-regulates E-cadherin and down-regulates Vimentin (**Figures 9D, F**). Similarly, E-cadherin-positive cells were increased and Vimentin-positive cells reduced after cinobufagin treatment, as determined by immunohistochemical analysis (**Figures 9E, G**). All these findings provide a critical clue that cinobufagin inhibits EMT *in vivo*.

DISCUSSION

IPF is a chronic lung disease of unknown cause, with a progressive course, fatal prognosis and comparative morbidity and mortality. In past decades, the pathogenesis of IPF has evolved from an earlier inflammatory hypothesis to a novel hypothesis of abnormal epithelial injury repair(Strieter, 2005). IPF is characterized by an abnormal and uncontrolled proliferation of fibroblasts and myofibroblasts, distortion of lung architecture due to repetitive chronic injury to the alveolar epithelial cells, and a subsequent disorganized repair process (Sgalla et al., 2016). Injured Type II alveolar epithelial cells repeatedly release a variety of mediators, cytokines and growth factors, which promote excessive activation of fibroblasts and eventually lead to imbalances in regenerative repair and scar repair, thereby causing IPF (Selman and Pardo, 2014). Therefore, inhibiting the activation of fibroblasts is important for inhibiting the occurrence of pulmonary fibrosis.

In the present study, we investigated the possible role of cinobufagin in pulmonary fibrosis *in vitro* and *in vivo*. We firstly evaluated the inhibition role of cinobufagin on TGF-β1 signaling pathway and found that cinobufagin could inhibit the TGF-β1/Smad3 signaling in dose-dependent manner. Further data showed that cinobufagin inhibited the migration and activation of mouse fibroblasts induced by TGF-β1 *in vitro*. Intriguingly, we showed that cinobufagin had no cytotoxicity effect on fibroblasts, which is consistent with previous research (Lu et al., 2017). Thus, cinobufagin treatment was relatively safe in normal cells. *In vivo* data showed that cinobufagin effectively inhibited ECM deposition and lung remodeling and restored loss of pulmonary function. Inflammation reaction was inhibited by cinobufagin as well in bleomycin-induced lung injury. Experimental results showed that cinobufagin attenuated the expression levels of p-Smad3, α-SMA, Col1a1 and Fn, indicating that cinobufagin treatment significantly maintained the balance between the degradation of ECM components in the local lung microenvironment, which is important for the amelioration of pulmonary fibrosis.

In addition to the proliferation and differentiation of resident lung fibroblasts, myofibroblasts may also be derived, in part, from EMT. EMT, accounting for approximately 33% of myofibroblasts, has been implicated in the development of fibrotic diseases. EMT-like changes play an important role in pulmonary fibrosis. Hence, we also investigated the effects of cinobufagin on EMT in this study. In this case, we used TGF-β1 to induce EMT-like changes in human alveolar epithelial cells. We found that TGF-β1 triggered the loss of epithelial markers, such as E-cadherin, in alveolar epithelial cells and the expression of Vimentin and N-cadherin, which are specific for mesenchymal cells, consistent with previous studies (Kasai et al., 2005; Willis et al., 2005; Cheng et al., 2012; Liu et al., 2014). Cinobufagin treatment inhibited the up-regulation of TGF-β1 induced EMT *in vitro* but also suppressed EMT phenotype *in vivo*, implying that the anti-fibrotic roles of cinobufagin are, at least in part, due to EMT inhibition. Earlier studies found that β-catenin is abnormally activated in the formation of pulmonary fibrosis (Konigshoff et al., 2008; Henderson et al., 2010). Subsequently, we found that cinobufagin reduced TGF-β1-induced β-catenin overexpression. This indicates that cinobufagin may interfere with the EMT process by inhibiting β-catenin expression. Collectively, these results suggest that cinobufagin antagonizes TGF-β-mediated Smad3 and β-catenin signaling to exhibit anti-fibrotic effects. Except for the TGF-β1/Smad3 signaling pathway, we also detect whether cinobufagin could intervene the non-Smad signaling pathway (data not shown). We found that cinobufagin could only influence the Smad3 pathway and had no effect on the non-canonical pathway of TGF-β1 signaling, which indicated that cinobufagin may regulate the core effector on the TGF-β1/Smad3 signaling pathway.

However, at present, we have not studied the detailed mechanism by which cinobufagin affects TGF-β-mediated Smad3 and β-catenin signaling. Therefore, we need to study the exact effect of cinobufagin on TGF-β signaling and whether cinobufagin may also impact other signaling pathways associated with pulmonary fibrosis.

In conclusion, our results indicate that cinobufagin inhibits TGF-β1/Smad3 signaling and subsequently suppresses fibroblast activation and differentiation, EMT and eventual ECM deposition. Furthermore, cinobufagin treatment leads to improved bleomycin-induced pulmonary fibrosis and inflammatory responses in mice. Based on these observations, we believe that cinobufagin has a variety of roles other than anti-tumor effects and may be used as an anti-fibrotic drug candidate. As a traditional Chinese medicine monomer, cinobufagin has better pharmacodynamic effect on IPF than Pirfenidone. In addition to inhibiting the activation of a series of fibroblasts induced by activated TGF-beta/smad3, cinobufagin can also reduce the source of myofibroblasts by resisting EMT and further improve pulmonary fibrosis. Therefore, on the one hand, we want to develop cinobufagin as a new indication of anti-pulmonary fibrosis, and at the same time, we hope that the mother nucleus of cinobufagin (i.e. effective group) can be used as a candidate for the development of new anti-pulmonary fibrosis compounds, so as to provide more drug options for clinical IPF patients.

ETHICS STATEMENT

All animal care and experimental procedures were complied with guidelines approved by the Institutional Animal Care and Use Committee (IACUC) of Nankai University (Permit No. SYXK 2014-0003). Animal studies are reported in compliance with the ARRIVE guidelines (Kliment and Oury, 2010; McGrath and Lilley, 2015).

AUTHOR CONTRIBUTIONS

CY, HZ, and TS contributed to the conception and design. XL, SL, ZB and MH contributed to the collection and assembly of data. JM, SG, and KH contributed to the data analysis and interpretation. YC contributed to the data revision. XL, ZB and SL contributed to the manuscript writing. JG and LL contributed to the administrative support. All authors read and approved the final manuscript.

SUPPLEMENTARY MATERIAL

FIGURE S1 | Cinobufagin inhibits TGF-β1/MAPK signaling in lung fibroblasts. Mlg cells were treated with TGF-β1 (5 ng·ml^{-1}) and cinobufagin (5 and 10 μM) for 1 h (n = 3 per group). The protein levels of ERK, P-ERK, JNK, P-JNK, P38, and P-P38 were analyzed by western blot. GAPDH was used as a loading control.

FIGURE S2 | Cinobufagin had no effect on the total levels of TGF-β1 and TGF-β receptor. **(A)** Western blot was used to analyze the protein levels of TGF-β1 in lung tissues. **(B)** Densitometric analysis of TGF-β1 in immunoblots using GAPDH as the internal reference. **(C)** Mlg cells were treated with TGF-β1 (5 ng·ml^{-1}) and cinobufagin (5 and 10 μM) for 24 h (n = 3 per group). The protein levels of TGF-β receptor I (TβRI) and TGF-β receptor II (TβRII) were analyzed by western blot. **(D, E)** Densitometric analysis of TβRI and TβRII in immunoblots using GAPDH as the internal reference.

FIGURE S3 | Cinobufagin inhibits TGF-β1/Smad3 signaling in alveolar epithelial cells. A549 cells were treated with TGF-β1 (5 ng·ml^{-1}) and cinobufagin (5 and 10 μM) for 1 h (n = 3 per group). The protein levels of **(A)** Smad3 and P-Smad3, **(B)** ERK, P-ERK, JNK, P-JNK, P38, and P-P38 were analyzed by western blot. GAPDH was used as a loading control.

FIGURE S4 | Cinobufagin inhibits LPS-induced expression of IL-6 and IL-1β in bone marrow derived macrophages. **(A, B)** Cultured bone marrow derived macrophages were treated with LPS (1 μg·ml^{-1}) and cinobufagin (5 and 10 μM) for 12 h (n = 3 per group). The RNA levels of IL-6 **(A)** and IL-1β **(B)** were analysed by RT-PCR. **(C, D)** Mlg cells were treated with TGF-β1 (5 ng·ml^{-1}) and cinobufagin (5 and 10 μM) for 12 h (n = 3 per group). The RNA levels of IL-6 **(C)** and IL-1β **(D)** were analysed by RT-PCR. Data are expressed as the means ± SD, *P < 0.05; ***P < 0.01.

REFERENCES

1. Alexander, S. P., Davenport, A. P., Kelly, E., Marrion, N., Peters, J. A., Benson, H. E., et al. (2015). The Concise Guide to PHARMACOLOGY 2015/16: G protein-coupled receptors. *Br. J. Pharmacol.* 172 (24), 5744–5869. doi: 10.1111/ bph.13348
2. Borensztajn, K., Crestani, B., and Kolb, M. (2013). Idiopathic pulmonary fibrosis: from epithelial injury to biomarkers — insights from the bench side. *Respiration* 86 (6), 441–452. doi: 10.1159/000357598
3. Chen, Y. L., Zhang, X., Bai, J., Gai, L., Ye, X. L., Zhang, L., et al. (2013). Sorafenib ameliorates bleomycin-induced pulmonary fibrosis: potential roles in the inhibition of epithelial-mesenchymal transition and fibroblast activation. *Cell Death Dis.* 4, e665. doi: 10.1038/cddis.2013.154
4. Cheng, J. C., Auersperg, N., and Leung, P. C. (2012). EGF-induced EMT and invasiveness in serous borderline ovarian tumor cells: a possible step in the transition to low-grade serous carcinoma cells? *PLoS One* 7 (3), e34071. doi: 10.1371/journal.pone.0034071
5. Coward, W. R., Saini, G., and Jenkins, G. (2010). The pathogenesis of idiopathic pulmonary fibrosis. *Ther. Adv. Respir. Dis.* 4 (6), 367–388. doi: 10.1177/17534658 10379801
6. Cui, X., Inagaki, Y., Wang, D., Gao, J., Qi, F., Gao, B., et al. (2014). The supercritical CO(2) extract from the skin of *Bufo bufo* gargarizans Cantor blocks hepatitis B virus antigen secretion in HepG2.2.15 cells. *Biosci. Trends* 8 (1), 38–44.
7. Cui, X., Inagaki, Y., Xu, H., Wang, D., Qi, F., Kokudo, N., et al. (2010). Anti-hepatitis B virus activities of cinobufacini and its active components bufalin and cinobufagin in HepG2.2.15 cells. *Biol. Pharm. Bull.* 33 (10), 1728–1732.
8. Curtis, M. J., Bond, R. A., Spina, D., Ahluwalia, A., Alexander, S. P., Giembycz, M. A., et al. (2015). Experimental design and analysis and their reporting: new guidance for publication in BJP. *Br. J. Pharmacol.* 172 (14), 3461–3471. doi: 10.1111/bph.12856
9. Dai, G., Zheng, D., Guo, W., Yang, J., and Cheng, A. Y. (2018). Cinobufagin induces apoptosis in osteosarcoma cells *via* the mitochondria-mediated apoptotic pathway. *Cell Physiol. Biochem.* 46 (3), 1134–1147. doi: 10.1159/000488842
10. Geng, Y., Dong, Y., Yu, M., Zhang, L., Yan, X., Sun, J., et al. (2011). Follistatin-like 1 (Fstl1) is a bone morphogenetic protein (BMP) 4 signaling antagonist in controlling mouse lung development. *Proc. Natl. Acad. Sci. U. S. A.* 108 (17), 7058–7063. doi: 10.1073/pnas.1007293108
11. Henderson, W. R., Jr., Chi, E. Y., Ye, X., Nguyen, C., Tien, Y. T., Zhou, B., et al. (2010). Inhibition of Wnt/beta-catenin/CREB binding protein (CBP) signaling reverses pulmonary fibrosis. *Proc. Natl. Acad. Sci. U. S. A.* 107 (32), 14309– 14314. doi: 10.1073/pnas.1001520107
12. Hisatomi, K., Mukae, H., Sakamoto, N., Ishimatsu, Y., Kakugawa, T., Hara, S., et al. (2012). Pirfenidone inhibits TGF-beta1-induced over-expression of collagen type I and heat shock protein 47 in A549 cells. *BMC Pulm. Med.* 12, 24. doi: 10.1186/1471-2466-12-24
13. Jiang, D., Liang, J., Hodge, J., Lu, B., Zhu, Z., Yu, S., et al. (2004). Regulation of pulmonary fibrosis by chemokine receptor CXCR3. *J. Clin. Invest.* 114 (2), 291–299. doi: 10.1172/JCI16861
14. Jenkins, R. G., Moore, B. B., Chambers, R. C., Eickelberg, O., Konigshoff, M., Kolb, M., et al. (2017). An official American Thoracic Society workshop report: use of animal models for the preclinical assessment of potential therapies for pulmonary fibrosis. *Am. J. Respir. Cell Mol. Biol.* 56 (5), 667–679. doi: 10.1165/ rcmb.2017-0096ST
15. Jo, H. E., Randhawa, S., Corte, T. J., and Moodley, Y. (2016). Idiopathic pulmonary fibrosis and the elderly: diagnosis and management considerations. *Drugs Aging* 33 (5), 321–334. doi: 10.1007/s40266-016-0366-1
16. Kasai, H., Allen, J. T., Mason, R. M., Kamimura, T., and Zhang, Z. (2005). TGF- beta1 induces human alveolar epithelial to mesenchymal cell transition (EMT). *Respir. Res.* 6, 56. doi: 10.1186/1465-9921-6-56
17. Kim, K., Lu, Z., and Hay, E. D. (2002). Direct evidence for a role of beta-catenin/ LEF-1 signaling pathway in induction of EMT. *Cell Biol. Int.* 26 (5), 463–476.
18. Kim, K. K., Kugler, M. C., Wolters, P. J., Robillard, L., Galvez, M. G., Brumwell, A. N., et al. (2006). Alveolar epithelial cell mesenchymal transition develops *in vivo* during pulmonary fibrosis and is regulated by the extracellular matrix. *Proc. Natl. Acad. Sci. U. S. A.* 103 (35), 13180–13185. doi: 10.1073/ pnas.0605669103
19. King, T. E., Jr., Bradford, W. Z., Castro-Bernardini, S., Fagan, E. A., Glaspole, I., Glassberg, M. K., et al. (2014). A phase 3 trial of pirfenidone in patients with idiopathic pulmonary fibrosis. *N. Engl. J. Med.* 370 (22), 2083–2092. doi: 10.1056/NEJMoa1402582
20. Kliment, C. R., and Oury, T. D. (2010). Oxidative stress, extracellular matrix targets, and idiopathic pulmonary fibrosis. *Free Radic. Biol. Med.* 49 (5), 707–717. doi: 10.1016/j.freeradbiomed.2010.04.036
21. Konigshoff, M., Balsara, N., Pfaff, E. M., Kramer, M., Chrobak, I., Seeger, W., et al. (2008). Functional Wnt signaling is increased in idiopathic pulmonary fibrosis. *PLoS One* 3 (5), e2142. doi: 10.1371/journal. pone.0002142
22. Li, F., Yang, R., Weng, Y., and Tang, X. (2009). Preparation and evaluation of lyophilized liposome-encapsulated bufadienolides. *Drug Dev. Ind. Pharm.* 35 (9), 1048–1058. doi: 10.1080/03639040902762987
23. Li, L., Li, D., Xu, L., Zhao, P., Deng, Z., Mo, X., et al. (2015). Total extract of Yupingfeng attenuates bleomycin-induced pulmonary fibrosis in rats. *Phytomedicine* 22 (1), 111–119. doi: 10.1016/j.phymed.2014.10.011
24. Liu, Z. C., Chen, X. H., Song, H. X., Wang, H. S., Zhang, G., Wang, H., et al. (2014). Snail regulated by PKC/GSK-3beta pathway is crucial for EGF-induced epithelial–mesenchymal transition (EMT) of cancer cells. *Cell Tissue Res.* 358 (2), 491–502. doi: 10.1007/s00441-014-1953-2
25. Maher, T. M. (2013). Beyond the diagnosis of idiopathic pulmonary fibrosis; the growing role of systems biology and stratified medicine. *Curr. Opin. Pulm. Med.* 19 (5), 460–465. doi: 10.1097/MCP.0b013e328363f4b7

26. Lu, X. S., Qiao, Y. B., Li, Y., Yang, B., Chen, M. B., and Xing, C. G. (2017). Preclinical study of cinobufagin as a promising anti-colorectal cancer agent. *Oncotarget* 8 (1), 988–998. doi: 10.18632/oncotarget.13519
27. McGrath, J. C., and Lilley, E. (2015). Implementing guidelines on reporting research using animals (ARRIVE etc.): new requirements for publication in BJP. *Br. J. Pharmacol.* 172 (13), 3189–3193. doi: 10.1111/bph.12955
28. Moustakas, A., and Heldin, C. H. (2007). Signaling networks guiding epithelial– mesenchymal transitions during embryogenesis and cancer progression. *Cancer Sci.* 98 (10), 1512–1520. doi: 10.1111/j.1349-7006.2007.00550.x
29. Ning, W., Li, C. J., Kaminski, N., Feghali-Bostwick, C. A., Alber, S. M., Di, Y. P., et al. (2004). Comprehensive gene expression profiles reveal pathways related to the pathogenesis of chronic obstructive pulmonary disease. *Proc. Natl. Acad. Sci. U. S. A.* 101 (41), 14895–14900. doi: 10.1073/pnas.0401168101
30. Ogura, T., Taniguchi, H., Azuma, A., Inoue, Y., Kondoh, Y., Hasegawa, Y., et al. (2015). Safety andpharmacokinetics of nintedanib andpirfenidone in idiopathic pulmonary fibrosis. *Eur. Respir. J.* 45 (5), 1382–1392. doi: 10.1183/09031936.00198013
31. Qi, F. H., Li, A. Y., Lv, H., Zhao, L., Li, J. J., Gao, B., et al. (2008). Apoptosis-inducing effect of cinobufacini, *Bufo bufo* gargarizans Cantor skin extract, on human hepatoma cell line BEL-7402. *Drug Discov. Ther.* 2 (6), 339–343.
32. Selman, M., and Pardo, A. (2014). Stochastic age-related epigenetic drift in the pathogenesis of idiopathic pulmonary fibrosis. *Am. J. Respir. Crit. Care Med.* 190 (12), 1328–1330. doi: 10.1164/rccm.201411-1953ED
33. Sgalla, G., Biffi, A., and Richeldi, L. (2016). Idiopathic pulmonary fibrosis: diagnosis, epidemiology and natural history. *Respirology* 21 (3), 427–437. doi: 10.1111/resp.12683
34. Southan, C., Sharman, J. L., Benson, H. E., Faccenda, E., Pawson, A. J., Alexander, S. P., et al. (2016). The IUPHAR/BPS Guide to PHARMACOLOGY in 2016: towards curated quantitative interactions between 1300 protein targets and 6000 ligands. *Nucleic Acids Res.* 44 (D1), D1054–D1068. doi: 10.1093/nar/ gkv1037
35. Strieter, R. M. (2005). Pathogenesis and natural history of usual interstitial pneumonia: the whole story or the last chapter of a long novel. *Chest* 128 (5 Suppl 1), 526S–532S. doi: 10.1378/chest.128.5_suppl_1.526S
36. Waiwut, P., Inujima, A., Inoue, H., Saiki, I., and Sakurai, H. (2012). Bufotalin sensitizes death receptor-induced apoptosis *via* Bid- and STAT1-dependent pathways. *Int. J. Oncol.* 40 (1), 203–208. doi: 10.3892/ijo.2011.1182
37. Wand, O., and Kremer, M. R. (2015). [Novel therapies for idiopathic pulmonary fibrosis]. *Harefuah* 154 (7), 446–450, 469, 468.
38. Wang, D. L., Qi, F. H., Xu, H. L., Inagaki, Y., Orihara, Y., Sekimizu, K., et al. (2010). Apoptosis-inducing activity of compounds screened and characterized from cinobufacini by bioassay-guided isolation. *Mol. Med. Rep.* 3 (4), 717–722. doi: 10.3892/mmr_00000323
39. Willis, B. C., and Borok, Z. (2007). TGF-beta-induced EMT: mechanisms and implications for fibrotic lung disease. *Am. J. Physiol. Lung Cell Mol. Physiol.* 293 (3), L525–L534. doi: 10.1152/ajplung.00163.2007
40. Willis, B. C., Liebler, J. M., Luby-Phelps, K., Nicholson, A. G., Crandall, E. D., du Bois, R. M., et al. (2005). Induction of epithelial–mesenchymal transition in alveolar epithelial cells by transforming growth factor-beta1: potential role in idiopathic pulmonary fibrosis. *Am. J. Pathol.* 166 (5), 1321–1332.
41. Zhai, X., Lu, J., Wang, Y., Fang, F., Li, B., and Gu, W. (2014). Reversal effect of bufalin on multidrug resistance in K562/VCR vincristine-resistant leukemia cell line. *J. Tradit. Chin. Med.* 34 (6), 678–683.
42. Zhang, J., Sun, Y., Liu, J. H., Yu, B. Y., and Xu, Q. (2007). Microbial transformation of three bufadienolides by Nocardia sp. and some insight for the cytotoxic structure-activity relationship (SAR). *Bioorg. Med. Chem. Lett.* 17 (22), 6062– 6065. doi: 10.1016/j.bmcl.2007.09.065
43. Zhang, Y., Lu, H., Ji, H., and Li, Y. (2015). Inflammatory pseudotumor of the liver: a case report and literature review. *Intractable Rare Dis. Res.* 4 (3), 155–158. doi: 10.5582/irdr.2015.01021
44. Zhou, X., Tang, L., Xu, Y., Zhou, G., and Wang, Z. (2014). Towards abetter understanding of medicinal uses of *Carthamus tinctorius* L. @ in traditional Chinese medicine: a phytochemical and pharmacological review. *J. Ethnopharmacol.* 151 (1), 27–43. doi: 10.1016/j.jep.2013.10.050

Permissions

All chapters in this book were first published by Frontiers; hereby published with permission under the Creative Commons Attribution License or equivalent. Every chapter published in this book has been scrutinized by our experts. Their significance has been extensively debated. The topics covered herein carry significant findings which will fuel the growth of the discipline. They may even be implemented as practical applications or may be referred to as a beginning point for another development.

The contributors of this book come from diverse backgrounds, making this book a truly international effort. This book will bring forth new frontiers with its revolutionizing research information and detailed analysis of the nascent developments around the world.

We would like to thank all the contributing authors for lending their expertise to make the book truly unique. They have played a crucial role in the development of this book. Without their invaluable contributions this book wouldn't have been possible. They have made vital efforts to compile up to date information on the varied aspects of this subject to make this book a valuable addition to the collection of many professionals and students.

This book was conceptualized with the vision of imparting up-to-date information and advanced data in this field. To ensure the same, a matchless editorial board was set up. Every individual on the board went through rigorous rounds of assessment to prove their worth. After which they invested a large part of their time researching and compiling the most relevant data for our readers.

The editorial board has been involved in producing this book since its inception. They have spent rigorous hours researching and exploring the diverse topics which have resulted in the successful publishing of this book. They have passed on their knowledge of decades through this book. To expedite this challenging task, the publisher supported the team at every step. A small team of assistant editors was also appointed to further simplify the editing procedure and attain best results for the readers.

Apart from the editorial board, the designing team has also invested a significant amount of their time in understanding the subject and creating the most relevant covers. They scrutinized every image to scout for the most suitable representation of the subject and create an appropriate cover for the book.

The publishing team has been an ardent support to the editorial, designing and production team. Their endless efforts to recruit the best for this project, has resulted in the accomplishment of this book. They are a veteran in the field of academics and their pool of knowledge is as vast as their experience in printing. Their expertise and guidance has proved useful at every step. Their uncompromising quality standards have made this book an exceptional effort. Their encouragement from time to time has been an inspiration for everyone.

The publisher and the editorial board hope that this book will prove to be a valuable piece of knowledge for researchers, students, practitioners and scholars across the globe.

List of Contributors

Milica Vukmirovic and Naftali Kaminski
Section of Pulmonary, Critical Care and Sleep Medicine, Precision Pulmonary Medicine Center (P2MED), Yale University School of Medicine, New Haven, CT, United States

Oliver Terwolbeck and Meike Müller
Fraunhofer Institute for Toxicology and Experimental Medicine, Hannover, Germany

Benedikt Jäger
Fraunhofer Institute for Toxicology and Experimental Medicine, Hannover, Germany
Department of Respiratory Medicine, University Medical Center, Freiburg, Germany
Faculty of Biology, Albert Ludwig University, Freiburg, Germany

Antje Prasse
Fraunhofer Institute for Toxicology and Experimental Medicine, Hannover, Germany
Department of Respiratory Medicine, University Medical Center, Freiburg, Germany
Department of Respiratory Medicine, Hannover Medical School and Biomedical Research in End-stage and Obstructive Lung Disease (BREATH), German Center for Lung Research (DZL), Hannover, Germany

Benjamin Seeliger and Tobias Welte
Department of Respiratory Medicine, Hannover Medical School and Biomedical Research in End-stage and Obstructive Lung Disease (BREATH), German Center for Lung Research (DZL), Hannover, Germany

Gregor Warnecke
Department of Heart, Thoracic, Transplantation and Vascular Surgery, Hannover Medical School, Hannover, Germany

Christian Bode
Department of Anesthesiology and Intensive Care Medicine, University Hospital Bonn, Bonn, Germany

Xianglin Zhou, Danhui Yang, Chengli Wei, Siqi LvQiu, Lin Wang, Yongkang Lin and Hong Luo
Department of Pulmonary and Critical Care Medicine, the Second Xiangya Hospital, Central South University, Changsha, China
Research Unit of Respiratory Disease, Central South University, Changsha, China
Hunan Diagnosis and Treatment Center of Respiratory Disease, Changsha, China

Xianglong Kong and Zhiguo Zhou
Respiratory Medicine, The First Hospital of Changsha, Changsha, China

Zhilan Yin
Department of Radiology, The Second Xiangya Hospital, Central South University, Changsha, China

Jun Tashiro, Gustavo A. Rubio and Sharon J. Elliot
Department of Surgery, University of Miami Miller School of Medicine, Miami, FL, United States

Andrew H. Limper
Department of Medicine, Mayo Clinic College of Medicine, Rochester, MN, United States

Kurt Williams
Department Pathobiology and Diagnostic Investigations, College of Veterinary Medicine, Michigan State University, East Lansing, MI, United States

Argyrios Tzouvelekis
Division of Immunology, Biomedical Sciences Research Center "Alexander Fleming", Athens, Greece
Department of Respiratory Medicine, School of Medicine, University of Patras, Patras, Greece

Marilyn K. Glassberg
Department of Surgery, University of Miami Miller School of Medicine, Miami, FL, United States
Department of Medicine, University of Miami Miller School of Medicine, Miami, FL, United States

Amit Kishore
Department of Pathological Physiology, Faculty of Medicine and Dentistry, Palacky University, Olomouc, Czechia
Accuscript Consultancy, Ludhiana, India

Martin Petrek
Department of Pathological Physiology, Faculty of Medicine and Dentistry, Palacky University, Olomouc, Czechia
Institute of Molecular and Translational Medicine, Faculty of Medicine and Dentistry, Palacky University, Olomouc, Czechia
Departments of Experimental Medicine, and Immunology, University Hospital Olomouc, Olomouc, Czechia

Vasilios Tzilas and Demosthenes Bouros
First Academic Department of Pneumonology, Hospital for Thoracic Diseases, "Sotiria", Medical School, National and Kapodistrian University of Athens, Athens, Greece

Argyris Tzouvelekis
First Academic Department of Pneumonology, Hospital for Thoracic Diseases, "Sotiria", Medical School, National and Kapodistrian University of Athens, Athens, Greece
Division of Immunology, Biomedical Sciences Research Center "Alexander Fleming", Athens, Greece

Serafim Chrysikos
5th Department of Pneumonology, Hospital for Thoracic Diseases, "Sotiria", Athens, Greece

Spyridon Papiris
2nd Pulmonary Medicine Department, Attikon University Hospital, Medical School, National and Kapodistrian University of Athens, Athens, Greece

Shengming Liu and Shanrui Li
Department of Rehabilitation Medicine, West China Hospital, Sichuan University, Chengdu, China
West China School of Pharmacy, Sichuan University, Chengdu, China

Konstantinos Ntatsoulis, Elli-Anna Stylianaki and Alexios N. Matralis
Institute of Bio-Innovation, Biomedical Sciences Research Center Alexander Fleming, Athens, Greece

Vassilis Aidinis
Institute of Bio-Innovation, Biomedical Sciences Research Center Alexander Fleming, Athens, Greece
Division of Immunology, Alexander Fleming Biomedical Sciences Research Center, Athens, Greece

Theodoros Karampitsakos
Department of Respiratory Medicine, School of Medicine, University of Patras, Patras, Greece

Daniel C. Zank
Division of Pulmonary, Allergy and Critical Care Medicine, University of Pittsburgh School of Medicine, Pittsburgh, PA, United States

Marta Bueno and Ana L. Mora
Division of Pulmonary, Allergy and Critical Care Medicine, University of Pittsburgh School of Medicine, Pittsburgh, PA, United States
Vascular Medicine Institute, University of Pittsburgh School of Medicine, Pittsburgh, PA, United States

Mauricio Rojas
Division of Pulmonary, Allergy and Critical Care Medicine, University of Pittsburgh School of Medicine, Pittsburgh, PA, United States
McGowan Institute of Regenerative Medicine, University of Pittsburgh School of Medicine, Pittsburgh, PA, United States
Dorothy P. & Richard P. Simmons Center for Interstitial Lung Disease, University of Pittsburgh School of Medicine, Pittsburgh, PA, United States

Qun Yu, Dewei Zhu, Yang Zou, Peili Rao and Yunhui Shen
School of Pharmacy, Shanghai University of Traditional Chinese Medicine, Shanghai, China

Kai Wang
Experiment Center for Science and Technology, Shanghai University of Traditional Chinese Medicine, Shanghai, China

Athina Trachalaki
Laboratory of Molecular and Cellular Pneumonology, Respiratory Medicine Department, School of Medicine, University of Crete, Heraklion, Greece
National Heart and Lung Institute, Imperial College London, London, United Kingdom
Royal Brompton Hospital, London, United Kingdom

Eliza Tsitoura, Semeli Mastrodimou, Eirini Vasarmidi, Eleni Bibaki, Nikolaos Tzanakis and Katerina Antoniou
Laboratory of Molecular and Cellular Pneumonology, Respiratory Medicine Department, School of Medicine, University of Crete, Heraklion, Greece

Rachele Invernizzi
National Heart and Lung Institute, Imperial College London, London, United Kingdom

Philip L. Molyneaux and Toby M. Maher
National Heart and Lung Institute, Imperial College London, London, United Kingdom
Royal Brompton Hospital, London, United Kingdom

Gabriela Leuschner
Department of Internal Medicine V, Ludwig Maximilians University, Comprehensive Pneumology Center (CPC-M), German Center for Lung Research (DZL), Munich, Germany

Jürgen Behr
Department of Internal Medicine V, Ludwig Maximilians University, Comprehensive Pneumology Center (CPC-M), German Center for Lung Research (DZL), Munich, Germany
Asklepios Fachkliniken München-Gauting, Gauting, Germany

Lloyd Tanner, Jesper Bergwik, Andrew B. Single, Ravi K. V. Bhongir and Arne Egesten
Respiratory Medicine, Allergology, and Palliative Medicine, Department of Clinical Sciences Lund, Lund University and Skåne University Hospital, Lund, Sweden

Jonas S. Erjefält
Unit of Airway Inflammation, Department of Experimental Medical Sciences, Lund University, Lund, Sweden

Paul Reynaud, Lucie Knabe, Carey Suehs, Isabelle Vachier, Jean Pierre Mallet and Anne Sophie Gamez
Department of Respiratory Diseases, Univ Montpellier, CHU Montpellier, Montpellier, France

Engi Ahmed, Charlotte Vernisse and Arnaud Bourdin
Department of Respiratory Diseases, Univ Montpellier, CHU Montpellier, Montpellier, France
PhyMedExp, Univ Montpellier, CNRS, INSERM, CHU Montpellier, Montpellier, France

Isabelle Serre
Department of Pathology, Univ Montpellier, CHU Montpellier, Montpellier, France

Sébastien Bommart
Department of Radiology, Univ Montpellier, CHU Montpellier, Montpellier, France

Jean Philippe Berthet
Pulmonology Unit, Ospedale Ca'Foncello, AULSS2 Marca Trevigiana, Trevise, Italy

Micaela Romagnoli
Department of Cardiac, Thoracic and Vascular Surgery, Univ Nice, CHU Nice, Nice, France

Hongbo Ma
Department of Rehabilitation Medicine, State Key Laboratory of Biotherapy and Cancer Center, National Clinical Research Center for Geriatrics, West China Hospital, Sichuan University, Chengdu, China
West China School of Pharmacy, Sichuan University, Chengdu, China

Xuyi Wu, Yi Li and Yong Xia
Department of Rehabilitation Medicine, State Key Laboratory of Biotherapy and Cancer Center, National Clinical Research Center for Geriatrics, West China Hospital, Sichuan University, Chengdu, China
Key Laboratory of Rehabilitation Medicine in Sichuan Province/Rehabilitation Medicine Research Institute, Chengdu, China

Ioanna Ninou and Christiana Magkrioti
Division of Immunology, Alexander Fleming Biomedical Sciences Research Center, Athens, Greece

Jia He, Yue Du, Gaopeng Li, Peng Xiao, Xingzheng Sun, Wenjun Song, Lihua Lai, Meng Xia and Qingqing Wang
Institute of Immunology, Zhejiang University School of Medicine, Hangzhou, China
The Key Laboratory for Immunity and Inflammatory Diseases of Zhejiang Province, Hangzhou, China

Jianhua Zhang
Department of Medical Laboratory, School of Medicine, Shaoxing University, Shaoxing, China

Jizhen Huang, Xiang Tong, Li Zhang, Lei Wang, Dongguang Wang, Shijie Zhang and Hong Fan
Department of Respiratory and Critical Care Medicine, West China Hospital/West China School of Medicine, Sichuan University, Chengdu, China

Yuan Zhang
Department of Ophthalmology, Renmin Hospital of Wuhan University, Wuhan, China

De Jin, Xuedong An, Yuqing Zhang, Liyun Duan, Fengmei Lian and Xiaolin Tong
Guang'anmen Hospital, China Academy of Chinese Medical Sciences, Beijing, China

Yingying Duan and Shenghui Zhao
Graduate School, Beijing University of Chinese Medicine, Beijing, China

Zhun Bi
State Key Laboratory of Medicinal Chemical Biology, College of Pharmacy and Tianjin Key Laboratory of Molecular Drug Research, Nankai University, Haihe Education Park, Tianjin, China

Lixin Li and Jingjing Gao
Tianjin Key Laboratory of Molecular Drug Research, Tianjin International Joint Academy of Biomedicine, Tianjin, China

Xiaohe Li, Shuaishuai Liu, Shaoyan Gao, Yunyao Cui, Kai Huang, Mengying Huang, Jiahe Mao, Tao Sun, Honggang Zhou and Cheng Yang
State Key Laboratory of Medicinal Chemical Biology, College of Pharmacy and Tianjin Key Laboratory of Molecular Drug Research, Nankai University, Haihe Education Park, Tianjin, China
Tianjin Key Laboratory of Molecular Drug Research, Tianjin International Joint Academy of Biomedicine, Tianjin, China

Index

www.ingramcontent.com/pod-product-compliance
Lightning Source LLC
LaVergne TN
LVHW082128200926
848484LV00008B/2021